APPROACHES TO THE STUDY OF MOTOR CONTROL AND LEARNING

ADVANCES IN PSYCHOLOGY

84

Editors:

G. E. STELMACH

P. A. VROON

NORTH-HOLLAND
AMSTERDAM • LONDON • NEW YORK • TOKYO

APPROACHES TO THE STUDY OF MOTOR CONTROL AND LEARNING

Edited by

Jeffery J. SUMMERS

Department of Psychology
University of Melbourne
Parkville, Victoria
Australia

1992

NORTH-HOLLAND
AMSTERDAM • LONDON • NEW YORK • TOKYO

NORTH-HOLLAND
ELSEVIER SCIENCE PUBLISHERS B.V.
Sara Burgerhartstraat 25
P.O. Box 211, 1000 AE Amsterdam, The Netherlands

Distributors for the United States and Canada:
ELSEVIER SCIENCE PUBLISHING COMPANY, INC.
655 Avenue of the Americas
New York, N.Y. 10010, U.S.A.

ISBN: 0 444 88455 6

Transferred to digital printing 2006

Preface

During the past two decades, there has been dramatic increase in interest in the study of motor behaviour. The aim of the present volume is to capture the diversity of topics, methods, and paradigms that currently characterise research in motor control and learning. The chapters cover the different approaches and different levels of analysis being adopted to examine the processes involved in the acquisition and control of a variety of skills, ranging from discrete arm movements to catching and handwriting.

In selecting contributors to the volume I aimed at a blend of authors with established reputations in the field and younger authors in the early stage of their research careers. The contributors were asked to review their research with particular emphasis on the methods and paradigms employed, the reasons for adopting a particular approach, and the future direction of their work. Contributors who have been working in a area for some time were also asked to discuss how their research methodology, and the questions being asked, have changed over time.

Within this general framework, authors were free to choose the contents of their chapters and the form of presentation. Some chose to address general issues in the field, some preferred to give an overview of their special area and/or a report of recent experimental work, others focused on theoretical issues.

The first section contains chapters examining general issues and trends in the study of motor control and learning, and chapters presenting an extensive overview of developments in a specific area. The next three sections contain chapters from scientists working in three broadly defined areas of interest: coordination and control; visuo-motor processes; and movement disorders. The chapters in each section provide a good overview of the research issues, theoretical frameworks, methods and paradigms developing in an area.

A number of people deserve sincere thanks for helping to produce this volume. Jenny Todd, my research assistant who spent countless hours, without complaint, formatting, proofreading, and preparing indexes for the chapters. It is largely due to her efforts that the volume is now in press. Rachel Benedict who also assisted with preparing the book for publication. John Butterfield and Alison Carter, the technical editors for the volume, provided encouragement and editorial suggestions. Samantha Albert for assistance with word processing.

Part of the preparation of this volume was completed while I was a fellow at the Netherlands Institute for Advanced Study (NIAS). I would like to thank Professor Dirk van de Kaa (Director) and the staff at NIAS for providing the perfect environment in which to read, write, think, and prepare edited volumes.

Finally, the contributors deserve utmost thanks for the quality of the chapters they prepared, their attempts to meet my deadlines, and their patience.

Melbourne *Jeffery J. Summers*

Table of Contents

Contributors

BRUCE ABERNETHY
Department of Human Movement Studies
University of Queensland
Queensland, 4072
Australia

J. GREG ANSON
School of Physical Education
University of Otago
P.O. Box 56
Dunedin
New Zealand

NICHOLAS C. BARRETT
School of Psychology
Curtin University
Perth
Western Australia, 6001
Australia

ROBIN BURGESS-LIMERICK
Department of Human Movement Studies
University of Queensland
Queensland, 4072
Australia

JUDITH L. CHARLTON
Faculty of Special Education and Disability Studies
Victoria College, Burwood Campus
221 Burwood Highway
Burwood
Victoria, 3125
Australia

DENIS J. GLENCROSS
School of Psychology
Curtin University
Perth
Western Australia, 6001
Australia

PATRICK HAGGARD
MRC Applied Psychology Unit
15 Chaucer Road
Cambridge CB2 2EF
England

DEBORAH HOARE
Department of Human Movement and Recreation Studies
University of Western Australia
Nedlands, Perth
Western Australia, 6009
Australia

GRAHAM K. KERR
University Laboratory of Physiology
Oxford University
Parks Road
Oxford OX1 3PT
England

DAWNE LARKIN
Department of Human Movement and Recreation Studies
University of Western Australia
Nedlands, Perth
Western Australia, 6009
Australia

JUDITH I. LASZLO
Department of Human Movement and Recreation Studies
University of Western Australia
Nedlands, Perth
Western Australia, 6009
Australia

PETER D. NEILSON
Clinical Research Unit for Anxiety Disorders
University of New South Wales
299 Forbes Street
Darlinghurst
New South Wales, 2010
Australia

MEGAN D. NEILSON
Clinical Research Unit for Anxiety Disorders
University of New South Wales
299 Forbes Street
Darlinghurst
New South Wales, 2010
Australia

NICHOLAS J. O'DWYER
Clinical Research Unit for Anxiety Disorders
University of New South Wales
299 Forbes Street
Darlinghurst
New South Wales, 2010
Australia

HELEN PARKER
Department of Human Movement and Recreation Studies
University of Western Australia
Nedlands, Perth
Western Australia, 6009
Australia

JAMES G. PHILLIPS
Department of Psychology
Monash University
Clayton
Victoria, 3168
Australia

J.R. PIJPERS
Faculty of Human Movement Sciences
Vrije Universiteit
Van der Boechorststraat 9
1081 BT Amsterdam
The Netherlands

GEERT J.P. SAVELSBERGH
Faculty of Human Movement Sciences
Vrije Universiteit
Van der Boechorststraat 9
1081 BT Amsterdam
The Netherlands

W.A. SPARROW
Faculty of Special Education and Disability Studies
Victoria College, Burwood Campus
221 Burwood Highway
Burwood
Victoria, 3125
Australia

GEORGE E. STELMACH
Exercise and Sport Science Institute
Psychobiology Section
Arizona State University
Tempe
Arizonia 85287
U.S.A.

ARNOLD J.W.M. THOMASSEN
NICI
P.O. Box 9104
6500 HE Nijmegen
The Netherlands

GERARD P. VAN GALEN
NICI
P.O. Box 9104
6500 HE Nijmegen
The Netherlands

BEATRIX VEREIJKEN
Faculty of Human Movement Sciences
Vrije Universiteit
Van der Boechorststraat 9
1081 BT Amsterdam
The Netherlands

STEFAN VOGT
Max-Planck-Institut für Psychologische Forschung
Leopoldstrasse 24
D-8000 Munchen 40
Germany

H.T.A.(JOHN) WHITING
Department of Psychology
University of York
Heslington
York Y01 5DD
England

L.R.T. WILLIAMS
Motor Learning and Control Laboratory
School of Physical Education
University of Otago
P.O. Box 56
Dunedin
New Zealand

PART I

MOTOR BEHAVIOUR RESEARCH: GENERAL ISSUES AND TRENDS

Approaches to the Study of Motor Control and Learning
J.J. Summers (Editor)

Chapter 1

THE RISE AND FALL OF DOMINANT PARADIGMS IN MOTOR BEHAVIOUR RESEARCH

Bruce Abernethy
University of Queensland.

W.A. Sparrow
Victoria College - Burwood.

In seminal work on the philosophy of science Kuhn (1962, 1970) demonstrated that knowledge advance in scientific fields is characterised by periods of normal science (in which a single paradigm and theoretical view dominates and guides the research effort of the field) interspersed with periods of paradigm crises (in which anomalous findings emerge which highlight faults and limitations in the prevailing theory) and revolutionary science (in which an alternative theoretical view rises to challenge and overthrow the prevailing view). In this paper we use content and citation analyses from the focal journal for motor control and learning research (the Journal of Motor Behavior) to trace historically the cycles of normal and revolutionary science in the motor control and learning field. Past dominant theoretical views are described in terms of the anomalous data that have contributed to their loss of favour. The current paradigm crisis between the so-called 'movement systems' and 'action systems' approaches to motor learning and control (Meijer & Roth, 1988) is considered in some detail and possible outcomes of the crisis (hybridisation vs. the emergence of a new dominant paradigm) are discussed in the light of the Kuhnian view of science.

Historically the research endeavour in the field of motor control and learning has been typified by tightly controlled laboratory studies focusing on simple but novel movements, movements largely atypical of those used in day-to-day activities (Whiting, 1980, 1982). This reductionist bias within motor behaviour research arises as a direct consequence of the heavy borrowing of research paradigms from experimental psychology (Wilberg, 1972). In turn, experimental psychology's acquisition of such normative methods has been directly from the physical and natural sciences of astronomy, physics, and chemistry, whose academic rigour and credibility experimental psychology ultimately seeks to replicate (Kendler, 1981). Despite the profound influence of the prevailing view of science upon both the type of research conducted and the kind of research questions which are addressed, researchers in many scientific fields, like motor control and learning, have, to date, shown surprisingly little interest in the philosophy of science. In this chapter we attempt to show how some simple and well established notions from the philosophy of science can be meaningfully applied to investigating the historical and contemporary development of theoretical perspectives in motor control and learning. In addition, we also seek to show how such notions can provide some prospective insight into both the kinds of research which are most likely to advance knowledge, and the possible direction for resolution of some current theoretical debates within the field.

Our presentation is in three major sections. In the first section we present in some detail Kuhn's (1962, 1970) notions regarding the role of normal science, revolutionary science, and paradigm crises in the development, advancement, and maturation of a field of study. Although Kuhn's views of science were developed more to account for developments in the physical than behavioural sciences,[1] are now somewhat dated, and are not without critique by other philosophers of science (e.g., see Bloor, 1971; Chalmers, 1982; Lakatos & Musgrave, 1970), the Kuhnian perspective is nevertheless adopted because of its considerable intuitive appeal and explanatory power. In this first section the Kuhnian view is used to explode the common misconception that knowledge and theory development through orthodox science is a linear, cumulative process. It is shown that a more realistic, historically accurate view of knowledge development in science is that of a non-cumulative process, punctuated and disrupted by periods of paradigm crisis and competition. The Kuhnian view of science is presented as a useful template for comparing historical developments in motor control and learning with normative developments in other fields. We argue that viewing historical developments

[1] Although Kuhn (1970, 1973) acknowledges this limitation in the scope of the examples used to formulate his original views his approach has nevertheless proven fruitful in the analysis of paradigm struggles in the behavioural sciences. (See Katahn & Koplin, 1968, Kendler, 1981, and Weimer & Palermo, 1973 for examples of application of Kuhn's views to the development of psychological theory and Martens, 1987 and Stelmach, 1987 for applications to sport psychology and skill acquisition).

in motor control and learning from a Kuhnian perspective is a useful means of both assessing the 'maturity' of the field relative to other areas of science and of putting current theoretical debates into an appropriate historical context.

In section two of this chapter we provide a necessarily brief history of important theoretical and paradigmatic developments in motor control and learning with an emphasis on contemporary developments. The basis and assumptions of four key theoretical propositions in the recent history of motor control and learning research are discussed along with descriptions of both the normal science they have supported and anomalous data which have led, or may lead, to their modification and/or rejection. The rise and fall of dominant paradigms in motor control and learning (i.e., the cycle from normal to revolutionary science) is traced using content and citation analyses from the predominant journal for motor control and learning, the *Journal of Motor Behavior*. The pervasiveness of different theoretical explanations is assessed in terms of the longevity of the normal science which has followed the presentation of each of the theories. Some secondary markers of normal science such as the development of specialist societies and journals are also considered.

The final section focuses on the current paradigm crisis between the so-called *movement systems* and *action systems* approaches to motor control and learning (Meijer & Roth, 1988). The points of divergence between the two approaches are briefly evaluated at a number of different levels of analysis. The question of whether the evolving dynamical action systems paradigm is likely to overthrow the incumbent information-processing movement systems paradigm is discussed, with particular attention given to the range of phenomena each approach can and cannot adequately accommodate. Lines of evidence in favour of a reconciled hybridisation of the two currently competing theoretical views are considered, although such a reconciliation is eventually deemed improbable. It is argued, with use of parallel examples from Kuhn's work, that the philosophical differences between the movement systems and action systems approaches are too great to readily support hybridisation, and that the viewpoints are sufficiently disparate and incompatible to indicate a period of protracted crises rather than rapid merger. Such a prediction is reached because the history of parallel problems for science and scientists is characterised by polarisation of theoretical views (Mahoney, 1976) and the resolution of paradigm crises through the eventual emergence of a dominant paradigm, rather than through any compromising of the assumptions underlying the competing views.

PROGRESS OF KNOWLEDGE THROUGH SCIENCE AND THE KUHNIAN NOTIONS OF NORMAL AND REVOLUTIONARY SCIENCE

Problems with the 'Textbook' View of Orthodox Science

The 'textbook' version of science (e.g., Bunge, 1967; Lachman, 1960) is that knowledge generation is a cumulative, linear process in which the body of available knowledge and theory is advanced through the continual derivation and testing of hypotheses derived from, and grounded in, current theory and knowledge (see also Martens, 1987). Knowledge is advanced through theory development with either observation providing the basis for the derivation of theory ('bottom-up' theory development) or existing theory guiding selective empirical testing and data collection which, in turn, leads to theory modification and enhancement ('top-down' theory development; Stelmach, 1987). Regardless of whether theory development proceeds in a 'bottom-up' or 'top-down' fashion it is generally conceived, within the orthodox view of science (cf. Martens, 1987), that knowledge develops in a given field through selective and continual refinement of theory, such that each new theory builds on that which has gone before and knowledge is accreted in a systematic, consistent fashion. Theory-testing is seen as a means of progressively explaining *more* of the phenomenon of interest in a given field (cf. Landers, 1983) to the extent that modern theory should be capable of explaining not only facts collected with that particular theoretical perspective in mind, but also all the preceding facts available from earlier study in the field (even when these 'facts' were collected with a different theoretical and perhaps ontological perspective in mind). The general belief is that science proceeds by building bigger and more exact theories with each theory including what has gone before plus extending the explanatory power to include new phenomena not previously explicable.

There are, however, a number of reasons why the scientific method cannot, or does not, operate in this fashion. One of the basic tenets of orthodox science is the tenet of objectivity - the operating concept that the scientist remains detached, impartial, and impersonal in the collection and interpretation of data, such that the same basic conclusions about the causes of given phenomena should eventually be revealed regardless of the personality characteristics, beliefs, etc. of the scientist making the observation. The objectivity tenet breaks down, perhaps surprisingly, not only in the "softer" sciences such as psychology but also in the so-called "harder" sciences such as physics and chemistry. Even in the "hard" sciences the interpretation of data varies substantially from scientist to scientist and is hence value-laden rather than value-free (Mahoney, 1976; Martens, 1987).[2] As a consequence the "laws" discovered in a given field are often largely a function of the particular scientist's "view of the world" and the paradigm from within which they operate. In many cases belief in a theory may cause blind adherence even when the theory is clearly contradicted by empirical data.

The Popperian view of science (Popper, 1959) is an attempt to alleviate the objectivity difficulties in science through systematic hypothesis testing of even the most accepted facts and theories. The well-known Popperian notion of falsification is grounded in the belief that any given theory can be disproved (or falsified) by contradictory data from a single empirical test and that one sound falsification should immediately result in refutation of the particular theory or hypothesis. From within this perspective direct proof of a given theory is impossible (thus creating a substantial logistical hurdle to rapid knowledge development; Henkel, 1976) but a theory's credibility can be measured in terms of the extent of collected evidence with which it is consistent.

Despite the persistence and popularity of the falsification view of theory development in most texts and formal curricula on *the* scientific method, analyses of the history of science, such as those performed by Kuhn (1962, 1970), suggest a rather different modus operandi for science in practice. Rather than science proceeding along the relatively smooth path to universal understanding that an orthodox scientific view would predict, the "progress" of science is characterised by far more discrete and disruptive periods of change. Falsification does not appear to operate in a definitive "all or none" fashion. Rather than the results of any particular empirical test being accepted outright (and theories being rejected on the basis of single contradictory results) the emphasis is usually primarily upon possible design, analysis, and interpretative flaws in the pivotal experiment that may have prevented the expected result from being obtained.

Kuhn's Notion of Normal Science and Scientific Revolutions

In reviewing the history of science, primarily in the fields of physics, chemistry, and astronomy, Kuhn (1962, 1970) observed that progress in these sciences occurred through a series of cycles marked by disruptive periods of paradigm crisis and revolution. Periods of marked debate and conflict between opposing

---

[2] In the so-called "hard" sciences the main factor undermining objectivity is inter-observer differences in data interpretation. In the behavioural sciences, where subject and observer interact, the characteristics of the scientist may influence not only the interpretation of data but also the nature of the collected data (e.g., see Barber, 1976; Rosenthal, 1966).

theoretical and conceptual views were inevitably resolved by new views and concepts emerging which completely displaced previously established views and orders. Contrary to the predictions of new theory development as a linear, cumulative process, new views and theoretical concepts rarely absorbed nor used as a foundation, the pre-existing theory. A dominant theory or concept at any point in the history of a given field achieves such status normally through *replacing* the previously dominant view rather than *emerging* from it.

Central to the Kuhnian view of science is the concept of the *paradigm*, somewhat loosely defined in Kuhn's original work as "...universally recognised scientific achievements that for a time provide model problems and solutions to a community of practitioners" (Kuhn, 1970, p. viii).[3] In an operational sense the term paradigm is perhaps most effective when used to describe a particular conceptual framework, its relevant problems, issues, and terms, its accepted methods and its associated theories with their (frequently implicit) views of the world and reality. Kuhn's principal thesis was that science is characterised by "...noncumulative developmental episodes in which an older paradigm is replaced in whole or in part by an incompatible new one," (Kuhn, 1962, p. 91) and that these 'developmental episodes' or cycles typically consist of stages identifiable as pre-science, normal science, crisis, and revolution. The major characteristics of each of these stages are described in the sections that follow.

Pre-Science. Kuhn used the term pre-science to describe that period in the early development of a research field in which the field is 'finding its feet' and delimiting its subject matter and scope. It is a period in which no single paradigm or theoretical position is sufficiently well accepted to guarantee a concerted research effort and, as a consequence, research activity proceeds in a somewhat 'piecemeal' manner. A diverse range of research topics are studied and these topics are linked in the most tenuous of manners, often more because the assorted subject matter does not fit pre-existing well-defined fields than because of common unifying theoretical themes. Early attempts at theory testing and development are frequently based almost entirely on theories imported from other fields (what Wilberg, 1972 has termed recipient paradigms) rather than developments intrinsic to the new field. The early days of motor control and learning research provides a good example of the use of such recipient paradigms in a "pre-science" period. In the period leading up to Henry and Rogers' (1960) memory drum theory, theories developed for verbal material in mainstream psychology, such as Thorndike's (1914) Law of Effect

---

[3] Kuhn's original definition of a paradigm was an inexact and potentially misleading one. In his 1970 revision of his original work a substantial portion of the postscript is dedicated to clarification of this problem.

or Hull's (1943) learning theory, were applied directly to the problems posed by the learning of motor skills.

Normal Science. Pre-science is replaced by what Kuhn (1962) has termed 'normal science' once the field of study matures to the point where there is some consensus and/or a dominant view which emerges regarding the appropriate problems, methods, and theories needed to understand the subject matter of the field. Kuhn equates normal science with paradigm-based research, defining normal science as "...research firmly based upon one or more past scientific achievements, achievements that some particular scientific community acknowledges for a time as supplying the foundation for its further practice" (1970, p. 10). Normal science is characterised by emergence of a single paradigm which has sufficient explanatory power, potential and past achievement to attract 'adherents' from other competing fields of scientific endeavour. At the same time the paradigm leaves a large number of specific problems (albeit necessarily drawn from a restricted range of topics) sufficiently 'open-ended' to present attractive problem-solving propositions for its followers.

The activities of normal science are quite distinct from those occurring during pre-science and during periods of paradigm crisis. The emphasis within normal science is upon empirical work undertaken to fully develop and articulate the theories of the dominant paradigm. This development involves the elimination of any residual ambiguities and the clarification of some of the 'grayer' areas of a given theory. The net purpose is to determine the full explanatory scope of the paradigm. The accumulation of 'facts' aimed to directly test predictions of the paradigm, but often with little or no value in their own right, occupies the majority of the time of scientists working within the dominant paradigm. As a result the majority of the research activities occurring during a period of normal science essentially involve "mopping up" operations with the bulk of published research involving relatively minor (arguably trivial) variations of the same basic paradigm. (An excellent example of this from within the motor control and learning field is the motor short-term memory work of the 1970s examining the relative role of distance and location cues; see Salmela, 1979). According to Kuhn (1970), normal science consists primarily of problem solving activities where the main motivating force for the scientist is the problem-solving act in itself,[4] rather than the drive to produce major conceptual advances in the field. During this phase the activities of the scientist adhere most closely to those specified in the doctrines of orthodox science (cf. Lachman, 1960) but with the important constraint that normal science does not,

---

[4] To this end Kuhn refers to the goal of research within a period of normal science being that of "...achieving the anticipated in a new way" (1970, p. 36).

as a principle of operation, search for novelties and ambiguities of fact or theory.

The development of normal science is an important maturational step in the development of any field and conversely the absence of a dominant research paradigm is indicative of immaturity in a field. The transition from pre-science to normal science in the field of motor control and learning arguably came as a direct result of the appearance of Henry and Rogers' (1960) memory drum theory of movement planning [5] - relevant work prior to this period being widely varied in both focus and method. Kuhn (1962, 1970) noted that the development of parallel professional activities, such as the formation of specialist journals and societies, and the attainment of a unique place in the curriculum of the specific or larger field are also indicators of the advent of normal science. In the case of the motor control and learning field such indicators would again point to the important role played by Franklin Henry. Although the development of a specialist journal cannot be linked directly to Henry,[6] he certainly played a central role in the development of a professional society (NASPSPA in 1966), the development of graduate education in motor control and learning, and the establishment of motor control and learning as an integral part of programs of kinaesiology and physical education (Brooks, 1981; Park, 1981; Schmidt, 1988a; Spirduso, 1981).

Paradigm Crises. Part of the activity of normal science involves seeking the "boundary conditions" (Greenwald, Pratkanis, Leippe, & Baumgardner, 1986) where a given paradigm can and, importantly, cannot, explain the data and established facts of the field. Adherents to normal science, in performing research within the dominant paradigm, end up, either advertently or inadvertently, pushing the existing paradigm to the extremes in order to see the total range of phenomena it is capable of explaining. As a consequence the explanatory bounds of the paradigm are eventually found beyond which the paradigm is incapable of satisfactorily predicting and describing observed phenomena. The consistent appearance of anomalous data sets in motion a chain of events which ultimately results in a paradigm crisis. Anomalous facts (i.e., facts inconsistent with the prevailing paradigm) are frequently overlooked

---

[5] For autobiographical accounts of the development of the memory drum theory and its ongoing capability to handle new data on movement planning see Henry (1981, 1986, in press).

[6] Although the *Research Quarterly* existed as an outlet for motor learning and control research from the 1930's, the establishment of specialist journals are attributable to Robert and Carol Ammons (with *Perceptual and Motor Skills* in the 1950's) and Richard Schmidt (with *Journal of Motor Behavior* in 1969).

in the initial development of many dominant paradigms yet, ironically, it is frequently such anomalies which eventually receive extended examination and which may ultimately serve to undermine and overthrow the dominant paradigm. [In the motor control and learning domain, for example, the notions underlying the mass-spring/equilibrium-point hypothesis pre-dated much of the normal science on motor programming which they ultimately aided in bringing under question. Similarly, Lashley's (1917) anecdotes on his de-afferented patient pre-dated much of the normal science inspired by Adams' (1971) closed-loop theory, yet such data ultimately aided in Adams' model being replaced by open-loop alternatives.] Kuhn (1962, 1970) points out that anomalous findings and flaws in the operating assumptions of the dominant paradigms are often overlooked due to human cognitive preference for congruity and parsimony (preferences consistent with the operating concepts of normal science) yet typically, and again somewhat ironically, once an anomaly in the existing paradigm is highlighted it becomes apparent to all scientists in the field.

The initial response to anomalous data is an attempt to adjust the existing dominant theory to accommodate the anomaly. This results in the proliferation of numerous *ad hoc* modifications to the original paradigm and this is one of the first indicators of an impending paradigm crisis. Divergent attempts at explaining the anomalous data results not only in *ad hoc* adjustments but the surfacing of a range of different enunciations of the existing 'normal' paradigm and theory, the questioning of some previously universally accepted explanations of common "standard" phenomena and a general loss of clarity regarding the fundamental premises of the dominant paradigm.[7] The proliferation of different forms of the mass-spring model in the early 80's (see Fel'dman, 1986) is perhaps a good motor control and learning example of the proliferation of versions of a common paradigm. A "full-blown" paradigm crisis is apparent when many of the eminent researchers in the field show sustained interest in the anomalous data.[8]

A particularly important response to a paradigm crisis, which is inconsistent with both the Baconian view of scientific objectivity and the Popperian view of theory rejection through falsification, is extreme resistance to change by those scientists who have "grown-up" with the prevailing dominant paradigm and who have substantial temporal and emotional investment in the paradigm

---

[7] It is important to note that such differences in interpretation of the dominant paradigm do not generally surface during periods of normal science.

[8] Arguably Schmidt's interest in the mass-spring model (e.g., Schmidt & McGown, 1980) and Newell's interest in dynamical perspectives of movement control (e.g., Newell, 1985; 1989) are indicative of some form of crisis for the motor programming paradigm.

(see Barber, 1961; de Grazzia, 1966; and Mitroff, 1974a, 1974b for examples). As early as 1936 Planck noted that changes in paradigms were not achieved on the basis of rational persuasion. He wrote later that "...a new scientific truth does not triumph by convincing its opponents and making them see the light, but rather because its opponents eventually die, and a new generation grows up that is familiar with it" (Planck, 1949, pp. 33-34). Similarly, Kendler (1981, p. 137), in discussing the Kuhnian view of science with particular respect to psychology, noted that "...the adherents of the existing paradigm learn to live with or, perhaps more properly speaking, to ignore the inconsistent results." With proponents of the existing normal science paradigm frequently occupying powerful gatekeeping roles through editorial and review positions in prominent journals (Mahoney, 1976), it is not surprising that paradigm change is a slow process and the resistance effects are so powerful. Long term dissatisfaction with the dominant paradigm and its failure to appropriately explain relevant data nevertheless inevitably results in an active search (usually by young scientists or those without an emotional interest in the preservation of the dominant paradigm) for new means of looking at the field and of explaining both pre-existing and anomalous data. These efforts may eventually result in the development of alternative paradigms which can compete for dominance, and in some cases overthrow, the existing paradigm.

There are three possible outcomes to a paradigm crisis. The prevailing dominant paradigm may prove capable, through *ad hoc* modification, of adequately handling the discrepant data responsible for triggering the crisis. In this case the field progresses in a cumulative manner, approaching the linear development predicted by an orthodox model of science. The paradigm crisis in this instance has the effect of improving the explanatory power of the dominant theory, although usually at the cost of increased complexity within the internal constructs used in the model.

A second possibility is that the prevailing paradigm may prove inadequate to cope with the discrepant data but no viable replacement emerges. Kuhn (1962, 1970) notes that in such cases the anomalous finding is placed in the 'too hard' basket and simply identified as an important issue for future generations to address. In such cases the history of the physical sciences reveals that the existing paradigm is retained even though it can be demonstrated to be both inadequate and patently incorrect. Contrary to the premises of falsification (Popper, 1959) contradictory data alone seems insufficient to displace an existing paradigm - a more attractive alternative must also be present. As Kuhn notes "the decision to reject one paradigm is always simultaneously the decision to accept another, and the judgement leading to that decision involves the comparison of both paradigms with nature *and* with each other." (1970, p. 77).

The final possible outcome of a paradigm crisis is the emergence of a new alternative paradigm and a subsequent period of protracted debate in which the old dominant paradigm and the new alternative 'revolutionary science' battle for acceptance as *the* best means of explaining existing knowledge and *the* best prospective direction for future gains in explanatory power.

Revolutionary Science. Revolutionary science consists of the period of battle between the competing paradigms and the emergence of a new paradigm to guide the future normal science activity of the field. The battle between paradigms (between the old normal science and the new revolutionary science) is eventually resolved because the majority of scientists in the field come to view one of the paradigms as progressive (in the terms of Lakatos, 1970a, b), providing opportunity for increased explanatory power for both the existing and the potential new facts of the field, and the other as recessive or degenerative, providing diminishing potential for furthering the field's search for explanation. To overthrow an existing paradigm a new paradigm must both resolve some outstanding, generally recognised problem and preserve a relatively large portion of the accrued knowledge from prior research activity in the field. The former requirement is probably the most important and demonstrations based on the comparative ability of the new and old paradigms to solve anomalous data in a logical and acceptable manner are usually at the cornerstone of resolution. New paradigms that permit "... the prediction of phenomena that had been entirely unsuspected while the old one prevailed" (Kuhn, 1970, p. 154) are particularly influential. The unexpected demonstration of the predictability of certain behavioural characteristics such as bimanual linkage, the entrainment of speech and manual activities, and phase transitions between different gait forms predictable from purely physical properties (e.g., Kelso, 1981; Kugler & Turvey, 1986) is, for example, some of the strongest evidence presented in favour of the dynamical models within the current movement systems-action systems debate. Likewise Kuhn (1970, p. 155) notes that new paradigms may also gain acceptance because they may be more pleasing than existing theories for more subjective reasons such as 'neatness', 'suitability', or 'simplicity'. The overthrow of Treisman's complex (1960) attenuation model of selective attention for Norman's (1968, 1969) neater and simpler pertinence-based model may be a good example of this. Such characteristics are also an initial attractive property of Gibson's (1979) ecological optics, and ecological psychology in general, although some of this apparent 'simplicity' and 'neatness' inevitably disappears as the paradigm develops and more details are provided.

The periods of debate between competing paradigms are typically the most important periods in shaping the long-term development of a particular field.[9]

---

[9] Studies requiring scientists to retrospectively classify landmark research (e.g., Diamond & Morton, 1978) typically reveal that studies which induce a paradigm change are the ones deemed most important.

A number of common features characterise a paradigm crisis regardless of the specifics of the field in which the crisis occurs. As the nature of the field, the kind of problems the field should endeavour to address, and the appropriate ontological view from within which to address such problems are frequently questioned during periods of paradigm crisis these periods of debate are frequently characterised by recourse to philosophical analysis. [The current debates between the movement systems and action systems approaches are certainly characterised by such debate at the philosophical level e.g., see Kugler, Kelso & Turvey's (1982) and Kugler's (1986) use of ecological realism as a central feature of the debate]. The debate between competing paradigms also results in a re-defining (at least by the emerging paradigm) of acceptable problems and key issues for the field, as well as the frequent re-defining of key terms and nomenclature. Revolutionary science often causes the emergence (or re-emergence) of problems that were either not considered previously or were considered trivial and these frequently become "...the archetypes of significant scientific achievement." (Kuhn, 1970, p. 103). [The emergence of the storage and novelty problems which caused a re-defining of Keele's (1968) original motor program notion (e.g., see Schmidt, 1982) or the focus on the problems of controlling large numbers of degrees of freedom and context-conditioned variability which Turvey (1977) brought to bear on the information processing model are examples of this shift in problem emphasis during times of paradigm crisis]. The re-defining of key terms of competing paradigms also inevitably results in some misunderstanding and difficulty in reaching the true issues in a given debate. In the current movement systems-action systems debate, for example, the concepts of "information" and "peripheral processes" have quite different meanings within the two competing paradigms.

Aside from the difficulties posed by terminology differences there are generally a number of more fundamental reasons why comparison between paradigms in a period of true paradigm crisis can never be complete. The principal problem is that competing paradigms very rarely ask identical questions and they are, therefore, in the majority of cases largely at cross-purposes. The nature of debate is often such that logical resolution is not possible because each paradigm practices science in a somewhat 'different world' to its opponent. As Kuhn (1970, p. 94) notes "...each group uses its own paradigm to argue in that paradigm's defence" and this makes empirical comparisons difficult, if not impossible. The frustrations in this regard noted by many of the participants in the movement systems-action systems debates (Meijer & Roth, 1988) are illustrative of this difficulty.

The inability, reluctance, or sheer impossibility of supporters of either competing paradigm giving up any of the basic assumptions or tenets that underlie their particular paradigm in order to facilitate direct empirical comparison with the alternative paradigm, also means that resolution of paradigm debates through integration of the two approaches is an unlikely result of a paradigm crisis. Counter to intuitive logic, compromise and the integration of the best features of competing views into a common, consolidated, hybrid paradigm rarely satisfactorily solves paradigm disputes (see also Dunnette, 1966). We will return to this point later in the chapter in discussing possible outcomes of the present motor learning and control debates between theorists grounding their views in information processing and a cybernetic model of man (the movement systems approach) and theorists grounding their views in modern physics and a philosophy of ecological realism (the action systems approach).

The Resolution of Paradigm Crises and the Emergence of New Normal Science. As noted previously, paradigm crises resolve through one of the competing paradigm's achieving dominance. The old paradigm of normal science is frequently superseded by the competing revolutionary paradigm which then, when it receives majority acceptance, takes on the mantle of the new normal science. It retains that status until new anomalous data emerges and the whole cycle of crisis and revolution is repeated.

It should be reiterated that those who induce a paradigm shift are typically those who are young to the field and/or have no emotional attachment to the existing paradigm. Kuhn noted that these are the people who, "...being little committed by prior practice to the traditional rules of normal science, are particularly likely to see that those rules no longer define a playable game and to conceive another set that can replace them" (1970, p. 90). Those who induce a paradigm shift often do so by importing to the field ideas and concepts already well developed in other, previously unrelated fields of science (Bartlett, 1958).[10] [Kugler's introduction of the principles of thermodynamics to the study of movement control (e.g., see Kugler, 1986) is a good example of such transporting of ideas]. Ironically it is those scientists who are instrumental in displacing the previous normal science who become the "gatekeepers" of the next era of normal science. These scientists are then typically as protective of their normal science and preservative of that paradigm as the predecessors they displaced.

Scientific revolutions, much like the political revolutions upon which their name was analogously based, are often disruptive, in the short-term, to the smooth normal science of a field but are nevertheless essential, in the long-term, to progress the field beyond the constraints of given frames of thinking and to refresh the means of looking at the problems of the field. Like the political analogue it is the expression of majority thought which is ultimately responsible

---

[10] See Abernethy (in press) for a more detailed consideration of the distinguishing characteristics of those scientists who have influenced the direction of research in the motor learning and control fields.

for the displacement of the 'old order'. The discontinuous and disruptive nature of scientific revolutions is typically lost in most texts, review chapters, and general reference material which attempt to summarise the current state of knowledge on a topic at a given point in time. Review papers and texts in search of unifying themes and continuity in their own presentation typically "re-write" the history of a field's development to make the gains in understanding appear more linear and cumulative than they are in reality. Such accounts contribute heavily to the "public" conception of science as an accumulative rather than as a "destroy and rebuild" kind of activity.

To accurately trace the cycles of normal and revolutionary science in a given field of study, therefore, requires use of sources other than texts, review chapters, and other retrospective summaries. In the next section we use a range of different tools to trace the cycles of normal and revolutionary science in the development of the motor learning and control field. Principally we rely on content and citation analyses from the *Journal of Motor Behavior* (arguably the most important and specialised journal for the publication of motor learning and control research) to trace major paradigms of normal science in motor learning and control.[11] In addition, where appropriate, we also refer to secondary effects suggested by Kuhn (1970, p. 19) (viz., the formation of specialist journals and societies and observable impacts on curricula) as additional markers of periods of normal science. We note throughout, as we have in this section, some examples of events which indicate that at least the recent history of motor learning and control research follows basically the Kuhnian notion. In particular, examples are given of the use of *ad hoc* modifications to preserve given theories; the reluctance of original adherents to abandon a given paradigm even when it is shown to be incorrect; the grounding of revolutionary science in many older notions and ambiguities overlooked by normal science; and the unique backgrounds and detachment from normal science of those inducing major paradigm changes.

---

[11] Kuhn (1970), in fact, suggests that such analyses may provide an appropriate means of indexing the onset of paradigm crises and revolutions. He suggests (p. 7) that "... a shift in the distribution of the technical literature cited in the footnotes to research reports ... ought to be studied as a possible index to the occurrence of revolutions."

PARADIGM CRISES AND CYCLES OF NORMAL AND REVOLUTIONARY SCIENCE IN THE HISTORY OF MOTOR LEARNING AND CONTROL RESEARCH

It is not our intent in this section to provide a detailed history of the motor learning and control field. Such histories of the field and reviews of major theories of motor learning and control (but presenting theory/knowledge development from a cumulative rather than a cyclical Kuhnian perspective) may be found in Dickinson and Goodman (1986), Kelso (1982), Rosenbaum (1985), Schmidt (1988a), Sheridan (1984), and Stelmach and Diggles (1982). It is rather our intent to trace the relatively recent rise and fall of dominant motor learning and control paradigms using an analysis of the content of published articles within the completed 20 year history of the *Journal of Motor Behavior*. The *Journal of Motor Behavior* was instigated in 1969 by Richard Schmidt in response to the recognised lack of a specialist journal for the publication of motor learning and control research. Since its instigation the journal has maintained regular quarterly issues with little major change in structure, format or purpose. Despite the growth of alternative publication outlets for motor learning and control research it remains the principal specialist journal in the field.

Although measures of the average number of articles published per annum which directly test a given theory or operate within the assumptions of a given paradigm provide only a rough indication of the popularity and dominance of a particular paradigm,[12] such measures may nevertheless be enlightening with respect to paradigm crises and the rise and fall of specific theories and paradigms. Figure 1 presents hypothetical data derivable from a journal content analysis to highlight potential relations between publication distributions and the rise (progression) and fall (degeneration) of different paradigms. In such a presentation the total number of papers directly addressing a given theoretical perspective is given by the area under the curve with the peak height of a given distribution representing the point of maximal interest in the particular paradigm and the horizontal spread providing an indication of the longevity of interest in the theory or paradigm.

The 20 year history of the *Journal of Motor Behavior* has been characterised primarily, but not exclusively, by research inspired by four major theoretical positions viz., the closed-loop theory of Adams (1971), the motor programming/schema theories arising from the works of Henry and Rogers

---

[12] Content analyses of this type are contaminated, among other things, by the variable delays and difficulties experienced in getting different types of research work into print and by the implicit equal weighting of importance assigned to all published articles in a given year.

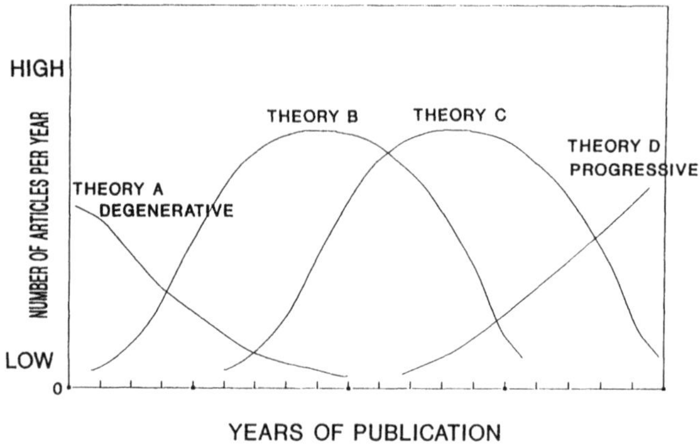

Figure 1. Hypothetical relationships between the distribution of published articles addressing a given theory and the rise (progression) and fall (degeneration) of that theory's claim for paradigmatic dominance.

(1960), Keele (1968), and Schmidt (1975, 1980), the impulse-variability theory of Schmidt, Zelaznik, Hawkins, Frank, and Quinn (1979) and the dynamical, oscillatory theories of motor control of Kelso, Kugler, and Turvey (e.g., Kelso, Holt, Rubin, & Kugler, 1981; Kugler, Kelso, & Turvey, 1982; Kugler & Turvey, 1986).[13] Figure 2 shows the number of articles per year (averaged over three year periods) which directly examine each of these theoretical propositions. It is apparent from even a cursory glance at Figure 2 that theory development in the motor learning and control field is not a continuous process but rather new theory emerges around the time existing theory is attracting peak research interest (usually inspired by the discovery of anomalous data). It is also readily apparent that each of the theoretical propositions presented to date differ markedly in their longevity and in their tendency toward progression or degeneration. In the text that follows we briefly describe the underlying assumptions and premises of each of these theories, the kind of normal science and experimentation they have supported and the key data resulting in the rise and demise of such propositions. In describing the current state of theorising

[13] The categorisation of some of these theoretical positions is somewhat arbitrary. A good case can be mounted, for example, for including the impulse-variability theory with theories of motor programming or for separating the schema theory from the notion of a generalised motor program.

in motor learning and control we arrive at the current paradigm crisis. The nature of the current crisis and its prospects for resolution are described in the final section of this paper.

Closed-Loop Theories of Motor Control and Learning

Although a role for feedback information in the ongoing control of movement had been posited at least by the time of Woodworth (1899), and later by Crossman and Goodeve (1963) in attempting to explain Fitts' Law (Fitts, 1954), the first consolidated theory of the role of feedback in both the control and learning of movement was provided by Adams (1971). Adams proposed that normal movement was controlled by continuous comparison between current afferent information arriving during the movement itself and a stored set of 'sensory consequences' arising from prior successful movements. This store of prior afferent information (what Adams termed the perceptual trace) was hypothesised to develop in the early (verbal-cognitive) stage of learning through the use of extrinsic knowledge of results (KR) but to become KR-independent at later (motor) stages of learning. The model was based on an engineering analog and was consistent with pre-existing knowledge on the role of feedback in learning and performance (e.g., Adams, 1968; Bilodeau, 1966) and on the operating principles of the simple stretch reflex.

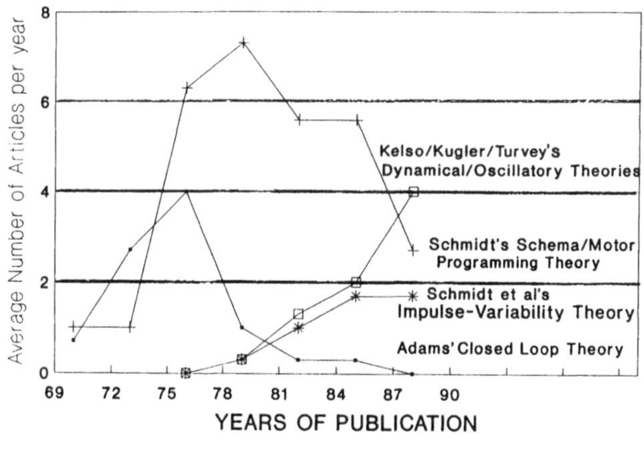

Figure 2. Average number of articles per year (averaged over 3 year periods) directly examining major motor control theories expressed as a function of the chronological history of the *Journal of Motor Behavior*.

Adams' theory gave rise to a body of normal science in which the predominant questions of interest revolved around tests of the importance of KR for learning (e.g., Newell, 1974; Newell & Chew, 1974; Wrisberg & Schmidt, 1975) and the nature of the error-detection mechanism (e.g., Adams & Goetz, 1973; Newell & Boucher, 1974; Schmidt & White, 1972) . Tests typically involved the use of slow linear positioning tasks and much of the evidence regarding KR importance, the presence of any error correction device, plus additional evidence from studies of feedback disruption (e.g., Glencross, 1977; Smith & Bowen, 1980) and the attention demands of positioning movements (e.g., Mcleod, 1978; Posner & Keele, 1969), was supportive. The anomalous data which ultimately undermined the closed loop theory's position of paradigmatic dominance was its limited explanatory power for the control of rapid actions (e.g., see Kelso & Stelmach, 1976). Particularly troublesome observations were related to the ability of subjects to control ballistic movements with duration less than feedback time (e.g., Lashley, 1951) and the ability of both human and animal subjects to continue to produce movement even in the complete absence of afferent information (e.g., Lashley, 1917; Taub, 1976). It is noteworthy that both these lines of anomalous data were in existence prior to the original formulation of Adams' theory.

Closed-loop theory attracted greatest interest in the period 1971 - 1976. Thereafter the paradigm was clearly recessive (see Figure 2) with tests of Adams' theory becoming less frequent as the normal science of the 1971-76 period lost its appeal. The rejection of closed-loop theory as *the* theory of motor control (even though it explains the control of slow positioning movements rather well) is a good example of the demise of a paradigm because of its limited explanatory scope and science's preference for all encompassing theories rather than task-specific ones.

Theories of Open-Loop Control, Motor Programs and Motor Schema

Precursors to an open-loop or centralised view of motor control date back as far as the writings of James (1890), Woodworth (1899), and Lashley (1917) for arm movements and even earlier for the control of saccadic eye movements (von Helmholtz, 1867). This, considered in conjunction with the intense and protracted interest in contemporary versions of centralised motor control (see Figure 2), portrays the notion of open-loop control and pre-planning as one of the more pervasive and persistent ideas within the motor control and learning field. In its long history the centralised control notion has undergone a series of extensions and refinements, many in the form of *ad hoc* adjustments to emergent anomalous data.

The early open-loop control notion championed by James (1890) and Lashley (1917) viewed the control of ballistic movements as involving the use of a set of pre-planned efferent commands that were executed essentially without modification by afference. The centralised control model was formalised into a testable theory by Henry and Rogers' (1960) memory drum theory, which was arguably the first formal theory of motor learning and control (see Henry, 1981, 1986; Spirduso, 1981). The memory drum theory hypothesised a relationship between reaction time (as an indicator of planning and initiation latency) and the complexity of movement and through its empirical basis both supported a range of normal science examining the RT-complexity relationship (e.g., Klapp, 1977, 1980) and incited some methodological debate (e.g., Klapp et al., 1979). Although the memory drum theory has been subsequently shown to need *ad hoc* modification to account for the unexpected mediating effects of movement type (Anson, 1982), this particular version of the central control model was largely superseded in the 1970s by the emergence of the computer metaphor and Keele's (1968) formalisation of the motor program as the vehicle for open-loop control.

Keele's original definition of the motor program was of a pre-structured set of centrally stored specific efferent normal commands which, when executed, allowed a desired movement pattern to be produced without reliance upon ongoing sensory information. The prediction of movement control independent of feedback information sparked a range of innovative experimental procedures and supported a new body of normal science. Not only was the program view consistent with pre-existing evidence (especially evidence demonstrating serial movement corrections with latencies less than reaction time (e.g., Pew, 1966) but it also proved consistent with evidence derived from a host of de-afferentation studies (e.g., Cross & McCloskey, 1973; Laszlo & Bairstow, 1971; Smith, Roberts, & Aitkens, 1972; Taub, 1976) and from a number of dual-task studies demonstrating elevated attention demand immediately prior to movement initiation (e.g., Posner & Keele, 1969). Less research attention was paid to the premise of pre-planning than to the premise of feedback independence, but nevertheless some empirical evidence has been presented demonstrating the 'running off' of pre-planned command sequences even when movement is unexpectedly blocked (Wadman, Denier van der Gon, Geuze, & Mol, 1979).

Typical of most periods of normal science the concentrated research focus upon the motor program concept unearthed some logical inconsistencies in Keele's program notion that necessitated some substantial *ad hoc* modifications to the original theory. Notable amongst the anomalies were the so-called *storage* and *novelty* problems (MacNeilage, 1970; Schmidt, 1982) which arose as a direct consequence of Keele's view that *specific* neural commands were stored in the motor program. This pair of problems dictated the need for a revised view of the motor program - one which needed reduced specificity and greater flexibility and one in which only the essential features needed to produce a wide range of variations of a given movement prototype were stored. In addition the original, strictly centralist view of the motor program suffered the antithesis of the problems encountered by closed-loop models (i.e., difficulty in explaining the ongoing correction of errors in long duration, slow velocity movements). Collectively these problems forced the field in the direction of the development of a hybrid model which retained the basic premise of central planning but which ensured that the program stored was general rather than specific and was developed and improved through the use of available feedback information. Such a model was provided in Schmidt's (1975) schema theory of motor learning and in his parallel development of the notion of the generalised motor program (Schmidt, 1976, 1985).[14] [In terms of the Kuhnian view of scientific development it is worth noting that Schmidt was in something of a unique position to reconcile both central and peripheral control positions. As a student of both Adams and Henry he had exposure to both perspectives but without a substantial commitment of time, energy or emotion into either of the competing paradigms].

Schema theory is based on the notion that task-specific experience results in the abstraction of the essential 'rules' specifying the relationship between the specific efferent commands (response specifications), environmental conditions, afferent information (in the form of sensory consequences), and movement outcome. These 'rules' provide the framework for a given class of movements and are stored in the control program. Schema theory has a learning emphasis and the so-called 'variability of practice' hypothesis it presents supported a tremendous amount of normal science in the late 1970s and early 1980s (e.g., McCracken & Stelmach, 1977; Moxley, 1979; see Schmidt, 1982 and Shapiro & Schmidt, 1982 for reviews). Despite its popularity as a theory for examination by normal science and its intuitive link with in practice trends in movement education, the evidence in favour of the theory is, at best, equivocal (e.g., van Rossum, 1989).

The persistent interest in the centralised control models is attributable more to the popularity of the generalised motor program concept than to the schema notion. The generalised motor program view (like the computer analogy upon which it is based) argues for the storage centrally of only those features of movement which remain invariant across a range of different task conditions. Those variable parameters which provide any given movement with its unique situation-specific characteristics are believed to be not stored but rather "mapped in" very late in the response organisation process. The generalised motor program notion adds, for the first time, an explicit commitment to the central *representation* of movement features as a key thrust within the centralist

---

[14] Although Schmidt's schema theory is the best known and most persistent hybrid view it is by no means the only attempt to integrate open and closed-loop control e.g., see Keele & Summers (1976) for a proposition on the specification of closed-loop reflex states within the motor program.

viewpoint (the stored features being those appearing as invariant in the movement kinematics). This has resulted in a whole gamut of normal science specifically concerned with the identification of invariant features of movement. In particular investigations of relative timing (e.g., Roth, 1988; Shapiro, 1978; Shapiro, Zernicke, Gregor, & Diestal, 1981; Viviani & Terzuolo, 1980) and relative force (e.g., Hollerbach, 1978) as potential invariant features of a range of motor skills remain popular, although the existence for such features seems less and less convincing (Gentner, 1987; Wann & Nimmo-Smith, 1990). Methodological debates regarding how invariants should be appropriately demonstrated are currently prominent (e.g., Corcos, Agarwal, & Gottlieb, 1985; Gentner, 1987; Heuer, 1988), serving as possible markers of an impending paradigm crisis. There is also a current move toward seeking evidence for invariant features through transfer studies (e.g., Heuer & Schmidt, 1988; see also Rosenbaum, 1977). This, along with parallel developments of computational models of the mind through cognitive science (e.g., Baron, 1987; Boden, 1988) ensures that interest in the central control/motor program view of movement control remains toward the forefront of current research activity.

Theories of Impulse-Variability

The impulse-variability models and theories proposed by Schmidt et al. (1978, 1979) were largely developed in an attempt to explain the well-known speed-accuracy trade-off described by Fitts' Law (Fitts, 1954). In contrast to the feedback-based explanations provided by Crossman and Goodeve (1963), the impulse-variability approach attempts to explain the effect in pre-programming terms and for this reason the work arising from the impulse-variability model should have perhaps been considered as part of the more general programming paradigm (at least with respect to the calculation of the data shown in Figure 2). The basis for considering the model separately was the expanded current scope of the model. It now supports a more general paradigm of normal science concerned with the effects of a diverse range of movement variables upon initial impulse variability (Schmidt, 1988a).

The impulse-variability model posits a direct relationship between the type of errors produced in motor tasks and the variability within the two components contributing to the initial impulse applied to a limb (viz., force and duration). The model has incited a range of normal science examining the effects of altered movement amplitude and duration upon initial impulse characteristics and upon resultant spatial and temporal errors (e.g., Newell, 1980; Newell, Carlton, & Hancock, 1984; see Hancock & Newell, 1985 and Schmidt, Sherwood, Zelaznik, & Leikind, 1985 for reviews). However, in a manner reminiscent of the difficulties encountered by closed-loop models, the explanatory power of the original model seems restricted to a given class of movements (viz., rapid, ballistic movements requiring a single initial impulse). Anomalous data emerges with more complex movements necessitating the need for *ad hoc* modifications of the original model (Meyer, Smith, & Wright, 1982; Meyer et al., 1988). The current version of the model (Meyer et al., 1988) bears some very strong parallels to some much older views of motor control (especially those of Woodworth, 1899), involving a hybridisation between open- and closed-loop views of control.

Dynamical, Emergent Perspective Theories of Motor-Control

In the case of the theories discussed to this point there has been considerable evidence of the effective use by motor control and learning theorists both of *ad hoc* amendments to existing theory and of the hybridisation of viewpoints from competing theoretical perspectives. In this sense the debates, particularly the centralist-peripheralist debates, which dominated the field from the late 1960s to the early 1980s, have not, in Kuhn's terms, resulted in revolutionary science *per se*. Anomalous data has been handled through *ad hoc* modification to existing theory and through abandonment of the search for a single, consolidated view of motor learning and control. Something of a stalemate situation was reached with the consensus that the differences in the control requirements for slow and fast movements could best be handled by different theories. The first evidence of a full scale paradigm crisis in the motor learning and control field originally emerged with the advent of conflicting consolidated theories of motor control and learning which do not afford the same prospect for reconciliation through ad hoc modification and/or hybridisation. This 'new' view of the problems of motor control and learning, coined as the 'action theory' approach (Meijer & Roth, 1988), has arisen largely out of the work of Turvey, Kugler, Kelso, and Reed (e.g., Kelso, 1981; Kelso & Schoner, 1988; Kelso et al, 1981; Kugler, 1986; Kugler, Kelso, & Turvey, 1982; Kugler & Turvey, 1986; Reed, 1982, 1988; Saltzman & Kelso, 1982) but has, in a relatively short period, attracted a considerable (and growing) following (Figure 2). The 'action systems' view is represented by a collection of theories which are grounded, *inter-alia,* in the belief that movement kinematics are *not* represented centrally (in a motor program, plan, schema, or any other form) but are rather an emergent property of the dynamics of the underlying motor system, and hence should be understood in terms of the collective physical properties of the functional muscle groups involved in any particular action.

Perhaps the first attempt to explain movement control in terms of the physical/dynamical properties of muscle was the equilibrium-point hypothesis of Fel'dman and Asatryan (Asatryan & Fel'dman, 1965; Fel'dman, 1966a, b), also known in slightly revised and more recent form as the mass-spring model (Bizzi, Polit, & Morasso, 1976; Polit & Bizzi, 1978). Typical of most radical departures in concept, this particular viewpoint on movement control was presented by researchers with backgrounds different from those previously involved in the field (they were physiologists rather than psychologists) and by researchers with no apparent attachment to the prevailing paradigm of the motor program/motor schema. The mass-spring model is based on the analogy of muscle to a weighted spring. It pre-supposes the use of critical set points (the points where the length-tension curves of opposing agonist and antagonist muscle groups are equal and opposite) as the basis for accurate movement localisation. The mass-spring model appears particularly advantageous in explaining the accurate reproduction of given spatial positions under conditions where starting position information is unreliable (hence disrupting the utility of any pre-established motor program) or ongoing afferent information is deprived [15] (hence preventing the operation of a closed-loop control model) (Polit & Bizzi, 1978, 1979). The mass-spring model supported an intense, though relatively short-lived, period of normal science in which some of the model's predictions were subjected to empirical scrutiny. These predictions included: superior recall accuracy for location rather than distance cues (e.g., Laabs, 1973); insensitivity to disruption of starting position information (e.g., Kelso & Holt, 1980); and effects upon movement time and spatial accuracy brought about by the addition of mass to a limb during both horizontal and vertical movements (e.g., Schmidt & McGown, 1980). These empirical tests of the mass spring-model typically involved unidirectional ballistic positioning tasks. In the long-term the model proved to have limited explanatory scope outside of these particular tasks. The presence of anomalous data arising from multi-directional movements (e.g., Schmidt, McGown, Quinn, & Hawkins, 1986) along with data indicating an important role for starting position information in movement recall accuracy (Fel'dman & Latash, 1982; Wallace, Frankeny, & Larish, 1982), argues that the model is probably too simple to readily explain either the control or learning of a wide range of motor skills (see also Hollerbach & Flash, 1982).

The mass-spring model (a *point attractor* system within the terminology of nonlinear dynamics) has been subsequently superseded by more complex dynamical models capable of accounting more easily for movement control in multi-directional, multi-joint movements. A favoured approach of action systems theorists (e.g., Kelso et al., 1981) is to consider the behaviour of the motor system as being that of an ensemble of limit cycle oscillators (*periodic attractors* in the nonlinear dynamics terms; Kelso & Kay, 1987; Kay, 1988) and

---

[15] The prediction of insensitivity to feedback information is one which would be reached from the mass-spring model but not from the earlier equilibrium-point hypothesis of Fel'dman and Asatryan. Fel'dman and Asatryan attributed a key role to feedback information from the muscle spindle in movement control (see Fel'dman, 1986).

to seek purely physical laws to account for selection of action categories and transitions between different forms or phases of inter-limb co-ordination (e.g., Kugler & Turvey, 1986; Turvey & Carello, 1986, 1988). The operating principles of the 'action systems' approach are derived from modern physics, and theoretical biology (e.g., Haken, 1977; Iberall, 1970; Rosen, 1978; Yates, 1979)[16] whilst the conceptual basis for these approaches involves a marriage of the views of Bernstein (1967) on co-ordination and Gibson (1961, 1979) on perception (Turvey, 1977). The conceptual origins dictate a commitment to Gibson's doctrine of ecological realism (the doctrine of reciprocity between perceiver and environment; Lombardo, 1987), and the concomitant rejection of cognitive representation, man-machine (and perceiver-environment) dualism and the basic operating principles of the information-processing model (Carello, Turvey, Kugler, & Shaw, 1984).

As a result of the philosophical differences between the action systems approach and the entrenched movement systems approach the type of data generated to support the action systems approach is necessarily quite different from that sought by adherents to the motor programming viewpoint. Normal science activities which have dominated the action systems approach have involved demonstrations of:

1. Bernstein's degrees of freedom problem and the problems posed to traditional computational models by the need for simultaneous control of a near infinite number of motor units (e.g., Turvey, Fitch, & Tuller, 1982).[17]
2. Cyclic stability and entrainment characteristics consistent with the expected properties of ensembled limit cycle oscillators (Kelso et al., 1981).
3. Global responses to perturbation of a specific joint consistent with a co-ordinative structures viewpoint (e.g., Abbs & Gracco, 1983; Kelso, Tuller, V-Bateson, & Fowler, 1984).
4. Phase transitions between different movement topologies which are predictable from physical scaling variables (Haken, Kelso, & Bunz,

---

[16] The important role of Peter Kugler in the advent of the dynamical theories should not be understated. Without attachment to any of the prevailing computational models of movement control but with a grounding in theoretical physics he was ideally positioned to import a new recipient paradigm (cf. Wilberg, 1972) to the motor learning and control field.

[17] Schmidt (1988b) points out quite correctly, however, that the degrees of freedom problem is more a difficulty for older views of the motor program (Keele, 1968) than it is for contemporary generalised motor program views.

1985; Kugler, 1986; Kugler et al., 1982; Kugler & Turvey, 1986; Thelen, Skala, & Kelso, 1987).

5. The availability of perceptual invariants specifying important co-ordinative information in units scaled to the dimensions of the perceiver and actor (Lee, 1976; Michaels, Prindle, & Turvey, 1985; Turvey & Carello, 1986, 1988; Warren, 1984).
6. Dynamic alternatives to cognitive/representational explanations of putative kinematic invariants, especially relative timing (Kelso, 1986; Kelso & Tuller, 1984; Kelso, V-Bateson, Saltzman, & Kay, 1985).

Figure 2 clearly indicates that interest in the action systems theories have emerged to the point where they now more than compete with the motor programming notion in terms of attractiveness to normal science,[18] suggesting that the motor control and learning field is now in the midst of a true paradigm crisis. Such a view is also supported by data from a citation analysis of the *Journal of Motor Behavior* undertaken by Sparrow and Sparrow (1990).

Those authors who are closely identified with motor programming theory would be expected to have received progressively fewer citations in the *Journal of Motor Behavior* as interest in the paradigm declined. Some evidence for this proposition is found in an analysis of the citation frequency in the *Journal of Motor Behavior* of various theorists over time. Steven Keele, for example, was cited 65 times between 1975 and 1979. From 1980 to 1984 he was cited 43 times and between 1985 and 1989 he received 21 citations from the contributors to the *Journal of Motor Behavior*. In contrast, those scholars who have promoted the action systems approach have enjoyed a corresponding increase in citation frequency. Over the same 4 year time intervals Scott Kelso obtained respectively 20, 73, and 76 citations. Peter Kugler made his first appearance in the Sparrows' multi-cited lists in the period 1985 to 1989, over these years he was the ninth most-cited author with 23 citations to articles in which he was the first or sole author. David Lee showed a similarly rapid emergence as a highly cited author by being fifth most-cited in the *Journal of Motor Behavior* between 1985 and 1987 with 33 citations. Once more Lee's citation history can be interpreted as evidence of growing support for the action systems paradigm.

It is noteworthy however, that some motor behaviour researchers have continued to be highly cited even though their work is supportive of a programming perspective rather than of the emerging action systems paradigm.

---

[18] For comparative purposes present activity in the motor programming view should perhaps be best approximated from Figure 2 by summating the number of articles per year examining the generalized motor programming theory *and* the impulse-variability theory.

Table 1. Dimensions of contrast between the 'Movement Systems' and 'Action Systems' approaches in motor control and learning.

DIMENSIONS OF CONTRAST	'MOVEMENT SYSTEMS' APPROACH	'ACTION SYSTEMS' APPROACH
Alternative Label	Information-processing approach Prescriptive approach Computational approach Representational approach	Dynamical approach Emergent approach Direct approach
Philosophical Origins	Belief in the man machine metaphor Implicit support of the actor-environment dualism	Belief in ecological realism Explicit support of actor environment synergy
Origin of Theoretical Explanation and Model	Computer Science and Engineering	Modern physics and Theoretical/Comparitive Biology
Direction of Explanatory Logic	Improved Explanatory Power by adding sophistication and intelligence to the computational model	Improved Explanatory power by seeking more fundamental processes
Nearest Psychology Sub-Discipline	Cognitive Psychology	Ecological Psychology
Movement Organisation and Control Mode	Top-down, hierachical control acting via prescription	Bottom up heterarchical control acting through coordinative structures
Solution to the control of Multiple Degrees of Freedom	Generalised motor programs structured and stored centrally	Coordinative structures which self assemble the dynamical properties of the motor system
Relationship of Control Mode to kinematics	A priori planning resulting in desired kinematics. Organisation and assembly prescribed from over-riding plan	Kinematics as an a posteriori consequence of the self organisation and self assembly of muscle collectives

Central Representation of Desired Movement	Present	Absent
Translation Mechanism	Essential to convert abstract plan to 'language' of muscle	Not necessary; All control is in common environmental units
Role of Muscle	Subserviently carries out control commands specified centrally	Determines movement form and phase interactions through dynamics
Temporal Organisation of Movement	Temporal features of kinematics metered out through an intrinsic time keeping device	Temporal features of kinematics arise as an emergent property through preservation of invariant phase angular relationships between effectors
Relationship to Perception	Independent serial processes with perception preceding action (Separate stages as revealed by Sternberg's addictive factors method)	Perception and action as tightly coupled processes, functionally and evolutionally inseparable. Perception in units of action and vice versa
Perceptual Model Supported	Computational model (e.g., Marr, 1982)	Direct Perception model of Gibson (1979)
Explanation of Learning	Improved information processing strategies (and, with development, increased processing capacities).	Increased attunement to essential invariants and control over context-conditioned variability
Role of Memory in Learning	Fundamental to improve strategy formation and long term skill acquisition	Minimal role in learning. Many deny memory processes per se because of necessity to invoke representation
Type of Experimental Paradigm Advocated	Laboratory work on contrived movements historically favoured but naturalistic work ultimately desirable	Ecological validity essential. Study of natural actions prescribed.
Units of Measurement	Information measured mathematically with respect to stimulus/task uncertainty and difficulty	Essential information desribed in units scaled to the actor

Richard Schmidt, for example, remained the most highly cited author in the *Journal of Motor Behavior* throughout each of the 1975-79, 1980-84 and 1985-89 time periods, indicating prolonged research interest in the theoretical premises he has presented. Stuart Klapp maintained third-ranked position in terms of citation frequency in both the 1980 to 1984 and 1985 to 1989 periods, despite an absolute fall in his citations numbers from 57 to 44. Likewise, Steve Keele continues to be highly cited. It might be argued from these citation data that there are strong "pockets of resistance" to the action systems advance with many groups of researchers maintaining an interest in motor programming and other theoretical perspectives.

In concluding this section the recent publication of research in other non-specialist motor control and learning journals (e.g., the publication in 1986 of a special issue on perception and action in *Acta Psychologica* and the frequent appearance of work on affordances following the publication in 1984 of Warren's work in the *Journal of Experimental Psychology: Human Perception and Performance*), and the emergence of a new society and journal (*Journal of Ecological Psychology*; first appearing in 1989) representing much of the emergent action systems viewpoint, should also be noted as additional indicators of what Kuhn (1962, 1970) would regard as a paradigm crisis. In the next and final section we discuss in more detail the nature of the existing paradigm crisis and use parallels from Kuhn's historical analysis of science to predict probable outcomes of the crisis.

THE CURRENT PARADIGMATIC CRISIS: THE MOVEMENT SYSTEMS-ACTION SYSTEMS CONTROVERSY

In contrast to the earlier, much publicised centralist-peripheralist (open loop - closed loop) debates in the motor learning and control field, where the principal point of contention related simply to the respective importance of pre-planned efferent commands and ongoing afferent information, the points of divergence between the movement systems and action systems are many and varied and do not lend themselves easily to reconciliation (Table 1).

The points of difference noted in Table 1 are by no means exhaustive and readings of the position papers of the leading protagonists in the current debates not only on the movement control front (e.g., Kelso, 1986 and Schmidt, 1988b) but also on the perception front (e.g., Michaels & Carello, 1981 and Ullman, 1980) indicate the presence of deep conceptual and philosophical differences in the two positions - differences atypical of the earlier centralist-peripheralist debate (Beek & Meijer, 1988). The presence of philosophy within a given debate in a scientific field is symptomatic of a paradigm crisis in Kuhnian terms and the current situation in the motor learning and control field appears to fit this description precisely. In the sub-sections that follow we consider briefly the options for resolution of the current crisis viz., the reconciliation of the differences between the two competing approaches and, in a manner reminiscent of the centralist-peripheralist debate, the emergence of a hybrid model or alternatively the onset of a period of protracted debate and revolutionary science resulting eventually in the emergence of a new dominant paradigm.

Grounds for a Movement Systems - Action Systems Reconciliation

Empirical work within the movement systems and action systems paradigms have typically involved the study of quite different things. The traditional information-processing approach has typically involved the testing of untrained subjects on contrived perceptual-motor tasks with relatively high cognitive demand while the action systems approach has focused upon overlearnt cyclic, natural actions often performed by experienced subjects. It is, therefore, tempting to suggest, as many have (e.g., Colley & Beech, 1988; Epstein, 1986; Roy, 1982, 1983; Schmidt, 1988b; Summers, 1986; van Wierengen, 1986, 1988), that the prevailing differences may be largely a function of differences in levels of analysis (Stelmach, 1987) and levels of skill automaticity. The well practised, automated natural actions examined by adherents to the action systems approach may well be controlled through use of the motor system dynamics in the absence, or near absence, of any type of *a priori* planning, cognitive representation, or cortical control. It may be equally true, however, that a higher, more attentionally demanding level of control (cf. Shiffrin & Schneider, 1977) involving planning, representation, and all manner of cognitive strategies may also exist. This mode of control might have a role in voluntarily initiating and, where necessary, overriding lower-level dynamic systems, especially during the early stages of learning. Such a system would more likely come under focus when the task being examined is a novel, cognitively-demanding task of the type typically used by adherents to the information-processing paradigm.

A number of pieces of evidence can be gathered together to support the hybrid view of a multi-levelled motor system (cf. Glencross, 1978), featuring, at one level, cognitive but attentionally-costly override of, at a lower level, an essentially automatic system composed of an ensemble of limit-cycle oscillators. Such supporting evidence would include :

1. Automatic gait control by sub-cortical mechanisms, but with dependence upon descending efference for pattern initiation (Grillner, 1975; Shik & Orlovskii, 1976)
2. Gait form transitions which are generally predictable from physical parameters such as mass and leg length (Hoyt & Taylor, 1981; Kugler & Turvey, 1986) but which can be voluntarily overridden, such as in the case of human race walkers (van Wierengen, 1986).

3. Tight spatial and temporal coupling of the two hands during early attempts at synchronous bimanual activity (Kelso, Southard, & Goodman, 1979) but an uncoupling of this with continued practice.
4. The presence of strict temporal entrainment properties of the two hands during polyrhythmical tapping by untrained subjects but an uncoupling of this bimanual dependence by trained subjects (musicians) (Summers, 1989).
5. An inability of dynamics alone to explain all variance observed in skilled (juggling) performance (Beek & Beek, 1988).

The attractive feature of a reconciled hybrid model of motor control is that it helps alleviate persistent anomalies for each of the competing paradigms. In particular the self-organising nature of dynamic control of cyclic (lower-level) activities provides a mechanism through which the computational demands of programmed control might be reduced to manageable levels. Likewise an acceptance of the possibility of some cognitive control processes allows the action systems approach to account more readily for learning effects, especially those taking place with the assistance of either verbal or visual instruction (for which some form of internal representation would appear likely). Such a hybridisation would not be without precedent with reasonably satisfactory intermeshing of 'top-down' and 'bottom-up' processing having been made in the past within cognitive psychology (e.g., Norman, 1968, 1969). The cerebellum with its unique design for accepting proprioceptive inputs from virtually all motor system receptors in one area and separate cortical inputs to another seems ideally designed to act as an integrator for both muscle-driven and cortically-driven information (Greer, 1984) and may well be an important neural correlate of any consolidated hybrid model of motor control.

The Case Against Reconciliation and the Prospect of Protracted Debate

Although the case for reconciliation of the two competing paradigms is superficially attractive, there are reasons to doubt whether a hybrid view would ever attract sufficient support from the adherents of either of the existing paradigms to form the basis of a new normal science. In particular it needs to be re-emphasised that, unlike earlier debates in the motor control and learning field which have, to some extent, been satisfactorily resolved through hybridisation, the current debate has all the characteristics of a true paradigm crisis. The history of science reveals that debates in such circumstances are rarely solved empirically because the competing paradigms have philosophical and conceptual differences. [Schmidt, 1988b and others in the movement systems - action systems debate (Meijer & Roth, 1988), for example, express clear frustration at the difficulty of finding sufficient common ground for empirical tests of the competing views]. Examination of Table 1 illustrates the extent of both the conceptual and philosophical differences between the two positions and the trend in recent debate (Meijer & Roth, 1988) has been for these differences to be increasing rather than diminishing. Standing firmly in the way of the acceptance of any hybrid model is the fact that no hybridisation can be meaningfully achieved without the basic tenets of one or both paradigms being undermined. For example, a multi-level hybrid model of the type proposed in the previous sub-section would require some form of cognitive representation to be included, yet to establish such an entity would directly violate the philosophical base of the action systems approach. A hybrid model is, therefore, unlikely to prove attractive to adherents of either competing paradigm and is hence unlikely to ever gain the necessary "majority view" to guide the ongoing normal science of the field.

In agreement with Beek and Meijer (1988) we believe that the current paradigm crisis is unlikely to be solved through reconciliation of the two views. Rather the motor learning and control field seems destined to enter a protracted period of paradigmatic debate and division. As to which view will eventually emerge as dominant is less clear. Support for the action systems approach, and ecological psychology in general, is clearly gaining impetus [19] and this is due among other things to the approach's aesthetic and intuitive appeal (e.g., the simplicity of many of the notions of ecological psychology are consistent with personal experience of many of the acts it describes); its attention to the operating mechanisms and language of muscle; and its interest in the study of natural 'real-world' actions.[20] However, the action systems approach is, at this point, far from committed to a clear unified theory of learning and this stands as a major hurdle to the demonstration of empirical adequacy and to the approach's emergence as a dominant paradigm capable of directing both the research and curriculum development activities of the field. Explaining learning adequately without recourse to cognitive constructs such as representation and memory is likely to prove extremely difficult. In addition, the presence of some

---

[19] The "defection" of influential figures in the field (such as Newell, 1989) to an 'action systems' perspective is a good example of growing acceptance of the emerging view.

[20] The ecological validity preference in itself should not be a deciding factor in the determination of the most appropriate paradigm, however. Although the prevailing information-processing paradigm of the movement systems theorists has usually involved contrived laboratory experiments there are nevertheless no structural limitations preventing the application of information processing principles to 'real world' motor control problems and indeed some good examples of this exist (e.g., McLeod, 1987; Roth,1988).

alarming facts for both current paradigms (such as the absence of kinematic features of true invariance; Gentner, 1987) suggests that some of the previous key problems for the field, especially Bernstein's (1967) degrees of freedom problem, may not as yet have had their final influence on the direction of the motor learning and control field. For whichever of the current views finally emerges as dominant from the current paradigm crisis there appear likely to be still further periods of turbulence ahead.

REFERENCES

Abbs, J.H., & Gracco, V.L. (1983). Sensorimotor actions in the control of multi-movement speech gestures. *Trends in Neuroscience*, *6*, 391-395.

Abernethy, B. (in press). Experimentation in action: A critique of the process of experimentation and the notion of the expert researcher. In C.W. Snyder, Jr., & B. Abernethy (Eds.), *Understanding human action through experimentation*. Champaign, IL: Human Kinetics.

Adams, J.A. (1968). Response feedback and learning. *Psychological Bulletin, 70*, 486-504.

Adams, J.A. (1971). A closed-loop theory of motor learning. *Journal of Motor Behavior, 3*, 111-150.

Adams, H.A. & Goetz, E.T. (1973). Feedback and practice as variables in error detection and correction. *Journal of Motor Behavior, 5*, 217-224.

Anson, J.G. (1982). Memory drum theory: Alternative tests and explanations for the complexity effects on simple reaction time. *Journal of Motor Behavior, 14*, 228-246.

Asatryan, D.G., & Fel'dman, A.G. (1965). Bio-physics of complex systems and mathematical models. Functional tuning of nervous system with control of movement or maintenance of a steady posture: I. Mechano-graphic analysis of the work of the joint on execution of a postural task. *Biophysics, 10*, 925-935.

Barber, B. (1961). Resistance by scientists to scientific discovery. *Science, 134*, 506-602.

Barber, T.X. (1976). *Pitfalls in human research: Ten pivotal points.* New York: Pergamon.

Baron, R.J. (1987). *The cerebral computer: An introduction to the computational structure of the human brain.* Hillsdale, NJ: Lawrence Erlbaum Associates.

Bartlett, F.C. (1958). *Thinking: An experimental and social study.* London: Unwin University Books.

Beek, P.J., & Beek, W.J. (1988). Tools for constructing dynamical models of rhythmic movement. *Human Movement Science*, 7, 301-342.

Beek, P.J., & Meijer, O.G. (1988). On the nature of 'the' motor-action controversy. In O.G. Meijer, & K. Roth (Eds.), *Complex movement behaviour: 'The' motor-action controversy* (pp. 157-185). Amsterdam: North-Holland.

Bernstein, N.A. (1967). *The co-ordination and regulation of movements.* Oxford: Pergamon Press.

Bilodeau, I.M. (1966). Information feedback. In E.A. Bilodeau (Ed.), *Acquisition of skill* (pp. 255-296). New York: Academic Press.

Bizzi, E., Polit, A., & Morasso, P. (1976). Mechanisms underlying achievement of final head position. *Journal of Neurophysiology, 39,* 435-444.

Bloor, D. (1971). Two paradigms of scientific knowledge? *Science Studies, 1,* 101-115.

Boden, M.A. (1988). *Computer models of mind: Computational approaches in theoretical psychology.* Cambridge: Cambridge University Press.

Brooks, G.A. (Ed.) (1981). *Perspectives on the academic discipline of physical education.* Champaign, IL: Human Kinetics.

Bunge, M. (1967). *Scientific research I: The search for system.* Berlin: Springer-Verlag.

Carello, C., Turvey, M.T., Kugler, P.N., & Shaw, R.E. (1984). Inadequacies in the computer metaphor. In M. Gazzaniga (Ed.), *Handbook of cognitive neuroscience* (pp. 229-248) New York: Plenum.

Chalmers, A.F. (1982). *What is this thing called science?* (2nd ed.). Brisbane, Australia: University of Queensland Press.

Colley, A.M. & Beech, J.R. (1988). Grounds for reconciliation: Some preliminary thoughts on cognition and action. In A.M. Colley & J.R. Beech (Eds.), *Cognition and action in skilled behaviour* (pp. 1-11). Amsterdam: North-Holland.

Corcos, D.M., Agarwal, G.C., & Gottlieb, G.L. (1985). A note on accepting the null hypothesis: Problems with respect to the mass-spring and pulse-step models of motor control. *Journal of Motor Behavior*, 17, 481-487.

Cross, M.J., & McCloskey, D.I. (1973). Position sense following surgical removal of joints in man. *Brain Research, 55,* 443-445.

Crossman, E.R.F.W., & Goodeve, P.J. (1983). Feedback control of hand movements and Fitts' law. *Quarterly Journal of Experimental Psychology, 35A*, 251-278. (Original work published 1963).

de Grazzia, A. (1966). The scientific reception system. In A. de Grazzia, R.E. Juergens, & L.C. Stecchini (Eds.), *The Velikovsky affair: Scientism vs. Science* (pp. 171-231). New Hyde Park, NY: University Books.

Diamond, S.S., & Morton, D.R. (1978). Empirical landmarks in social psychology. *Personality and Social Psychology Bulletin, 4*, 217-221.

Dickinson, J., & Goodman, D. (1986). Perspectives on motor learning theory and motor control. In L.D. Zaichkowsky & C.Z. Fuchs (Eds.), *The psychology of motor behavior: Development, control, learning and performance* (pp. 29-48). Ithaca, NY: Mouvement Publications.

Dunnette, M. D. (1966). Fads, fashions, and folderol in psychology. *American Psychologist, 21*, 343-352.

Epstein, W. (1986). Contrasting conceptions of perception and action. *Acta Psychologica, 63*, 103-115.

Fel'dman, A.G. (1966a). Functional tuning of the nervous system with control of movement or maintenance of a steady posture: II. Controllable parameters of the muscles. *Biophysics, 11*, 565-578.

Fel'dman, A.G. (1966b). Functional tuning of the nervous system with control of movement or maintenance of a steady posture: III. Mechanographic analysis of the execution by man of the simplest motor tasks. *Biophysics, 11*, 667-675.

Fel'dman, A.G. (1986). Once more on the equilibrium point hypothesis (model) for motor control. *Journal of Motor Behavior, 18*, 17-54.

Fel'dman, A.G., & Latash, M.L. (1982). Interaction of efferent and afferent signals underlying joint position sense: Empirical and theoretical approaches. *Journal of Motor Behavior, 14*, 174-193.

Fitts, P.M. (1954). The information capacity of the human motor system in controlling the amplitude of movement. *Journal of Experimental Psychology, 47*, 381-391.

Gentner, D.R. (1987). Timing of skilled motor performance: Tests of the proportional duration model. *Psychological Review, 94*, 255-276.

Gibson, J.J. (1961). Ecological optics. *Vision Research, 1*, 253-262.

Gibson, J.J. (1979). *The ecological approach to visual perception*. Boston, MA: Houghton-Mifflin.

Glencross, D.J. (1977). Control of skilled movement. *Psychological Bulletin, 84*, 14-29.

Glencross, D.J. (1978). Cognitive structure and the acquisition of skill. In D.J. Glencross (Ed.), *Psychology and sport* (pp. 97-119). Sydney: McGraw-Hill.

Greenwald, A.G., Pratkanis, A.R., Leippe, M.R., & Baumgardner, M.H. (1986). Under what condition does theory obstruct research progress? *Psychological Review, 93*, 216-229.

Greer, K. (1984). Physiology of motor control. In M.M. Smyth & A.M. Wing (Eds.). *The psychology of human movement* (pp. 17-46). London: Academic Press.

Grillner, S. (1975). Locomotion in vertebrates: Central mechanisms and reflex interaction. *Physiological Reviews, 55*, 247-304.

Haken, H. (1977). *Synergetics: An introduction*. Heidelberg: Springer-Verlag.

Haken, H., Kelso, J.A.S., & Bunz, H. (1985). A theoretical model of phase transitions in human hand movements. *Biological Cybernetics, 51*, 347-356.

Hancock, P.A., & Newell, K.M. (1985). The movement speed-accuracy relationship in space-time. In H. Heuer, U. Kleinbeck, & K.-H. Schmidt

(Eds.), *Motor behavior: Programming, control, and acquisition* (pp. 153-188). Berlin: Springer-Verlag.

Henkel, R.E. (1976). *Tests of significance*. Beverley Hills, CA: Sage Publications.

Henry, F.M. (1981). The evolution of the memory drum theory of neuromotor reaction. In G.A. Brooks (Ed.), *Perspectives on the academic discipline of physical education* (pp. 301-322). Champaign, IL: Human Kinetics.

Henry, F.M. (1986). Development of the motor memory trace and control program. *Journal of Motor Behavior, 18*, 77-100.

Henry, F.M. (in press). Perspectives on the development of the memory drum theory. In C.W.Snyder, Jr., & B.Abernethy (Eds.), *Understanding human action through experimentation*. Champaign, IL: Human Kinetics.

Henry, F.M. & Rogers, D.E. (1960). Increased response latency for complicated movements and a 'memory drum' theory of neuromotor reaction. *Research Quarterly, 31*, 448-458.

Heuer, H. (1988). Testing the invariance of relative timing: Comment on Gentner (1987). *Journal of Experimental Psychology: Human Perception and Performance, 95*, 552-557.

Heuer, H., & Schmidt, R.A. (1988). Transfer of learning among motor patterns with different relative timing. *Journal of Experimental Psychology: Human Perception and Performance, 14*, 241-252.

Hollerbach, J.M. (1978). *A study of human motor control through analysis and synthesis of handwriting*. Unpublished doctoral dissertation, Massachusetts Institute of Technology, Cambridge.

Hollerbach, J.M., & Flash, T. (1982). Dynamic interactions between limb segments during planar arm movement. *Biological Cybernetics, 44*, 67-77.

Hoyt, D.F., & Taylor, C.R. (1981). Gait and the energetics of locomotion in horses. *Nature*, 292, 239-240.

Hull, C.L. (1943). *Principles of behavior*. New York: Appleton-Century-Crofts.

Iberall, A. (1970). Periodic phenomena in organisms seen as non-linear systems. *Theoria to Theory, 4*, 40-53.

James, W. (1890). *The principles of psychology* (Vol.1) New York: Holt.

Katahn, M., & Koplin, J.H. (1968). Paradigm clash: Comment on "Some recent criticisms of behaviorism and learning theory with special reference to Breger and McGough and to Chomsky". *Psychological Bulletin, 69*, 147-148.

Kay, B. (1988). The dimensionality of movement trajectories and the degrees of freedom problem: A tutorial. *Human Movement Science, 7*, 343-364.

Keele, S.W. (1968). Movement control in skilled motor performance. *Psychological Bulletin, 70*, 387-403.

Keele, S.W., & Summers, J.J. (1976). The structure of motor programs. In G.E. Stelmach (Ed.), *Motor control: Issues and trends* (pp. 109-142). New York: Academic Press.

Kelso, J.A.S. (1981). Contrasting perspectives on order and regulation in movement. In J. Long, & A. Baddeley (Eds.), *Attention and Performance IX* (pp. 437-458). Hillsdale, NJ: Lawrence Erlbaum Associates.

Kelso, J.A.S. (1982). The process approach to understanding human motor behavior: An introduction. In J.A.S. Kelso (Ed.), *Human motor behavior: An introduction* (pp. 3-19). Hillsdale, NJ: Lawrence Erlbaum Associates.

Kelso, J.A.S. (1986). Pattern formation in multi-degree of freedom speech and limb movements. *Experimental Brain Research Supplement, 15*, 105-128.

Kelso, J.A.S., & Holt, K.G. (1980). Exploring the vibratory systems analysis of human movement production. *Journal of Neurophysiology, 43*, 1183-1196.

Kelso, J.A.S., Holt, K.G., Rubin, P., & Kugler, P.N. (1981). Patterns of human interlimb coordination emerge from the properties of nonlinear, limit-cycle oscillatory processes: Theory and data. *Journal of Motor Behavior, 13*, 226-261.

Kelso, J.A.S., & Kay, B.A. (1987). Information and control: A macroscopic analysis of perception-action coupling. In H. Heuer & A.F. Sanders (Eds.), *Perspectives on perception and action* (pp. 3-32). Hillsdale, NJ: Lawrence Erlbaum Associates.

Kelso, J.A.S., & Schoner, G. (1988). Self-organization of coordinative movement patterns. *Human Movement Science, 7*, 27-46.

Kelso, J.A.S., Southard, D.L., & Goodman, D. (1979). On the coordination of two handed movements. *Journal of Experimental Psychology: Human Perception and Performance, 5*, 229-238.

Kelso, J.A.S., & Stelmach, G.E. (1976). Central and peripheral mechanisms in motor control. In G.E. Stelmach (Ed.), *Motor control: Issues and trends* (pp. 1-40). New York: Academic Press.

Kelso, J.A.S., & Tuller, B. (1984). Converging evidence in support of common dynamical principles for speech and movement coordination. *American Journal of Physiology, 246*, R928-R395.

Kelso, J.A.S., Tuller, B., V-Bateson, E., & Fowler, C.A. (1984). Functionally specific articulatory cooperation following jaw perturbations during speech: Evidence for coordinative structures. *Journal of Experimental Psychology: Human Perception and Performance, 10*, 812-832.

Kelso, J.A.S., V-Bateson, E., Saltzman, E.L., & Kay, B. (1985). A qualitative dynamic analysis of reiterant speech production: Phase portraits, kinematics and dynamic modeling. *Journal of the Acoustical Society of America, 77*, 266-280.

Kendler, H.H. (1981). *Psychology: A science in conflict*. New York: Oxford University Press.

Klapp, S.T. (1977). Reaction time analysis of programmed control. *Exercise and Sport Sciences Reviews, 5*, 231-253.

Klapp, S.T. (1980). The memory drum theory after twenty years: Comments on Henry's note. *Journal of Motor Behavior, 12*, 169-171.

Klapp, S.T., Abbott, J., Coffman, K., Greim, D., Snider, R., & Young, F. (1979). Simple and choice reaction time methods in the study of motor programming. *Journal of Motor Behavior, 11*, 91-101.

Kugler, P.N. (1986). A morphological perspective on the origin and evolution of movement patterns. In M.G. Wade, & H.T.A. Whiting (Eds.), *Motor development in children: Aspects of coordination and control* (pp. 459-525). Dordrecht: Martinus Nijhoff.

Kugler, P.N., Kelso, J.A.S., & Turvey, M.T. (1982). On coordination and control in naturally developing systems. In J.A.S. Kelso, & J.E. Clark (Eds.), *The development of movement control and coordination* (pp. 5-78). New York: Wiley.

Kugler, P.N., & Turvey, M.T. (1986). *Information, natural law and the self-assembly of rhythmic movement*. Hillsdale, N.J: Lawrence Erlbaum Associates.

Kuhn, T.S. (1962). *The structure of scientific revolutions*. Chicago: University of Chicago Press.

Kuhn, T.S. (1970). *The structure of scientific revolutions* (2nd edition). Chicago: University of Chicago Press.

Kuhn, T.S. (1973). Second thoughts on paradigms. In F. Suppe (Ed.), *The structure of scientific theories* (pp. 459-482). Urbana, IL: University of Illinios Press.

Laabs, G.J. (1973). Retention characteristics of different reproduction cues in motor short-term memory. *Journal of Experimental Psychology, 100*, 168-177.

Lachman, S.J. (1960). *The foundations of science*. New York: Vantage Press.

Lakatos, I. (1970a). History of science and its rational reconstruction. In R.C. Buck, & R.S. Cohen (Eds.), *Boston studies in the philosophy of science* (Vol. 8). Dordrecht, Netherlands: Reidel.

Lakatos, I. (1970b). Falsification and the methodology of scientific research programmes. In I. Lakatos, & A. Musgrave (Eds.), *Criticism and the growth of knowledge* (pp. 91-196). Cambridge: Cambridge University Press.

Lakatos, I., & Musgrave, A. (Eds.), (1970). *Criticism and the growth of knowledge*. Cambridge: Cambridge University Press.

Landers, D.M. (1983). Whatever happened to theory testing in sport psychology? *Journal of Sport Psychology, 5*, 135-158.

Lashley, K.S. (1917). The accuracy of movement in the absence of excitation from the moving organ. *The American Journal of Physiology, 43*, 169-194.

Lashley, K.S. (1951). The problem of serial order behavior. In L.A. Jeffress (Ed.), *Cerebral mechanisms in behavior: The Hixon Symposium*. New York: Wiley.

Laszlo, J.I., & Bairstow, P.J. (1971). Accuracy of movement, peripheral feedback and efference copy. *Journal of Motor Behavior, 3*, 241-252.

Lee, D.N., (1976). A theory of visual control of braking based on information about time-to-collision. *Perception, 5,* 437-459.

Lombardo, T.J. (1987). *The reciprocity of perceiver and environment: The evolution of James J. Gibson's ecological psychology.* Hillsdale, NJ: Lawrence Erlbaum Associates.

MacNeilage, P.F. (1970). Motor control of serial ordering of speech. *Psychological Review, 77,* 182-196.

Mahoney, M.J. (1976). *Scientist as subject: The psychological imperative.* Cambridge, MA: Ballinger.

Martens, R. (1987). Science, knowledge, and sport psychology. *The Sport Psychologist, 1,* 29-55.

McCracken, H.D., & Stelmach, G.E. (1977). A test of the schema theory of discrete motor learning. *Journal of Motor Behavior, 9,* 193-201.

McLeod, P. (1978). Does probe RT measure central processing demand? *Quarterly Journal of Experimental Psychology, 30,* 83-89.

McLeod, P. (1987). Visual reaction time and high-speed ballgames. *Perception, 16,* 49-59.

Meijer, O.G., & Roth, K. (Eds.) (1988). *Complex movement behaviour: 'The' motor-action controversy.* Amsterdam: North-Holland.

Meyer, D.E., Abrams, R.A., Kornblum, S., Wright, C.E., & Smith, J.E.K. (1988). Optimality in human motor performance: Ideal control of rapid aimed movement. *Psychological Review, 95,* 340-370.

Meyer, D.E., Smith, J.E.K., & Wright, C.E. (1982). Models for the speed and accuracy of aimed movements. *Psychological Review, 89,* 449-482.

Michaels, C.F., & Carello, C. (1981). *Direct perception.* Englewood Cliffs, NJ: Prentice-Hall.

Michaels, C.F., Prindle, S., & Turvey, M.T. (1985). A note on the natural basis of action categories: The catching distance of mantids. *Journal of Motor Behavior, 17,* 255-264.

Mitroff, I.I. (1974a). *The subjective side of science.* New York: Elsevier.

Mitroff, I.I. (1974b). Norms and counter-norms in a select group of the Apollo moon scientists: A case study of the ambivalence of scientists. *American Sociological Review, 39,* 579-595.

Moxley, S.E. (1979). Schema: the variability of practice hypothesis. *Journal of Motor Behavior, 11,* 65-70.

Newell, K.M. (1974). Knowledge of results and motor learning. *Journal of Motor Behavior, 6,* 235-244.

Newell, K.M. (1980). The speed-accuracy paradox in movement control: Errors of time and space. In G.E. Stelmach (Ed.), *Tutorials in motor behavior* (pp. 501-510). Amsterdam: North-Holland.

Newell, K.M. (1985). Coordination, control and skill. In D. Goodman, R.B. Wilberg, & I.M. Franks (Eds.), *Differing perspectives in motor learning, memory, and control* (pp. 295-317). Amsterdam: North-Holland.

Newell, K.M. (1989). On task and theory specificity. *Journal of Motor Behavior, 21,* 92-96.
Newell, K.M., & Boucher, J-L.P. (1974). Motor response recognition: Two processes. *Journal of Motor Behavior, 6,* 81-86.
Newell, K.M., Carlton, L.G., & Hancock, P.A. (1984). Kinetic analysis of response variability. *Psychological Bulletin, 96,* 133-151.
Newell, K.M., & Chew, R.A. (1974). Recall and recognition in motor learning. *Journal of Motor Behavior, 6,* 245-253.
Norman, D.A. (1968). Toward a theory of memory and attention. *Psychological Review, 75,* 522-536.
Norman, D.A. (1969). *Memory and attention.* New York: Wiley.
Park, R.J. (1981). The emergence of the academic discipline of physical education in the United States. In G.A. Brooks (Ed.), *Perspectives on the academic discipline of physical education* (pp. 20-45). Champaign, IL: Human Kinetics.
Pew, R.W. (1966). Acquisition of hierarchical control over the temporal organization of a skill. *Journal of Experimental Psychology, 71,* 764-771.
Planck, M. (1949). Scientific autobiography and other papers. (Trans. F. Gaynor). New York.
Polit, A., & Bizzi, E. (1978). Processes controlling arm movements in monkeys. *Science, 201,* 1235-1237.
Polit, A. & Bizzi, E. (1979). Characteristics of motor programs underlying arm movements in monkeys. *Journal of Neurophysiology, 42,* 183-194.
Popper, K. (1959). *The logic of scientific discovery.* New York: Harper & Row.
Posner, M.I., & Keele, S.W. (1969). Attentional demands of movement. *Proceedings of the 16th Congress of Applied Psychology.* Amsterdam: Swets and Zeitlinger.
Reed, E.S. (1982). An outline of a theory of action systems. *Journal of Motor Behavior, 14,* 98-134.
Reed, E.S. (1988). Applying the theory of action systems to the study of motor skills. In O.G. Meijer & K. Roth (Eds.), *Complex motor behaviour: 'The' motor-action controversy* (pp. 45-86). Amsterdam: North-Holland.
Rosen, R. (1978). *Fundamentals of measurement and representation of natural systems.* New York: North-Holland.
Rosenbaum, D.A. (1977). Selective adaptation of "command neurons" in the human motor system. *Neuropsychologia, 15,* 81-92.
Rosenbaum, D.A. (1985). Motor programming: A review and scheduling theory. In H. Heuer, U. Kleinbeck & K.-H. Schmidt (Eds.), Motor behavior: *Programming, control, and acquisition* (pp. 1-33). Berlin: Springer-Verlag.
Rosenthal, R. (1966). *Experimental effects in behavioral research.* New York: Appleton-Century-Crofts.
Roth, K. (1988). Investigations on the basis of the generalized motor programme hypothesis. In O.G. Meijer, & K. Roth (Eds.), *Complex movement*

behaviour: 'The' motor-action controversy (pp. 261-288). Amsterdam: North-Holland.

Roy, E.A. (1982). Action and performance. In A. Ellis (Ed.), *Normality and pathology in cognitive function*. London: Academic Press.

Roy, E.A. (1983). Neuropsychological perspectives on apraxia and related disorders. In R.A. Magill (Ed.), *Memory and control of action* (pp. 293-320). Amsterdam: North-Holland.

Salmela, J.H. (1979). Psychology and sport: Fear of applying. In P. Klavora, & J.V. Daniel (Eds.), *Coach, athlete and the sport psychologist* (pp. 13-21). Toronto, Ontario: University of Toronto.

Saltzman, E., & Kelso, J.A.S. (1982). Skilled actions: A task dynamic approach. *Psychological Review, 94,* 84-106.

Schmidt, R.A. (1975). A schema theory of discrete motor skill learning. *Psychological Review, 82,* 225-260.

Schmidt, R.A. (1976). Control processes in motor skills. *Exercise and Sport Sciences Reviews, 4,* 229-261.

Schmidt, R.A. (1980). Past and future issues in motor programming. *Research Quarterly for Exercise and Sport, 51,* 122-140.

Schmidt, R.A. (1982). The schema concept. In J.A.S. Kelso (Ed.), *Human motor behavior: An introduction* (pp. 219-235). Hillsdale, NJ: Lawrence Erlbaum Associates.

Schmidt, R.A. (1985). The search for invariance in skilled movement behavior. *Research Quarterly for Exercise and Sport, 56,* 188-200.

Schmidt, R.A. (1988a). *Motor control and learning: A behavioral emphasis* (2nd ed.). Champaign, IL: Human Kinetics.

Schmidt, R.A. (1988b). Motor and action perspectives on motor behavior. In O.G. Meijer & K. Roth (Eds.), *Complex movement behaviour: 'The' motor-action controversy* (pp. 3-44). Amsterdam: North-Holland.

Schmidt, R.A., & McGown, C.M. (1980). Terminal accuracy of unexpectedly loaded rapid movements: Evidence for a mass-spring mechanism in programming. *Journal of Motor Behavior, 12,* 149-161.

Schmidt, R.A., McGown, C., Quinn, J.T., & Hawkins, B. (1986). Unexpected inertial loading in rapid reversal movements: Violations of equifinality. *Human Movement Science, 5,* 263-273.

Schmidt, R.A., Sherwood, D.E., Zelaznik, H.N., & Leikind, B.J. (1985). Speed-accuracy trade-offs in motor behavior: Theories of impulse variability. In H. Heuer, U. Kleinbeck, & K.-H. Schmidt (Eds.), *Motor behavior: Programming, control, and acquisition* (pp. 79-123). Berlin: Springer-Verlag.

Schmidt, R.A., & White, J.L. (1972). Evidence for an error detection mechanism in motor skills: A test of Adams' closed-loop theory. *Journal of Motor Behavior, 4,* 143-153.

Schmidt, R.A., & Wrisberg, C.A. (1973). Further tests of Adams' closed-loop theory: Response-produced feedback and the error detection mechanism. *Journal of Motor Behavior, 5,* 155-164.

Schmidt, R.A., Zelaznik, H.N., & Frank, J.S. (1978). Sources of inaccuracy in rapid movement. In G.E. Stelmach (Ed.), *Information processing in motor control and learning* (pp. 183-203). New York: Academic Press.

Schmidt, R.A., Zelaznik, H.N., Hawkins, B., Frank, J.S., & Quinn, J.T. (1979). Motor-output variability: A theory for the accuracy of rapid motor acts. *Psychological Review, 86,* 415-451.

Shapiro, D.C. (1978). *The learning of generalized motor programs.* Unpublished doctoral dissertation, University of Southern California, Los Angeles.

Shapiro, D.C. & Schmidt, R.A. (1982). The schema theory: Recent evidence and developmental implications. In J.A.S. Kelso, & J.E. Clark (Eds.), *The development of movement control and co-ordination* (pp. 113-150). Chichester: John Wiley.

Shapiro, D.C., Zernicke, R.F., Gregor, R.J. & Diestel, J.D. (1981). Evidence for generalized motor programs using gait-pattern analysis. *Journal of Motor Behavior, 13,* 33-47.

Sheridan, M.R. (1984). Planning and controlling simple movements. In M.M. Smyth, & A.M. Wing (Eds.), *The psychology of human movement* (pp. 47-82). London: Academic Press.

Shiffrin, R.M., & Schneider, W. (1977). Controlled and automatic human information processing. II. Perceptual learning, automatic attending, and a general theory. *Psychological Review, 84,* 127-190.

Shik, M.L., & Orlovskii, G.N. (1976). Neurophysiology of a locomotor automatism. *Physiological Reviews, 56,* 465-501.

Smith, J.L., Roberts, E.M., & Atkins, E. (1972). Fusimotor neuron block and voluntary arm movement in man. *American Journal of Physical Medicine, 5,* 225-239.

Smith, W.M., & Bowen, K.F. (1980). The effects of delayed and displaced visual feedback on motor control. *Journal of Motor Behavior, 12,* 91-101.

Sparrow, W.A., & Sparrow, H.T. (1990). *The Journal of Motor Behavior from 1970 to 1989: Its contributors, most cited authors and most cited journals.* Manuscript submitted for publication.

Spirduso, W.W. (1981). The emergence of research on motor control and learning. In G.A. Brooks (Ed.), *Perspectives on the academic discipline of physical education* (pp. 255-272). Champaign, IL: Human Kinetics.

Stelmach, G.E. (1987). The cutting edge of research in physical education and exercise science: The search for understanding. In M.J. Safrit, & H.M. Eckert (Eds.), *The cutting edge in physical education and exercise science research* (pp. 8-25). Champaign, IL: Human Kinetics.

Stelmach, G.E., & Diggles, V.A. (1982). Control theories in motor behavior. *Acta Psychologica, 50*, 83-105.

Summers, J.J. (June, 1986). *Timing of human movement.* Paper presented at the 21st International Congress of Applied Psychology, Jerusalem, Israel.

Summers, J.J. (1989). Temporal constraints in the performance of bimanual tasks. In D. Vickers, & P.L. Smith (Eds.), *Human information processing: Measures, mechanisms and models* (pp. 155-168). Amsterdam: Elsevier.

Taub, E. (1976). Movements in nonhuman primates deprived of somatosensory feedback. *Exercise and Sport Sciences Reviews, 4,* 335-374.

Thelen, E., Skala, K.A., & Kelso, J.A.S. (1987). The dynamic nature of early coordination: Evidence from bilateral leg movements in young infants. *Developmental Psychology, 23,* 179-186.

Thorndike, E.L. (1914). *Educational psychology.* New York: Columbia University.

Treisman, A.M. (1960). Contextual cues in selective listening. *Quarterly Journal of Experimental Psychology, 12,* 242-248.

Turvey, M.T. (1977). Preliminaries to a theory of action with reference to vision. In R. Shaw, & J. Bransford (Eds.), *Perceiving, acting and knowing* (pp. 211-263). Hillsdale, NJ: Lawrence Erlbaum Associates.

Turvey, M.T., & Carello, C. (1986). The ecological approach to perceiving-acting: A pictorial essay. *Acta Psychologica, 63,* 133-155.

Turvey, M.T., & Carello, C. (1988). Exploring a law-based ecological approach to skilled action. In A.M. Colley & J.R. Beech (Eds.), *Cognition and action in skilled behaviour* (pp. 191-203). Amsterdam: North-Holland.

Turvey, M.T., Fitch, H.L., & Tuller, B. (1982). The Bernstein perspective: I. The problems of degrees of freedom and context conditioned variability. In J.A.S. Kelso (Ed.), *Human motor behavior: An introduction* (pp. 239-252). Hillsdale, NJ: Lawrence Erlbaum Associates.

Ullman, S. (1980). Against direct perception. *Behavioral and Brain Sciences, 3,* 373-415.

van Rossum, J.H.A. (1989). *Motor development and practice: The variability of practice hypothesis in perspective.* Amsterdam: Free University Press.

van Wieringen, P.C.W. (1986). Motor coordination: Constraints and cognition. In M.G. Wade & H.T.A. Whiting (Ed.) *Motor development in children: Aspects of coordination and control* (pp. 361-371). Dordrecht: Martinus Nijhoff.

van Wieringen, P.C.W. (1988). Discussion: Self-organization or representation? Let's have both! In A.M. Colley & J.R. Beech (Eds.), *Cognition and action in skilled behavior* (pp. 247-253). Amsterdam: North Holland.

Viviani, P., & Terzuolo, C. (1980). Space-time invariance in learned motor skills. In G.E. Stelmach & J. Requin (Eds.), *Tutorials in motor behavior* (pp. 525-533). Amsterdam: North-Holland.

von Helmholtz, H. (1867). *Handbuch der physiologischen optik.* Leipzig: Voss.

Wadman, W.J., Denier van der Gon, J.J., Geuze, R.H., & Mol, C.R. (1979). Control of fast goal-directed arm movements. *Journal of Human Movement Studies, 5,* 3-17.

Wallace, S.A., Frankeny, J.R., & Larish, D.D. (1982). Effects of initial limb position on the accuracy, reaction time and electromyographic patterns of rapid movements. *Human Movement Science, 1,* 215-231.

Wann, J.P. & Nimmo-Smith, I. (1990). Evidence against the relative invariance of timing in handwriting. *Quarterly Journal of Experimental Psychology, 42A,* 105-117.

Warren, W.H., Jr. (1984). Perceiving affordances: Visual guidance of stair climbing. *Journal of Experimental Psychology: Human Perception and Performance, 10,* 683-703.

Warren, W.H., Jr. (1988). Action modes and laws of control for the visual guidance of action. In O.G. Meijer, & K. Roth (Eds.), *Complex movement behavior: 'The' motor-action controversy* (pp. 339-380). Amsterdam: North-Holland.

Weimer, W.B., & Palermo, D.S. (1973). Paradigms and normal science in psychology. *Science Studies, 3,* 211-244.

Whiting, H.T.A. (1980). Dimensions of control in motor learning. In G.E.Stelmach, & J. Requin (Eds.), *Tutorials in motor behavior* (pp. 537-550). Amsterdam: North-Holland.

Whiting, H.T.A. (1982). Skill in sport - a descriptive and prescriptive appraisal. In J.H. Salmela, J.T. Partington, & T. Orlick (Eds.), *New paths of sport learning and excellence* (pp. 7-13). Ottawa, Ontario: Sport in Perspective Inc.

Wilberg, R.B. (1972). A suggested direction for the study of motor performance by physical educators. *Research Quarterly, 43,* 387-393.

Woodworth, R.S. (1899). The accuracy of voluntary movement. *Psychological Review, 3* (Suppl. 2).

Wrisberg, C.A., & Schmidt, R.A. (1975). A note on motor learning without post-response knowledge of results. *Journal of Motor Behavior, 7,* 221-225.

Yates, F.E. (1979). Physical biology: A basis for modeling living systems. *Journal of Cybernetics and Information Science, 2,* 57-70.

Approaches to the Study of Motor Control and Learning
J.J. Summers (Editor)

Chapter 2

MOTOR CONTROL AND LEARNING: HOW FAR DO THE EXPERIMENTAL TASKS RESTRICT OUR THEORETICAL INSIGHT?

Judith I. Laszlo
The University of Western Australia

A review of unidimensional movement and reaction time studies is presented. The review focuses on three aspects of the experimental work: the questions asked; experimental controls introduced; and the contribution to theoretical knowledge of motor control and learning. Molecular and molar approaches are compared and the advantages of using complex tasks are discussed in terms of advancing our knowledge of the interaction between the perceptuo-motor processes and in building a comprehensive theory of movement control.

Throughout life, motor control is exercised continuously. In an unbroken chain, whether awake or asleep, animals and humans make postural adjustments and/or perform purposive movements.

This continuous stream of changing muscular balance is unceasingly and intimately monitored through kinaesthetic information. No motor event, however minute, is free of concomitant change in kinaesthetic input. Thus motor behaviour is best considered in conjunction with sensory, or perceptual function, hence, perceptuo-motor behaviour is the preferred descriptive label for motor behaviour. Welford, in his 1988 article says: "The study of skills, integrating cognitive and motor performance, which rose to prominence in the 1940s, has as yet mainly tackled simple tasks. Despite substantial achievements, many problems remain." (p. 458). Welford does not mention perception but does refer to cognition. Important as cognition is in some motor tasks, it is not a necessary, or essential part of all motor acts. In posture, in basic locomotor acts, or when we perform highly practised complex skills, there is no need to think about the task. It is often said that thinking about the next step we take will make us stumble. On the other hand, when we learn to drive a car we certainly use cognitive abilities. There is a continuum from cognitive-perceptuo-motor to perceptuo-motor skills.

A number of disciplines are relevant to motor function: Anatomy, physiology, psychology, human movement science, bioengineering, education, neurology, paediatrics, and sport medicine are some which come to mind. The academic background of the researcher will, to a large extent, determine the choice of the problem investigated, the experimental design used, and the technique employed. While some of us can bridge two disciplines - probably none of us have the knowledge across the entire spectrum of fields relevant to motor function.

Let me illustrate this problem of demarcation by taking physiological and psychological non-communication as an example. In 1972 Matthews published his book in which he reviewed the properties of the kinaesthetic receptors, and their physiological-functional characteristics, and the contribution of various receptor types to the global perception of kinaesthesis. Later studies vary from single receptor work (Ferrell, 1985; Gregory & Proske, 1979; Vallbo, 1974) to the role of kinaesthesis in the whole animal (Taub, 1976; Wylie & Tyner, 1981). Experimentation on human subjects include acute deafferentation (Laszlo, Baguley, & Bairstow, 1970; Laszlo & Bairstow, 1971), exposure of the tendon in the experimenter's big toe (McCloskey, Macefield, Gandevia, & Burke, 1987), passive movement of the middle finger (McCloskey, Cross, Honner, & Potter, 1984), and using tendon, vibration (Lackner, 1985), to study the role of global kinaesthesis, tendon, and muscle receptors.

In addition, it had been established, some 20 years ago (Brooks, 1969; Evarts & Fromm, 1977), that the classical view of strict separation of motor and sensory areas in the cortex was incorrect. Indeed, areas designated as motor or as sensory serve both functions and hence must be considered as motor-sensory or sensory-motor areas. Co-ordinated sensory-motor function has been found in the cerebellum as well (Brooks & Thach, 1981). These findings, relevant to kinaesthesis and central nervous system functions are, by and large, not taken into account by psychologists working in the field of motor control. Yet, ultimately, we will need to amalgamate the findings from all research areas if we are to arrive at a unified body of knowledge of how movements are controlled and skills acquired, and guard against the promulgation of theories in our own discipline which conflict with facts which have been established outside our own field.

Even within a single discipline, psychology, the type of research we undertake is governed by factors which we could describe as differences in personality and intellectual curiosity.

There are various options open to us when we choose our research questions and methods. Some of us like 'let's see what happens' questions, others want short, sharp, well defined queries. We might engage in studies in which we try to observe every-day behaviour, or we might set up highly controlled laboratory tasks. There are researchers who accept scores indicative of an outcome, others who are not happy unless they can obtain hard numerical values to the fourth decimal point in mm, sec, or whatever. Some embark on studies with large number of subjects because they are curious how a big slice of humanity functions, while others restrict the number of subjects and are happy to look at a restricted population. There are workers who feel comfortable in attaching the subject to a computer, or those who feel a need to have personal communication with each subject. There is no value judgment implied here. We carry out research which best satisfies our curiosity or for which we can attract research funds.

Further divisions can be observed between those workers who concentrate on behavioural manifestations without worrying about the processes underlying them, and those who adopt a theory and consider behaviour as indicative of the processes which are the building blocks of the theory.

Another classification relates to the molecular versus molar approach. In the molecular approach small, well defined bits of behaviour are examined, while molar research is focused on broadly based ‘representative’ chunks of behaviour. Both, molecular and molar studies have advantages and difficulties.

In the molecular approach the researcher is able to fall back on well tried tasks, such as unidimensional lever positioning or reaction time tasks. He or she might improve on instrumentation, and be assured of obtaining precise measurements. The researcher will be able to draw on an established body of findings, and will be able to publish the work with relative ease, as due to previous publications the task gained ‘respectability’. In short: molecular research is SAFE.

In the molar approach the choice of suitable tasks is the first hurdle. Finding every-day tasks seems a reasonable aim, but how are every-day tasks defined? Behaviour which occurs in the normal environment can be observed, but is difficult to quantify. Once isolated and transplanted into the laboratory, in order to allow experimental manipulations and reliable measurements, it is likely to lose its every-day character, as happened in the Howard and Henderson study (1989) in which perceptual problems of normal and cerebral palsied children were investigated in a "Real World Example". The children were asked to judge, from a three or six meter distance, whether they could get through an opening surrounded by curtains. This task was thought to be equivalent with judging whether they could get through an open door. Getting through a door opening is a "real-life" task, but guessing whether one could get through an opening surrounded with a soft curtain is certainly not the same task even if it is superficially similar. The other difficulty with every-day tasks is, that unless the choice is guided by theoretical considerations, it is likely to be rather an arbitrary, and often an idiosyncratic choice. For example, in the

McCarthy Scales of Children's Abilities (1972) drawing ability includes the item of drawing a straight line and a cross simultaneously with the two hands. Apart from the fact that this task is near impossible to perform, it is hardly a task required under every-day conditions. It takes a lot of thought, and trial and error, before ecologically valid, and scoreable tasks can be found. Finally, the more novel the task, the more difficult it is to get the work accepted for publication.

On the positive side, well chosen, complex tasks, related to every-day function are often more interesting and motivating for subjects than repetitious, 'classic' tasks (Lintern, 1989). The task of intercepting moving targets, be it catching balls, or crossing targets on a video-screen, can be fun. For example, in a study adults, normal children, and children with perceptuo-motor dysfunction were tested on the video task, in which a hit was rewarded by an 'explosion' of the target into concentric lines (Bairstow, 1987, 1989; Bairstow & Laszlo, 1989). The task was so popular that subjects asked for additional trials at the end of an already demanding session.

One further point in favour of choosing complex tasks is that individual differences are more pronounced here than in simple tasks. This is an important point - individual differences are not only interesting, but are the essence of diagnosis and treatment of motor dysfunction and of educational psychology.

In the following sections of this chapter I will review investigations falling into the categories of molecular and molar research. I will try to assess the advances made within these frameworks in our knowledge of motor control and learning - as I see it. At this point I need to foreshadow, what some readers might consider a serious omission in my deliberations. I will make no distinction between motor control and motor learning. The reason for this seeming negligence is that I see these two processes as inseparable. Ongoing motor control is necessary in all situations, in postural adjustment, in the performance of well practised skills, and during the learning of a skill. Conversely, learning does not stop at a predestined point in skill acquisition. Even the greatest ballet dancers keep on learning and improving through practice. The Olympic athletes practise to achieve a 0.01 sec reduction in running time, and typists try for increased speed and accuracy throughout their career - especially if they are after promotion. It is not possible to determine when the highest level of the skill has been reached in any one task by any one individual (Fitts & Posner, 1967). Not only is it impossible to pinpoint the transition from learning to control, but within the theoretical framework I have adopted, the information processing closed-loop model, the same processes underlie both learning and performance.

I need to make one final point before I start the review of the literature. My selection of examples will, by necessity, be somewhat arbitrary. I am an avid collector of reprints, and I will be working from my collection of some 5500 papers. In my filing system one of the categories is: experimental task. There are 1,275 papers which could be classified according to task. For interest, I will give the breakdown below:

Task	*Number of papers*	*Percentage/1,275*
Tracking	33	2.59
Lever	405	31.76
Serial and complex	161	12.63
Pattern perception/ reproduction	84	6.89
Force control	112	8.78
Posture	50	3.92
Handwriting/ drawing	61	4.78
Reaction time	369	28.94

It is unlikely that I was biased in favour of lever and reaction time tasks as my main interest lies in complex skills.

From the above figures it becomes obvious that I cannot review all the papers from my collection. I will endeavour to select as representative and unbiased a sample as I can when illustrating a point.

I have chosen unidimensional movements and reaction time studies in terms of their contribution to our understanding of motor behaviour and their role in theory construction. I will also discuss some studies using complex skills, for comparison.

UNIDIMENSIONAL LEVER STUDIES

My personal introduction to the LEVER took place in 1972 at the University of Michigan, in R. A. Schmidt's laboratory. It was a simple piece of equipment built of wood and placed on a table. The subject held on to a fair sized, round wooden handle, only occasionally taking bits of the apparatus with her in the form of a splinter embedded in her palm. From humble beginnings, the new generations of levers have been developed. The advanced models are on line with computers both for stimulus delivery and data recording. It is now possible to control torque, or inject sudden changes of resistance against the movement. Yet the basic task remains unchanged - the lever is moved to a predetermined location or along a preset length.

The first question one might ask regarding lever positioning studies is whether the task can be accepted as representative of motor tasks in general. To translate this into present day jargon: is the lever positioning task ecologically valid? One might harbour some doubts as to an affirmative answer if one considers the highly integrated and complex nature of the perceptuo-motor system and the artificial and simplified nature of the lever task. There is no every-day skill that resembles lever positioning. The nearest one would be sliding a finger on the string of a string instrument. However, in this case the player has to terminate the movement with accuracy, while the lever is often moved to a physical stop.

Moving to a stop introduces a significant, though unacknowledged, problem. In the active condition, the subject moves the lever to a stop which defines the extent of the required movement, or its end-location. In the response condition the stop is not present. It is assumed, if only tacitly, that the stimulus and response movements rely on the same perceptuo-motor processes. This assumption is not valid. When moving to a stop the subject programs one movement parameter only, that is: move along the channel. There is no need to program for braking of the movement, the stop will define the end-point. Kinaesthetic, or kinaesthetic and visual feedback informs the subject where the stop is, without the need for generating corresponding corollary discharge (Laszlo & Ward, 1978; Wiesendanger, 1969). The motor program, and hence the corollary discharge, when moving to the stop, includes the activation of the agonist and synergist muscles, but not the activation of the antagonist muscles which are necessary for active movement termination (Wierzbicka, Wiegner, & Shahani, 1986). Matters are further complicated as in the stimulus condition corollary discharge and kinaesthetic feedback are in contradiction with each other. While the subject programs a movement of indefinite length, kinaesthetic feedback is suddenly received, giving information about the unscheduled termination of the movement (Bairstow & Laszlo, 1980). In the response condition the subject must program the termination of the movement, and this program must be based on the previously conflicting corollary discharge and kinaesthetic information. Finally, in the passive stimulus presentation condition, where the subject's arm is moved by the experimenter, corollary discharge is absent, but kinaesthetic feedback is generated.

Keeping in mind these problems inherent in the lever studies, it is of interest to look at the questions which are addressed by researchers using this task. Four major areas are investigated: coding of distance versus location; retention and interference in motor memory; the role of vision versus kinaesthesis in recall; and the role of knowledge of results.

Extent Versus Location: Which is Coded More Accurately?

The dichotomy of distance moved versus location reached is clearly defined in the unidimensional positioning studies. The differences are based on experimental manipulations and instructions to the subject. The task is performed in the absence of vision. In their lever study on kinaesthetic judgment of direction, location, and extent, Bradshaw, Bradshaw, & Nettleton (1989, p. 1139) state that: "Motor memory refers to our ability accurately to reproduce a criterion extent without vision." It follows that if distance and location are coded in different ways, the kinaesthetic signals generated by these two tasks must differ. Whether the subject aims to reproduce a set distance or location, in a movement unidimensionally constrained, the kinaesthetic feedback is similar. In both cases gradual increase in length of the antagonist muscles is signalled, along with shortening of the agonist and synergist muscles. This is followed by a sudden reversal in relative length of the muscle compartments in the braking phase generating its own feedback configuration. This feedback pattern during reproduction of the stimulus movement is based on recall of feedback from the stimulus movement. During the stimulus presentation feedback is generated from the gradual length change only, as the braking phase is absent in both moving to a stop and in passive movement.

The assumption that extent and location differ in terms of kinaesthetic signals cannot be supported on physiological grounds. There is no mechanism which would bring into play different receptor classes depending on the goal of the movement, - moving a certain distance or to a set location. Some authors have suggested (e.g., Adams, 1977) that joint receptors respond in the location task, while other receptors are brought into play in distance coding. This assumption cannot be supported. Firstly, joint position and length of the muscles bridging the joint are directly related. Joint angle cannot be changed without concomitant change in the length of the muscles. Thus whenever a joint position is changed all classes of kinaesthetic receptors are affected. Secondly, joint receptors lost their functional importance quite some decades ago (Skoglund, 1956) while muscle spindles became the leaders in the kinaesthetic field (Burgess & Clark, 1969; McCloskey, 1978; Matthews, 1964, 1972; Proske, Schaible & Schmidt, 1988; to list just a few).

While a physiological basis for the separation of extent and location coding cannot be found, it is obvious that in the lever experiments the difference can be defined. Is this distinction upheld in every-day tasks? If one wants to reach an end-location, such as a teapot, one can achieve this goal in many different ways, taking a direct or indirect route, hence varying movement length. On the other hand, when one plays the piano, moving from one key to the other certainly demands accurate distance control. But when we draw a geometric figure, do we aim for a certain length of line or do we aim for a corner? It is likely that in most situations location and distance are both included in the planning and programming of the movement, and that these two aspects of movement control are interrelated.

Within the restriction imposed by the lever task, did a clear distinction emerge between movement extent and end-location? In the most basic condition, location and distance coding was measured without introducing delay or interference between the criterion and test movements. Vision of the apparatus was eliminated by blindfold (Duffy, Montague, & Laabs, 1975; Laabs, 1973; Roy & Diewert, 1978), partial blindfold (Diewert, 1975), by chin-rest (Laabs, 1974, 1976), or by asking the subjects to close their eyes (Corlett & Dickinson, 1983 a,b).

The fact that in all the studies vision was eliminated during trials, albeit not with equal rigour, implied that the researcher was interested in the kinaesthetic coding of the dependent variables. It was acknowledged that the two modalities, vision and kinaesthesis differ in the type of information they convey. Vision is an externally referenced sense, locating stimuli in the external environment, while kinaesthesis, internally referenced, relates the position of body and body parts to each other, irrespective of the external environment. The blindfolded subject, presented with the criterion movement, could rest at the stop for 1 s (Duffy et al., 1975), 2 s (Marteniuk, 1973, 1977), or 3 s (Diewert, 1975; Laabs, 1974). Thus the subject was given the opportunity to relate hand position to an environmental landmark seen either before vision was eliminated, or imagined as related to the apparatus such as the edge of the table. During reproduction of the end-location both the visual and kinaesthetic memory traces could be used. In contrast, distance travelled, or movement extent, was less dependent on external landmarks and hence visual memory traces were not helpful. Generally, the results of the studies showed that location is recalled more accurately than extent, though the reasons given did not include the above argument. The study of Newell and Chew (1975) was the only one in which the criterion movement was presented in full view, while visual presentation of the test movements was systematically varied. That is, the subject could rely not only on remembered landmarks but could see the length of the movement to be reproduced. The results are in contradiction to all other studies. Visual information favoured distance over location, supporting the argument that in the design used in most studies, landmarks influence the results.

Once delay between criterion and test movement was introduced the results were not uniform. Delays varied from 10 s (Marteniuk, 1973) to 45 s (Duffy et al., 1975) and the interval was unfilled (Laabs, 1973, 1974, 1976; Marteniuk, 1977; Roy, 1977), filled with mental activity unrelated to the task (Laabs, 1973;

Marteniuk, 1973; Roy, 1977), mental rehearsal (Duffy et al., 1975; Laabs, 1976; Marteniuk, 1973), or interfering movements (Duffy et al., 1975; Laabs, 1973). Unfilled intervals affected distance reproduction only (Laabs, 1973; Roy, 1977), or location only (Diewert, 1975). Mental activity hindered reproduction of distance (Diewert, 1975; Marteniuk, 1973; Roy, 1977) or location (Laabs, 1973). Mental rehearsal (Diewert, 1975; Marteniuk, 1973) and interfering movements (Diewert, 1975; Laabs, 1974) reduced reproduction accuracy of length only. Overall, the majority favours distance as more susceptible to forgetting compared to location. One could argue that visual memory for landmarks, easily translated into verbal labels, are relatively resistant to decay and interference, and that these verbal labels are useful in location, while labelling of distance in length units is not (McCloskey, 1978). It follows that location is more resistant to forgetting than extent.

In some of the studies, (Marteniuk, 1977; Roy, 1977; Roy & Diewert, 1978; Stelmach, Kelso, & McCullagh, 1976) rather than moving to the stop, subjects were asked to preselect the criterion movement. That is, the subject programmed the entire movement instead of the general movement direction alone. Stelmach (1977) found that preselected criterion movements were recalled with greater accuracy than movements to a stop or passive movements. This superiority in recall, for both extent and location (Roy & Diewert, 1978), or location alone (Roy, 1977) was tentatively explained by Stelmach (1977) as being due to lessening the need for feedback during recall. It is more likely that corollary discharge and kinaesthetic feedback congruence in programmed movements leads to better performance in preselected movements, compared to conflict of these factors in constrained active movements, and lack of program generated corollary discharge in passive movements. These factors have been discussed previously.

One of the puzzling aspects of this group of studies is the diversity of the level at which the independent variables were chosen. One such variable was the length of the criterion movement. Overall, it was found that long movements were recalled shorter, while short movements were recalled longer (Diewert, 1975; Duffy et al., 1975; Laabs, 1974; Marteniuk, 1977; Marteniuk, Shields, & Campbell, 1972). It is unclear what constitutes a short versus a long movement. Distances varied from 10 cm (Duffy et al., 1975) to 50 cm (Diewert, 1975), from 10 ° (Laabs, 1973) to 125 ° (Marteniuk et al., 1972). Even within the studies by the same author, considerable variations occurred. Laabs in 1974 used 20 °, 25 °, and 30 ° as short, 40 °, 45 °, and 50 ° as long distances, while in 1976, 35 °, 40 °, and 45 ° were compared with 50 °, 55 °, and 60 °, which makes 40 °- 45 ° long in 1974, short in 1976. The difference between adjacent stimuli were as little as 5 ° (Laabs, 1973, 1974, 1976), or as large as 50 ° (Marteniuk et al., 1972). The 5 ° between stimuli raises a question: could subjects tell the adjacent stimuli apart? Intuitively, 5 ° seems a small step indeed, especially if one considers the size of an adult fist and if one takes into account that in preselected movements plus or minus 5 cm error was acceptable (Marteniuk, 1977). Magill and Parks' (1983) study, measuring just noticeable differences, tends to counterindicate the choice of these small differences.

Lastly, the statistical measures applied could be looked at. The dependent variable can be treated by algebraic, constant, and variable error, AE, CE, and VE, respectively. Roy (1976) advocated the use of all three measures in all studies. Authors cited, on the other hand, seem to have chosen one, two, or three of these error measures. Significant results, at $p< .05$ were obtained with one measure or another. The importance of one significant value amongst the many nonsignificant ones is rather difficult to evaluate.

The Importance of Vision and Kinaesthesis in Recall of Movement

The question of whether movements encoded visually or kinaesthetically are recalled with greater accuracy has been investigated in many experimental settings, including unidimensional lever studies. These two modalities are compared in terms of information carrying capacity and retrieval characteristics. Intra- and cross- modal comparisons were used in these studies. A rich variety of independent variables have been introduced by the authors. These included differences in criterion movement delivery, length and number of exposures, and sensory enhancement. Visual presentation included static visual displays, such as showing a rod painted along a predetermined length (Connolly & Jones, 1970; Hulme, Biggerstaff, Moran, & Mckinlay, 1982; Hulme, Smart, Moran, & Raine, 1983; Jones & Connolly, 1970; Marteniuk & Rodney, 1979), visual exposure of the stop (Faust-Adams, 1975), or visual sequential presentation where a light was moved along the set distance (Adams & Goetz, 1973; Chew, 1976; Diewert & Stelmach, 1977; Jones, 1973; Newell, Shapiro, & Carlton, 1979). In all the studies reviewed, subjects had an opportunity to see the room in which the testing was conducted. Thus visual information was available at three levels: in the kinaesthetic condition stored visual traces of environmental cues were available; in the sequential stimulus presentation visual information was received along a temporal sequence similar to that found in kinaesthesis, and with visual landmarks present; while in static visual display the entire stimulus could be visually scanned, without temporal dispersion, and against environmental landmarks.

Viewing of the room is not taken into consideration, though visual memory traces of environmental cues might aid kinaesthetic recall. Nor do authors take into account the difference between sequential versus static visual stimulus presentation when comparing results across studies. It has been shown (Bairstow & Laszlo, 1979; Laszlo & Broderick, 1985) that static and sequential visual stimuli are recalled differently. Kinaesthetic information was generated by criterion movements to a stop in all studies, except when the movement was passive (Diewert & Stelmach, 1977). Kinaesthesis was said to be enhanced by spring-loading the lever (Adams & Goetz, 1973, Adams, Marshall, & Goetz, 1972). While increased resistance to movement would certainly alter the kinaesthetic picture, this change in input could not be considered as enhancement. In any case, this 'enhanced' kinaesthetic input was equated with normal visual and auditory input. Kinaesthetic information generated by moving the unloaded lever, in contrast, was compared with the criterion movement given in the absence of visual cues, and/or white noise masked auditory information.

Here, as in previously discussed studies, the length of the criterion movement was varied in a seemingly arbitrary fashion. The shortest criterion movement was 5 cm (Jones, 1973), the longest 50 cm (Diewert & Stelmach, 1977), and within studies criterion movements differed from each other by 2.5 cm (Adams & Goetz, 1973) or 5 cm (Connolly & Jones, 1970; Faust-Adams, 1975; Hulme et al., 1982; Hulme et al., 1983; Jones, 1973; Jones & Connolly, 1970).

There was scant uniformity across studies regarding the recall conditions. In most cases visual recall (V) involved the subject watching the experimenter's movement and giving verbal indication when the response was equivalent to the criterion movement length, except where the subject had to choose between two responses made to stops (Adams & Goetz, 1973; Faust-Adams, 1975). Kinaesthetic (K) recall was made to a self-selected end point or a choice from two stops was asked for (Adams & Goetz, 1973; Faust-Adams, 1975).

Some authors compared filled with unfilled retention intervals of 10 s (Jones & Connolly, 1970) or 20 s (Marteniuk & Rodney, 1979) duration. Unfilled retention intervals were as long as 90 s in Adams, Marshall, & Goetz's (1972) study. Newell et al., (1979) varied the time, within the 10 s retention interval, when the subject was informed of the modality condition under which recall was to be made. Effect of practice was investigated by Faust-Adams (1975). In children, intra- versus cross-modal function was assessed as an index of kinaesthetic development (Hulme et al., 1982) and this kinaesthetic index was correlated with motor skills (Hulme et al., 1983), a somewhat unexpected use of the lever task.

All three measures, AE, CE, and VE were included in some, AE alone in other studies, while percentage of error was used by Adams & Goetz (1973). Overall superiority of intra-modal over cross-modal recall was found in two cases only (Connolly & Jones, 1970; Marteniuk & Rodney, 1979). In all other studies the results were influenced by the various and varied manipulations of the independent variables such as movement length, length of retention intervals, practice, and age of the subjects. That is, the results were relevant to one specific combination of experimental conditions only. For instance, Diewert & Stelmach (1977) reported that V-V and K-K did not differ from each other significantly at the 20, 35, and 50 cm criterion lengths. Intra- versus cross-modal recall differed from each other at 50 cm only, at which length V-V was most accurate overall. In general V-K was better than K-V, and V-K favoured 20 over 50 cm. The K-V condition was superior at 20 and 35 cm compared to 50 cm.

It appears that the question addressed in these studies (i.e., is vision or kinaesthesis more adept at encoding and retaining unidimensional movement information) has not been answered. While each author has advanced theoretical explanations for their own findings, one cannot amalgamate these into a unitary explanation, even within the confines of the lever task, let alone propose a theoretical frame-work for the role of vision and kinaesthesis in general motor control.

The Importance of Knowledge of Results

Schmidt (1982), writing about knowledge of results (KR), says: "....most writers agree that such information (KR) is the single, most important variable, except of course for practice itself, for determining motor learning and performance" (p. 527). KR has been accepted as essential in motor learning since Adams' closed-loop theory of motor control was published in 1971. Adams based his model on findings of lever studies. Authors conducting lever studies did not question the role of KR in acquisition, rather they used KR to explore the importance of kinaesthesis versus vision (Adams, Gopher, & Lintern, 1977; Adams, Marshall, & Goetz, 1972; Johnson, 1980; Reeve, Mackey, & Fober, 1986; Reeve & Mainor, 1983; Smyth, 1978), the effect of interference (Johnson, 1980; Shea & Upton, 1976), whether sequential or random order of presentation of various stimuli would enhance learning (Stelmach & Szendrovits, 1981), and whether passive or active movements are learned more accurately (Lee & Magill, 1985).

A common feature in the studies reviewed is the availability of verbal KR during acquisition trials, except in one case (Smyth, 1978), where KR was given visually, not verbally. However, in every other respect the studies varied from each other in, yet again, a seemingly random fashion. The choice of experimental variables was explained, but reason was not given for the number of trials used in acquisition and retention, nor was the choice of the specific type of KR information justified. For example, the number of acquisition trials varied between studies from 15 (Johnson, 1980) to 50 (Stelmach & Szendrovits, 1981), and within studies from 15-50 (Adams, Goetz & Marshall, 1972, Adams et al., 1977). The number of retention trials, where KR was withdrawn, was spread widely from five trials (Smyth, 1978) to 50 (Adams, Goetz & Marshall, 1972, Adams et al., 1977). Precision of KR was given to subjects varying from 1 mm (Shea & Upton, 1976), 3 mm (Adams et al., 1972), 5 mm (Lee & Magill, 1985; Stelmach & Szendrovits, 1981), in 0.35 cm 'units', though the subjects were not given the actual 'unit' size (Johnson, 1980), or as directional, but non-quantified error information (Reeve & Mainor, 1983; Reeve et al., 1986). Yet, if amount of practice and type of KR are as important in learning as we are made to believe (e.g., Schmidt, 1982), variations in the number of acquisition trials with KR and precision of KR information must have an important influence on the results of the studies in their own rights, and could over-shadow the effects of the main experimental variable, such as relative modality contribution to recall. Further, it would make comparisons between studies, focusing on similar questions, difficult indeed.

It is not surprising that the results do not yield a clear, overall picture, especially as here again a combination of AE, CE, and VE scores were used in the data analyses. The role of kinaesthesis versus vision in motor learning does not appear to have been clarified any further than was reported in the previous section. The results of the Adams' studies (Adams et al., 1972; Adams et al., 1977), for example, showed that the amount of practice with KR was significant, but feedback manipulations were not. Withdrawal of KR did not affect recall performance adversely when augmented feedback was present in both acquisition and recall trials, and kinaesthetic manipulations alone failed to lead to significant differences in the acquisition trials. When kinaesthetic conditions were changed between acquisition and recall trials significant differences were found, however. In contrast, Reeve et al. (1986) have found that acquisition under kinaesthetic feedback conditions, with KR present, led to superior recall in the absence of KR, than when acquisition was under visual or visual plus kinaesthetic input.

Direction of movement, relevant to body midline, did not emerge as a significant variable in the Reeve and Mainor (1983) series of studies. Learning two interfering movements, without KR, did lower accuracy in the retention trials, showing that even in the absence of KR, some trace of the interfering movement was retained (Shea & Upton, 1976). Passive versus active movements did not differ from each other in acquisition, but did in retention trials, if, and only if, subjects changed from one movement condition to the other between acquisition and recall (Lee & Magill, 1985). Finally vision was shown to be an effective mode of KR delivery (Smyth, 1978).

General conclusions as to the importance of verbal KR, from these studies would be difficult to reach, and a strong unified theoretical structure built on the results, even for unidimensional lever movements alone, does not emerge.

Unidimensional Movements Without a Lever; the Mass-Spring Theory

While unidimensional lever studies allow but one degree of freedom in movement execution (i.e., where to stop, or how far to move), they do not aim to restrict the number of joints involved in the movement. Mass-spring theorists, on the other hand, have chosen to investigate single joint movements. In monkeys, elbow joint movements (Bizzi, 1980; Polit & Bizzi, 1978, 1979), in man, the movements of the interphalangeal joint of the index finger (Kelso & Holt, 1980) were studied in the performance of unidimensional aiming tasks. Mass-spring theory is based on the proposition that the muscles act as springs, and that these control the muscle-joint assemblies. The physical property of the muscle is said to be sufficient as the unifying explanatory concept in general motor control. In support of this theory it is claimed that even in the total absence of feedback, and despite random perturbation introduced during the movement, the required end-location is reached with precision. The data presented do not substantiate this claim, however. For instance, in the Bizzi papers (Bizzi, 1980; Polit & Bizzi, 1978, 1979) accuracy was defined in a rather curious way. The monkey's task was to move the elbow joint in order to point at one light in a row of lights which were 5 ° apart. The error tolerance was 10 °, thus including three lights. It transpires from the description of the performance of the monkeys that some lights were more often pointed to than others, depending on their location and hence anatomical accessibility. In addition, the accuracy of pointing appeared to be reduced in the deafferented animals, when perturbation was introduced, compared to performance of the non-deafferented animals, or to performance in the absence of perturbation (Figure 1, Polit & Bizzi, 1978). The task of the human subjects (Kelso & Holt, 1980) was to reach a 30 ° extension of the index finger under the various experimental conditions. This accuracy demand coincided with the anatomical restriction imposed on the joint. That is, 30 ° extension can be defined as maximal extension, rather than a point around which finger extension is selected when aiming for a set end-location.

Predictably, criticism of the mass-spring theory is not difficult to find (e.g., Bullock & Grossberg, 1988; Corcos, Agarwal, & Gottlieb, 1985; Nichols, 1985; Sanes, 1986) What is surprising is that authors, who carried out lever studies (Schmidt & McGown, 1980; Stelmach, Kelso, & McCullagh, 1976; Stelmach & Kelso, 1977) could reconcile the mass-spring theory and theories generated by the lever studies. If mass-spring theory is accepted, the questions addressed by the lever studies become irrelevant or redundant. If motor control depends on the physical properties of the muscles alone, and muscles are responsible for reaching predetermined end-locations, how is the question of end-location versus extent of movement to be discussed? If feedback is not necessary to reach end-location, then neither vision, nor kinaesthesis are of relevance, and trying to define their relative contribution is meaningless. Furthermore, what is motor memory in terms of mass-spring? Do muscles, which act like springs, remember and forget? If so, Nureyev's statement gains scientific support. Nureyev, when asked why he needs to practice ballet for eight hours every day answered, that without practice his muscles forget! Finally, does verbal KR affect the spring in the muscle?

The degree of reductionism advocated by the mass-spring theorists leads to a mechanical view-point which is in stark contrast to the observed plasticity of motor behaviour.

REACTION TIME STUDIES: QUESTIONS ABOUT QUESTIONS

Measurement of reaction time (RT) is used widely in psychology, beside it being a favourite in motor skill research. I will look only at studies within the motor area. Even within this area I will concentrate on works carried out in the 1980s, and will include earlier studies only when they form the springboard for the later experiments. While unidimensional lever studies could be grouped around a number of questions, the majority of RT studies focus on one theoretical objective, elucidation of the nature of motor programming. The RT paradigm, including simple and choice RT designs, is used in an attempt to define programming parameters and to delineate those parameters which can be preprogrammed, that is, programmed prior to the delivery of the imperative stimulus rather than during the RT interval.

What are the programming parameters which are nominated as being formed independently from other parameters? Perhaps one of the most classic queries is whether accuracy demand and/or complexity of the response have an effect on RT duration and hence, on programming. The classic studies (e.g., Henry & Rogers, 1960; Henry, 1961; Klapp, 1975) were presented as irrefutable evidence that gradual increase in accuracy demand or response complexity leads to gradual lengthening of RT, indicating that both simple and complex programs are generated during the RT period. Some evidence contradicting, or at least qualifying, the classical viewpoint did emerge (Laszlo & Bairstow, 1974; Laszlo & Livesey, 1977). It was shown that significant increase in RT occurs between responses with and without accuracy demands, even when the two responses required identical movements. However, further gradual increase in accuracy and response complexity had no additional effect on RT. Phillips and Glencross in 1985 claimed that their results support the relationship between gradual increase in response complexity and RT. The next move came from Canic and Franks (1989). Reviewing the literature, they came to the conclusion that the complexity issue has not been unequivocally resolved and hence they embarked on the 'definitive' study to get the final answer. Response complexity, in their experiment, was equated with the number of response units, using simple reaction time (SRT) and no uncertainty. Whether number of discrete response units are indeed indicative of complexity, such as aiming for one or two targets in a continuous movement on moving paper (Laszlo & Livesey, 1977), is arguable. In any case, Canic and Franks did find that SRT increased linearly as a function of the number of response units.

The next programming parameter is related to the selection of muscles, digits, or limbs. Representative papers include: Klapp (1977) and Zelaznik, Shapiro, and Carter (1982), giving some limited support for digit selection as a programming parameter. Rosenbaum and Saltzman (1985) found a relationship between RT and choice of limb, though Zelaznik and Hahn (1985) could not arrive at an unambiguous answer, while Heuer (1986) argued that specific parameters can be set independently for the two hands, albeit some common parameters can be found as well. It appears that there is some room for argument regarding whether muscle, digit, or hand selection can be included in the list of programming parameters.

Timing is a strong candidate for nomination as an independent programming parameter following Klapp's dit-dah studies (1977a,b). Klapp stated that timing is programmed in general. Zelaznik et al. (1982) support Klapp's notion, advancing the idea that duration of the response can be programmed independently from digit selection, provided duration uncertainty is eliminated. Some three years later Zelaznik and Hahn, (1985) qualified this stand, arguing that the variables involved in motor control are not sufficiently understood to allow us to establish the order in which the programming variables are selected. On the other hand, Carlton, Carlton, and Newell (1987) came to the conclusion that timing cannot be accepted, without constraints, as an independent programming parameter because response dynamics (i.e., force control) are also involved in duration control. Overall the emerging picture on timing is somewhat complicated.

Spatial parameters, extent and direction of movement and target location, are variables engaging workers in both the lever and RT studies. Using the RT paradigm, Megaw (1972) considered that direction is the primary programming parameter, while extent can be considered as a modification of the generalised program. Kerr (1976) disagreed with Megaw. Indeed she raised the question whether it was at all logical to accept direction and extent as separate processes. My argument, advanced in the previous section, relevant to lever studies, certainly supports Kerr's viewpoint, showing that in physiological terms extent and direction cannot be taken as independent programming factors. Zelaznik et al. (1982) joined this stand by expressing doubt whether these variables are even appropriate to the language of motor control. A different opinion was expressed by Larish and Frekany (1985) who claimed that direction can be reprogrammed, while extent and selection of the limb are changed selectively. Even mass-spring theory puts in an appearance in the RT field. Girouard, Proteau, Laurencelle, and Black (1987) maintained that target location is of primary importance in programming. Finally, it was argued (Dornier & Reeve, 1988) that direction is an independent parameter, while extent and selection of limb interact. It would be somewhat unrealistic to say that the question of relative contribution of the spatial programming parameters has been answered clearly.

On the theoretical plane, authors propose three possible ways in which parameters are selected for programming: in parallel, in series, or hierarchically. Each of these modes have their advocates. Parallel programming was advanced by Klapp (1977), but Heuer (1986) proposed that common parameters cannot be prepared simultaneously and put forward the continuity hypothesis. Zelaznik and Hahn (1985) argued that it is premature to try and establish the order in which the parameters are selected for programming until a better understanding of the variables involved in motor control has been established. This is a somewhat different view from that which Zelaznik expressed earlier (Zelaznik et al., 1982) where Schmidt's (1980) generalised programming theory was called into question, yet implying support for the notion of in series selection of parameters, saying that the subject should be able to select parameters in any order. The hierarchical model was favoured by Larish and Frekany (1985), but rejected by Rosenbaum and Saltzman (1984) who supported the Motor-Program Editor Model.

Perhaps the most difficult concept to come to terms with is preprogramming. Within Schmidt's definition preprogramming is the preparation of a response prior to the appearance of the imperative stimulus, provided the specific response demanded is known in advance. Phillips and Glencross (1985) took the stand that some aspects of a program are preprepared, while others are not. Larish and Frekany (1985) came to the conclusion that all alternatives can be preprogrammed - a stand which extends preprogramming beyond Schmidt's definition, and one which necessitates postulation of reprogramming. Spijkers (1987) stated, categorically, that all movement parameters can be preprogrammed. On the other hand, Zelaznik and Hahn (1985) were definitely against preprogramming. Again, a far from clear picture!

Experimental designs are more uniform in RT studies than were encountered in the lever experiments. In most recent RT work a precuing technique is used in order to manipulate uncertainty (Canic & Franks, 1989; Dornier & Reeve, 1988; Girouard et al., 1987; Heuer,1986; Larish & Frekany, 1985; Zelaznik et al., 1982; Zelaznik & Hahn, 1985). Thus the reason for discordant theoretical stands and contradictions are not likely to be due to differing control of experimental variables. Reasons other than experimental controls must have led some authors to express doubts about the efficacy of RT experiments as an adequate paradigm in measuring motor processes. For instance, Siegel (1985) queried the usefulness, reliability, and validity of RT as a measure of motor processes. He speculated that while RT is a relatively simple measure, the processes which underlie RT are complex, and thus a direct relationship between RT and underlying processes cannot be expected. Lee and Elliott (1986, p. 174) did go one step further in their criticism, saying that: "...what is used to define programming complexity (i.e., RT) is also being used to measure programming complexity." In other words, the principles underlying RT studies are based on circular reasoning. Canic and Franks (1989) did not call into question the usefulness of the RT paradigm, yet they did ask the question why subjects should wait for the signal to implement a selected program if there is no uncertainty and there are no catch trials. That is, why is a planned movement not executed immediately on receiving the stimulus when both the response and the time when it should be omitted are known in advance. Although they found evidence to support Sternberg, Monsell, Knoll, and Wright's (1978) model, the very question undermines the rationale of the RT studies by weakening the triggering role of the imperative stimulus. Indeed, the fact that there is linear increase in RT with increase in response units shows that the programs for consecutive response units cannot be lined up neatly, awaiting their turn.

This brief overview of RT studies presents a gloomy picture. Why is it that a well controlled, relatively simple, and well instrumented experimental method, used and used again, should not yield a clear, coherent theoretical answer to the questions asked?

I argued that the lever task is artificial and does not present the perceptuo-motor system with a situation it was developed to handle. Could that be the case with RT also? In everyday parlance 'reaction time' is used freely, while unidimensional movement is not. Some people are described as being good drivers because they have fast RTs, or bad because they have slow RTs. Nobody, outside psychology, ever talks of lever tasks! Schmidt (1980) gives cautious support to RT as an everyday task. The example described by him is of a child suddenly appearing in front of a car. He stresses that the similarity of the experimental RT paradigm to everyday sudden response situations can be accepted only if we make a number of qualifying assumptions. He mentions the fact that there is opposition to the acceptance of the laboratory RT task being a true representation of everyday situations. There are some apparent and possibly important differences between The Subject (in the laboratory) and The Driver (on the road). The Subject's behaviour is demarcated as starting with the warning signal, being triggered by the imperative stimulus, and being terminated (I mean the behaviour, not the Subject) when the response is completed. That is the Subject is a passive, empty shell before the start and after completion of the response. In contrast, the Driver is active before the imperative stimulus, the child, makes his or her appearance. He/she does not change from a passively waiting human to an active one, but initiates a change in activity. I would like to argue that the difference between Subject and Driver is one of degree, not of kind. The Subject might appear passive and idle before being 'activated', but at least, he or she is actively engaged in maintaining postural control, partly to conform with experimental demands and partly to maintain some degree of comfort. Thus it seems unlikely that the experimental RT situation is divorced from normal perceptuo-motor demands.

If it is not the artificiality of the experimental set-up, could it be that the questions asked are not appropriate? The target process to be clarified is programming: what is programmed, when is the program constructed, how much of the program is preprepared? Let me consider, first of all, what is meant by a motor program. In physiological terms (Carlton et al., 1987; Freund, H.-J., 1983) programming is defined as the selection and activation of a set of motor units (MU). Activation of a MU consists of action potentials being transmitted along a motor nerve fibre, followed by an all-or-none contraction of all muscle fibres served by the particular motor nerve fibre, (i.e., by the muscular response). Hence, once the program is generated isometric and/or isotonic contraction follows inevitably. When the psychologists talk about the delay between the stimulus and the response as being due to programming, they cannot refer to MU activation. Once a program is triggered it must run its course, it cannot be delayed or stored. Motor programs are not preset, unchangeable sets of commands to predetermined MUs. The 'Programmer' does not pull out the appropriate computer program or even subprogram. There are no set programs in terms of preselected specific MUs for specific movements. Overtly identical movements are achieved by different combinations of MUs chosen from the available MU pool. The choices depend on prevailing posture, environmental conditions, and preceding activity. In short, no two movements are identical in programming terms (Paillard, 1960). It follows that rather than programming, the process which occurs during the RT period would be motor planning (Freund, 1985; Girouard et al., 1987; Roland, Skinhoj, Lassen, & Larsen, 1980). Planning is regarded as the precursor of programming, dependent on the goal of the movement and previous experience (Rosenbaum & Saltzman, 1984). It is the motor plan which is then translated into the specific motor program. The difference between planning and programming can be illustrated by the results of a study in which the task requirements, and hence the goal, differed, yet the movements were the same (Laszlo & Bairstow, 1974). The goal was either a fast index finger movement without a set endpoint, or the same movement to a target which was placed exactly at the point where the movement would be terminated if the target would not be present. RT was longer for the target condition - the planning was more complex, more time consuming when an accuracy demand was present than without it, albeit the two programs did not differ in complexity.

Is it possible that the lack of coherent theory on motor programming, as investigated by the RT paradigm is due to the fact that the process which underlies RT is not programming? If it is not programming it is hardly surprising that programming parameters cannot be separated. As for which parameters of the response are planned independently from each other, and in which order, becomes a non-question. Planning is goal directed, and as far as the goal of the movement is concerned all parameters must be incorporated in the plan as it is hardly possible to separate one aspect of the goal from any other. One last word on theoretical considerations. If, as is argued, it is planning, not programming which is the process investigated in RT studies, the question of whether, or which parameters can be preprogrammed should be reformulated. Can a movement be planned before the imperative stimulus? If it is known what the response should be, it can be planned, if there is uncertainty, planning must be postponed. Thus responses would be preplanned in simple RT, planned in choice RT. A rather simple solution to a knotty problem.

There are some intriguing questions relevant to the absolute values of RT. Obviously, the absolute times recorded will depend on the sensitivity of the equipment, the more sensitive the instrument the quicker it will register the change from resting to movement. This is not a real problem as instrumentation remains the same within each experiment across conditions and absolute values need not be compared across experiments. Yet, if one looks at the figures in studies where motor time is measured, one encounters significant differences between conditions as short as 10 ms (Heuer, 1986). Now, 10 ms is within the limits of delay across one synapse in the Central Nervous System. In a pathway as complex as the sensory-motor pathway it is rather amazing to find that a 10 ms difference is sufficient to distinguish between, lets say, spatial and temporal programming characteristics.

It could be argued that we should consider studies which break RT into premotor and motor components, measuring central evoked responses and EMG, in addition to the initial mechanical response (e.g., Anson, this volume; Carlton, Robertson, Carlton, & Newell, 1985; Haagh & Brunia, 1985) It is unlikely, however, that a review of these investigations could clarify the issues raised above, as a one - to - one relationship within premotor measures, and between premotor and motor indices has not been established (Haagh & Brunia, 1985).

Finally, one last question could be posed. Taking into account the unsolved theoretical issues and contradictory arguments generated by the RT studies, is it reasonable to investigate age related RT differences in order to define changes in motor processes with age. Indeed the reasons advanced for the slowing of RT - and by extrapolation - of motor function with age are numerous, (e.g., Rabbitt, 1981). But there are non-motor explanations, which might be equally acceptable, such as Smith and Brewer's (1985) explanation of a shift from speed to accuracy, or Era, Jokela, and Heikkinen (1986) who tender as reasons for the increase of between subject variance with advanced age, cognitive factors, length of education, and perceived health.

Do RT studies contribute significantly to our understanding of perceptuo-motor function? Are they more appropriate than lever studies in leading to a generalisable perceptuo-motor theory? Overall, I would lean towards answering both questions in the negative. It is clear that the RT task is not as far removed from everyday functional demands as the lever studies. But the RT paradigm suffers from one important shortcoming - it isolates a molecule of behaviour, yet is used to define not the behaviour of the molecule, but of the entire system of which the molecule is but one minute part. In other words, the RT situation is an artificially simplified, rigid behavioural model, yet the questions set to be answered by the RT studies relate to global and plastic processes. The experimental paradigm and the theoretical questions have their roots in different strata of behaviour and hence they do not amalgamate.

FROM MOLECULAR TO MOLAR RESEARCH

From the foregoing the reader might have gained the impression that I am not a wholehearted supporter of molecular research as represented by unidimensional aiming and RT studies. Perhaps Henderson's statement (1975, p. 184) expresses my doubts raised in the most concise way. She writes: "....one might ask whether the analysis of lever positioning responses contributes at all to our understanding of complex skills - perhaps pulling a lever is the 'nonsense syllable' of motor skills."

A comparison of unidimensional movement tasks and aiming tasks in which the subjects are free to choose the mode of response could highlight the advantages of working within a relatively natural, and plastic frame-work. Space restricts even a cursory review of aiming studies. Only a few, arbitrarily chosen, examples will be mentioned to highlight the distinctions between the two approaches.

The first difference between free aiming tasks and lever studies is in the questions each experimental paradigm generates. The controversy of end-location versus extent coding, occupying an important place in the lever literature is 'ignored' in the aiming studies. This is not an oversight. The kinaesthetic receptors cannot differentiate between these task demands, nor is there a clear distinction between location and distance in every-day tasks. If one wants to reach an object (end-location), one may reach for it from any number of starting positions (varying movement extent). It would place an enormous burden on the motor control system if each reach for the object would have to be acquired one by one and the memory for each response were to be stored, just in case one encountered identical conditions in the future; identical that is, in terms of end-location relevant to starting distance and direction from the object. Rather than memorising individual programs, the appropriate motor plan is formulated, which in turn is translated into the MU activation pattern or motor program.

The role of verbal KR is seldom investigated in free aiming studies. In aiming, in contrast to the lever situation, KR is available as a matter of course. We know when we make contact with the object we were reaching for, we can see where the aimed ball or dart has landed. Thus in many aiming tasks verbal KR would be redundant.

In the lever studies, the relative importance of kinaesthesis and vision are compared, without arriving at an unambiguous answer. In the aiming studies, rather than focusing on a direct comparison between the senses, vision can be examined in terms of its functional role during acquisition, or performance, or as a source of KR. For instance, it has been found (Henderson, 1975, 1977) that the absence of vision, while practising dart throwing, does not eliminate improvement in accuracy in unskilled subjects, nor does it prevent the subject from judging where the dart has landed. In a discrete task (Carlton, 1981) it was found that seeing the stylus is more helpful than seeing the target, that is, monitoring the movement visually is more important than looking at the stationary end-location. The timing of the movement was, however, not influenced by the presence or absence of vision.

Importantly, individual differences can be investigated in aiming studies, though they are not taken into account in lever studies. Examples of studies looking at individual differences include Henderson's (1975) work where skilled versus unskilled dart throwers were compared and Bairstow's studies (Bairstow, 1987, 1989; Bairstow & Laszlo, 1989) on aiming for moving targets. Here individual styles in spatial and temporal programming were established in adults, normal children, and children with perceptuo-motor dysfunction, respectively.

An advantage of the free aiming tasks over the lever set-up is that one is able to investigate free aiming in children as young as a few weeks (Mathew & Cook, 1989; Stack, Muir, Sherriff, & Roman, 1989; Von Hofsten & Lindhagen, 1979; Von Hofsten, 1980; Von Hofsten & Fazel-Zandy, 1984), while the lower age limit in lever studies seems to be five years (Corlett & Dickinson, 1983a,b). A number of aspects of perceptuo-motor development have been studied using free aiming tasks. The importance of vision (Stack et al., 1989; Von Hofsten & Rosblad, 1988), development of spatial programming (Von Hofsten & Fazel-Zandy, 1984), and spatial-temporal movement parameters (Mathew & Cook, 1989) have been examined. Regarding vision, age related trends on the reliance of vision could be studied from four years of age (Whiting & Cockerill, 1972; Von Hofsten & Rosblad, 1988). In both these studies a vision by age interaction was found, with older children depending less on vision than younger ones. Indeed, Von Hofsten and Fazel-Zandy (1984) claimed that reliance on vision and kinaesthetic development are interrelated.

Finally, in the lever studies variations in task parameters introduce differences in results and hinder direct comparisons between studies. In the aiming experiments, differences in task characteristics do not restrict evaluation across studies. Could the reason be that the questions asked in the aiming studies can relate to general motor control principles, while the questions addressed in the lever studies must conform to the narrow task imposed limits; limits which do not form natural boundaries in every-day motor function.

Can investigations using a restrictive and mechanistic task lead to an understanding of a complex and plastic process? Can RT studies lead to insight into the nature of the motor program?

The RT task is a variant of the aiming paradigm. In the RT situation the subject aims for a target, as is the case in the lever situation, but the spatial aspect of the response in RT studies is not measured, the dependent variable is time. Yet when planning the movement both spatial and temporal requirements of the response are taken into account, and only in programming are the two movement parameters independent from each other to a certain degree (Brooks, 1981; Georgopuolos, Schwartz, & Kettner, 1986). Considering only the spatial, or only the temporal aspect of a movement could give an impoverished picture of the functional characteristics of movement control.

I have chosen two experiments in support of the molar approach, one by Bairstow and Laszlo (1989) and one by Pew (1974). The Bairstow and Laszlo (1989) study formed part of a project in which perceptuo-motor dysfunction (PMD; clumsiness) was investigated (Laszlo, Bairstow, Bartrip, & Rolfe, 1988; Laszlo, 1990). The process-orientated Perceptual-Motor Abilities Test (PMAT; Laszlo & Bairstow, 1985) was used to diagnose specific process dysfunction in 7 - 12 year old children. The PMAT assesses kinaesthetic sensitivity, spatial and temporal programming, and motor planning. Most test items resemble everyday tasks and games. Treatment consisted of improving, through training, the process or processes in which the children failed to reach age appropriate levels. Inadequate kinaesthetic sensitivity was the most frequent cause of PMD (i.e., 75% of the children were dyskinaesthetic). Training in the defective process or processes significantly alleviated the motor difficulties and related secondary symptoms were relieved. The Bairstow and Laszlo (1989) study compared the performance of the PMD children before and after treatment, using an aiming task for moving targets, the "video-game", referred to earlier. Each response, from home position to moving target, was analysed according to the following variables: movement initiation time, movement duration, initial acceleration, peak speed, location of peak speed, speed units (how often the hand accelerated and decelerated), and terminal speed were the temporal measures; onset angle, prediction angle, direction units and terminal error were the spatial indices. The results of the study showed large individual differences in coping strategies used by the PMD children in performing the task, both in the spatial and temporal variables. Further, it was established that adequate kinaesthetic ability is necessary for rapid initiation and effective braking of the movement. Thus, by selecting a task which is free of artificial restrictions, the interrelated perceptuo-motor processes could be investigated concurrently.

Pew's 1974 study is an outstanding example of the molar approach focused on the characteristics of the motor program. He used pursuit tracking as the experimental task. The target moved in a random pattern throughout the 65 s trials. In the middle, 20 s segment the same random pattern was repeated in all trials. However, the subjects did not know, and did not become aware of the repetition. I tried out this task over a number of trials and although I knew that in the middle of each trial I would be presented with the same pattern, I could not detect where the repetition occurred. Thus as far as the subject was concerned in each trial a new tracking pattern was used. With practice, tracking accuracy, measured as integrated absolute error, increased for all segments. However, the improvement of the middle, repeated segment, was significantly greater than that of the other, non-repeated segments. It could have been argued that the repetition of the same movement pattern would lead to a rigidly constructed motor program which is called into action at the appropriate time, resulting in better performance than for the non-repeated segment where new motor programs had to be generated at every trial. That this was not the case was shown when an ingenious experimental manipulation was introduced, i.e. the repeated segment was exactly inverted. Movements to the left were now changed to movements to the right, and right to the left, consequently the motor program had to be altered completely. If the original improvement would be due to the development of a set program, inversion of the pattern would be expected to lead to a considerable performance decrement. This was not the case. Although after inversion the repeated segment was tracked less accurately than prior to inversion, it nevertheless maintained superiority over the non-repeated segments. Before the trials in which the middle segment was inverted, Pew introduced a secondary, attention demanding, non-motor task during tracking. A pre-set motor program would be less affected by the secondary task than when programming of a new movement is necessary. Yet accuracy in the repeated segment decreased to a greater extent than in the non-repeated segments, and significantly more errors occurred in the secondary task during performance of the repeated segment than in the others. In other words, 'automation' of the movements was not found, though this would be expected if a rigid pre-set program was available. Pew concludes (p. 393) that: "What we observe in human skilled behaviour is the rich intermingling of (these) various levels of control as a function of the task demands, the state of learning of the subject and the constraints imposed on the task and the subject by the environment." This statement is supported by his elegant experimental work and is an excellent summary of the non-reductionist standpoint.

REFERENCES

Adams, J.A. (1971). A closed - loop theory of motor learning. *Journal of Motor Behavior, 3,* 111-150.

Adams, J.A. (1977). Feedback theory of how joint receptors regulate the timing and positioning of a limb. *Psychological Review, 84,* 504-523.

Adams, J.A. (1988). Historical review and appraisal of research on the learning, retention, and transfer of human motor skills. *Psychological Bulletin, 101,* 41-74.

Adams, J.A., & Goetz, E.T. (1973). Feedback and practice as variables in error detection and correction. *Journal of Motor Behavior, 5,* 217-224.

Adams, J.A., Goetz, E.T., & Marshall, P.H. (1972). Response feedback and motor learning. *Journal of Experimental Psychology, 92,* 391-397.

Adams, J.A., Gopher, D. & Lintern, G. (1977). Effects of visual and proprioceptive feedback on motor learning. *Journal of Motor Behavior, 9,* 11-22.

Adams, J.A., Marshall, P.J., & Goetz, E.T. (1972). Response feedback and short-term motor retention. *Journal of Experimental Psychology, 92,* 92-95.

Bairstow, P.J. (1987). Analysis of hand movement to moving targets. *Human Movement Science, 6,* 205-231.

Bairstow, P.J. (1989). Development of planning and control of hand movement to moving targets. *British Journal of Developmental Psychology, 7,* 29-42.

Bairstow, P.J., & Laszlo, J.I. (1979). Perception of size of movement patterns. *Journal of Motor Behavior, 11,* 167-178.

Bairstow, P.J., & Laszlo, J.I. (1980). Motor commands and the perception of movement patterns. *Journal of Experimental Psychology: Human Perception and Performance 16,* 1-12.

Bairstow, P.J., & Laszlo, J.I. (1989). Deficits in the planning, control and recall of hand movements in children with perceptuo-motor dysfunction. *British Journal of Developmental Psychology*, 7, 251-273.

Bizzi, E. (1980). Central and peripheral mechanisms in motor control. In G.E. Stelmach and J. Requin (Eds.), *Tutorials in motor behavior* (pp. 231-143). Amsterdam: North-Holland.

Bradshaw, J.L., Bradshaw, J.A., & Nettleton, N.C. (1989). Direction and location of movement in kinasthesis judgements of extent. *Neuropsycholgia, 27,* 1139-1151.

Brooks, V.B. (1969). Information processing in the motorsensory cortex. In Leibovic, K.N. (Ed), *Information processing in the nervous system* (pp. 231-243). New York: Springer-Verlag.

Brooks, V.B. (1981). Task related cell assemblies. In Pompeiano, O., & Masan, C.A. (Eds.), *Brain mechanisms and perceptual awareness.* New York: Raven Press.

Brooks, V.B. and Thach, W.T. (1981). Cerebellar control of posture and movement. In Brooks, V.D. (Ed.), *Handbook of physiology: Section I: The nervous system, Vol.II. Motor control* (pp. 877-946). Baltimore: American Physiological Society.

Bullock, D., & Grossberg, S. (1988). Neural dynamics of planned arm movements: Emergent invariants and speed - accuracy properties during trajectory formation. *Psychological Review, 95,* 49-90.

Burgess, P.R., & Clark, J.F. (1969). Characteristics of knee joint receptors in the cat. *Journal of Physiology, 203*, 317-335

Burwitz, L. (1974). Proactive interference and directed forgetting in short-term motor memory. *Journal of Experimental Psychology, 102,* 799-805.

Canic, M.J., & Franks, I.M. (1989). Response preparation and latency in patterns of tapping movements. *Human Movement Science, 8,* 123-139.

Carlton, L.G. (1981). Visual Information: The control of aiming movements. *Quarterly Journal of Experimental Psychology, 33A,* 87-93.

Carlton, L.G., Carlton, M.J., & Newell, K.M. (1987). Reaction time and response dynamics. *Quarterly Journal of Experimental Psychology, 39A,* 337-360.

Carlton, M.J., Robertson, R.N., Carlton, L.G., & Newell, K.M. (1985). Response timing variability: Coherence of kinematic, and EMG parameters. *Journal of Motor Behavior, 17,* 301-319.

Chew, R.A. (1976). Verbal, visual and kinesthetic error feedback in the learning of a simple motor task. *Research Quarterly, 47*, 254-259.

Connolly, K.,& Jones, B. (1970). A developmental study of afferent - reafferent integration. *British Journal of Psychology, 61,* 259-266.

Corcos, D.M., Agarwal, G.C., & Gottlieb, G.L. (1985). A note on accepting the null hypothesis: Problems with respect to the mass-spring and pulse-step models of movement control. *Journal of Motor Behavior, 17,* 481-488.

Corlett, J.T., & Dickinson, J. (1983a). Proactive and retroactive interference in children's motor short-term memory. *Journal of Human Movement Studies, 9,* 21-29.

Corlett, J.T., & Dickinson, J. (1983b). The effect of distance and location cues on linear arm positioning by children. *Journal of Psychology, 113,* 47-51.

Craft, J.L. (1976). Rehearsal of kinaesthetic information in motor short-term memory. *Perceptual and Motor Skills, 42*, 99-104.

Craft, J.L., & Hinricks, J.V. (1971). Short-term retention of simple motor responses: Similarity of prior and succeeding responses. *Journal of Experimental Psychology, 87,* 297-302.

Diewert, G.I. (1975). Retention and coding in motor short term memory: A comparison of storage codes for distance and location information. *Journal of Motor Behavior, 7,* 183-190.

Diewert, G.L., & Stelmach, G.E. (1977). Intramodal and intermodal transfer of movement information. *Acta Psychologica, 41,* 119-128.

Dornier, L.A., & Reeve, T.G. (1988). Evaluation of the temporal anticipation within the movement - precuing procedure. *Journal of Human Movement Studies, 15,* 91-100.

Duffy, T.M., Montague, W.E., & Laabs, G.J. (1975). The effect of overt rehearsal on motor short-term memory. *Journal of Motor Behavior, 7,* 59-63.

Era, P., Jokela, J., & Heikkinen, E. (1986). Reaction and movement times in men of different ages. *Perceptual and Motor Skills, 63, 111-130.*

Evarts, E.V. & Fromm, C. (1977). Sensory responses in motor cortex neurons during precise motor control. *Neuroscience Letters, 5,* 267-272.

Faust-Adams, A.S. (1975). The role of visual feedback in short-term motor memory. *Journal of Motor Behavior, 7,* 275-280.

Ferrell, W.R. (1985). The response of slowly adapting mechano receptors in the cat knee joint to tetanic contraction of hind limb muscles. *Quarterly Journal of Experimental Physiology, 70,* 337-345.

Fitts, P.M., & Posner, M.I. (1967). *Human performance*. California: Brooks/Cole Publishing Company.

Freund, H.J. (1983) Motor unit and muscle activity in voluntary motor control. *Physiological Review, 63*, 387-436.

Freund, H. J. (1985). Clinical aspects of premotor function. *Behavioral Brain Research, 18,* 187-191.

Georgopoulos, A. P., Schwartz, A.B., & Kettner, R.E. (1986) Neuronal population coding of movement direction. *Science, 233*, 1416-1419.

Girouard, Y., Proteau, L., Laurencelle, L., & Black, P.A. (1987). A demonstration that target information is used during movement planification. *Journal of Human Movement Studies, 13,* 107-133.

Gregory, J.E., & Proske, V. (1979). The responses of Golgi tendon organs to stimulation of different combinations of motor units. *Journal of Physiology, 295,* 251-261.

Haagh, S.A.V.M., & Brunia, C.H.M. (1985). Anticipatory response - relevant muscle activity, CNV amplitude and simple reaction-time. *Electro encephalography and Clinical Neurophysiology, 61,* 30-39.

Henderson, S.E. (1975). Predicting the accuracy of a throw without visual feedback. *Journal of Human Movement Studies, 1,* 183-189.

Henderson, S.E. (1977). Role of feedback in the development and maintenance of a complex skill. *Journal of Experimental Psychology: Human Perception and Performance. 3,* 224-233.

Henry, F.M. (1961). Stimulus complexity, movement complexity, age and sex in relation to reaction latency and speed in limb movements. *Research Quarterly, 32, 253-266.*

Henry, F.M. & Rogers, D.E. (1960). Increased response latency for complicated movements and a "Memory Drum Theory" of neuromotor reaction. *Research Quarterly, 31,* 448-458.

Heuer, H. (1986). Intermanual interactions during programming of aimed movements: Converging evidence on common and specific parameters of control. *Psychological Research 48,* 37-46.

Howard, E.M. & Henderson, S.E.. (1989). Perceptual problems in cerebal-palsied children: A real world Example. *Human Movement Science, 8,* 141-160.

Hulme, C., Biggerstaff, A., Moran, G., & McKinlay, I. (1982). Visual, kinaesthetic and cross-modal judgements of length by normal and clumsy children. *Developmental Medicine and Child Neurology, 24,* 461-471.

Hulme, C., Smart, A., Moran, G., & Raine, A. (1983). Visual, kinaesthetic and cross-modal development: Relationships to motor skill development. *Perception, 12,* 477-483.

Johnson, P. (1980). The relative weightings of visual and nonvisual coding in a simple motor learning task. *Journal of Motor Behavior, 12,* 281-291.

Jones, B. (1973). When are vision and kinaesthesis comparable? *British Journal of Psychology, 64,* 587-591.

Jones, B., & Connolly, K. (1970). Memory effects in cross-modal matching. *British Journal of Psychology, 61,* 267-270.

Kelso, J.A.S., & Holt, K.G. (1980). Exploring a vibratory systems analysis of human movement production. *Journal of Neurophysiology, 43,* 1183-1196.

Kerr, B. (1976). Decision about movement direction and extent. *Journal of Human Movement Studies, 3,* 199-213.

Klapp, S.T. (1977a). Feedback versus motor programming in the control of aimed movements. *Journal of Experimental Psychology: Human Perception and Performance, 104,* 147-153.

Klapp, S.T. (1977b). Response programming, as assessed by reaction time, does not establish commands from particular muscles. *Journal of Motor Behavior, 9,* 301-312.

Klapp, S.T. (1977). Reaction time analysis of programmed control. *Exercise and Sport Science Reviews, 5,* 231-253.

Laabs, G.J. (1973). Retention characteristics of different reproduction cues in motor short-term memory. *Journal of Experimental Psychology, 100,* 168-177.

Laabs, G.J. (1974). The effect of interpolated motor activity on the short-term retention of movement distance and end-location. *Journal of Motor Behavior, 6,* 279-288.

Laabs, G.J. (1976). A note concerning the effect of a kinaesthetic memory load on the retention of movement and location. *Journal of Motor Behavior, 8,* 313-316.

Lackner, J.R. (1984). Some influences of tonic vibration reflexes on the position sense of the contralateral limb. *Experimental Neurology, 85,* 107-113.

Larish, D.D., & Frekany, G.A. (1985). Planning and preparing expected and unexpected movements: Reexamining the relationships of arm, direction and extent of movement. *Journal of Motor Behavior, 17,* 168-169.

Laszlo, J.I. (1990). Child perceptuo-motor development: Normal and abnormal development of skilled behaviour. In C.A. Hauert (Ed.), *Developmental psychology: Cognitive, perceptuo-motor, and neuropsychological perspectives* (pp. 273-308). Amsterdam: North-Holland.

Laszlo, J.I., Baguley, R.A., & Bairstow, P.J. (1970). Bilateral transfer in tapping skill in the absence of peripheral information. *Journal of Motor Behavior, 2,* 261-271.

Laszlo, J.I., & Bairstow, P.J. (1971). Accuracy of movement, peripheral feedback and efference copy. *Journal of Motor Behavior, 3,* 241-252.

Laszlo, J.I., & Bairstow, P.J. (1974). Sensory control of short duration movements. *Proceedings of the Australian Physiological and Pharmacological Society, 5,* 87.

Laszlo, J.I., & Bairstow, P.J. (1985). *Perceptual-motor behaviour: Developmental assessment and therapy.* London: Holt, Rinehart, & Winston.

Laszlo, J.I., Bairstow, P.J., Bartrip, J., & Rolfe, U.T. (1988). Clumsiness or perceptuo-motor dysfunction? In A.M. Colley, & J.R. Beech (Eds.), *Cognition and action in skilled behaviour* (pp. 293-310). Amsterdam: North-Holland.

Laszlo, J.I., & Broderick, P. (1985). The size illusion: Visual and kinaesthetic information in size perception. *Perception, 14,* 285-291.

Laszlo, J.I., & Livesey, J.P. (1977). Task complexity accuracy, and reaction time. *Journal of Motor Behavior, 9,* 171-177.

Laszlo, J.I., & Ward, G.R. (1978). Vision, proprioception and corollary discharge in a movement recall task. *Acta Psychologica, 42,* 477-493.

Lee, T.D., & Elliott, D. (1986) Probing the motor program: Effects of output competition during movement preparation. *Human Movement Science, 5,* 173-183

Lee, T.D., & Magill, R.A. (1985). On the nature of movement representation in memory. *British Journal of Psychology, 76,* 175-182.

Lintern, G. (1989). The learning strategies program. Concluding remarks. *Acta Psychologica, 71,* 301-309.

McCarthy, D. (1972). *McCarthy scales of children's abilities.* New York: The Psychological Corporation.

McCloskey, D.I. (1978). Kinaesthetic sensibility. *Physiological Review, 58,* 763-873.

McCloskey, D.I., Cross, M.J., Honner, R., & Potter, E.K. (1983). Sensory effects of pulling or vibrating exposed tendons in man. *Brain, 106,* 21-37.

McCloskey, D.I., Macefield, G., Gandevia, S.C., & Burke, D. (1987). Sensing position and movements of the fingers. *NIPS, 2,* 226-230.

Magill, R.A., & Dowell, M.N. (1977). Serial - position effects in motor short-term memory. *Journal of Motor Behavior, 9,* 319-323.

Magill, R.A., & Parks, P.F. (1983). The psychophysics of kinesthesis for positioning response: the physical stimulus - psychological response relationship. *Research Quarterly for Exercise and Sport, 55,* 346-351.

Marteniuk, R.G. (1973). Retention characteristics of motor short-term memory. *Journal of Motor Behavior, 5,* 249-259.

Martenuik, R.G. (1977). Motor short-term memory measures as a function of methodology. *Journal of Motor Behavior, 9,* 247-250.

Marteniuk, R.G. & Rodney, M. (1979). Modality and retention effects in intra and cross- modal judgements of kinaesthetic and visual information. *British Journal of Psychology, 70,* 405-412.

Marteniuk, R.G., Shields, K.W., & Campbell, S. (1972). Amplitude, position, timing and velocity cues in reproduction of movement. *Perceptual and Motor Skills, 35,* 51-58.

Mathew, A., & Cook, M. (1989). The nature of control mechanisms in reaching by young infants. In D. Vickers and P.L. Smith (Eds.), *Human information processing: Measures, mechanisms, and models* (pp. 169-186). Amsterdam: North-Holland.

Matthews, P.B.C. (1964). Muscle spindles and their motor control. *Physiological Review, 44,* 219-288.

Matthews, P.B.C. (1972). *Mammalian muscle receptors and their central actions.* London: Edward Arnold.

Megaw, E.D. (1972) Direction and extent uncertainty in step-input tracking. *Journal of Motor Behavior, 4,* 171-186.

Newell, K.M., & Boucher, J-L, P. (1974). Motor response recognition: Two processes. *Journal of Motor Behavior, 6,* 81-86.

Newell, K.M., & Chew, R.A. (1975). Visual feedback and positioning movements. *Journal of Motor Behavior, 7,* 153-158.

Newell, K.M., Shapiro, D.C., & Carlton, M.J. (1979). Coordinating visual and kinaesthetic memory codes. *British Journal of Psychology, 70,* 87-96.

Nichols, T.R. (1985). Is "The Mass-Spring Model" a testable hypothesis? *Journal of Motor Behavior, 17,* 499-500.

Paillard, J. (1960). The patterning of skilled movements. *Handbook of physiology,* I. *Neurophysiology, Vol III* (pp. 1679-1708). American Physiological Society.

Patrick, J. (1971). The effect of interpolated motor activities in short-term motor memory. *Journal of Motor Behavior, 3,* 39-48.

Pew, R.W. (1974). Levels of analysis in motor control. *Brain Research, 71,* 393-400.

Phillips, J., & Glencross, D. (1985). The interdependence of reaction time and movement time in programmed movements. *Acta Psychologica, 59,* 209-225.

Polit, A., & Bizzi, E. (1978). Processes controlling arm movements in monkeys *Science, 201,* 1235-1237.

Polit, A., & Bizzi, E. (1979). Characteristics of motor programs underlying arm movements in monkeys. *Journal of Neurophysiology, 42,* 183-194.

Proske, V., Schaible, H.G., & Schmidt, R.F. (1988). Joint receptors and kinaesthesia. *Experimental Brain Research, 72,* 219-224.

Rabbitt, P.M.A. (1981) Sequential reactions. In D. Holding (Ed.), *Human skills* (pp. 153-175). New York: Wiley.

Reeve, T.G., & Mainor Jr., R. (1983). Effects of movement context on the encoding of kinaesthetic spatial information. *Research Quarterly for Exercise and Sport, 54,* 352-363.

Reeve, T.G., Mackey, L.J. & Fober, G.W. (1986). Visual dominance in the cross-modal kinesthetic to kinesthetic plus visual feedback condition. *Perceptual and Motor Skills, 62,* 243-252.

Roland, P.G., Skinhoj, E., Lassen, N.A., & Larsen, B. (1980). Different critical areas in man in organisation of voluntary movements in extrapersonal space. *Journal of Neurophysiology, 43,* 137-150.

Rosenbaum, D.A., & Saltzman, E. (1984). A motor-program editor. In Prinz, E., & Sanders, A.F. (Eds.), *Cognitive and motor processes* (pp. 51-61). Berlin: Springer-Verlag.

Roy, E.A. (1976). Measuring change in motor memory. *Journal of Motor Behavior, 8,* 283-288.

Roy, E.A. (1977). Spatial cues in memory for movement. *Journal of Motor Behavior, 9,* 151-156.

Roy, E.A., & Davenport, W.G. (1972). Factors in motor short-term memory: The interference effect of interpolated activity. *Journal of Experimental Psychology, 96,* 134-137.

Roy, E.A., & Diewert, G.L. (1978). The coding of movement extent information. *Journal of Human Movement Studies, 4,* 94-101.

Sanes, J.N. (1986). Kinematics and end-point control of arm movements are modified by unexpected changes in viscous loading. *Journal of Neuroscience, 6,* 3120-3127.

Schmidt, R.A. (1980). Past and future issues in motor programming. *Research Quarterly for Exercise and Sport, 51,* 122-140.

Schmidt, R.A. (1982). *Motor control and learning*. Champaign, Illinois: Human Kinetics Publishers.

Schmidt, R.A., & Ascoli, K.M. (1970). Attention demand during storage of traces in motor short-term memory. *Acta Psychologica, 34,* 497-504.

Schmidt, R.A., & McGown, C.M. (1980). Terminal accuracy of unexpectedly loaded rapid movements: Evidence for a mass-spring mechanism in programming. *Journal of Motor Behavior, 12,* 149-161.

Shea, J.B., & Upton, G. (1976). The effects on skill acquisition of an interpolated motor short-term memory task during the KR-delay interval. *Journal of Motor Behavior, 8,* 277-281.

Siegel, S. (1985). Information processing abilities and performance on two perceptual-motor tasks. *Perceptual and Motor Skills, 60,* 459-466.

Skoglund, S. (1956). Anatomical and physiological studies of knee joint innervation in the cat. *Acta Physiologica Scandinavia. 36,* suppl. 124, 1-101.

Smith, G.A., & Brewer, N. (1985). Age and individual differences in correct and error reaction times. *British Journal of Psychology, 76,* 199-203.

Smyth, M.M. (1978). Attention to visual feedback in motor learning. *Journal of Motor Behavior, 10,* 185-190.

Spijkers, W.A.C. (1987). Programming of direction and velocity of an aiming movement: The effect of probability and response - specificity. *Acta Psychologica, 65,* 285-304.

Stack, D.M., Muir, D.W., Sherriff, F., & Roman, J. (1989). Development of infant reaching in the dark to luminous objects and 'invisible sounds'. *Perception, 18,* 69-82.

Stelmach, G.E. (1969). Prior positioning responses as a factor in short-term retention of a simple motor task. *Journal of Experimental Psychology, 81,* 523-526.

Stelmach, G.E. (1970). Kinaesthetic recall and information reduction activity. *Journal of Motor Behavior, 3,* 183-194.

Stelmach, G.E. (1977). Prior organization in motor control. *Journal of Human Movement Studies, 3,* 157-168.

Stelmach, G.E., & Kelso, J.A.S. (1977). Memory processes in motor control. In S.Dorric (Ed.), *Attention and performance, VI.* (pp. 719-739). Hillsdale, NJ: Lawrence Erlbaum Associates.

Stelmach, G.E., Kelso, J.A.S., & McCullagh, P.D. (1976). Preselection and response biasing in short-term motor memory. *Memory & Cognition, 4,* 62-66.

Stelmach, G.E., & Szendrovits, L.D. (1981). Error detection and correction in a structured movement task. *Journal of Motor Behavior, 13,* 132-143.

Stelmach, G.E. & Walsh, M.F. (1973). The temporal placement of interpolated movements in short-term motor memory. *Journal of Motor Behavior, 5,* 165-173.

Stelmach, G.E., & Wilson, M. (1970). Kinaesthetic retention, movement extent and information processing. *Journal of Experimental Psychology, 85,* 425-430.

Sternberg, S., Monsell, S., Knoll, R.L., & Wright, C.E. (1978). The latency and duration of rapid movement sequences: Comparisons of speech and typewriting. In Stelmach, G.E. (Ed.), *Information processing in motor control and learning* (pp. 117-152). New York: Academic Press.

Taub, E. (1976). Motor Behavior following deafferentation in the developing and motorically mature monkey. In Herman, R.M., Grillner, S., Stein, P.S.G., & Stuart, D.G. (Eds.), *Neural control of locomotion* (pp. 675-705). New York: Plenum Publishing Corp.

Vallbo, A.B. (1974). Afferent discharge from human muscle spindles in non-contracting muscles. Steady state impulse frequency as a function of joint angle. *Acta Physiology Scandinavia, 90,* 303-318.

Von Hofsten, C., (1980). Predictive reaching for moving objects by human infants. *Journal of Experimental Child Psychology, 30,* 369-382.

Von Hofsten, C., & Fazell-Zandy, S. (1984). Development of visually guided hand orientation in reaching. *Journal of Experimental Child Psychology, 38,* 208-219.

Von Hofsten, C., & Lindhagen, K. (1979). Observations on the development of reaching for moving objects. *Journal of Experimental Child Psychology, 28,* 158-173.

Von Hofsten, C., & Rosblad, B. (1988). The integration of sensory information in the development of precise manual pointing. *Neuropsychologia, 26,* 805-821.

Welford, A.T. (1988). Acquiring skill: some experiences. *Journal of Motor Behavior, 20,* 458-461.

Whiting, H.T.A., & Cockerill, I.M. (1972). The development of a simple ballistic skill with and without visual control. *Journal of Motor Behavior, 4,* 155-162.

Wierzbicka, M.M., Wiegner, A.W., & Shanani, B.T. (1986). Role of agonist and antagonist muscles in fast arm movements in man. *Experimental Brain Research, 63,* 331-340.

Wiesendanger, M. (1969). The pyramidal tract, recent investigations on its morphology and function. *Ergebnisse der Physiologie, Biologischen Chemie and Experimenetellen Pharmacalogie, 61,* 72-136.

Wylie, R.M., & Tyner, C.F. (1981). Weight-lifting by normal and deafferented monkeys: Evidence for compensatory changes in ongoing movements. *Brain Research, 219,* 172-177.

Zelaznik, H.N., & Hahn, R. (1985). Reaction time methods in the study of motor programming: The precuing of hand, digit and duration. *Journal of Motor Behavior, 17,* 190-218.

Zelaznik, H.N., Shapiro, D.C., & Carter, M.C. (1982). The specification of digit and duration during motor programming: A new method of precuing. *Journal of Motor Behavior, 14,* 57-68.

Approaches to the Study of Motor Control and Learning
J.J. Summers (Editor)

Chapter 3

HUMAN SKILL AND MOTOR CONTROL: SOME ASPECTS OF THE MOTOR CONTROL - MOTOR LEARNING RELATION

H.T.A. (John) Whiting
University of York

Stefan Vogt
Max-Planck-Institute for Psychological Research

Beatrix Vereijken
Free University Amsterdam

The chapter is divided into two parts. In the theoretical part the steps from research on motor control to problems of skill acquisition and training are explored. The presentation is organised around two polarities - motor control/motor learning and prescriptive/emergent theories. Within the latter two frameworks, the changing conceptualisation and contrasts of motor control/motor learning are traced and compared. The paper concludes with an experimental section in which original experiments on motor control and learning, from both a computational and an ecological perspective, are presented and discussed.

INTRODUCTION

While the step from research on motor control to problems of skill acquisition and training is not entirely a step in the dark, it is a difficult one to make since such applications are more implicit than explicit. Indeed, Schmidt (1986), who has a long association with the fields of motor control and learning, paints a sombre picture of the contributions made by these fields to meaningful questions posed by teachers and trainers.

Also within the two theoretical subfields of control and learning, transfer of concepts and mutual stimulation has been limited. In this respect, movement scientists seem to have shared cognitive psychology's credo that "if performance is not well understood, it is somewhat premature to study learning" (Newell & Simon, 1972, p. 8). Since the early 1970's, research interest in movement science has shifted away from skill acquisition toward more elementary control processes (Salmoni, 1989; see also Abernethy & Sparrow, this volume). However, while the analyses of expert performance in cognitive psychology are currently preparing the way for a "reemergence of learning theory within instructional research" (Glaser, 1990, p. 29), movement science still seems to be preoccupied with problems of motor control. The aim of the present chapter is to recapitulate some of the changes in perspective that have taken place in this field and to discuss their value for an integrative perspective on motor control and psychomotor skill acquisition.

At the outset, it has to be recognised that there is no real consensus of opinion between theories of motor control; it is a dynamic field and explanations tend to be polarised with the debate continuing at many different levels of analysis. Implications for the acquisition and training of skill might, therefore, be expected to differ - and might even be seen to be contradictory - depending on which particular approach is embraced. Broadly speaking, the polarisation to which reference has been made is reflected in two clusters of motor control theory that can be distinguished on the basis of the extent to which computational processes are deemed to play a role. Following Bullock and Grossberg (1988), amongst others, two extreme positions can be identified:

1. Theories that posit the existence of a high-level stage involving explicit computation and internal representation of the invariant(s) which, in turn, is used as a basis for performing the desired action (e.g., the minimum jerk theory of Hogan and his colleagues - Flash & Hogan, 1985; Hogan, 1984).
2. Theories in which the need for explicit computation and representation of the invariant(s) is denied. Instead, the action pattern emerges as the result of (i.e., is constrained by) 'events distributed across many interacting sensory, neural, and muscular loci' (see also Kelso & Tuller, 1984; Kugler, 1986).

In motor developmental terms these positions have been polarised as 'pre-ordered prescriptions' as against 'dynamic constraints' (Paillard, 1986). It is interesting, therefore, - in terms of the discussion to follow - that Paillard, at least, is of the opinion that the two explanations are clearly not mutually exclusive but patently complementary. Also Pew and Rosenbaum (1988), in their review on motor control, argue for complementarity by attributing the two apparently exclusive perspectives to different explanatory levels in Marr's

(1982) sense. There is, however, a problem here in that proponents of pre-ordered prescriptions are faced with the need to account - *a priori* - for the effect of interactions that originate in resource dynamic components that have not been considered, traditionally, to constrain movement organisation (Bingham, Schmidt, Turvey, & Rosenblum, 1991).

The problem that is quickly encountered in exploring these polarised approaches is one of definition. Before we can proceed from motor control to motor learning, we have to know to what extent there is agreement amongst the different theoreticians about the concept of motor control *per se*. In order to do this, it would be sensible to explore, at least superficially, the historical context of the concept in order to bring into focus the changes that have taken place, both in conceptualisation and empirical justification, for the differing standpoints adopted. Only then can the links between motor control, motor learning, and training be brought into perspective. The difficulty of this latter step should not be underestimated, clouded, as it is, by the fact that motor control theories are oriented toward the 'here and now' (performance), whereas interest in training lies in future outcomes - 'becoming'. While it is not impossible that theories of motor control directed to expert performance may have relevance for motor control in the relatively inexpert, this should not necessarily be taken for granted. Any teacher of human skill knows how difficult it is to extrapolate from what the expert does to what the inexpert ought to do. The problem is signalled in a different way in a recent critique by Paillard (1989) of a target article by van Ingen Schenau (1989), addressed to the topic of constraints on multi-joint movements and the unique action of bi-articular muscles. What he questions is the universality of such constraints. He suggests that the analysis presented by van Ingen Schenau refers to restricted conditions - extreme performance. The 'universal principle', he maintains, seems to vanish in the perplexing versatility of the functioning system in its normal physiological range which, in the last resort, is what we really have to understand. Such statements should caution against the assumption that the necessary direction of events is from expert motor control to motor learning. It might well be that knowledge about how skills are learned might have much to offer to theorists of motor control.

In the following section, we turn to definitions of motor control and, thereafter, a short historical perspective is presented of recent motor control/motor learning approaches. Subsequently, we will explore the motor control tenets of a selection of theories under the two categories outlined above. In doing so, we will attempt to discover what suggestions are made about motor learning and how it might be facilitated. In the absence of explicit information, in this respect, we will attempt to speculate on the basis of available evidence. Finally, we will briefly discuss two lines of experimental work from our laboratories which try to accommodate some of the changing concepts of control and skill acquisition.

DEFINITION OF MOTOR CONTROL

It has first to be reiterated that motor control is concerned with the 'here and now', with the question of how the movements involved in solving an immediate motor problem posed by the environment are produced. It is not surprising, therefore, that most current neurophysiological studies of motor control "have used overlearned stabilised motor performance in order to reduce variability in the search for correlations between behavioural and neural parameters" (Paillard, 1986, p. 426). Care has to be taken, therefore, in extrapolating from motor control theories conceived in the context of artificially isolated limb systems to how people operate in their natural environment. The interesting question (already signalled) that arises has to do with less skilful performance - is there talk here of a lack or absence of motor control? Clearly, any all-embracing theory of motor control has to provide explanations not only for the control of expert performance but also of performance at lower levels of expertise. Of course, it is not a question of either/or, since at any point in time the organism may be considered to be more or less competent depending on the particular problem which it is required to solve. This is all too apparent in behavioural development. While the human infant at birth is generally immature in terms of much of its behaviour, some of its systems are capable of very competent and precise actions - for example, the control of sucking movements and tracking a moving object with the eyes (Connolly, 1986).

While movement coordination and control are often seen to be synonymous, some workers make a clear distinction. Kugler, Kelso, and Turvey (1980), for example, see coordination as the process that constrains the system's free variables into a behavioural unit and see control as being the process by which values are assigned to that behavioural unit. This unit may be looked upon as the 'organisational invariant', the dynamic variables of which (e.g., stiffness, damping) have to be parameterised to meet the demands of each new problem situation.

In this respect, note should be taken of Roberton's (1986) contention that few contemporary motor development researchers take the opportunity to study age change (as opposed to age differences) and few actually study either the act or the process of 'becoming coordinated'. Coordination she sees as the evolving concatenation in space and time of the movements of body parts to accomplish a given task.

CHANGING CONCEPTUALISATIONS

Current theories of motor control exhibit - despite their contrasting styles of explanation - increasing agreement about what needs to be explained, namely the well coordinated and temporally ordered movement patterns of humans and animals in spite of the multitude of degrees of freedom available to them. Two contrasting perspectives on this control problem have been hinted at above. These two perspectives have recently been addressed by Kugler (1986) - a proponent of natural-physical approaches to motor control and learning. Kugler sees the so-called motor systems approach as stemming from artefactual machine analogies in which the effective control of the behaviour of a multivariable system (the degrees of freedom problem) is seen as a mechanical (engineering) problem, while the natural/physical approach is centred around the geometrical principles that determine the origin and evolution of form and the physics of symmetry-breaking instabilities that bring about changes in form. In the machine analogy - Kugler points out - degrees of freedom *per se* are seen to be a curse while in the natural-physical approach they are regarded as a necessity to be exploited.

These two contrasting approaches bring with them different sets of assumptions and hence interpretations of the way in which movements are controlled and coordinated. The artificial-machine perspective assumes the presence of devices within the CNS that, when activated, produce coordinated movements, that is, the emphasis is on more or less detailed prescriptions for control giving rise to conceptual metaphors like 'schemas' and 'motor programs' or to the identification of neural substrates, such as central pattern generators (Kugler, 1986). In contrast, from a natural-physical perspective, the emphasis is on self-organising systems - on intrinsic symmetries (patterns of invariance) and how they are sustained under some scale changes and broken under others (Kugler, 1986). To operationalise these two approaches in a more specific way, the presence of relative timing invariance which, at least in the not too distant past, has been used to characterise a particular movement form, can serve as an example. While a motor systems approach would account for this invariance by postulating an internal timer, such as a motor program, a natural/physical approach would see this invariant characteristic as emerging as a consequence of a 'playing-out' of the dynamics of the system (Kelso & Tuller, 1984). The coordinative structure, whose presence may be signalled by the invariant timing, is a "temporary marshalling of many degrees of freedom into a task-specific functional unit" (Kelso, Tuller, Vatikiotis-Bateson, & Fowler, 1984, p. 828). While what has become to be known (since Bernstein, 1967) as the 'degrees of freedom problem' has been one of the explicit departure points of ecological theories about motor control and coordination, the computational approach has moved in this direction via a series of reconceptualisations - often in response to critique from theorists of another persuasion. Before turning to the contributions that both perspectives made to the field of skill acquisition, it is useful to briefly sketch the developments in this motor systems or computational approach since it has, in the literature, the longest history.

Motor Programs and Motor Control

Up to the early 1970's, motor programs were invoked as an ontological specification of the centralists' position within the debate centred around central versus peripheral motor control. Accordingly, the main characterisations of a motor program were its preparation before movement initiation and its execution in the absence of peripheral feedback (Keele, 1968). In comparison, the interest in constraints on the movement form in a particular task was only marginal. The degrees of freedom problem was not perceived as a problem *per se* at that time and the definition of a program as directly specifying neuromuscular activity was seen to be unproblematic within the issues considered central.

In the mid 1970's, on the basis of critique related to problems of storage, the production of novel movements, and the interaction between inflow and outflow information, questions began to be asked about the nature of such central representations. What precisely were their attributes? Were they completely prescriptive in the sense of specifying every detail of a particular movement, or were they only responsible for the invariant (topological characteristics) of a particular class of movement? The emphasis was seen to shift from the specification of detail to the *abstract* nature of motor programs (for overviews, see Keele, 1981, 1986; Kelso, 1981; Rosenbaum, 1985; Schmidt, 1988; Summers, 1989) exemplified best, perhaps, by Schmidt's (1975) concept and terminology of generalised motor programs (GMP's), the parameters of which could be tuned to fit the current situation.

In the present context, two aspects of this revised conceptualisation of motor control should be stressed: First, interest in spatio-temporal characteristics of movements generally increased and a variety of skills were studied under the common theoretical aim of identifying the 'language' of the presumed abstract memory structure. Second, empirical findings - such as relative timing invariance - were frequently taken as direct indicators of the underlying program structure. Thus, the fundamental ambiguity of behavioural phenomena with respect to the possibly underlying generative principles remained a blind spot in theorising, and the concept of abstract, *explicit* representations crept in without serious attempts at empirical evaluation. Furthermore, as long as this working assumption was accepted, the origin of a particular temporal order was still not perceived as an outstanding research problem.

More recently, a second major redefinition of the program concept is underway (e.g., Pew, 1984) and while it may be too early to specify its nature in any precise way, some trends can certainly be signalled. In the first place, the notion of relative timing as a potential candidate for the invariant characteristic of a GMP has been called into question on the basis of a re-evaluation of previous findings as well as by new empirical data (e.g., Gentner, 1987; Zelaznik, Schmidt, & Gielen, 1986). Thus, the empirical basis of the assumed memory structure turns out to be more vulnerable than previously thought. As a consequence, it is attractive to search for higher-order invariants beyond the (absolute or relational) metrics of a performance - as was foreshadowed in Bernstein's (1967, p. 42) concept of higher-order topological properties. Yet, even here, the steps to be taken from describing behavioural phenomena of stability and adaptability to statements about (for example) features of a 'program' should be seen as anything but trivial. Furthermore, if metrical constancies turn out to be only a special case of normally non-metrical invariances in performance, a set of generative principles must be looked for which explain the metrical variability and, at the same time, account for the preserved unity of skilled performance (e.g., Vogt, Stadler, & Kruse, 1988). Accordingly, Pew (1984), among others, underlines the distributed nature of motor control, which means that the kinematic pattern is seen as a result of a variety of contributing levels with each level exhibiting a quasi-autonomous status.

Recent views on distributed processing (Rumelhart & McClelland, 1986) would also caution against taking the all too obvious step from behavioural phenomena to statements about central representations. While a description of a system's behaviour as 'schema' or 'program' controlled may be useful at a particular early stage of analysis, one may ultimately be forced into modelling the system's organisation in a way which explains the reliable generation of a movement pattern without recourse to an explicit representation or schema:

> Because the schema is in reality the theorist's interpretation of the system configuration, and because the system configures itself differently according to the sum of all the influences upon it, each new invocation of a schema may differ from the previous invocations. Thus, the system behaves *as if* there were prototypical schemas, but where the prototype is constructed anew for each occasion by combining past experiences with the biases and activation levels resulting from the current experience and the context in which it occurs (Norman, in McClelland & Rumelhart, 1986, p. 537; italics our own).

Such an interpretation has at least a certain face validity when one considers the flexibility with which the human organism organises itself even when solving motor problems of the same kind. It also rhymes well with those who see coordinative structures as *temporary* assemblies of muscle complexes designed to solve a particular problem *at that time*.

To summarise this section, a number of concepts of a motor program have been discussed progressing from the prescriptive to the emergent. The latter, resulting from questioning the (implicit) assumption of explicit representation of kinetic or kinematic parameters in skilled actions, has led to new standpoints about the organismical basis for the generation of complex movement patterns.

This process has to be seen as constructive and creative, involving the participation of a variety of neural subsystems and not as a passive retrieval of a uniform stored copy of the movement.

Computational Theories of Motor Learning

One of the reasons why theories of motor control have had little to say about motor learning *per se* has to do with the fact that while theories of motor control tend to be neurophysiological in nature, theories that have to do with skill acquisition have been of much more interest to psychologists. This is exemplified in the classic psychological text of Bilodeau and Bilodeau (1969) on the principles of skill acquisition in which the topic of motor control is not even indexed. The distinction between these two concepts of control and learning is reflected in Fitts' (1964) earlier definition of a skilled response as "one in which receptor-effector-feedback processes are highly organised, both spatially and temporally", thus embracing both coordination and control, here and now. In contrast, the study of skill learning is the study of "how such organisation or patterning comes about" (p. 244).

More recently, in his overview on motor learning, Adams (1987) explicitly excludes motor control from consideration, arguing that the present disciplines of motor control, neurophysiology and information-processing show little interest in learning as such. In a similar way, Newell (1981) expresses his scepticism about the isolated study of motor control:

> ...if we wait to understand the processing of information and the control of movement, as a prerequisite to introducing into our conceptual frameworks the process of learning, we are likely to wait a very long time indeed (p. 216).

It is, perhaps, not contradictory that the same author (Newell, 1985) proclaims a view of skilled behaviour tied more directly to concepts derived from motor control as being 'long overdue' - at the same time making clear that the step from motor control to learning has to be an active and creative one.

However, before turning to related current developments, let us briefly recapitulate some of the earlier attempts to link motor learning to concepts from motor control. Here, the learning theories of Adams (1971) and Schmidt (1975) can be considered as prototypical examples - both making explicit use of concepts from cybernetics and (motor) control theory. The problems inherent in these approaches to learning can be demonstrated in Schmidt's (1976) variability of practice hypothesis - one example of the way in which externally imposed constraints might be used to optimally promote the development of a motor program. There are, however, fundamental problems in this respect apart from the question as to what evidence exists for the efficacy of such practice - of which there would appear to be very little (van Rossum, 1987).

Essentially, the proposition is that the more variable the practice within a given movement class, the greater the strength of the recall schema so established. Strength would seem to refer to the potential to generate appropriate new movements within the same class. The problem, in this respect, is the lack of clarity about the stage(s) of learning for which variable (as against constant) practice might be relevant. This problem is extenuated by Shapiro and Schmidt's (1982) contention that while schema development is dependent upon the prior existence of generalised motor program, it is not intended to explain how such program come into being. The direct consequence of such a standpoint is that the applicability of schema theory, if at all, is restricted to the later stages of skill learning when such generalised program have become established. In the terms used by Whiting (1984), it has to do with the *attunement* of already existing GMP's rather than with *adaptation*, the acquisition of new patterns of coordination. Thus, in considering Schmidt's theory as a theory of motor learning, one either has to limit motor learning to the attunement of already existing GMP's or, more fundamentally, to ask 'where do the GMP's come from?'. A number of (incomplete) answers have been provided to such a question. For example, Zanone and Hauert (1987, p. 122) adopt the standpoint that "the neonate has a finite catalogue of 'archaic' generalised motor programs" at his disposal. A number of reactions can be made to this standpoint (Whiting, 1987). In the first place, as Prechtl (1986) points out, the neonatal repertoire does not appear *de novo* at birth but is preceded by a prenatal developmental course. Thus, exponents of a motor program approach would want to maintain that GMP's were also available at that stage. Such a regression would eventually lead to the conclusion that representations for all classes of movement (coordinations) were already present *in utero* and simply had to be attuned to existing problem situations. While one might come a long way with such an argument when restricting explanations to phylogenetic skills, ontogenetic skills (in which coordinations are often very unnatural) would give rise to more overt problems.

Concerning the acquisition of new coordinations, one of the few contributions from an information processing perspective is the assumption of a *template* or *internal model* which is thought to be formed prior to overt performance and to be used as a reference for developing an adequate motor program (Keele, 1973, 1986; Keele & Summers, 1976; Summers, 1989). A crucial question, in this context, is in what respect delegating responsibility to another theoretical construct could facilitate our understanding of the emergence of novel behaviour. The original concept of a template as comprising detailed sensory consequences of the novel movement pattern may not bring us much further here, because one would now have to ask where the new template comes from. An explanation in terms, for example, of mere exposure to an external model must be seen as simplistic, as it ignores firstly, the question what *specific information* can be detected in a modelling situation, and secondly, the equivocal results for the use of demonstrations in the learning of new skills (see Scully & Newell, 1985).

In alternative interpretations, the *selective* and *abstract* nature of internal models is emphasised, for example, in the concepts of 'action prototypes' (Annett, 1983), 'amodal invariants' (Neisser, 1985) and of an 'image of the act' (Whiting & den Brinker, 1982; Whiting, 1988) - these concepts refer to qualitative features of movements. On the one hand, these interpretations of an internal model come closer to our phenomenal experience in approaching an unfamiliar task, on the other, the functional role of such abstract entities in the immediate control of *inexpert* performance may appear obscure from an information processing point of view.

A testable assumption, at least, is that internal models can be acquired independent of overt performance (e.g., in a modelling situation, by providing alternative and more detailed descriptions of a task, or by mental practice), but the situation becomes more complex if we consider the widely varying effects of such procedures in different tasks. For conceptualising these differences, a viable framework has been put forward by Whiting and den Brinker (1982) in their distinction between the 'image of the act' and the 'image of achievement'. The former is construed to be the qualitative (topological) form of a movement - a coordination problem - and the latter as the pattern of external (metric) forces to be overcome - a control problem. When faced with a new motor task for the first time that requires adaptive behaviour, the learner is confronted with two problems: how to coordinate his movements in order to meet the demands of the new situation and, how to meet the requirements of the environmental constraints. In attempting to complete the motor task an answer has to be provided to both of these problems. It would not be surprising if the learner, in concentrating his or her attention on the one (e.g., the new coordination pattern) would have less attention for the other (e.g., meeting the external demands). Successful performance at a particular task may then depend on the degree to which the formation of an adequate image of achievement represents a separate problem, which must be solved during extensive practice, or whether the step from an image of the act to the generation of an image of achievement can be done on the basis of prior generalised experience of the learner, as, for example, in complex uniarticular movements.

In sum, we feel that the concept of an internal model offers some interesting research perspectives - it remains to be seen, however, whether a narrow information processing framework could handle the non-prescriptive, high-level character which makes this concept attractive or whether a different theoretical framework will provide a better context for this presently under-researched area.

We now turn to alternative approaches to 'motor learning' provided by proponents of ecological psychological approaches.

Ecological Psychological Approaches

Under this umbrella term are subsumed the so-called action theory and natural physics approaches signalled previously. Such theories find their origin in the earlier work of Bernstein (1967) on the control and coordination of movement and in Gibson's (1979) theory of direct perception. Different exponents of the ecological approach, while generally embracing one another's conceptual framework, choose in their empirical work to place more emphasis on the one rather than the other, that is, on environmental as against organismic and task constraints (to use the categories enunciated by Newell, 1986). This has to be seen as having more to do with the complexity of the problem *per se*, that is, the explanation of the control and coordination of human actions rather than any essential difference of opinion as to the relative importance of the one as against the other. In fact, in recognising the essential perception-action coupling that pervades all human actions, they see any separation of action from perception as being artificial. This idea expresses itself in what Bootsma (1988), for example, refers to as the principle of compensatory variability - fluctuations in one execution variable being compensated for by fluctuations in another. Whether, for example, an act is performed a little faster or initiated somewhat earlier appears to be inconsequential as long as a coupling between perceptual and movement variables is sustained - a phenomenon well exemplified in Kelso, Saltzman, and Tuller's (1986) study on speech production under perturbation.

It has to be said, once again, that the major focus of attention - as in all theories of motor control - has been on the 'here and now' and, at this stage of development of the ecological psychological approach, little (explicit) attention has been given to motor learning (recent exceptions being Jeka & Kelso, 1989; Kelso, 1990; Newell, Kugler, van Emmerik, & McDonald, 1989; Vereijken, Whiting, & Beek, 1990). In fact, in as far as the latter term implies the learning of movements *per se*, exponents of the ecological approach might want to question the validity of such a departure point and to think more in terms of solutions to motor problems posed by the environment during which movement patterns emerge as a result of organism-environment interaction.

This apparent neglect of motor learning (however conceived) is understandable and may reflect nothing more than a question of priorities. Although working from another perspective (control theory), Doyle (1987) in his analysis of the skill of riding a bicycle makes the point that the specification of a control system must be preceded by a precise specification of the system to be controlled, thereby providing a possible reason why learning *per se* has, until now, been given a low priority.

To date, there have been few such specifications (however, see Beek, 1989; Doyle, 1987; Vereijken et al., 1990). More recently, Kelso (1990) has pointed to the necessity to clarify the nature of the intrinsic dynamics of a task - the order parameter dynamics that arise as a result of non-specific changes in control parameters [1] - in order to know what is modified or what is learned before determining how new patterns of movement are acquired. The reason why this is so important has been made explicit by Beek (1989) in his detailed analysis of the dynamics of the skill of juggling:

> Once the laws and regularities of a skill are known, a 'reference frame' becomes available relative to which the changes in a learning process can be interpreted (p. 190).

Beek (1989) went on to demonstrate the spatial and temporal constraints that organise the act of juggling and, hence, to provide a principled description of the parameters which guide its learning. In this context, the word 'constraint' refers to any reduction in the degrees of freedom irrespective of the mechanism of reduction. Such a usage encompasses not only restrictions on action that are not themselves responsible for the production of action, but also physical principles of dynamical self-organisation from which coordination may arise.

Most theories and approaches to motor skill, as suggested above, use terms like 'control', 'coordination' and 'skill' interchangeably. Ecological theorists, in contrast, make explicit distinctions between the terms. In short, they define coordination as the way in which a person constrains his/her degrees of freedom into coordinative structures (temporary assemblages of muscle synergies) so that only a few 'free' parameters remain. The manipulation of the 'free' parameters is what is referred to as control. Skill is the optimal assignment of values to the controlled variables (Newell, 1985). Thus, unlike traditional motor systems approaches, the ways in which patterns of coordination are acquired is of fundamental importance to exponents of this line of thinking.

Implicit in this approach is that the action system, through its (task) dynamics, becomes autonomously self-organised in providing its solution to a particular motor problem. The high dimensionality of the musculature is reduced to a few order parameters assembled from the most relevant quantities (which tend to be few in number), expressing the extent of system order in the transition from one stable coordination mode to another (see Kelso, 1990 and Turvey, 1990 for further explication and examples).

---

[1] The order parameter or 'collective variable' is the defining characteristic of a particular pattern by which qualitative changes in that pattern are indexed as a system by which qualitative changes in that pattern are indexed as a system is led by the control parameter through a series of pattern changes. Control parameters are non-specific to the resulting patterns, that is, they are responsible for the pattern changes but do not contribute towards their form.

> On this view, motor organisation is accounted for as an *a posteriori* consequence of the dynamics of the action system in accordance with general principles of self-organisation, rather than assumed *a priori* (Warren, 1987, p. 200).

It is clear that, for ecological psychologists, the problem of motor learning (perhaps more appropriately labelled skill acquisition) can better, or perhaps more veridically, be considered to be the problem of how both coordination and control of the system, in providing solutions to a particular problem posed by the environment, are achieved. The departure point, in this respect, is the essential role of the continuous stream of perceptual - especially visual and haptic - information. Turvey (1990), in a general way, points to the complementarity between the multivariable movement system and the multivariable environment which mutually constrain their respective degrees of freedom resulting in attenuation rather than amplification of dimensionality. It is, perhaps, for this reason that von Hofsten (1986) sees perception and action as evolving together rather than being tacked on to one another - an increase in the sophistication of the one, resulting, reciprocally, in an increase in the sophistication of the other.

The early stage of (new) skill acquisition consists primarily of acquiring the appropriate (optimal) topological characteristics of the body and limbs. Although this search for optimality has been ongoing - particularly in the field of biomechanics - specific successes have been sparse. Bernstein (1967), however, provides more general insights in pointing out that in exercises in sports and gymnastics, the motor structure (referred to as style) is incorporated as an integral part in the meaningful aspect of the given problem. "For this reason it is one of the primary objects of the trainer to achieve as determinate a formulation and as rapid a stabilisation of the motor structure as is possible for his pupil..."(p. 134). Further practice leads to refined scaling of the relative motions with optimal scaling reflecting skilled performance. Of course, such a standpoint says nothing about how training to such an end would be organised, but speculations in this respect can be put forward - speculations that, in retrospect, give substance to Bernstein's contention that skill training involves repetition without repetition, that is, subjects do not repeat the same movements but try, instead, to solve the motor problem presented in ways which are refined from occasion to occasion.

Newell et al. (1989), for example, centre their ecological approach to the learning of coordination and control on 'search strategies' used by subjects to explore and locate the gradient and equilibrium regions (specified by low energy requirements) of the dynamical properties of the perceptual-motor work space. In this way, they hope to arrive at a principled basis for a theory of the acquisition of coordination that is general to all activity classes. By search strategies, they mean the way in which an organism explores (perceptually) the work-space of the organism-environment interaction in order to 'solve the motor problem'. Exploration of the work-space (by, for example, exploratory movements), they claim, both creates and annihilates critical regions in the field, giving rise to a variety of information states. Turvey, Carello, and Kim (1990) were able to show that such 'exploratory behaviour' is highly structured and effective, rather than being random or trial and error. Such an approach nicely encompasses the traditional need to have information not only about the actions which should be carried out but also about those that are less desirable (in the sense that they give rise to unnecessary energy expenditure). By this means, the subject 'learns' not only what information is relevant but also what is less relevant (Rabbitt, 1967) - the latter, in Beek's (1989) terms, serving as a reference frame. This return to the concept of exploration - discovery learning (Vereijken & Whiting, 1990) - is an interesting one implying, as it does, that the learner is constrained to discover for himself or herself an optimal solution by the way in which the environment is structured at that time or that a teacher so organises the environment that the learner is constrained to conform to particular task requirements that he/she has in mind (e.g., the way in which a striking implement is held and manipulated or the way in which the 'forcing' of some external piece of apparatus - such as an ice skate - is brought about). In so doing, the learner is able to provide solutions appropriate to his/her body configurations. The similarity here with the professional approach of the movement educationist is striking. But, as is often the case, practice cannot await theory for its implementation. These earlier insights and experience of the teacher of movement skills, if listened to, might have provided insights for the researcher that would have precipitated this line of approach.

This return to the concept of discovery learning has led Shaw and Alley (1985) to characterise the ecological approach to the issues of learning as the learning of the laws (by acquaintance) in contrast to the traditional learning theory approach which has attempted to define the laws of learning.

The ideas embodied in this section have given rise to a variety of approaches by the present authors to the problem of skill learning from an ecological psychological point of view. In the following, short overviews of two of these lines of research will be given, both of which were concerned with control and learning issues and thus illustrate kinds of interplay between these two fields. Furthermore, both research lines exemplify transitions from more traditional approaches toward incorporating concepts and methods from ecological psychology. Given the current interest in this 'alternative' approach to 'motor learning', a rapid increase in the number of such studies, with a corresponding refinement of concepts and methodologies is to be expected.

EXPERIMENTAL STUDIES

Motor Control and Learning in the Pattern Reproduction Task

Our first example of experimental work comes from a pattern reproduction task, in which subjects are asked to learn to reproduce from memory a visually displayed movement pattern by moving a lever with the right arm - basically a movement imitation task.

The history of this experimental paradigm mirrors, on a small scale, the above-mentioned shift toward control studies during the last two decades, since only the initial studies by Armstrong and Pew (see Pew, 1974) were explicitly concerned with the effect of different training methods. Later studies were either directed toward observable changes in motor control with practice (e.g., Marteniuk & Romanow, 1983) or tested specific hypotheses about motor control and representation using transfer paradigms (e.g., Bamford & Marteniuk, 1988; Heuer & Schmidt, 1988).

The initial motivation for the experiments described in the following (cf., Vogt, 1988) was to test a particular model of central representation of complex movement sequences, the *Fourier coding analogy* (Gallistel, 1980). Here, the basic assumption is that a movement trajectory is internally represented in terms of sine wave components. The pattern reproduction task was chosen as it provided an economical way of testing our predictions and, additionally, as it allowed comparisons with concurrent models - such as serial chaining or relative timing invariance - to be made. Furthermore, the earlier studies by Franks and Wilberg (1982) and Marteniuk and Romanow (1983) had already shown systematic changes in the spectral density function with practice. Thus, the objective of the first experiment was to proceed from this descriptive stage - which did not allow strict conclusions about the underlying control structure to be drawn - to specific hypothesis testing. The main prediction was that learning a particular pattern should facilitate the transfer to a pattern with the same constituent frequency components (but with shifted relative phases), and that the transfer to a pattern with different frequencies and phases should be smaller. Accordingly, a transfer paradigm was used in which three groups of 10 subjects each had to learn one out of three patterns (see Figure 1) for 80 trials and were tested on the other two patterns for another 2 x 8 trials in a pre- and post test.

However, while an analysis of the learning trials revealed an increase in the higher harmonics with practice, as observed in the previous studies, no selective positive transfer between the two patterns with identical frequency components was found (see Figure 2). In fact, the only positive transfer effect observed was between the two patterns with a similar movement form but with different frequency components (patterns B and C). A second hypothesis stating that the reproductions in the early learning stage should mirror the criterion pattern

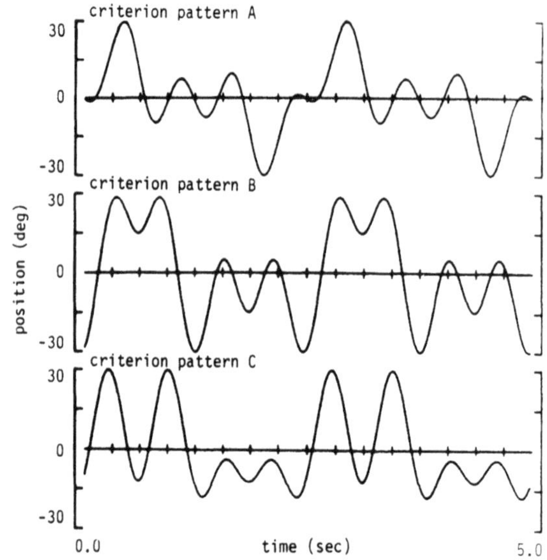

Figure 1. Position time curves of the three criterion patterns used in Experiment 1. Patterns A and B were generated from identical frequency components (0.4, 0.8 and 1.6 Hz) with different relative phases, in pattern C the second frequency component was replaced by 1.2 Hz.

primarily with respect to spectral similarity (as opposed to spatio-temporal similarity) could not be confirmed either (see Vogt, 1988).

Thus, in the first stage of the research project, a promising model comprising both skilled performance and learning (the latter as a resonance-like process) could not be supported by the results. In retrospect it can be added that a recent study by Stanley and Franks (1990), testing the same hypothesis, also revealed no evidence to support the Fourier model of trajectory representation.

A second step in the experimental analysis was initiated by an unexpected finding concerning the temporal microstructure of the reproductions. The basic finding was a pronounced covariation of cycle duration with the amplitude of the cycle - a finding which pointed to a limited generality of the 'isochrony principle' (Viviani, 1986) and contradicted a corresponding clock-like control model as proposed by Heuer and Schmidt (1988) in the context of their pattern reproduction experiments. In sum, the consecutive experiments (Vogt, Stadler, & Kruse, 1988) revealed that the (co-)variations of cycle time covered a ratio of about 1 : 1.5 for small and large movement amplitudes even after a larger number of practice trials (n = 176) and irrespective of equal cycle times in the criterion pattern. Furthermore, the resulting *relative timing* changed

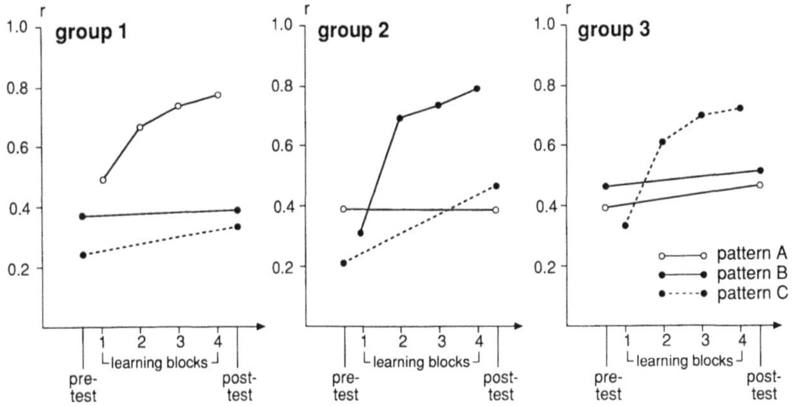

Figure 2. Correlations between criterion pattern and reproductions in 10 learning blocks of 8 trials and in the pre- and post tests on two non-learned patterns. The only significant increase from pre- to post test is in group 2 for pattern C.

spontaneously in eight consecutive transfer trials with a longer execution time (8.5 sec instead of 5 sec). The results raised further doubts about models which assume the explicit representation of time or time ratios as an universal alphabet of motor memory as, for example, in the model of generalised motor programs. Instead, the results suggested a motor control model with at least two separable levels, first, a more abstract representation of the movement form (in the sense of an 'image of the act' as mentioned earlier) and, second, some lower-level generative principles of trajectory formation, of which the exploitation of available kinetic energy appeared to be an important one (cf. Vogt et al., 1988).

After this step into a pure motor control issue, we decided to return to the question of representation or what actually had been learned in the task. On the one hand, neither the Fourier coding analogy nor the concept of invariant relative timing were in line with our foregoing observations; on the other hand, it was difficult to imagine how a movement form could be represented in any other way than concrete spatio-temporal (or spectral) coordinates. How could the notion of an 'abstract representation' be filled for the present task? In this situation, attention was turned toward the initial learning stage, that is, toward the first attempts of subjects to reproduce the given criterion pattern. The rationale of this step was that studying the learning history might provide some new ideas about the kind of representation. Since the quantitative analyses of these trials had mainly shown high inter-trial-variabilities and only small correlations with the criterion pattern, visual inspection of the position-time-curves was chosen as an additional means for detecting any kind of consistency within these early 'reproductions'.

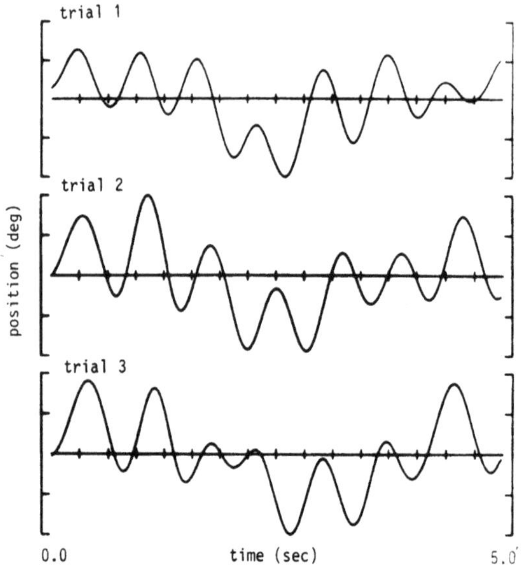

Figure 3. The first 3 performances of a subject with pattern A as criterion pattern. Trial 3 exhibits a segregation into large and small cycles and a centring around the mid axis.

A respective qualitative analysis of the first 8 reproductions of 15 subjects of pattern A (as shown in Figure 1) revealed a small number of similarity criteria between the criterion pattern and the reproductions (see also Vogt, in press). While nearly all 120 performances corresponded to the cycle time and global movement size of the criterion pattern, a first improvement could be defined by the appearance of large and small movement cycles, irrespective of their temporal order, and by a *centring* of these cycles around the mid axis of the screen. Figure 3 shows three consecutive trials which demonstrate this progression.

A second improvement consisted in the appearance of a correct sequence of the large movement cycles (irrespective of the sequence of the small cycles), that is, an *alternation* of direction of the large cycles. Figure 4 shows four consecutive trials of another subject demonstrating this second step. From trial 1 to trial 8, the occurrence of this type of performance increased from 20% to 90% of cases.

To summarise, the initial learning stage could be described as the successive incorporation of a number of qualitative features into the performance. A dominant characteristic of these features is that they do not refer to single

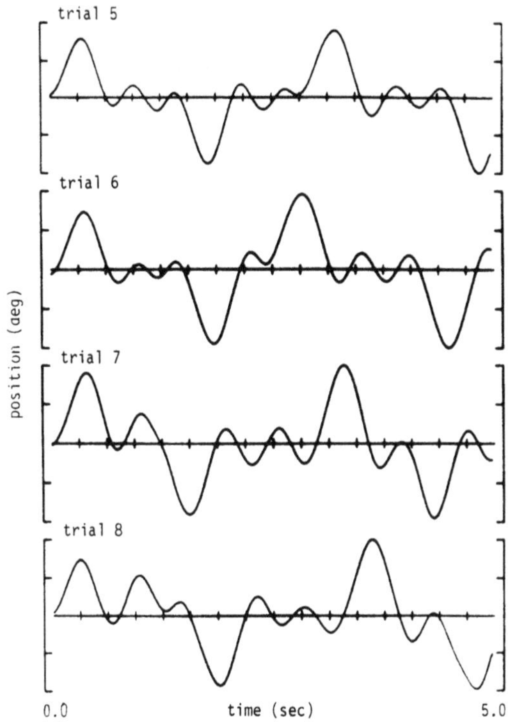

Figure 4. Trials 5 to 8 of another subject trying to reproduce pattern A. Note the instable number of the small movement cycles even after a correct performance in trial 6.

positions of movement elements within a sequence (in the sense of a serial chaining model of learning), moreover they refer to *global* and mainly spatial aspects of the movement sequence, for example, the 'centring around the midline', the 'segregation into large and small cycles', or the 'alternation of direction of the large cycles'. *Sequencing,* then, can be seen as the result of a *parallel articulation of these global, higher-order invariants* and would no longer need an explanation in terms of an explicit serial representation. Thus, while this line of study is just beginning and does not yet allow definitive conclusions, the analysis opens up an alternative view of representation of movement sequences, which is well in line with current theorising about parallel and multi-level processing as discussed previously.

Reviewing the course of this research line in the present context, we can summarise that issues of motor control (representation and principles of trajectory formation) were clearly dominant here and that learning trials were introduced basically as a means for achieving stable performances and as a basis for transfer procedures. Only in the latest stage of the project were the (unstable) initial reproductions examined as a phenomenon *per se*, and the respective analyses revealed a new hypothesis about the characteristics of a central representation and its formation during learning. Thus, the results may be seen as an example of how studying the initial learning stage and its variability can provide valuable clues about skilled motor control.

Future experimental work will be concerned with testing specific predictions from this alternative view of representation, for example, by studying transfer of 'higher-order invariants' as described above. Secondly, alternative ways of teaching will be studied in which the invariants discovered in unguided learning situations are introduced successively in a 'learning program'. Thirdly, perceptual and performance-dependent contributions in acquiring a movement form will be examined in different tasks, such as dancing and pattern reproduction, which research will hopefully lead to questions about skill acquisition and training more closely tied to actual problems of the learner and, at the same time, based on our advanced knowledge about motor control.

Learning Slalom Ski-type Movements

Our second example comes from a line of research focused on the learning of slalom ski-type movements. It provides a demonstration for a shift from a traditional approach to a dynamical approach. Furthermore, although this line of research is concerned in the first place with how the *learning* of a novel motor task involving multiple degrees of freedom can be understood and - eventually - facilitated, along its progression it also showed interesting excursions into the field of motor control.

The general paradigm for this series of studies involved subjects learning to make slalom ski-type movements on a ski-apparatus (Figure 5; see den Brinker & van Hekken, 1982 for details of this apparatus). In all experiments performed on this apparatus, training was continued for a period of four to five consecutive days. Each day consisted of two measurement trials interspersed with six training periods under a variety of conditions. Dependent variables - shown in a previous study to be good indices of learning (den Brinker & van Hekken, 1982) - were the amplitude, frequency, and fluency of the movements of the ski-apparatus platform (for an example of performance curves, see Figure 6).

In a first series of experiments, utilising traditional motor learning paradigms, was studied how the process of learning - as indexed by changes in performance - could be manipulated by imposing a variety of constraints. These imposed constraints included training at five different prescribed

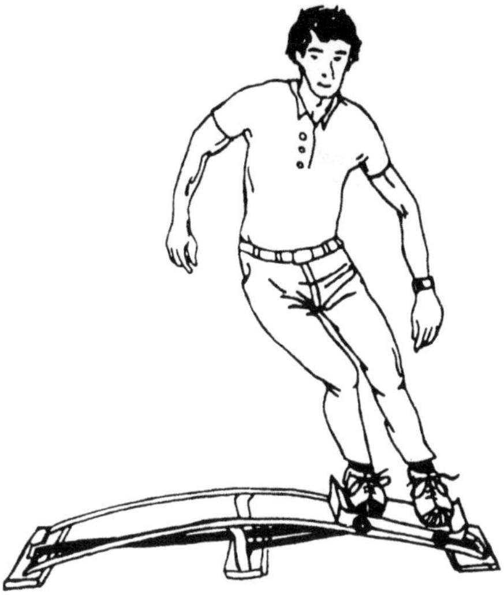

Figure 5. The ski-apparatus.

frequencies (van Emmerik, den Brinker, Vereijken, & Whiting, 1989), training under augmented feedback conditions (den Brinker, Stäbler, Whiting, & van Wieringen, 1986), and training with or without the availability of a video model (Whiting, Bijlard, & den Brinker, 1987).

The requirement to move at different *prescribed* frequencies during training resulted in sub-optimal learning for subjects required to train at a high frequency (i.e., 21% above preferred frequency) and particularly poor progress - on the criteria maintained - for subjects required to train at a low frequency (i.e., 21% below preferred frequency) (van Emmerik et al., 1989).

In the second experiment of the series, subjects receiving feedback about, and being required to pay attention to, the amplitude of the movement of the ski-apparatus were shown to be superior to those required to perform in a similar way while receiving feedback about either frequency or fluency of platform movement. The former led to inferior amplitude and the latter to inferior frequency (den Brinker et al., 1986). None of the experimental groups, however, showed superior performance on any of the variables used than a control group that received no augmented feedback (Vereijken & Whiting, 1990). Figure 6 shows, as an example, the performance curves for the different groups on the parameter amplitude. The results thus indicated that augmented feedback in the learning of this task is not crucial, in that the control group who

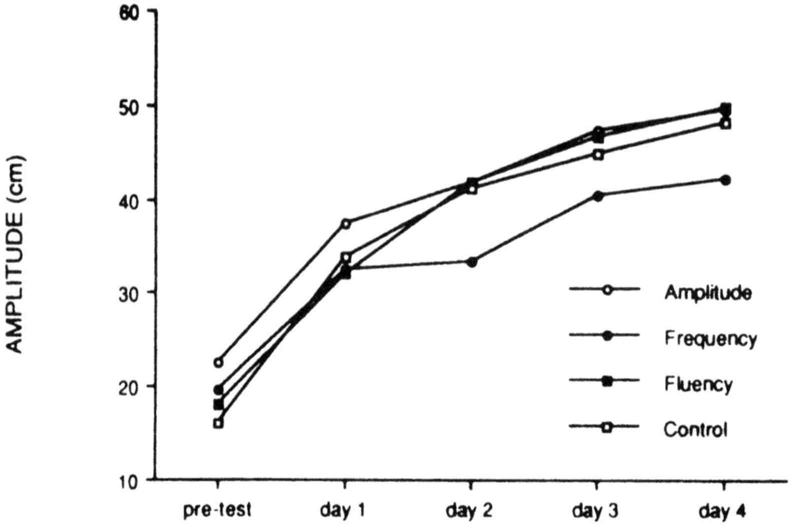

Figure 6. Means over days and conditions for the parameter amplitude of platform movements.

had to rely on discovery learning achieves the same, or a higher performance level, on the criteria maintained.

The third imposed constraint in this series involved learning with or without the availability of a video model of an expert performer while actually learningto perform the slalom ski-type movements. Here, the subjects who had the advantage of the availability of a video model showed superior learning on the parameter fluency only (Whiting et al., 1987).

It is significant in the context of the present paper to note that none of the above constraint manipulations resulted in superior learning - after a period of four training days - on the parameters amplitude and frequency of platform movements than 'discovery learning' per se. A qualification does, however, have to be made since in no case was a dependent variable used which would reflect the endeavours of the subjects per se. Such a statement suggests caution in accepting, for example, that the dependent variables used to date are really those which reflect learning *changes* rather than merely being indices of learning. After all, it is well recognised that the relation kinetic-kinematic is a many to few: knowledge about the externally defined kinematic outcome does not uncover how underlying internal dynamics relate to this outcome. With this in mind, it was decided to adopt an approach that would give credence to the kinetic changes that underlie the surface kinematic manifestations. Departure point in this approach was the contention that one first has to know *what* is

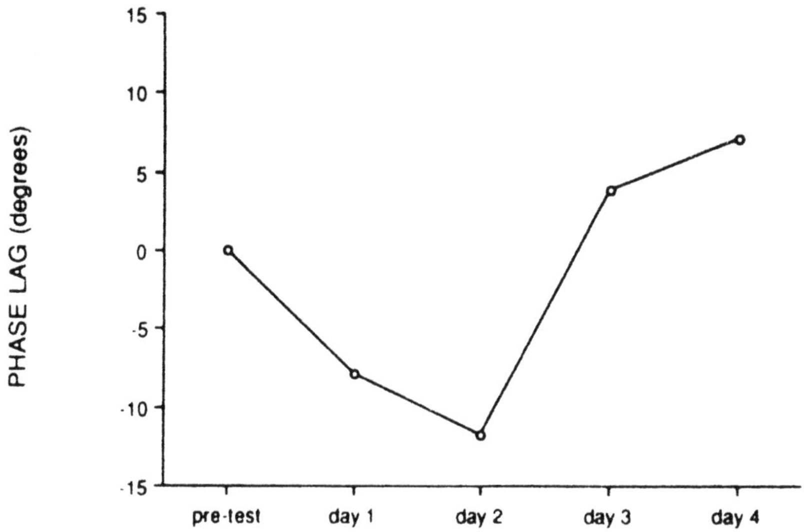

Figure 7. Mean phase lag over days for a discovery learning group.

being learned (a clear motor control question) before one can begin to come to terms with the question as to *how* learning takes place (Beek, 1989). What the subject is required to do will be heavily influenced by the dynamic characteristics of the ski-apparatus itself. Since the subject will have to discover and eventually exploit these apparatus constraints, recourse was made to a dynamical description of the subject apparatus system in which such constraints can become operationalised (Vereijken, Whiting, & Beek, 1990). This description involved two stages: modelling of the ski-apparatus when loaded with passive weights and modelling when a subject is operating. The first stage resulted in a full quantitative description of stiffness and damping as functions of displacement, angular velocity, and mass. Non-linearity was observed because of spring elasticity and its characteristic relaxation time.

A subject standing on the platform - stage two - can only influence the oscillation of the platform by changing his or her moment of inertia (i.e., translating -raising or lowering - the centre of mass and rotating the centre of mass around the point of support). Incorporating these inertia terms into the equation of motion of the platform it was possible to deduce the main characteristics of the subject's motion (i.e., centre of mass, its rate of change and its phase lag with the platform oscillations). The latter variable, the phase lag between the oscillations of the centre of mass and the platform oscillations, indicates when the subject exerts force on the platform. A negative phase lag means that the subject exerts force *before* the platform passes through the centre of the apparatus. On the contrary, a positive phase lag indicates that the subject manages to postpone the forcing of the platform until *after* having passed the centre. The phase lag thus characterises the relation between subject and apparatus and as such received our special attention as a possible additional parameter in our work on motor learning.

After having derived theoretically the phase lag parameter, return was made to our earlier motor learning paradigm. In a subsequent experiment, one group of subjects trained for four days in a discovery learning condition using the general paradigm outlined above. From the combined results of amplitude, frequency, and phase lag, the learning process can be described as follows:

Subjects, while learning to maximise amplitude and frequency, initially move out of phase with the platform. Before crossing the centre of the ski-apparatus they force the platform instead of exploiting the elasticity of the stretched springs. This is indicated by a high negative phase lag (see Figure 7). Shortly thereafter, this phase lag becomes minimised. From the second day onwards, displacement increases to its maximum, achieved by an increase of translational and rotational motion. The better subjects, eventually, succeed in bringing the phase lag between the motion of their centre of mass and that of the platform to above zero (i.e., they ride the system as long as possible, thus utilising the energy that is stored in the springs).

Pursuing this line of inquiry, the efficacy of the different kinds of constraints invoked in the abovementioned earlier experiments carried out on the ski-apparatus was re-examined (Vereijken et al., 1990). The phase lag parameter was shown to be able to differentiate between experimental groups that could not be differentiated on the basis of the earlier kinematic variables alone. On the basis thereof it was concluded that the phase lag parameter has additional explanatory power about the fundamental relation between the subject and the apparatus, information that was not available on the basis of the previous kinematic outcome variables alone. Future research will continue investigating this phase lag parameter and its possible contributions to understanding the problems of teaching in general and of the learner in particular.

In sum, the following can be seen from the two examples of experimental work: The experimental work on pattern reproductions, although predominantly concerned with motor control, found on its way interesting motor learning issues that in turn led to alternative hypotheses about motor control issues such as central representation and its formation. The work on the ski-apparatus, on the contrary, while emphasising motor learning, made excursions into the field of motor control in order to understand what is involved in performing a certain task. Both lines of research thus show that it is not so much the dominant focus on either motor control or learning but rather the flexible interplay between methods and lines of thinking characteristic to either area that leads to ideas and interpretations that otherwise might not have been taken into consideration.

CONCLUDING REMARKS

In essence, the present Chapter was organised around two polarities - motor control vs. motor learning, and 'prescriptive' vs. 'emergent' theories. The two clusters of theoretical approaches, which form the focus of the discussion, can be characterised as having a common emphasis on motor control and a related neglect of learning issues. It was illustrated how theories of motor programming are becoming more sensitive to problems that confronted, at the outset, those adopting an ecological psychological approach. This provides the future possibility, with respect to motor control, of a convergence between these approaches rather than a further polarisation.

In our discussion of computational theories of motor learning, the undefined origin of a program - the acquisition of coordination - was seen to be one of the major blind spots in theorising. Traditionally, the concept of an internal model has been introduced here and thus links to higher cognitive processes are strived for. It remains to be seen, however, if the problem of *novelty* can find a principled answer in a recourse to such mental operations. The point was consistently made that research on motor control directed to the 'inexpert' rather than the 'expert' has been largely neglected in computational approaches which, given the important contribution that such studies might make to the understanding of skill acquisition, was to be regretted. At the same time it was emphasised that the benefit in this respect might be reciprocal.

While the themes of inexpert performance and learning have also received limited attention in ecological ('emergent') approaches - which are primarily addressed to actor-environment compatibilities and not to eventual discrepancies - some research efforts in this field can currently be observed. The perspective, here, is to describe the transitions in skill level as a pattern formation process (an evolution of form), which increasingly conforms to, and exploits, physical constraints and minimum regions within a given task without invoking explanatory concepts such as internal cognitive representations.

In this respect, prescriptive and emergent approaches might initially encounter even sharper contrasts of theoretical perspective in the field of learning than in pure motor control. However, the prospect of an integrative view of motor control and learning, embracing the physical as well as cultural aspects of human skill, should be worth the battle!

REFERENCES

Adams, J.A. (1971). A closed-loop theory of motor learning. *Journal of Motor Behavior, 3, 111-150.*

Adams, J.A. (1987). Historical review and appraisal of research on the learning, retention, and transfer of human motor skills. *Psychological Bulletin, 101*, 41-74.

Annett, J. (1983). Motor learning: A cognitive psychological viewpoint. In H. Rieder, K. Bös, K. Reischle, & H. Mechling (Eds.), *Motorik und Bewegungsforschung: Ein Beitrag zum Lernen im Sport* (pp. 220-230). Schorndorf: Hofmann.

Bamford, R.B., & Marteniuk, R.G. (1988). Visual feedback, movement learning, and the representation of movement. *Human Movement Science, 7,* 1-26.

Beek, P.J. (1989). *Juggling dynamics.* Amsterdam: Free University Press.

Bernstein, N.A. (1967). *The co-ordination and regulation of movements.* Oxford: Pergamon Press.

Bilodeau, E.A., & Bilodeau, I.McD. (1969, Eds.). *Principles of skill acquisition.* New York: Academic Press.

Bingham, G.P., Schmidt, R.C., Turvey, M.T., & Rosenblum, L.D. (1991). Task dynamics and resource dynamics in the assembly of a coordinated rhythmic activity. *Journal of Experimental Psychology: Human Perception and Performance, 17*, 359-381.

Bootsma, R.J. (1988). *The timing of rapid interceptive actions.* Amsterdam: Free University Press.

Brinker, B.P.L.M. den, & Hekken, M.F. van (1982). The analysis of slalom-ski movements using a ski-simulator apparatus. *Human Movement Science, 1*, 91-108.

Brinker, B.P.L.M. den, Stäbler, J.R.L.W., Whiting, H.T.A., & Wieringen, P.C.W. van (1986). The effect of manipulating knowledge of results on the learning of slalom-type ski movements. *Ergonomics, 29*, 31-40.

Bullock, D., & Grossberg, S. (1988). Neural dynamics of planned arm movements: Emergent invariants and speed-accuracy properties during trajectory formation. *Psychological Review, 95,* 49-90.

Connolly, K.J. (1986). A perspective on motor development. In M.G. Wade & H.T.A. Whiting (Eds.), *Motor development in children: Aspects of coordination and control* (pp. 3-21). Dordrecht: Martinus Nijhoff.

Doyle, A.J.R. (1987). *Bicycle riding skills.* Unpublished Ph.D. thesis, University of Sheffield, Department of Psychology.

Emmerik, R.E.A. van, Brinker, B.P.L.M. den, Vereijken, B., & Whiting, H.T.A. (1989). Preferred tempo in the learning of a gross cyclical action. *The Quarterly Journal of Experimental Psychology, 41*, 251-262.

Fitts, P.M. (1964). Perceptual-motor skills learning. In A.W. Melton (Ed.), *Categories of human learning* (pp. 243-285) New York: Academic Press.

Flash, T., & Hogan, N. (1985). The coordination of arm movements: An experimentally confirmed mathematical model. *Journal of Neuroscience, 5,* 1688-1703.

Franks, I.M., & Wilberg, R.B. (1982). The generation of movement patterns during the acquisition of a pursuit tracking task. *Human Movement Science, 1,* 251-272.

Gallistel, C.R. (1980). *The organization of action: A new synthesis.* Hillsdale, NJ: Lawrence Erlbaum Associates.

Gentner, D.R. (1987). Timing of skilled motor performance: Test of the proportional duration model. *Psychological Review, 94,* 255-276.

Gibson, J.J. (1979). *The ecological approach to visual perception.* Boston: Houghton Mifflin.

Glaser, R. (1990). The reemergence of learning theory within instructional research. *American Psychologist, 45,* 29-39.

Heuer, H., & Schmidt, R.A. (1988). Transfer of learning among motor patterns with different relative timing. *Journal of Experimental Psychology: Human Perception and Performance, 14,* 241-252.

Hofsten, C. von (1986). The emergence of manual skills. In M.G. Wade & H.T.A. Whiting (Eds.), *Motor development in children: Aspects of coordination and control* (pp. 167-185). Dordrecht: Martinus Nijhoff.

Hogan, N. (1984). An organizing principle for a class of voluntary movements. *Journal of Neuroscience, 4,* 2745-2754.

Ingen Schenau, G.J. van (1989). From rotation to translation: Constraints on multi-joint movements and the unique action of bi-articular muscles. *Human Movement Science, 8,* 301-337.

Jeka, J.J., & Kelso, J.A.S. (1989). The dynamic pattern appproach to coordinated behavior: A tutorial review. In S.A. Wallace (Ed.), *Perspectives on the coordination of movement* (pp. 3-45) Amsterdam: North-Holland.

Keele, S.W. (1968). Movement control in skilled motor performance. *Psychological Bulletin, 70,* 387-403.

Keele, S.W. (1973). *Attention and human performance.* Pacific Palisades, CA: Goodyear.

Keele, S.W. (1981). Behavioral analysis of motor control. In V.B. Brooks (Ed.), *Handbook of physiology, Section 1, Vol. 2: Motor control* (pp. 1391-1413). Bethesda, MD: American Physiological Society.

Keele, S.W. (1986). Motor control. In K.R. Boff, L. Kaufman, & J.P. Thomas (Eds.), *Handbook of perception and human performance, Vol. 2.* (pp. 1-60). New York: Wiley.

Keele, S.W., & Summers, J.J. (1976). The structure of motor programs. In G.E. Stelmach (Ed.), *Motor control: Issues and trends* (pp. 109-142). New York: Academic Press.

Kelso, J.A.S. (1981). Contrasting perspectives on order and regulation in movement. In J.B. Long & A.D. Baddeley (Eds.), *Attention and performance IX* (pp. 437-457). Hillsdale, NJ: Lawrence Erlbaum Associates.

Kelso, J.A.S. (1990). Phase transitions: Foundations of behavior. In H. Haken & M. Stadler (Eds.), *Synergetics of cognition* (pp. 249-268). Berlin: Springer.

Kelso, J.A.S., Saltzman, E., & Tuller, B. (1986). The dynamical perspective in speech production: Data and theory. *Journal of Phonetics, 14,* 29-60.

Kelso, J.A.S., & Tuller, B. (1984). A dynamical basis for action systems. In M. Gazzaniga (Ed.), *Handbook of cognitive neuroscience* (pp. 321-356). New York: Plenum.

Kelso, J.A.S., Tuller, B., Vatikiotis-Bateson, E., & Fowler, C. (1984). Functionally specific articulatory cooperation following jaw perturbations during speech: Evidence for coordinative structures. *Journal of Experimental Psychology: Human Perception and Performance, 10,* 812-832.

Kugler, P.N. (1986). A morphological perspective on the origin and evolution of movement patterns. In M.G. Wade & H.T.A. Whiting (Eds.), *Motor development in children: Aspects of coordination and control* (pp. 459-525). Dordrecht: Martinus Nijhoff.

Kugler, P.N., Kelso, J.A.S., & Turvey, M.T. (1980). On the concept of coordinative structures as dissipative structures: I. Theoretical lines of convergence. In G.E. Stelmach & J. Requin (Eds.), *Tutorials in motor behavior* (pp. 3-47). Amsterdam: North-Holland.

Marr, D. (1982). *Vision.* San Francisco: Freeman.

Marteniuk, R.G., & Romanow, S.K.E. (1983). Human movement organization and learning as revealed by variability of movement, use of kinematic information, and Fourier analysis. In R.A. Magill (Ed.), *Memory and control of action* (pp. 167-197). Amsterdam: North-Holland.

McClelland, J.R., & Rumelhart, D.E. (1986). *Parallel distributed processing. Explorations in the microstructure of cognition, Vol.* 2. Cambridge, MA: MIT Press.

Neisser, U. (1985). The role of invariant structures in the control of movement. In M. Frese & J. Sabini (Eds.), *Goal-directed behavior: The concept of action in psychology* (pp. 97-108). Hillsdale, NJ: Lawrence Erlbaum Associates.

Newell, A., & Simon, H.A. (1972). *Human problem solving.* Englewood Cliffs, NJ: Prentice Hall.

Newell, K.M. (1981). Skill learning. In D.H. Holding (Ed.), *Human skills* (pp. 203-226). Chichester: Wiley.

Newell, K.M. (1985). Coordination, control and skill. In D. Goodman, R.B. Wilberg, & I.M. Franks (Eds.), *Differing perspectives in motor learning, memory, and control* (pp. 295-317). Amsterdam: North-Holland.

Newell, K.M. (1986). Constraints on the development of coordination. In M.G. Wade & H.T.A. Whiting (Eds.), *Motor development in children: Aspects of coordination and control* (pp. 341-360). Dordrecht: Martinus Nijhoff.

Newell, K.M., Kugler, P.N., Emmerik, R.E.A. van, & McDonald, P.V. (1989). Search strategies and the acquisition of coordination. In S.A. Wallace (Ed.), *Perspectives on the coordination of movement* (pp. 85-122). Amsterdam: North-Holland.

Paillard, J. (1986). Development and acquisition of motor skills: A challenging prospect for neuroscience. In M.G. Wade & H.T.A. Whiting (Eds.), *Motor development in children: Aspects of coordination and control* (pp. 415-441). Dordrecht: Martinus Nijhoff.

Paillard, J. (1989). Living systems as organizing organizations. *Human Movement Science, 8,* 411-413.

Pew, R.W. (1974). Levels of analysis in motor control. *Brain Research, 71,* 393-400.

Pew, R.W. (1984). A distributed processing view of human motor control. In W. Prinz & A.F. Sanders (Eds.), *Cognition and motor processes* (pp. 19-27). Berlin: Springer.

Pew, R.W., & Rosenbaum, D.A. (1988). Human movement control: Computation, representation, and implementation. In R.C. Atkinson, R.J. Herrnstein, G. Lindzey, & R.D. Luce (Eds.), *Stevens' handbook of experimental psychology, 2nd edition. Volume 2: Learning and cognition* (pp. 473-509). New York: Wiley.

Prechtl, H.F.R. (1986). Prenatal motor development. In M.G. Wade & H.T.A. Whiting (Eds.), *Motor development in children: Aspects of coordination and control* (pp. 53-64). Dordrecht: Martinus Nijhoff.

Rabbitt, P. (1967). Learning to ignore irrelevant information. *American Journal of Psychology, 80,* 1-13.

Roberton, M.A. (1986). Developmental changes in the relative timing of locomotion. In H.T.A. Whiting & M.G. Wade (Eds.), *Themes in motor development* (pp. 279-293). Dordrecht: Martinus Nijhoff.

Rosenbaum, D.A. (1985). Motor programming: A review and scheduling theory. In H. Heuer, U. Kleinbeck, & K.-H. Schmidt (Eds.), *Motor behavior: Programming, control and acquisition* (pp. 1-33). Berlin: Springer.

Rossum, J.H.A. van (1987). *Motor development and practice: The variability of practice hypothesis in perspective.* Amsterdam: Free University Press.

Rumelhart, D.E., & McClelland, J.L. (1986). *Parallel distributed processing. Explorations in the microstructure of cognition, Vol. 1.* Cambridge, MA: MIT Press.

Salmoni, A.W. (1989). Motor skill learning. In D.H. Holding (Ed.), *Human skills, 2nd edition* (pp. 197-227). Chichester: Wiley.

Schmidt, R.A. (1975). A schema theory of discrete motor skill learning. *Psychological Review, 82,* 225-260.

Schmidt, R.A. (1976). The schema as a solution to some persistent problems in motor learning theory. In G.E. Stelmach (Ed.), *Motor control: Issues and trends* (pp. 41-65). New York: Academic Press.

Schmidt, R.A. (1986). *Toward a better understanding of the acquisition of skill: Theoretical and practical contributions of the task approach.* Paper presented at the symposium 'Future directions in exercise and sport research'. Exercise and Sport Science Institute, Arizona State University, January 9-12.

Schmidt, R.A. (1988). *Motor control and learning: A behavioral emphasis.* Champaign, IL: Human Kinetics.

Scully, D.M., & Newell, K.M. (1985). Observational learning and the acquisition of motor skills: Toward a visual perception perspective. *Journal of Human Movement Studies, 11,* 169-186.

Shapiro, D.C., & Schmidt, R.A. (1982). The schema theory: Recent evidence developmental implications. In J.A.S. Kelso & J.E. Clark (Eds.), *The development of movement control and coordination* (pp. 113-150). New York: Wiley.

Shaw, R.E., & Alley, J.R. (1985). How to draw learning curves: Their use and justification. In T.D. Johnston & A.T. Pietrewicz (Eds.), *Issues in the ecological study of learning* (pp. 275-304). Hillsdale, NJ: Lawrence Erlbaum Associates.

Stanley, M.L., & Franks, I.M. (1990). *Learning to organize the frequency components of a perceptual motor skill.* Paper submitted for publication.

Summers, J.J. (1989). Motor Programs. In D.H. Holding (Ed.), *Human skills, 2nd edition* (pp. 49-69). Chichester: Wiley.

Turvey, M.T. (1990). Coordination. *American Psychologist, 45,* 938-953.

Turvey, M.T., Carello, C., & Kim, N.G. (1990). Links between active perception and the control of action. In H. Haken & M. Stadler (Eds.), *Synergetics of cognition* (pp. 269-295). Berlin: Springer.

Vereijken, B., & Whiting, H.T.A. (1990). In defence of discovery learning. *Canadian Journal of Sports Sciences, 15,* 99-106.

Vereijken, B., Whiting, H.T.A., & Beek, W.J. (1990). *Phase lag as an order parameter in the learning of a complex skill.* Paper submitted for publication.

Viviani, P. (1986). Do units of motor action realls exist? In H. Heuer & C. Fromm (Eds.), *Generation and modulation of action patterns* (pp. 201-216). Berlin: Springer.

Vogt, S. (1988). Einige gestaltpsychologische Aspekte der zeitlichen Organisation zyklischer Bewegungsabläufe. *Bremer Beiträge zur Psychologie, 77.*

Vogt, S. (in press). Invariantenbildung im Reproduktionsversuch - Ein empirischer Ansatz zu Genese und Struktur bewegungsleitender Repräsentationen. *Proceedings of the International Symposium 'Motorik und Bewegungsforschung',* Saarbrücken, 1989.

Vogt, S., Stadler, M., & Kruse, P. (1988). Self-organization aspects in the temporal formation of movement gestalts. *Human Movement Science, 7,* 365-406.

Warren, W.H. (1987). An ecological conception of action. *Cahiers de Psychologie Cognitive, 7,* 199-203.

Whiting, H.T.A. (1984). The concepts of 'adaptation' and 'attunement' in skill learning. In O.G. Selfridge, E.L. Rissland, & M.A. Arbib (Eds.), *Adaptive control of ill-defined systems* (pp. 187-205). New York: Plenum.

Whiting, H.T.A. (1987). A 'cog' in the 'motor' or a spanner in the works? *Cahiers de Psychologie Cognitive, 7,* 204-210.

Whiting, H.T.A. (1988). Imitation and the learning of complex cyclical actions. In O.G. Meijer & K. Roth (Eds.), *Complex movement behavior: The motor-action controversy* (pp. 381-401). Amsterdam: North-Holland.

Whiting, H.T.A., Bijlard, M.J., & Brinker, B.P.L.M. den (1987). The effect of the availabiity of a dynamic model on the acquisition of a complex cyclical action. *The Quarterly Journal of Experimental Psychology, 39,* 43-59.

Whiting, H.T.A., & Brinker, B.P.L.M. den (1982). Image of the act. In J.P. Das, R.F. Mulcahy, & A.E. Wall (Eds.), *Theory and research in learning disabilities* (pp. 217-235). New York: Plenum.

Zanone, P.G., & Hauert, C.A. (1987). For a cognitive conception of motor processes: A provocative standpoint. *Cahiers de Psychologie Cognitive, 7,* 109-129.

Zelaznik, H.N., Schmidt, R.A., & Gielen, S.C.A.M. (1986). Kinematic properties of rapid aimed hand movements. *Journal of Motor Behavior, 18,* 353-372.

Approaches to the Study of Motor Control and Learning
J.J. Summers (Editor)

Chapter 4

HANDWRITING AS A MOTOR TASK: EXPERIMENTATION, MODELLING, AND SIMULATION

Arnold J.W.M. Thomassen and Gerard P. van Galen
University of Nijmegen

The paper reviews some of the experimental and theoretical research in the field of handwriting, where an increased activity has been displayed over the past two decades. First, attention is paid to the specific features of the current research methodology and of handwriting as a motor task, including its effector-anatomy and geometry aspects. The theoretical framework into which most of the research findings are accommodated is a multi-stage model with a mixed hierarchical and parallel architecture. A separate section is devoted to the constraints determining the selection of stroke sequences in graphic action when copying unfamiliar patterns. The paper is concluded with a discussion of computational approaches. These are concerned not only with the simulation of handwriting production, but also with the automatic recognition of cursive script, an extremely difficult task which requires support from insights in the motor aspects of handwriting generation.

The past decade has witnessed a growing activity in the quantitative research of handwriting and drawing. This increased interest is due to an improvement in our understanding of motor control, human performance and complex action and their neurological basis, as well as to major developments in electronic hardware and computer software for the recording and analysis of graphic behaviour. Moreover, the present computer age also gave impetus to investigators in various disciplines to approach motor organisation, including handwriting and drawing, in computational terms. On the applied side, furthermore, there is a growing need for instruction methods of handwriting based on insights into the process, and for a proper use of modern computer facilities in handwriting education. Understanding the representation, learning, and performance aspects of handwriting is a condition for applying adequate educational and technological tools to support the mastering of the skill. Finally, the automatic processing of handwriting and sketched graphics opens up many possibilities for on-line and off-line interaction with computers, as well as for the automatic classification of pieces of handwriting for specific tasks ranging from palaeographic to security and police work. These developments have led to a better understanding of the handwriting process and to the exchange of views between disciplines. This situation is clearly reflected by the contents of a series of multidisciplinary conferences on handwriting (Thomassen, Keuss, & Van Galen, 1984; Kao, Van Galen & Hoosain, 1986; Plamondon, Suen, & Simner, 1989; Wann, Wing, & Sovik, 1990; Plamondon & Leedham, 1990), a series which is expected to be continued. It goes without saying that experimental psychology, cognitive science, and computer science have contributions to make to this multidisciplinary field.

This chapter intends to review some of the experimental, modelling, and computational work conducted in the area; there will be a certain bias towards approaches followed at the authors' Department at NICI, where the study of the motor aspects of handwriting occupies an important place. Handwriting may be seen not only as a linguistic production task, but also as a special type of motor task in which the writer prepares and executes specific sequences of spatial patterns over time. The latter viewpoint will be adopted in this chapter; the semantic and syntactic components of the written message will be left in the background. This does not imply that we reject the idea that there are important interactions between these components and the motor aspects of handwriting. For one thing, we will see that a typical feature of handwriting is its relatively low rate as a linguistic output modality; this may impose constraints on the linguistic processes and on the format of their outcome. Such interactions, however, will hardly be discussed here. The review will concentrate on the motor aspects. After a brief historical introduction, it will discuss experimental techniques, data and modelling first, followed by a brief review of rule-governed aspects of graphic behaviour, and it will be concluded by a discussion of computational approaches.

HISTORICAL AND CULTURAL BASIS OF HANDWRITING

As long as thirty-thousand years ago, our ancestors started to make inscriptions on rocks and paintings on the walls of caves, presumably as an element of their social rites (Putman, 1989). Handwriting, as the skill to produce stylised signs in a formalised manner to convey language, certainly shares with prehistoric art the cognitive capability to represent meaning by graphic products. The differences, however, are also very large. Gelb (1952) pointed out that, in contrast to the pictorial and descriptive forerunners of script, writing is characterised by the use of conventional and stylised signs. Following the principle of economy, early as well as modern writings use simple, recurrent forms selected from a limited repertoire. A second, inherent feature of writing is its close relation to spoken language. Contrary to what is often thought, all major writings of the world, and among them Egyptian hieroglyphs as well as ancient and modern Chinese characters, refer to units of spoken language (Gelb, 1952). This role of phonological carrier played by handwriting should not be confused with the principle of phonetisation. Through this principle the phonological representation of a word is parsed as to its constituent phonetic elements and then replaced, element by element, by syllabic or alphabetic signs. This device is a characteristic feature of so-called alphabetic writing systems as contrasted with pictographic writings like Chinese. The invention of this phonological-graphemic device made it possible to represent the enormous richness of spoken words by a limited number of conventional signs.

The present Latin system of writing as used in the Western world is a direct descendant of the alphabetical script brought to Italy by the Greeks. These in turn (around 900 B.C.) had perfected what they learned from the Phoenicians, who are commonly considered to be the first to have introduced a purely sound-based script which contrasted with the Egyptian and Sumerian systems. The latter, and older, writings were mixtures of logographic (i.e., each sign stands for a word) and phonetic styles of writing (i.e., each sign stands for a sound). Because in many languages the spelling rules have not kept pace with the development of their pronunciation, it is ironic to see that history has endowed the modern writer with an alphabetic system which on many occasions is used in a nearby pictographic manner. Recent views on the relationship between the human brain, writing systems, and handwriting movements may be found in Sirat, Irigoin, and Poulle, (1990) and De Kerckhove and Lumsden (1988). The English word 'write' is related to the Old Norse 'rita', which means to incise, to carve. The same meaning is present in the Greek word 'graphein' from which modern words originate like 'graphics' and 'graph'. Apparently, writing has originally been associated with incising marks on objects. The production of such marks (or rather 'signs' because the other significant aspect of writing is that it conveys meaning) obviously involves a complex motor skill.

Following our small excursion into the cultural and historical aspects of writing, how should we characterise the skill of writing from a motor point of view? To regard handwriting as a motor skill places its research in the perspective of human performance. The experimental work to be described will indeed reflect the tradition in that area. Before discussing a few experimental and theoretical issues, we will briefly mention some features of the research techniques and analysis procedures.

RESEARCH TECHNIQUES AND ANALYSIS PROCEDURES

Motor aspects of handwriting may be studied in a variety of ways. For example, the writing trajectory can be related fruitfully to the arm's muscle activity (EMG; Vredenbregt & Koster, 1971), or to the angles of the joints in shoulder, elbow, wrist, and fingers (Van Emmerik & Newell, 1989). A relatively simple technique, however, currently adopted by most research groups as their principal method, concerns the recording of the pen-point movements across the paper. Apart from the simple fact that commercially available digitisers are highly suitable for this purpose, there is another argument for looking at the pen-point trajectory: At its most relevant, abstract level, the motor system does not appear to organise excursions in the horizontal plane in terms of muscles and joints, but rather in terms of spatial trajectories (e.g., Abend, Bizzi, & Morasso, 1982). Seen in this light, the movements of the pen point should reflect essential kinematic information.

The digitiser (e.g., Calcomp 9000) is a flat board which records the pen's position when it is in contact with the paper; moreover, its vertical projection onto the writing surface may be recorded as well, although the error increases with the distance from the paper. Sampling is done with great precision (0.2 mm) and at a high rate (100 Hz), so that the spatial and temporal features of the moving pen can be known accurately. This is, of course, also essential for the derivation of velocity, acceleration, and jerk estimates at any locus along the writing trace. A special facility is the acquisition of axial pen-pressure data at the same sampling frequency.

The writing signal entering the computer thus comprises 100 planar (X,Y) coordinate pairs and 100 pressure (Z) estimates per second. The laboratory-made electronic ball-point pen does not differ much from a normal pen, except that its pressure-sensing device (if present) may add slightly to the weight and the dimensions of the barrel. From the top of the latter emanates a thin, flexible wire, leading to the far end of the digitiser, which is connected to the computer (e.g., VAX-11/750, VAX workstation, or IBM PC). The instructions and the stimuli are generally presented on a tachistoscopic display (Vector General). This screen can also be used by the experimenter to check the adequacy of the subject's performance, or to display features of the recorded signal, so that certain parts of the trace or of its derivatives may be studied or selected by means of cursors for finer analysis. Finally, the display is often used to provide the subject with feedback of some kind or other. The most important data concern reaction time, movement duration, velocity, acceleration, jerk, size, curvature, and pressure. Software for these and many other analysis purposes (to some extent also suitable to be run on a PC) has been developed in the NICI Department. For technical details of signal processing, we refer to the literature (Maarse, 1987; Teulings, 1988; Teulings & Maarse, 1984; Teulings & Thomassen, 1979; Thomassen, Teulings, Schomaker, & Morasso,

1988). The analysis of the dynamic or static writing trace often requires its segmentation into manageable and meaningful units. Obviously, larger units may be whole pages or lines of cursive script, which allow the derivation of highly informative global features (e.g., Maarse, Schomaker, & Teulings, 1988). Smaller units, which have been shown to be relevant from a motor viewpoint (see below), are single letters and single strokes. From a kinematic point of view, strokes are considered to be the smallest relevant units of the writing movement. Normally, they are performed 'ballistically', so that they are characterised by a single-peaked velocity profile (Maarse, 1987); they have a typical duration of 100 ms. Moreover, strokes are usually delimited by loci of low velocity and high curvature in the writing trace, which most often occur at the top or at the bottom of low-curvature near-vertical segments. In the analysis a distinction is made between up strokes and down strokes. It appears that up strokes, which include connecting strokes between letters, are considerably more variable than down strokes (Maarse & Thomassen, 1983).

SOME RELEVANT FEATURES OF HANDWRITING AS A MOTOR TASK

From a motor point of view, fluent, cursive handwriting is an interesting task because it is composed of a set of different motor components. Firstly, the use of a pen is typically a distal task for the most delicate muscles of the hand and fingers. In an individual's life the capability to hold a pen with the required precision, and the skill to produce characters accurately develops much later than locomotion, reaching, and grasping (Connolly & Elliott, 1972), and indeed much later than speech. A second interesting aspect of writing is that it requires the joint operation of form production and spatial adjustment processes. Letter forms are steered internally: The generation of a specific letter in its appropriate case is the outcome of a cognitive process in which the writer uses his or her stored motor knowledge. But at the same time, subsequent letters have to be ordered along lines with a specific spacing and lineation. The latter feature of the task is a typical spatial demand that asks for a high degree of eye-hand coordination. Writers also learn to keep letter forms, and their slant and size, constant across lines and pages. Such constancy is possible only if the motor system can compensate for the large biomechanical differences which arise when the hand flexes and extends within words, moves from left to right along the line, and from the top to the bottom of the page. One can easily observe that the muscular contractions involved in the production of a specific letter are highly dependent upon the position of the hand. The high degree of constancy of letter shapes within a person's script, even if written with different limbs, has served as evidence for the existence of abstract motor programs (Merton, 1972). The essence of this idea is that motor knowledge is not stored in the brain in the form of concrete instructions to specific muscles but in that of a more general, probably spatial code, which is used to generate specific muscle commands only in a final output stage where the current biophysical context is taken into account. To this ability of the motor system to attain constant goals in a varying context and with varying means, which is commonly named 'motor constancy' or 'motor equivalence' (Bernstein, 1967), we will refer repeatedly in this chapter.

A further feature that makes handwriting interesting for a theory of motor behaviour is the combination of a typically serial production mode with an apparently parallel programming architecture. The serial mode is directly clear from the observation of writing. Sentences are produced word by word, words originate letter by letter, and letters grow stroke by stroke. The production rate is highly dependent on writing style, age of the writer, and content of the message. It has been shown that adult writing speed is achieved only at the age of 15 (Sassoon, Nimmo-Smith, & Wing, 1986). Individual strokes, which as we saw are often considered to be the basic elements at the motor output level, are seldom faster than 80 to 100 ms (Teulings & Thomassen, 1979). The production of script at a rate of two or three letters per second, is thus considerably lower than speech and typing. For a motor theory of writing it is important to note that its slower production makes it much more likely in handwriting than in speech that motor programs relating to subsequent parts of a message are retrieved and unpacked concurrently with the real-time production of earlier parts of the utterance. Hulstijn and Van Galen (1988) tested whether the hierarchical model of speech production formulated by Sternberg, Monsell, Knoll, and Wright (1978) also applies to handwriting tasks. In short, the Sternberg model assumes that the overall motor structure of an utterance, as defined by the number of stress groups, is prepared in advance of the initiation of the first phoneme to be spoken. This relative abstract representation of the motor program is temporarily buffered in a short-term motor buffer which functions as a working memory from where, on-line with task performance, separate stress groups are retrieved for real-time execution. Because the retrieval of syllables from a longer string in the motor buffer should take more time, it is furthermore predicted by Sternberg's model that performance time per syllable also increases with the length of the utterance.

Hulstijn and Van Galen (1988) compared data of several studies on the effect of sequence length on reaction time and movement time in handwriting and drawing tasks. The general conclusion from their study was that handwriting does not obey the Sternberg subprogram-retrieval model. Reaction time did not increase consistently with the number of elements, and for those experiments where an increase was found, the slope of the RT-function appeared to be highly dependent on the level of training. Moreover, writing time per letter (or per 'grapheme', because many different writing and drawing patterns were used in their experiments) did not increase with sequence length. The authors noted a hierarchical feature in the preparation of handwriting tasks in the sense that more abstract aspects of the task appeared to be manifest during the reaction-time period, whereas more concrete motor aspects had an influence on the duration of preceding strokes or on the intervals between the production of successive graphemes. These data disagreed with Sternberg et al. (1978) as regards the strictly serial character of subprogram-retrieval processes. Thus, the authors proposed that, due to the relative low production rate of handwriting, the cognitive and motor preparation of forthcoming task elements is continued during real-time execution. As a result, cognitive and motor features of a handwriting task are considered important determinants of the writing times of subsequent segments of the task.

As mentioned, time functions describing the formation of stroke trajectories can easily be derived (Teulings & Maarse, 1984; Teulings & Thomassen, 1979), and detailed mathematical descriptions of trajectory formation in handwriting are presently available (e.g., Maarse, Van Galen, & Thomassen, 1989). At the same time, however, such detailed observations of duration, length, and fluency, and of other parameters of letter trajectories, have also revealed the parallel nature of writing, in which forthcoming elements of the writing task are prepared concurrently with the real-time execution of earlier writing segments. For example, in a study by Van der Plaats and Van Galen (1990) it has been shown that when subjects arrive at the start of a word with a difficult letter (in this experiment this was the letter *m* , which is difficult due to the repetition of similar strokes) they need more time for the spacing between the preceding word and the word starting with *m*. In the same study, the effect of word length on the initiation of writing was investigated. Also this variable appeared to prolong the duration of the spacing movement preceding the longer words. It thus appeared that task demands of different kinds affected the same response segment, and that both demands (difficult letter, longer word) exerted their influence in advance of the real-time execution. The authors explained the prolongations of writing time as reflecting the increased processing load involved in the preparation of more demanding, forthcoming writing segments. They favoured a multi-stage, parallel-architecture handwriting model, as proposed by Van Galen, Smyth, Meulenbroek, and Hylkema, (1989). A more detailed account of this model will be given below.

Clearly, handwriting is a complex and compound motor task with roots in linguistics as well as in biomechanics. To give a comprehensive account of all the research that has contributed to our current understanding of the skill goes beyond the scope of this chapter. Main themes, however, can be pointed out. In the following paragraphs we will sketch some of the major issues which seem to form corner stones for a comprehensive theory. These issues are concerned with the role of the anatomy of the writing hand and the geometrical dimensions of script, with the discovery of cognitive and motor processes contributing to writing performance, and with the functional architecture of these processes. This part of the chapter will be concluded by a summary of the handwriting model as recently formulated by one of the authors (Van Galen, 1991). Following the description of the model we will touch upon a recent line of theorising in the field of handwriting (i.e., the role of grammars of action). Like many complex skills handwriting is not only the outcome of a specific organisation of processing stages. Action strategies play an important role as well. The final part of the chapter is devoted to a new and exciting means to study human behaviour: In that section we will discuss the simulation of handwriting production by computer algorithms. It will become clear that all of the elements of a cognitive and motor theory are necessary to mimic cursive script.

Effector Anatomy and the Geometry of Handwriting

Very early in this century McAllister (1900) observed that the duration of back-and-forth movements made with a pencil is related to the direction of movement. Strokes performed with the right hand in a right-upward direction (i.e., wrist-joint movements) were written most rapidly and took 30% less time than the relatively slow movements in a perpendicular direction (i.e., movements of the thumb-and-finger system). Strokes in the in-between directions had intermediate movement durations. The finding of such an orthogonally structured vector space for writing movements, together with the obviously different roles of wrist and finger movements in the production of script, has inspired several authors to consider the generation of letters as originating from two independent movement systems. One of these would (in righthanders) be locked to the right-upward diagonal and would represent the wrist system. The other would represent the right-downward diagonal and correspond to the thumb-and-finger system. Vredenbregt and Koster (1971) designed a handwriting simulator illustrating the potential role of two such independent muscle systems in the formation of letter shapes. In their simulation of the letter generation process they used a carriage enabling movements of a pen in up-down and left-right directions across a sheet of paper (Figure 1). Two pairs of electric motors were used to produce movements in these two directions. Pen strokes of different lengths were produced by applying a constant voltage for varying amounts of time. To obtain diagonal pen strokes, two motors, one from each pair, were driven simultaneously. Mechanical inertia and viscosity in the system were simulated through the fact that the motors functioned as generators of electrical energy as long as they were passively moved by their inertia or by their active counterpart. This led to a smoothing of abrupt transitions of direction. Thus, the dynamics of the system were instrumental in shaping the control provided by the sequence of

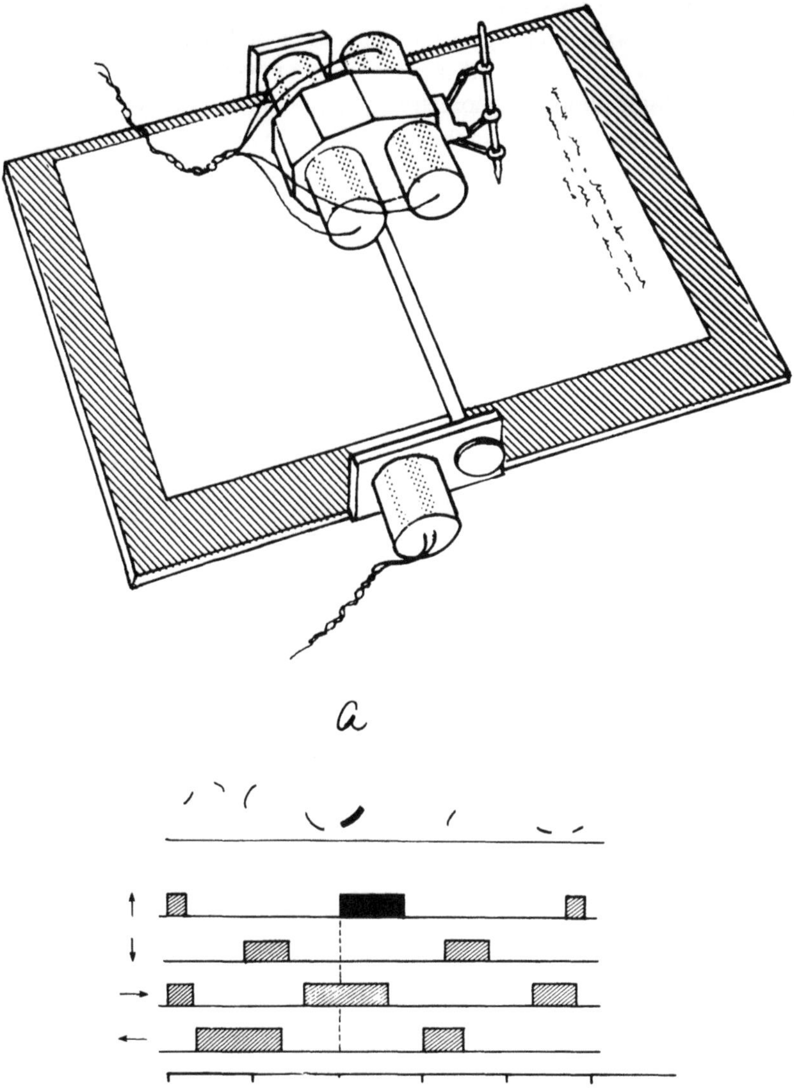

Figure 1. Mechanical apparatus (upper part) and vertical and horizontal pulse durations to simulate the production of the lowercase cursive-script letter *a* (lower part), as used by Vredenbregt and Koster (1971). (Adapted from Van Galen & Wing, 1984).

voltage pulses, just as in human-limb dynamics the physical properties of muscles and joints make a significant contribution to the movement trajectories. The notion of main axes underlying the generation of letter forms and other aspects of script has appealed to other researchers as well. Hollerbach (1981) applied the same logic about the geometry of finger and hand movements in his oscillator model of handwriting. In this model a periodical, 'oscillating' nature of handwriting movements is assumed. Letter forms are thought to be the result of paired oscillating movements in two perpendicular directions superimposed on a constant left-to-right shift. Hollerbach showed that varying amplitude and phasing of these oscillators yields the letter forms of cursive script.

An account of handwriting in terms of main axes was attempted by Teulings, Thomassen, and Maarse (1989). They identified two orthogonal main axes, one corresponding to wrist-joint movements, and one to finger movements. It was noted, however, that neither of these axes corresponds to the 'main' directions of writing inherent in the horizontal baseline and in the near-vertical slant of script. The authors concluded that the notion of main axes in handwriting may be useful for trajectory-description purposes, but is inappropriate to picture essential features of the representation of handwriting.

At the level of the hand and finger joints, Maarse, Schomaker, and Thomassen (1986) demonstrated that the biomechanical changes involved in the abduction of the hand during the writing of a word were not accompanied by corresponding changes in writing slant. Instead, as production progressed from left to right, the fingers tended to take over very flexibly more and more of the performance, keeping writing slant relatively constant. The authors interpreted these findings as evidence of a centrally organised system responsible for writing slant, rather than the simple, biomechanically based system which they had proposed earlier (Maarse & Thomassen, 1983). The combined data from these experiments point out that a one-to-one relationship between anatomical or biophysical structures and the geometry of handwriting does not exist, and that shape and slant constancy in performance must be accounted for by a more intricate, abstract control mechanism. In this context it is of interest that more recently, evidence was found that two independent spatial reference systems may be used in the production of even very simple writing patterns (Meulenbroek & Thomassen, 1991). The writers in this study made small back-and-forth movements in prescribed and in spontaneously adopted directions under different forearm positions, with and without vision. The dependent variables involved performance accuracy of instructed directions, frequencies of (spontaneously adopted) preferred directions, as well as video analyses of finger and hand movements. One of the supposed systems appeared to be determined by the anatomical structure of the arm-hand-fingers effector; the orientation of this system is dependent on that of the writing arm; the system is involved most in oblique movement directions. The second reference system is of a more abstract kind; it corresponds to geometrically orthogonal coordinates and it is mainly responsible for horizontal and vertical movements. It is probably associated with perception as much as with movement control, and it is relatively unaffected by changes in arm posture.

The earliest models of handwriting involving two independent movement directions in handwriting have as a specific feature that these components operate entirely in a time-based fashion. Letter shapes depend on the accurate timing of onset and offset of each of the components. Such a strict temporal control of the generation of letter forms has, however, been seriously questioned (e.g., Teulings, Thomassen, & Van Galen, 1986; Thomassen & Teulings, 1983, 1985). The latter experiment will be discussed in the next section; its outcome is that characters are probably not represented at the central level in terms of timing relationships but in a spatial code. Earlier it had been demonstrated by Thomassen and Teulings (1985) that size changes in letters may indeed be achieved by different means (force or duration increase, or both), depending on the type of context. These findings also replicated the results of Wing (1980). Taking together the recent evidence of anatomical, biomechanical factors on the one hand and of timing factors on the other, it appears that letter shapes and their features such as slant do not result in a one-to-one fashion from a concrete, pre-existing structure, nor from detailed motor codes or commands stored in the brain. Rather, also in these respects, handwriting is characterised by motor equivalence. Its movements appear to be prepared much more ad hoc, transforming abstract codes into concrete movement instructions, than could possibly be accounted for by such permanent representation. The features of each real-time adaptation to a spatio-temporal context may probably be regarded as emergent properties of the well-trained system operating under the spatial constraints which are a typically imposed by the requirement of legibility of cursive script.

A GENERAL FRAMEWORK AND SOME EXPERIMENTAL RESULTS

In recent years, a multi-stage model of handwriting has been proposed and modified by Van Galen (1980; Van Galen & Teulings, 1983; Teulings, Thomassen, & Van Galen, 1983). Irrespective of its precise form in each study, the model always involves long-term storage, memory retrieval, movement preparation, and motor execution. We will now pay some attention to each of these stages and report some experimental results pertaining to each of them. On a priori grounds it may be assumed that motor information concerning the units of handwriting, whatever their extent or format, is stored permanently in motor programs. Since we use different allographs, or writing patterns, for a single grapheme (e.g., *e* and *E* for /e/), the stored representations are allographic rather than graphemic (see also Wing, Lewis, & Baddeley, 1979). It may be argued that only the general 'topological' structure of writing movements is stored, perhaps together with the global sequence and directions of their strokes (Van Galen & Teulings, 1983). Parameters like size, slant, roundedness, and speed are most likely adjusted only at a later processing stage. The theoretically relevant question regarding the format of long-term storage has been investigated by Teulings (1988; Teulings, Thomassen, & Van Galen, 1986). Is its representation coded primarily in terms of spatial, temporal, or force attributes? Teulings found that the spatial features of handwritten patterns show systematically less variability over replications and conditions than its duration and force characteristics do. Moreover, it was shown that invariant spatial distances in handwriting are achieved by a flexible trade-off between force level and duration. The conclusion was that spatial attributes are dominant in the central representation.

Another relevant question is concerned with the nature of the units retrieved from long-term storage. Do these processing units have the extent of allographs, or are they of a smaller or bigger size? Again, Teulings (1988; Teulings, Thomassen, & Van Galen, 1983) performed some revealing experiments, using two-letter tasks in an RT paradigm. He based the research on the fact that repeated access to the same memory representation is achieved more rapidly than successively accessing two different representations (Klapp & Wyatt, 1976). Now, if the units of processing have the extent of strokes, repeated access to the same stroke representation (in non-identical similar allographs, having identical strokes) should result in a reduction of RT. However, if not strokes, but whole allographs constitute the units of processing, repeated access to an identical allograph representation should yield shorter RTs, whereas access to two different allograph representations should not lead to such a reduction. Moreover, it should make no difference whether these allographs are similar (having common strokes) or dissimilar. Exactly the latter results were obtained in the RT experiments by Teulings. Thus, in the two-letter tasks studied, allograph representations appeared to be the units of processing in memory retrieval.

In order to prepare the actual writing movements, the retrieved allograph representations are assumed to be buffered temporarily. Repeated allographs are known to be represented in this buffer more than once, which is a source of interference during their readout (cf. Sternberg, Monsell, Knoll, & Wright, 1978) and to lead to a slower execution once the movement has started. In the experiments by Teulings, it was shown that movement duration (MT) indeed increased for identical allograph pairs but not for different pairs, irrespective of their similarity (i.e., their having identical strokes). Thus, in the buffer stage also, allograph representations appeared to be the processing units.

The abstract representation concerning the global shape and stroking sequence of the allographs needs to be transformed into a set of well-timed muscle contractions adapted to the current postural and environmental circumstances. In principle, cursive script is produced by arm, hand, and finger effectors, each with their own task during the performance, but also with a high degree of flexibility (see e.g., Maarse, Schomaker, & Thomassen, 1986). As we saw above, the existence of two principal axes in handwriting execution has been established (Teulings, Thomassen, & Maarse, 1989), but as we have also seen, there is no evidence that these axes (which do not coincide with visible features in the writing trace) play a role in the central representation of writing movements. Summing up, the experimental evidence supports the notion that, at least in the two-letter tasks used, spatially coded allographs (specific letter forms) are most likely the units that are both stored permanently and processed during handwriting preparation and initiation. The actual execution of these allographs, which is done stroke-by-stroke in a ballistic mode, is left to a multi-joint effector system which flexibly exploits its many degrees of freedom.

Thus far, we have relied on RT experiments involving the execution of single, brief messages. Real-life writing, however, implies the parallel processing of semantic, syntactic, lexical, orthographic, and graphemic information concerning parts of the message closer or farther ahead of the allograph that is presently being retrieved, buffered, and initiated. Recent work by Van Galen and his coworkers has shown that the transformations at several of these levels can be traced by reduced pen velocities at specific moments in time. As we will see, this approach constitutes a promising example of integrating the stage-analysis approach with the study of parallel processing in complex, continuous task performance.

The Handwriting Task Seen as a Succession of Stages

Our discussion of the motor aspects of handwriting has shown that handwriting is a compound and complex task involving many cognitive and motor processes. Through the availability of electronic equipment to study in detail response-initiation times, pen-stroke trajectories, and interstroke latencies, experimental psychologists were challenged to disentangle the complex script-production process as to its components. Above, we referred to the observation by Merton (1972) which was suggestive of a distinction between an abstract stage of motor programming and a concrete movement-initiation stage which translates the spatial letter codes into muscular commands appropriate in the biophysical context. Required letter size is such a context. An early attempt to provide experimental evidence for a differentiation between motor control of letter form and letter size control processes has been made by Wing (1980). In his experiment subjects wrote words like *elegy* at different sizes. Wing found evidence for a dissociation between the production of height variations within and between words. Within-word height variations, as between *e* and *l*, seemed to be realised predominantly by an adjustment of the duration of the agonist force burst. Between-word height variation, as in the word *elegy* written small or large, could be attributed to a variation of the time interval between agonist and antagonist onset. Wing suggested that overall writing size, and stroke size used to discriminate letter forms, were controlled by two different mechanisms. As indicated above, Thomassen and Teulings (1985), who studied factors in letter production as a function of form and size, thereby distinguishing between macro, meso, and micro context, came to a similar conclusion.

Van Galen and Teulings (1983) applied the additive factor logic of Sternberg (1969) to strengthen their view that the generation of letter forms (named 'motor programming' in their model), the control of letter size (named 'parameterisation'), and the final adaptation to the current biophysical context (named 'muscular initiation') represent three independent motor-processing stages in handwriting. The logic of the method is based on the assumption that reaction times are summed processing times which originate from a limited number of successive processing stages through which a task stimulus is processed on its way from sensory input to the elicitation by the motor system of the corresponding response. According to the theory it is further assumed that if two experimental variables each contribute in a statistically independent manner to the variance in reaction-time measurements, one is justified to relate each variable to a different processing stage. In their experiment, Van Galen and Teulings varied novelty of a writing pattern, its overall size, and the musculature to draw the first stroke of the pattern. According to their three-stage theory of motor programming, each of these three experimental variables corresponds to a different process. Novelty should relate to access to long-term motor memory which stores abstract representations of motor patterns. Size should be modulated by a parameterisation stage, which applies an overall-force parameter to the muscular system in order to produce the pattern at its required size. The activation of the most appropriate motor units to initiate a task is assigned to a third, muscle-initiation process, assumed to be dependent on the anatomical constraints in a given task situation. The experiment, designed according to the additive factor methodology of Sternberg (1969), generally proved the independence of variables related to form, scale, and anatomy involved in the task. Meulenbroek and Van Galen (1988) replicated these findings with line-drawing tasks.

Further support for the independent status of size and muscular control was provided by Pick and Teulings (1983). These authors studied whether subjects are able to modify geometrical aspects of their handwriting. It appeared that writers can easily alter the orientation of the writing line, and they can also vary the slant of their script without disruption of other parameters. It appears to be extremely difficult, however, to modify independently within letters the size of the horizontal and the vertical component of letter forms. In correspondence with the conclusion reached by Van Galen and Teulings (1983), the authors suggested that size and geometrical orientation of script are controlled by different processes. Size seems to involve a parameter applied to the motor instructions for a letter as a whole, whereas slant and orientation are varied through the relative contribution of wrist and finger musculature in movement execution.

The experiments reported thus far have led to the proposition of a modular model of handwriting by Van Galen (1991). A distinctive feature of this model, as compared to models on trajectory formation, is that handwriting is seen as the end product of several cooperating processing stages, each of which is involved in the preparation and monitoring of a different aspect of the task. The modules are engaged in a hierarchical organisation in such a manner that 'higher' stages are involved in the processing of more abstract features of the task (e.g., linguistic content of the message, spelling of words) whereas 'lower' processors are more directly concerned with the production of motor output (letter-form retrieval, size control, muscular adjustment, in that order).

Corroborative evidence for a modular view of handwriting comes from neuropsychological studies. Ellis (1982, 1988) has presented data, from writing errors in normal subjects as well as from so-called double-dissociation manifestations in neurological patients, which support the view that separate cognitive and motor processes are involved in the skill of handwriting. The discrimination between the monitoring of form and scale factors was supported further by observations made by Margolin and Wing (1983) who observed differential effects of brain stroke and Parkinson's disease upon handwriting. Stroke patients were characterised by disturbances of the letter formation process, whereas Parkinsonian patients lost control of the overall size of letters.

The model of Van Galen (1991) is depicted in Figure 2. Before explaining it in more detail, however, we have to dwell for a while on another important finding providing evidence not for sequential, but for parallel processing in handwriting.

Towards a Hierarchical and Parallel Functional Architecture

We mentioned several studies from which it appears that writing times in natural handwriting tasks reflect processing demands of different kinds, often related to forthcoming task segments. We will refer to a few other studies which were performed along the same lines. Brown et al. (1988, 1989), in a study on the written production of discourse, demonstrated a trade-off relation between language production and motor control as measured by writing speed and legibility. The authors suggested that formulation, motor-execution and output-monitoring processes, although separate processes, run in parallel and draw on a common source of processing capacity. Van Galen et al. (1986) analysed the effects of word length, letter position, and letter length on reaction times and writing times. It appeared that the initiation of words took 12 ms longer for one syllable length increase, but once writing had started, longer words led to a speeding up of the writing process. This increased speed was attributed to a strategic adaptation to longer response sequences which is a more general motor strategy effect in handwriting (Van der Plaats & Van Galen, 1990), similar to that in speech (Nooteboom, 1972). However, when writing times for identical letters were studied at varying letter positions, it appeared that a letter-position effect was found independently from the overall speeding-up effect. The same letter was written more slowly when it occurred at an earlier position in the task word. It was concluded that, following the installation of a phonological code and a speed-setting process at word level, a letter-by-letter grapheme-selection process is responsible for lexical and motor processing at letter level. The increase of writing speed towards the end of a word was attributed to the shrinking content of the phonological store entailing a decreasing retrieval load for letters at later positions.

Van Galen et al. (1989) replicated the effect of letter position on writing time. In this study also independent effects of repetition at the letter level and at the stroke level were found. Repeated letters led to a decrease in writing time of the letter preceding the repetition, which was analogous to the finding of a reduced initiation time for words with a repeating syllable structure (Van Galen, 1990). But the writing time of the double letter pair itself was increased as compared to non-repeating letter pairs. The latter finding of a facilitatory effect of repetition before the initiation of writing on the one hand, and an inhibitory effect during writing performance on the other, has been demonstrated with the repetition of phonologically identical syllables as well.

The combined effects of the phonological structure of a word and the motor complexity of separate letters were studied by Van Galen (1990). The movement-time data in this study showed a global slowing down of the writing movements at word level as a function of the phonological similarity of consecutive syllables of task words. This effect was independent of a local effect at letter level of a repetitive stroking structure (as in the letter *m*). Again, these findings support modular and hierarchical processing during real-time word production. Preceding the initiation of writing movements a phonological code is presumably placed into short-term memory. The construction of such a code is less demanding for a phonologically repetitive structure as is evidenced by the shorter latencies for words with a repeating syllable structure. During the writing of a word, however, the retrieval of phonologically similar elements represents the more difficult condition. This effect is additive with respect to a stroke-repetition effect at letter level. The latter increase of writing time for similar segments in *m* as compared to *n* was attributed to the non-shrinking feature of the motor buffer.

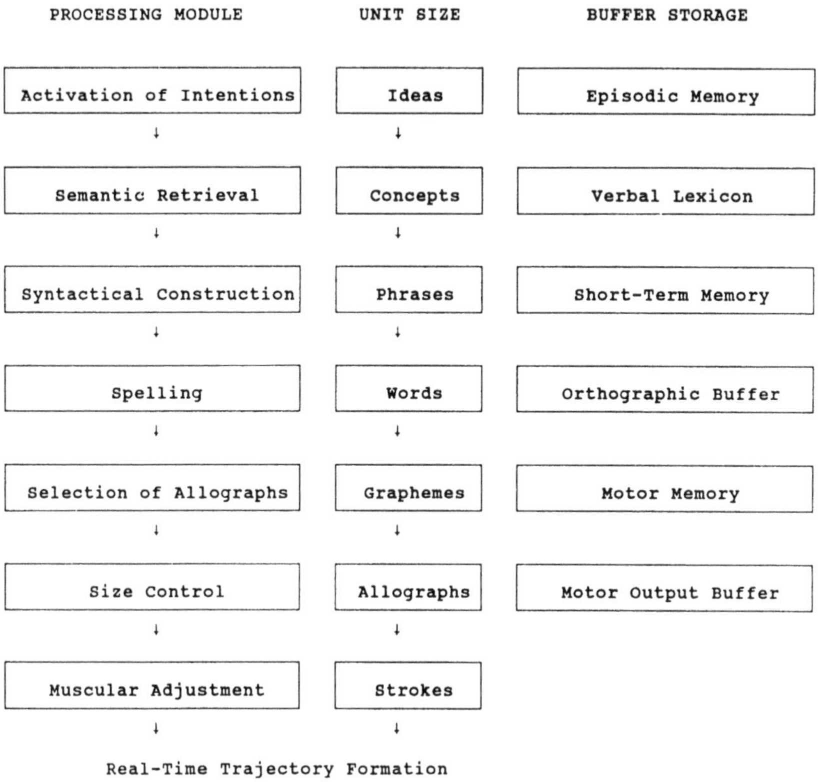

Figure 2. Architecture of processing stages (left-hand column), processing units (central column), and mediating memory stores (right-hand column) for the production of handwriting, as proposed by Van Galen (1991).

OUTLINE OF A MODEL OF HANDWRITING

The analysis of real-time writing processes has produced several elements for the specification of a model of handwriting (see Figure 2). Most importantly, handwriting has been shown to be a typical parallel task. There is ample evidence that demands of different kinds have summed effects on the duration of handwriting trajectories. At the same time, however, a specific hierarchy of the manifestation of task demands has been demonstrated. Effects related to larger task units (e.g., words) affect the production speed of earlier task segments more remote relative to the real-time realisation of the demanding units. At an intermediate level (letters), repetition and letter length influence writing trajectories one or two letter positions ahead of the demanding structure. At the lowest level studied (strokes), it appears that repetitions and difficult stroke alternations leads to an increase in writing time of the difficult strokes themselves (Van Galen et al., 1989). In the latter task elements, movement organisation and real-time production presumably coincide.

A graphic representation of the model of handwriting as sketched in Van Galen (1991) is presented in Figure 2. In the lefthand column of the figure, separate processing modules are mentioned for which an independent status seems to be justified. The vertical organisation of the modules corresponds to their assumed hierarchical ordering relating to the real-time performance of a written message. Arrows between neighbouring stages indicate that the output from a higher stage constitutes the input for the next-lower stage. In the righthand column of Figure 2, the mediating role of storage buffers is indicated. In the model it is assumed that the output from each stage is transiently stored in working memories which are typical for the corresponding stage. The role of these temporal storage nodes is twofold. Firstly, they accommodate for time frictions between information processing activities in different modules. Secondly, it is assumed that a processor lower in the hierarchy can read information from the buffer with a unit size which is appropriate for that stage. In the central column of the figure, we have identified the hypothetical nature of the unit size which each stage uses when importing information from the next-higher stage. It should be noted that the number of different processing modules may not be considered as a unique solution for the current empirical data. The top three, most abstract, processors we borrowed from the psycholinguistic literature (Levelt, 1989).

Handwriting enters the focus of our model at the spelling module. Spelling is the process through which elements of an utterance are substituted by their corresponding graphemic codes. In the handwriting literature it is commonly held that we have two different routes for the activation of a graphemic representation of a word. One process makes use of phoneme-to-grapheme conversion rules. Through the other, lexical route, writers have direct access to stored knowledge about the spelling of written words. The reliance on one or the other of these alternative routes is thought to be dependent on the type of units to be spelled (words or non-words) and on the regularity of the spelling of specific words in a specific language. Evidence for strong versions of the dual-route theory, implying complete independence, comes from clinical studies of neurological patients with spelling difficulties (Ellis, 1982; Margolin, 1984), and from studies on reading. In the latter research area, the independence of both routes has been questioned (Humphreys & Evett, 1985). We have, therefore, and for reasons of simplicity, opted for a single, undifferentiated spelling module.

In the model, motor processes play a role below the spelling module. From this level onwards, the model discriminates between selection of specific letter forms, or allographs, size control, and muscular adjustment. The selection of allographs should be seen as the activation of motor programs or engrams corresponding to the graphemic representation in the orthographic buffer and to the instructed writing mode (e.g., lower case, upper case, manuscript style, cursive-script style). In essence, the selection of an allographic motor pattern is a two-step process. The current writing mode (e.g., cursive script) activates the long-term motor repertoire that should be applied in the second, grapheme-to-allograph conversion step. Evidence for a distinct status of repertoires for upper-case and lower-case forms of letters has recently been produced in a clinical study by Patterson and Wing (1989). In the model it is assumed that letter forms (i.e., allographs) are stored and retrieved as spatial codes for the guidance of writing movements. Although actually further variations of letter forms ('graphs') exist, they probably arise as a result of biophysical influences on the generation of the real-time writing trajectory. Since such variations, together with the trajectories of letter-connection strokes, may be seen as emergent features of the writing process (Van der Plaats & Van Galen, 1990) it is not necessary to have such graphic motor patterns stored in long term memory. Writing size and speed are proposed to be monitored at a separate stage. Size control, in the model, is linked to the letter level and not to separate letter strokes. The final stage as described by the model is thought to represent the recruitment of synergies of agonist and antagonist muscle forces necessary for the realisation of a writing trajectory in a given biophysical context.

Finally, an essential feature of the handwriting model depicted in Figure 2 is the hierarchical organisation of the modules. From the experiments on task demands during writing performance it was concluded that higher processors operate at a longer distance (in time) from real-time execution. Although this type of hierarchy might be considered as indicative of the serial architecture of the model, it must be stressed that, from a functional point of view, the model has a parallel character. This is possible because processors higher in the hierarchy, continue to process information related to forthcoming parts of the message simultaneously with the spelling out of the details of the current output segments by the lower-order processors.

A GRAMMAR OF GRAPHIC ACTION

In the next few paragraphs, we will pay attention to some highly relevant principles of sequencing in graphic behaviour. We will be concerned with 'rules' governing the selection of stroke order and stroke direction in graphic behaviour. In formally taught cursive script these rules may be hidden under shape or precision requirements, or may be overlearned as features of alphabetical characters, so that the autonomous way in which they generally operate does not always appear at the surface. For research purposes, therefore, one most often reverts to the copying of geometrical patterns. Thus far, the origin and nature of the rules are by no means clear, but we are gradually getting more grip on them by defining the conditions under which they operate, the degree to which they interact and depend on biomechanical factors, and to what extent they are reflected by other behavioural variables such as reaction time and kinematic characteristics of the performed trajectories.

The graphic skills of writing, copying, and drawing involve the efficient sequential production of the segments of the intended spatial patterns. In general terms, such patterns, either imagined or perceived as instantaneous spatial structures, have to be 'linearised' (i.e., produced in a temporal sequence). Each segment in the sequence must not only receive a place in the temporal ordering, but must also be drawn in one of mostly two possible directions. In other words, the stroke order, the starting points, and stroke directions must be specified. The selection of a suitable (economical, accurate) sequence appears to be subject to a number of cultural, cognitive, physical, and mechanical constraints, including biases based on (actual or generalised) preferences related to effector properties, on opportunities for visual inspection and guidance, on prior learning and acquired skill in graphic tasks.

The first paper, by Goodnow and Levine (1973), who used Bruner's phrase 'grammar of action' to emphasise the rule-bound nature of the behavioural tendencies, demonstrated developmental trends in obeying rules such as 'start at the top of the pattern', and 'draw segments from left to right'. Further developmental, educational, and cultural control and performance aspects have been investigated by various authors. It has also been shown that the organisation principles at different levels may interact (Thomassen & Tibosch, 1991). Van Sommers (1984) presented an interesting set of new data and a global cognitive-psychological framework for its interpretation. For a given set of patterns, the strength of each of the rules may be estimated (Thomassen, Tibosch, & Meulenbroek, 1989). In general it appears that keeping the pen on paper while connecting one segment to the next ('threading') is a very dominant rule. Drawing rightwards (by righthanders) is a slightly stronger tendency than the rule of drawing downwards. Accuracy requirements are often met by starting at a later segment from a point on an earlier one ('anchoring'). The operation of the graphic production rules is reflected by the latencies and the kinematics of the movements. If a rule is appropriate, its application facilitates both the preparation and the execution of the segments involved. Rules operating at a higher level in the hierarchy (such as planning an anchored sequence) tend to be reflected by longer latencies and shorter movement times (Thomassen, Meulenbroek, & Tibosch, 1991).

In a recent study (Thomassen, Meulenbroek, & Hoofs, in press) it was shown that drawing equal-length parallel segments is often done in immediate succession and in the same direction. Here the subject obviously takes advantage of using the same motor specifications ('program') more than once. The opportunity to do so often appears to determine the organisation of the movements in the entire (four-stroke) pattern, even though the parallel performance can be realised only late in the sequence. It was concluded by these authors that the economy of repeated program use is anticipated: Such anticipation involves setting the stage for its implementation, which is accompanied by a slight delay. A further finding in the latter study was that subjects tend to draw especially the terminal segment of the pattern in a preferred direction (rightwards, downwards), such that the completion of the graphic action is associated with relaxation. Probably this is an instance of a general principle of complex action (see e.g., Rosenbaum & Jorgensen, in press).

Further general principles which have hardly been studied so far, may be observed in actual handwriting. An example is the tendency of a progressive decrease of movement amplitudes within words. It has been suggested that this size decline may be due to the increased stiffness of the effector system as the hand rotates outward during the writing of a word. The increasing difficulty of keeping movement amplitudes constant across a word might then be traded off against the decreasing linguistic information content within that word (Maarse, Schomaker, & Thomassen, 1986). Such a bias may then generalise over situations where stiffness does not play a part whatsoever. Other graphic production rules or biases of writing may similarly be associated with linguistic and orthographic features, such as the frequent occurrence of words starting with an upper-case letter and continuing with (smaller) lower-case letters. This may exert a strong generalised influence on writing performance also outside linguistic contexts (e.g., Van der Plaats, Van Galen, & Thomassen, in preparation).

It is most likely that the 'grammar of graphic action' defining these rules is a subcategory of a more general grammar of action concerned with the organisation of complex movement sequences involved in our everyday interaction in the real world. Unfortunately, such sequences have not yet been studied at all systematically. However, some elementary principles are becoming clear. They are often concerned with the selection of effectors and movement segments and their spatio-temporal ordering as a fundamental problem in more or less complex situations or tasks. In such tasks, the physical constraints and opportunities of the action space are exploited, while the mechanical properties of the effectors and the inherent dynamics of the appropriate systems may be used to the full. Higher-order solutions may also be sought, such as taking advantage of the option to quote motor programs or specifications repeatedly in immediate succession. This opportunistic strategy may be subsumed under the single leading principle which has recently been given the name 'optimality' of movement organisation.

COMPUTATIONAL APPROACHES TO THE STUDY OF HANDWRITING

The modelling of cursive script has repeatedly been attempted during the past decades. Early models aimed at the production of pieces of handwriting by mechanical devices (Denier van der Gon, Thuring, & Strackee, 1962; Vredenbregt & Koster, 1971). The more recent computer simulation attempts were concerned with the specification of strokes and allographs and their combinations, and with entire words (e.g., Dooijes, 1984; Edelman & Flash, 1987; Hollerbach, 1981; Maarse, 1987; Morasso, 1986; Morasso & Mussa Ivaldi, 1982; Plamondon & Maarse, 1989). Simulating handwriting at the stroke level is concerned with the regeneration and concatenation of small segments of script on the basis of parsimoniously coded features of these segments in the target script. Maarse (1987) demonstrated that asymmetrical triangular velocity distributions in the X and Y directions yield the best approximation of the stroke's amplitude and shape. Morasso (1986) showed that mixed models involving spatial, velocity, and acceleration features are also promising. The ultimate, comprehensive computer model capable of generating handwriting in a 'realistic', psychologically plausible way should (if we constrain the model to the motor domain outlined above) translate a sequence of symbols representing the character shapes (allographs) into a sequence of muscle commands. While doing so, it should also specify the relations between the letter forms and the kinematics of the movements producing them in natural handwriting.

A model of cursive-script generation has recently been developed at the NICI Department (Schomaker, Thomassen, & Teulings, 1989). The model is concerned with the production of connected, fluent handwriting on the basis of general motor principles of handwriting as well as of specific features that characterise the writing sample from a male adult individual whose handwriting is being simulated. The general principles are concerned with the flow of information through stages of processing that lead from the highest cognitive representation of the intended message down to the movements that guide the pen tip in and above the writing plane. The model's output simulates both the spatial and the temporal characteristics of the writing trace during its production.

In general, a parsimonious parameterisation is adopted, even though the model is ultimately designed to simulate a wide range of handwriting-production phenomena. The model is characterised by two distinct levels. At the symbolic level it represents allographs and allograph connections by sets of symbols making up abstract codes; in the case of connecting strokes, these codes are generated by a cursive-connections grammar. At the quantitative level, the symbols are transformed into sequences of ballistic stroke movements, parameterised in the spatial and velocity domains.

The primary theoretical basis of the model lies in motor theory as developed in the human-performance tradition in experimental psychology as reviewed above, and of biophysics, and as supported by empirical findings in these disciplines of the type similarly outlined above. An example of human-performance evidence is that the unit of planning in handwriting is not smaller than a single letter (allograph) and not larger than a few allographs (Hulstijn & Van Galen, 1988; Teulings, Thomassen, & Van Galen, 1983). A finding from biodynamics research is that in a broad range of movement classes, to which also handwriting belongs, movements are planned and organised in three-dimensional Cartesian space rather than in joint space (Abend, Bizzi, & Morasso, 1982; Hollerbach & Flash, 1981; Morasso, 1986).

Furthermore, the model operates within the following theoretical framework. At the highest, semantic level, a writer's intended message is conceived. At syntactic and lexical levels the message is phrased and worded. Selection of orthographically prescribed letters is done at the level of graphemes; their specific shapes are determined at the next-lower, allographic level by a formal allograph selection syntax which specifies the allographs satisfying certain typographical or topological requirements, e.g., at the beginning of a sentence ('upper case'), or in the context of surrounding allographs.

In the model itself, the selected allograph, which has a permanently stored spatial representation, is transformed into its spatio-temporal representation in terms of the appropriate sequence of strokes. The latter transformation is assumed to be automatised for each allograph, with its fixed topological structure. The successive allographs in a 'word', however, must be concatenated by means of connecting strokes or by movements above the paper. The model specifies these connections in terms of a trajectory in three-dimensional space. The conversions of the latter trajectory to n-dimensional joint space and to the movement-execution levels are not dealt with by the model. Because of the ballistic nature and the short duration of stroke production, current strokes are unaffected by feedback. However, a feedback loop concerning lineation information may result in adjusting the programming of subsequent strokes.

An essential characteristic of the model is that it treats handwriting sequences as built up of allograph and connecting strokes. Ballistically produced stroke segments with their characteristic velocity profiles make up the letters and their interconnections. A stroke is defined in the velocity domain by two sinusoidal momentum impulses, one for its horizontal and one for its vertical component. Presently, the third dimension is represented merely by a binary code (pen-up/pen-down) although it was shown recently that pressure is related to the writing trace in an intricate, subject-dependent fashion (Schomaker & Plamondon, 1990). The geometrical direction, length, and shape of a stroke are represented by the displacement dX, dY in space and by a shape parameter C defining the stroke's ending in terms of the relatively longer duration (Tx, Ty)

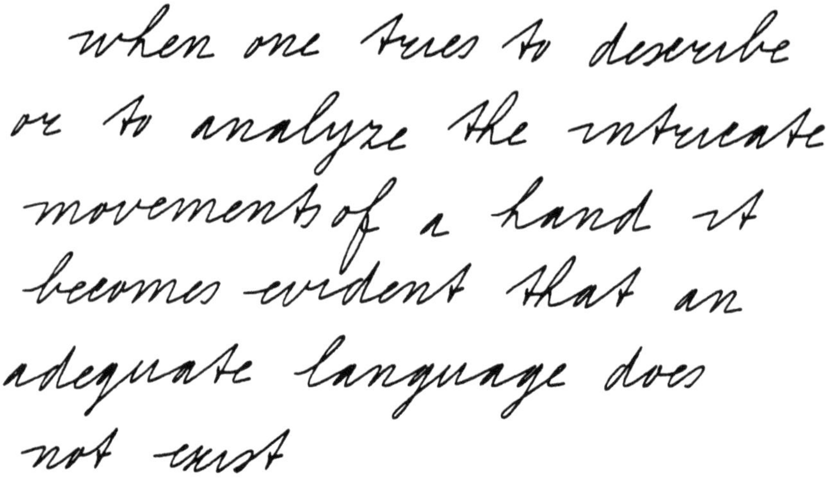

Figure 3. Some lines of an adult person's handwriting simulated by Schomaker's model. Note that the text itself was never written by this person (From Schomaker, Thomassen, & Teulings, 1989).

of the X or Y component. The resulting shape features at the stroke's ending (blunt or sharp; clockwise or counterclockwise) determine the curve direction of the next stroke's beginning.

In the terminology of data structures and data-processing modules, the model's stages are the following. First, for the chain of allograph symbols, the connecting strokes and pen lifts between successive pairs of allographs are determined through reference by a cursive connections grammar to a symbolic letter description. The cursive connections grammar is a formal description of the behaviour of the association processes that are supposedly active in the allograph-allograph transitions. The resulting symbol chain is subsequently converted into a sequence of stroke parameters through reference by a stroke parameterisation module to a quantitative letter description. Tempo, size, and further shape factors (slant, roundedness) exert a global influence upon these parameters. Finally, a stroke generator distributes the available time over the X and Y momentum impulses corresponding to the specified size and shape of the stroke. Error correction of subsequent strokes occurs if the output, which is continually monitored, produces deviations greater than a criterion distance from the lineation reference available in the symbolic letter descriptions.

The model's achievements are promising. At present, the model is capable of a reasonable spatial as well as temporal approximation of the cursive script of the target writer simulated. See Figure 3. This is certainly striking in view of the parsimonious coding format adopted. A vertical grid of nine classes of vertical stroke size appears to be satisfactory. The horizontal grid, involving only three classes of horizontal connecting-stroke size, may need a further refinement, however. Moreover, extensions of the range of the model, such as by a module taking care of a context-dependent selection of the allographs, would add to the naturalness of the model's performance. The cursive connections grammar as a formal module may be replaced by an associative network.

The model obviously has a restricted scope in the sense that it specifies neither the highest nor the lowest stages of planning: It takes as its input the selected allograph strings and its output defines the spatio-temporal movement of the pen tip, leaving unspecified the intricate biomechanical system which selects the muscles and their force levels, and which produces the actual movements. Such a specification was not the intention of the model, and in fact has not been the intention of any of the existing handwriting models known to the authors. In a recent model, which implements the specification of the kinematics of handwritten characters in relatively simple terms, given their symbolic description (Edelman & Flash, 1987), such a specification of the effectors was likewise omitted. The results of the latter study make it plausible that the central nervous system specifies handwriting at a fairly high, topological or symbolic level indeed, leaving the concrete effectors and the resulting exact shape and its kinematics to lower parts of the motor system.

Some final comments are concerned with the role of the present computational model in the automatic analysis and interpretation of cursive script. The various stages of preparing and generating cursive script as specified earlier in this chapter and in the present model, which transform symbolic and abstract information into concrete and quantitative information, are roughly also present in an on-line analysis system being developed by Teulings and Schomaker at the NICI Department. The latter algorithm is largely based on knowledge of the motor system producing handwriting. The order of the modules in the analysis system is of course reversed in comparison to the order in the synthesis model discussed. (For a brief outline of the system, see Thomassen, Teulings, Schomaker, Morasso, & Kennedy, 1988). The on-line recognition of cursive script is indeed concerned with the interpretation of concrete time-bound pen displacements as intended strings of abstract characters, or words. Thus, to the extent that the present model implements human handwriting generation, the cursive-script analysis system, which may be seen as the inverse of the latter, promises to be a useful algorithm for the extremely difficult (and as yet unaccomplished) task of automatically 'understanding' cursive script. It involves a sequence of basic operations performed by relatively independent modules. Segmentation is, likewise, mainly concerned with ballistic strokes. One of the most essential modules is specialised in coding the segmented strokes in approximately the terms of the starting and ending positions and shape features outlined above.

Given our increased understanding of the handwriting process and, more specifically, of the intrinsic relationships between the dynamic features of that process and their static consequences in the handwriting trace, it is feasible that, in the more distant future, dynamic features will contribute even to the automatic off-line recognition of handwriting products. In the case of human handwriting recognition, such a dynamic appreciation of static allographs is likely to occur. Recently, Freyd (1987) provided evidence that the human recognition of static handwriting may indeed take place by reference to the implicit dynamics (order and directions) of the strokes produced sequentially when the characters were being formed.

CONCLUSION

Having made our tour along a considerable number of aspects of handwriting research, reviewing larger as well as smaller topics of investigation, we must still note the limited scope of the present chapter. Neither did we pay attention to the development and maturation of handwriting, nor to the neuropsychological correlates of handwriting and its disturbances. Also neglected were the role of perceptual guidance and the function of training in the representation and performance of units of handwriting. In all these areas relevant research has been reported over the past decade. From the research we did review, however, it appears that the experimental and computational approaches made to handwriting are capable of gradually improving our fundamental knowledge of relevant aspects of the handwriting process as a motor skill. Its pure results may be expected to support the applied research in different disciplines that were mentioned in the introduction. Most of the problems, though, are far from solved at this stage. Considerable further research is needed here to arrive, for example, at the 'best' method for handwriting instruction to children, including an optimal model alphabet, or to achieve the 'best' classification of handwriting features in forensic science and in palaeography. Even though these potential contributions by themselves require a greatly increased body of fundamental knowledge in the handwriting process, its most complete and crucial test seems to be the automatic recognition of unconstrained cursive script. The adequacy of such a recognition system, which is based on our knowledge of the process, and which for the data-driven part of its analysis, makes use (either on-line or, more ambitiously, off-line) of the dynamic features in the trajectory, will teach us in due course how far we have stretched not only our imagination, but also our understanding of the multifaceted process of handwriting.

ACKNOWLEDGMENTS

This chapter was written whilst both authors were Fellows at the Netherlands Institute of Advanced Study (NIAS) at Wassenaar. The research reviewed was supported in part by NWO and by ESPRIT.

REFERENCES

Abend, W., Bizzi, E., & Morasso, P. (1982). Human arm trajectory formation. *Brain, 105*, 331-348.

Bernstein, N. (1967). *The coordination and regulation of movements*. New York: Pergamon.

Brown, J.S., Carr, Th. H., Brown, T.L., McDonald, J.L., Charalambous, A., & West, E. (1989). Coordinating language generation and motor control in discourse production via handwriting. In R. Plamondon, C.Y.Suen & M.L. Simner (Eds.), *Computer recognition and human production of handwriting* (pp. 299-316). Singapore: World Scientific.

Brown, J.S., McDonald, J.L., Brown, T.L., & Carr, T.H. (1988). Adapting to processing demands in discourse production: The case of handwriting. *Journal of Experimental Psychology: Human Perception and Performance, 14*, 45-59.

Connolly, K., & Elliott, J. (1972). The evolution and ontogeny of hand function. In N. Blurton Jones (Ed.), *Ethological studies of child behavior* (pp. 329-371). Cambridge: Cambridge University Press.

De Kerckhove, D., & Lumsden, C.J. (Eds.) (1988). *The alphabet and the brain: The lateralization of writing*. Berlin: Springer.

Denier van der Gon, J.J., Thuring, J.P., & Strackee, J. (1962). A handwriting simulator. *Physics in Medicine and Biology, 3*, 407-413.

Dooijes, E.H. (1984). *Analysis of handwriting*. Ph.D. Thesis, University of Amsterdam.

Edelman, S., & Flash, T. (1987). A model of handwriting. *Biological Cybernetics, 57*, 25-36.

Ellis, A.W. (1982). Spelling and writing (and reading and speaking). In A.W. Ellis (Ed.), *Normality and pathology in cognitive functions* (pp. 113-146). London: Academic Press.

Ellis. A.W. (1988). Normal writing processes and peripheral acquired dysgraphias. *Language and Cognitive Processes, 3*, 99-127.

Freyd, J.J. (1987). Dynamic mental representations. *Psychological Review, 94*, 427-438.

Gelb, I.J.(1952). *A study of writing*. Chicago: University of Chicago Press.

Goodnow, J.J., & Levine, R.A. (1973). The grammar of action: Sequence and syntax in children's copying. *Cognitive Psychology, 4*, 82-98.

Hollerbach, J.M. (1981). An oscillation theory of handwriting. *Biological Cybernetics, 39*, 139-156.

Hollerbach, J.M., & Flash, T. (1981). *Dynamic interactions between limb segments during planar arm movement.* AI Memo No. 635. Cambridge, Mass.: MIT-AI Lab. November.

Hulstijn, W., & Van Galen, G.P. (1988). Levels of motor programming in writing familiar and unfamiliar symbols. In A.M. Colley and J.R. Beech (Eds.), *Cognition and action in skilled behaviour* (pp. 65-85). Amsterdam: Elsevier Science Publishers.

Humphreys, G.W., & Evett, L.J. (1985). Are there independent lexical and nonlexical routes in word processing? An evaluation of the dual-route theory of reading. *The Behavioral and Brain Sciences, 8,* 689-740.

Kao, H.S.R., Van Galen, G.P., & Hoosain, R. (Eds.) (1986). *Graphonomics: Contemporary research in handwriting.* Amsterdam: North-Holland.

Klapp, S.T., Wyatt, E.P. (1976). Motor programming within a sequence of responses. *Journal of Motor Behavior, 8*, 19-26.

Levelt, W.J.M. (1989). *Speaking: From intention to articulation.* Cambridge, Mass.: MIT Press.

Maarse, F.J. (1987). *The study of handwriting: Peripheral models and signal processing techniques.* Ph.D. Thesis Nijmegen. Lisse: Swets & Zeitlinger.

Maarse, F.J., Schomaker, L.R.B., & Teulings, H.-L. (1988). Automatic identification of writers. In G. Mulder & G. van der Veer (Eds.), *Human-computer interaction.* Berlin: Springer.

Maarse, F.J., Schomaker, L.R.B., & Thomassen, A.J.W.M. (1986). The influence of changes in the effector coordinate system on handwriting movements. In H.S.R. Kao, G.P. van Galen, & R. Hoosain (Eds.), *Graphonomics: Contemporary research in handwriting* (pp. 33-46). Amsterdam: North-Holland.

Maarse, F.J., & Thomassen, A.J.W.M. (1983). Produced and perceived writing slant: Difference between up and down strokes. *Acta Psychologica, 54*, 131-147.

Maarse, F.J., Van Galen, G.P., & Thomassen, A.J.W.M. (1989). Models for the generation of writing units in handwriting under variations of size, slant, and orientation. *Human Movement Science, 8*, 271-288.

Margolin, D.I. (1984). The neuropsychology of writing and spelling: Semantic, phonological, motor, and spelling processes. *Quarterly Journal of Experimental Psychology, 36A*, 459-489.

Margolin, D.I., & Wing, A.M. (1983). Agraphia and micrographia: Clinical manifestations of motor programming and performance disorders. *Acta Psychologica, 54*, 263-283.

McAllister, C.N. (1900). Researches on movements used in handwriting. *Studies from the Yale Psychological Laboratory, 8*, 21-63.

Merton, P.A. (1972). How we control the contraction of our muscles. *Scientific American, 226*, 30-37.

Meulenbroek, R.G.J., & Thomassen, A.J.W.M. (1991). Stroke-direction preferences in drawing and handwriting. *Human Movement Science, 10*, 247-270.

Meulenbroek, R. G. J., & Van Galen, G. P. (1988). Foreperiod duration and the analysis of motor stages in a line drawing task. *Acta Psychologica, 69*, 19-33.

Morasso, P. (1986). Trajectory formation. In P. Morasso & V. Tagliasco (Eds.). *Human movement understanding* (pp. 9-58). Amsterdam: North-Holland.

Morasso, P., & Mussa Ivaldi, F.A. (1982). Trajectory formation and handwriting: A computational model. *Biological Cybernetics, 45*, 131-142.

Nooteboom, S.G. (1972). *Production and perception of vowel durations: A study of durational properties of vowels in Dutch*. PhD Thesis, University of Utrecht.

Patterson, K., & Wing, A. (1989). Processes in handwriting: A case for case. *Cognitive Neuropsychology, 6*, 1-23.

Pick, H.L., & Teulings, H.-L. (1983). Geometric transformations of handwriting as a function of instruction and feedback. *Acta Psychologica, 54*, 327-340.

Plamondon, R., & Leedham, G. (Eds.) (1990). *Computer processing of handwriting*. Singapore: World Scientific.

Plamondon, R., & Maarse, F.J. (1989). An evaluation of motor models of handwriting. *IEEE Transactions on Systems, Man, and Cybernetics, 19*, 1060-1072.

Plamondon, R, Suen, C.Y., & Simner, M.L. (Eds.) (1989). *Computer recognition and human production of handwriting*. Singapore: World Scientific.

Putman. J.J. (1989). The search for modern humans. *National Geographic, 174*, 438-477.

Rosenbaum, D.A., & Jorgensen, M.J. (in press). Planning macroscopic aspects of manual control. *Human Movement Science*.

Sassoon, R, Nimmo-Smith, I, & Wing, A.M. (1986). An analysis of children's penholds. In H.S.R. Kao, G.P. van Galen, & R. Hoosain (Eds.), *Graphonomics: Contemporary research in handwriting* (pp. 93-106). Amsterdam: North-Holland.

Schomaker, L.R.B., & Plamondon, R. (1990). The relation between pen force and pen-point kinematics in handwriting. *Biological Cybernetics, 63*, 277-289.

Schomaker, L.R.B., Thomassen, A.J.W.M., & Teulings, H.L. (1989). A computational model of cursive handwriting. In R. Plamondon, C.Y.Suen & M.L.Simner (Eds.), *Computer recognition and human production of handwriting* (pp. 153-178). Singapore: World Scientific.

Sirat, C., Irigoin., J., & Poulle, E. (Eds.) (1990). *L'ecriture: Le Cerveau, l'oeil et la main*. Turnhout: Brepols.

Sternberg, S. (1969). The discovery of processing stages: Extensions of Donders' method. In W.G. Koster (Ed.), *Attention and performance II* (pp. 276-315). Amsterdam: North-Holland.

Sternberg, S., Monsell, S., Knoll, R.L., & Wright, C.E. (1978). The latency and duration of rapid movement sequences: Comparisons of speech and typewriting. In G.E. Stelmach (Ed.), *Information processing in motor control and learning* (pp. 118-150). New York: Academic Press.

Teulings, H.-L. (1988). *Handwriting-movement control: Research into different levels of the motor system*. PhD Thesis, University of Nijmegen.

Teulings, H.-L., & Maarse, F.J. (1984). Digital recording and processing of handwriting movements. *Human Movement Science, 3*, 193-217.

Teulings, H-.L., & Thomassen, A.J.W.M. (1979). Computer-aided analysis of handwriting movement. *Visible Language, 13*, 219-231.

Teulings, H.-L., Thomassen, A.J.W.M., & Maarse, F.J. (1989). A description of handwriting in terms of main axes. In R. Plamondon, C.Y. Suen, and M.L. Simner (Eds.), *Computer recognition and human production of handwriting* (pp. 193-211). Singapore: World Scientific.

Teulings, H.-L., Thomassen, A.J.W.M., & Van Galen, G.P. (1983). Preparation of partly precued handwriting movements: The size of movement units of handwriting. *Acta Psychologica, 54*, 165-177.

Teulings, H.-L., Thomassen, A.J.W.M., & Van Galen, G.P. (1986). Invariants in handwriting: The information contained in a motor program. In H.S.R. Kao, G.P. Van Galen & R. Hoosain (Eds.), *Graphonomics: Contemporary research in handwriting* (pp. 305-315). Amsterdam: North-Holland.

Thomassen, A.J.W.M., Keuss, P.J.G., & Van Galen, G.P. (Eds.) (1984). *Motor aspects of handwriting: Approaches to movement in graphic behavior*. Amsterdam: North-Holland.

Thomassen, A.J.W.M., Meulenbroek, R.G.J. & Hoofs, M.P.E. (in press). Economy and anticipation in graphic stroke sequences. *Human Movement Science*.

Thomassen, A.J.W.M., Meulenbroek, R.G.J.,& Tibosch, H.J.C.M. (1991). Latencies and kinematics reflect graphic production rules. *Human Movement Science, 10,* 271-290.

Thomassen, A.J.W.M., & Teulings, H.L. (1983). Constancy in stationary and progressive handwriting. *Acta Psychologica, 54*, 179-196.

Thomassen, A.J.W.M., & Teulings, H.L. (1985). Time, size and shape in handwriting: Exploring spatio-temporal relationships at different levels. In J.A. Michon & J.L. Jackson (Eds.), *Time, mind and behavior* (pp. 253-263). Berlin: Springer.

Thomassen, A.J.W.M., Teulings, H.-L., Schomaker, L.R.B., & Morasso, P. (1988). *Experimentation and modelling in the study of cursive script*. Report ESPRIT Project 419.

Thomassen, A.J.W.M., Teulings, H.-L., Schomaker, L.R.B., Morasso, P., & Kennedy, J. (1988). Towards the implementation of cursive-script understanding in an on-line handwriting-recognition system. In C.E.C., D.G.XIII (Eds.), *ESPRIT '88: Putting the technology to use*. Part I (pp. 628-639). Amsterdam: North-Holland.

Thomassen, A.J.W.M., & Tibosch, H.J.C.M., (1991). A quantitative model of graphic production. In J. Requin and G. E. Stelmach (Eds.), *Tutorials in motor neuroscience*. Dordrecht: Kluwer.

Thomassen, A.J.W.M., Tibosch, H.J.C.M., & Maarse, F.J. (1989). The effect of context on stroke direction and strike order in handwriting. In R. Plamondon, C.Y. Suen, & M. Simner (Eds.), *Computer recognition and human production of handwriting* (pp. 213-230). Singapore: World Scientific.

Van der Plaats, R.E., & Van Galen, G.P. (in press). Effects of spatial and motor demands in handwriting. *Journal of Motor Behavior*.

Van der Plaats, R.E., Van Galen, G.P., & Thomassen, A.J.W.M. (in preparation). *Allographic choice and parameterization processes in handwriting: Evidence for rule-governed processing*.

Van Emmerik, R.E.A., & Newell, K.M. (1989). The relationship between pen-point and joint kinematics in handwriting and drawing. In R. Plamondon, C.Y. Suen, & M.L. Simner (Eds.), *Computer recognition and human production of handwriting* (pp 231-248). Singapore: World Scientific Publishing Co.

Van Galen, G.P. (1980). Storage and retrieval of handwriting patterns: A two-stage model of complex motor behavior. In G.E. Stelmach & J. Requin (Eds.), *Tutorials in motor behavior* (pp. 567-578). Amsterdam: North-Holland.

Van Galen, G.P. (1991). Handwriting: Issues for a psychomotor theory. *Human Movement Science, 10,* 165-192.

Van Galen, G.P. (in press b). Phonological and motoric demands in handwriting: Evidence for discrete transmission of information. *Acta Psychologica*.

Van Galen, G.P., Meulenbroek, R.G.J., & Hylkema, H. (1986). On the simultaneous processing of words, letters and strokes in handwriting: Evidence for a mixed linear and parallel model. In H.S.R. Kao., G.P. van Galen., & R. Hoosain (Eds.), *Graphonomics: Contemporary research in handwriting* (pp. 5-20). Amsterdam: North-Holland.

Van Galen, G.P., Smyth, M.M., Meulenbroek, R.G.J., & Hylkema, H. (1989). The role of short-term memory and the motor buffer in handwriting under visual and non-visual guidance. In R. Plamondon, C.Y.Suen & M.L.Simner (Eds.), *Computer recognition and human production of handwriting* (pp. 253-272). Singapore: World Scientific.

Van Galen, G.P., & Teulings, H.-L. (1983). The independent monitoring of form and scale factors in handwriting. *Acta Psychologica, 54*, 9-22.

Van Galen, G.P., & Wing, A.M. (1984). The sequencing of movements. In M.M. Smyth & A.M. Wing (Eds.), *The psychology of human movement* (pp. 153-182). London: Academic Press.

Van Sommers, P. (1984). *Drawing and cognition: Descriptive and experimental studies of graphic production processes*. Cambridge: Cambridge University Press.

Vredenbregt, J., & Koster, W.G. (1971). Analysis and synthesis of handwriting. *Philips Technical Review, 32*, 73-78.

Wann, J., Wing, A.M., & Sovik, N. (Eds.) (1990). *The development of graphic skills: Research perspectives and educational implications*. London: Academic Press.

Wing, A.M. (1980). The height of handwriting. *Acta Psychologica, 46*, 141-151.

Wing, A.M., Lewis, V.J., & Baddeley, A.D. (1979). The slowing of handwriting by letter repetition. *Journal of Human Movement Studies, 5*, 182-188.

PART II

COORDINATION AND CONTROL

Approaches to the Study of Motor Control and Learning
J.J. Summers (Editor)

Chapter 5

MEASURING CHANGES IN COORDINATION AND CONTROL

W.A. Sparrow
Victoria College, Burwood

Dependent measures for assessing changes in coordination and control as a function of practice and associated variables are presented. Examples are drawn from the literature on gait, sports skills, and laboratory aiming tasks to illustrate how coordination and control have been operationally defined. Some suggestions are made as to how the magnitude of change in coordination can be evaluated. Finally, it is proposed that single-case research designs should be considered by motor behaviour researchers as an alternative to large between-subject designs.

In recent years researchers in the motor behaviour field have become increasingly concerned with measuring changes in movement patterns due to practice and associated variables, such as recovery from injury, physical growth, and various forms of information feedback. Future research on changes in coordination and control with practice will be productive only if two requirements are satisfied. One is that the hypothesised changes in coordination and control with practice should derive from some general principles or theory with which to explain those changes. The future of such endeavour, however, appears grim in an intellectual climate where even the need for hypotheses in motor control research is being questioned (see Winter, 1987). A second requirement for progress on the effects of practice is that coordination can be accurately measured and *changes* in the movement pattern reliably identified. It is the second of the above requirements that is the focus of this paper. Some advice will be offered on the measurement of movement patterns, and alternative research designs for learning and coordination experiments will be presented because traditional between-subject designs may be impractical when detailed movement pattern measures are required. In terms of measuring movement patterns let us first consider the types of dependent variables that can be used to evaluate changes in coordination and control.

DEPENDENT VARIABLES

Coordination and Control

Usage of the terms "coordination" and "control" has increased as motor behaviour researchers have become more familiar with the work of Kugler and co-workers. Newell (1985), for example, draws on Kugler, Kelso, and Turvey (1980) to provide operational definitions of coordination, control, and skill. A liberal interpretation of Newell's (1985) definitions is as follows. Coordination can be defined as the relationship between either the movements of limb segments of the same limb, what we can refer to as "intra-limb coordination", or the relationship between the movements of two different limbs (or the segments of different limbs) which can be referred to as "inter-limb coordination". Intra-limb coordination therefore defines the topology of a single limb's movement, whereas inter-limb coordination defines how two or more limbs maintain a temporal and spatial relationship to each other.

Control refers to the absolute magnitude of the limb or limb segment movement. For example, the amplitude, velocity, acceleration, or force of the movement would dictate the degree of control. The goal of the task specifies an optimum or target value of one of these variables and a "well-controlled" movement is one which satisfactorily approximates the optimum or target outcome. Furthermore, if kinetic or kinematic measures over time are used as dependent measures they are still indicative of control because they do not specify directly the pattern of limb or limb segment movements. They should not, therefore, be referred to as measures of coordination. Thus, coordination and control can be independent in the execution of a skill and the overall goal of the task could be achieved by changing coordination, control, or both. By way of illustration the game of golf presents an unusual case in which the coordination (the topology of the swing) and control (how hard the ball is hit) can remain constant while the outcome, the final position of the ball, will vary according to the angle of the head on the chosen club. "Skill", therefore, can be defined operationally in terms of the ability to correctly coordinate and control the movement to achieve the overall goal of the task.

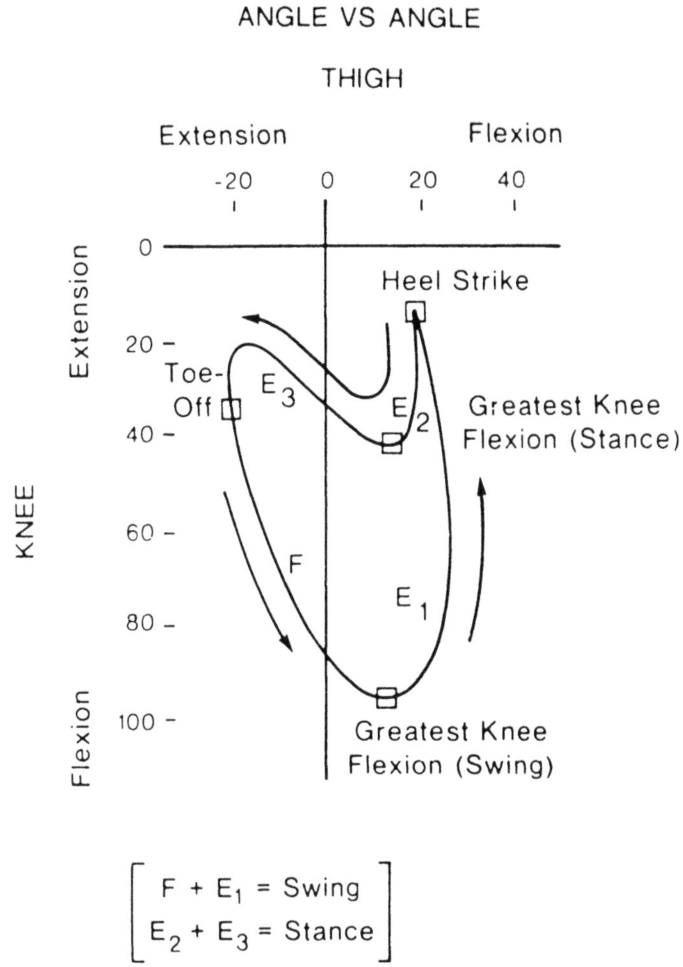

Figure 1. Angle-angle diagram of one step cycle. The diagram should be read counterclockwise from the point of heel strike, the beginning of E_2. Note that the rectangles positioned about the perimeter of the enclosed pattern demarcate the time and spatial boundaries of the four phases of the Phillippson step cycle; the phases start with E_2 and sequentially move to E_3, F, and E_1. (From "Evidence for generalized motor programs using gait pattern analysis" by Shapiro, D.C. et al., (1981) *Journal of Motor Behavior, 13*, p. 40. Reprinted with permission of the Helen Dwight Reid Educational Foundation. Published by Heldref Publications, 4000 Albemarle St., N.W., Washington, D.C. 20016. Copyright (c) 1981).

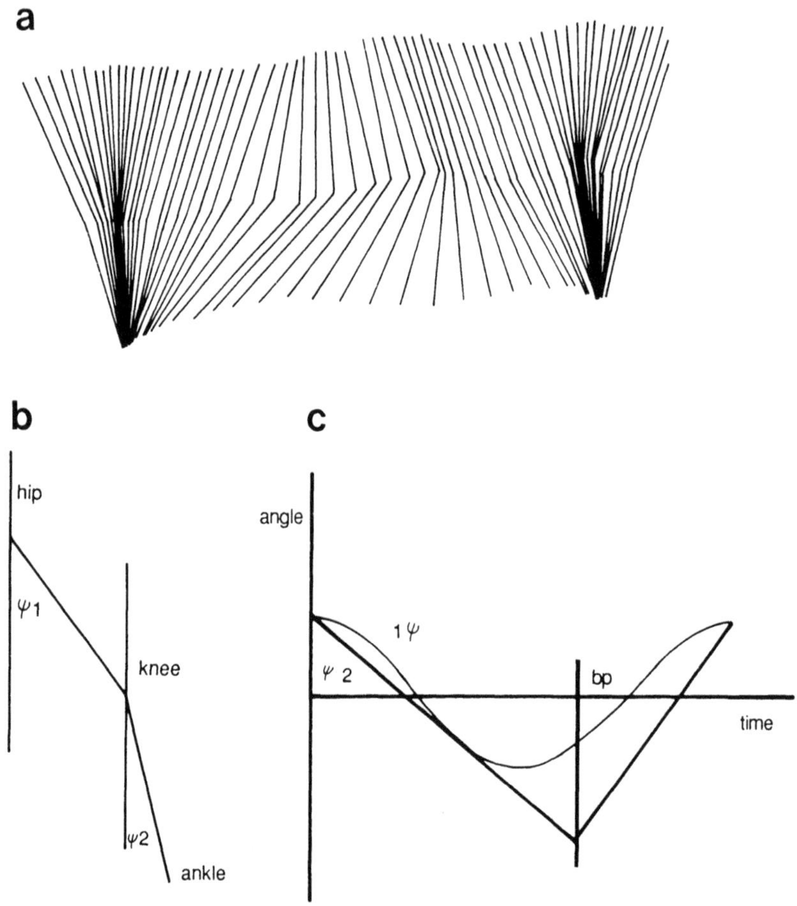

Figure 2. Schematic of leg movement during locomotion; a) recorded movement; b) convention for the measurement of the angles; c) variation in time of the angular displacement of the upper and lower leg, approximated as a sinusoid and a sawtooth like function. bp is the breakpoint of the sawtooth function. (From "Perceptual cues that determine the labelling of human gait" by Hoenkamp, E., (1978), *Journal of Human Movement Studies, 4*, p. 61. Reprinted by permission).

Intra-limb Coordination

Work in the area of human gait analysis provides some valuable methods for quantifying both intra-limb and inter-limb coordination. Intra-limb coordination is conveniently described using an angle-angle diagram to show the change in spatial and temporal relationships of limb segments over a movement cycle.

Figure 1 shows an angle-angle diagram for human gait with step-cycle phases as indicated. Note that the relative motion of the limb segments over time is, as it were, "taken out" by this technique such that it is necessary to identify the joint angles at significant discrete points in time such as Toe-off and Heel strike. One method of overcoming this problem of losing the time at which certain events occur is by plotting the joint angles over time, the diagram below (Figure 2) shows how this is done. The angles plotted over time in diagram C of Figure 2 are not empirical data but approximations of the actual data to a sinusoidal and sawtooth function. The breakpoint (bp) of the sawtooth function is where there is a reversal of the direction of change in the magnitude of the joint angles.

As Newell (1985) indicates, angle-angle diagrams can be used to describe discrete short duration actions as well as in the more common application to

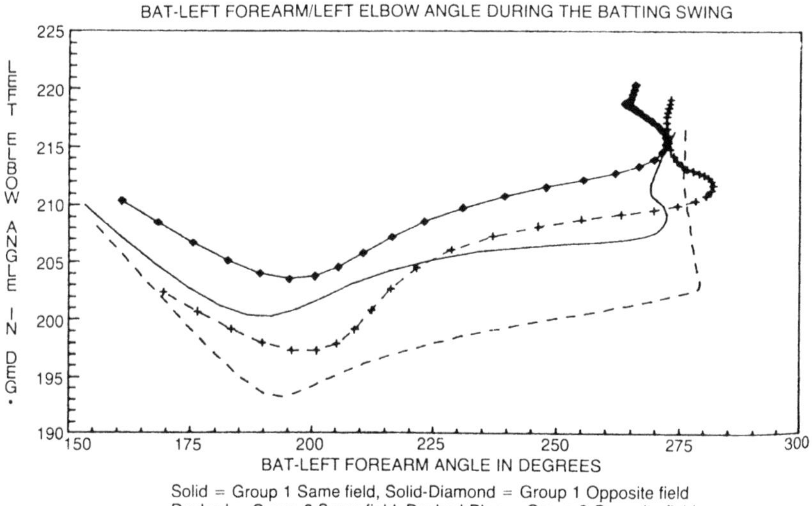

Figure 3. Angle-angle diagram of the elbow angle and bat-left forearm angle during a baseball batting swing to either the same field or the opposite field by ineffective (Group 1) or effective (Group 2) opposite field hitters. (From "A kinematic analysis of the baseball batting swing involved in opposite-field and same-field hitting" by McIntyre, D.R. & Pfautsch, E.W. (1982). *Research Quarterly for Exercise and Sport, 53*, p. 212. Copyright 1982 by the American Alliance for Health, Physical Education, Recreation and Dance. Reprinted by permission).

cyclical activities such as locomotion. In cyclical activities the limbs return to their relative position at the start of the cycle, giving the familiar closed-shaped diagram. Newell (1985) presented an example of an angle-angle diagram being used to describe the relative motion of a baseball bat, forearm, and lower arm during swings by performers designated by their coach as ineffective opposite field hitters (Group 1) or effective opposite field hitters (Group 2), this is shown in Figure 3. Fundamental differences in the coordination pattern of the two groups can be observed. For example, the Group 1 batters show a greater similarity in the coordination pattern of their swings to the same field and to the opposite field than do the Group 2 batters. The angle-angle plots also demonstrate differences between the groups with respect to the magnitude of the joint angles when hits to the same side of the field are compared.

Inter-Limb Coordination

Students of gait have developed various techniques for describing the relationship between the movements of limbs. One technique is the support phase diagram which has been used to describe developmental changes in infant creeping patterns (Burnside, 1927; Sparrow, 1989) and changes in adult creeping patterns over trials (Sparrow & Zrizarry-Lopez, 1987). The infant creeping diagrams in Figure 4 show that often the contralateral knee and hand moved almost simultaneously, as in subject MJH at 12 months, 12 days, whereas in other diagrams one of the contralateral pair moved in advance of its partner, as in the relationship between the right knee and left hand for subject DWC at 13 months, 9 days. These support phase diagrams show, therefore, both the proportion of the stride cycle that the limb is in swing or support and the relative timing of swing and support phases of each limb.

Another way in which inter-limb coordination in creeping has been described quantitatively is by means of a support graph such as that devised by Hildebrand (1967). Sparrow (1989) used this technique to compare creeping patterns of human adults and infants, the result was Figure 5. The ordinate shows precisely the temporal relationship between the right hand and the right foot or knee. Using this system human creeping gaits can also be classified according to conventions established for quadrupedal species. It is interesting to note in reference to Newell's (1985) interest in nominal categories of skills, that a distinction between walk and run is made using the criterion of 50% of stride interval for right hindlimb contact. Similarly, the relative timing of ipsilateral right side limbs dictates the labelling of the gait pattern as "diagonal sequence" or "lateral sequence". This is an example of a fairly arbitrary labelling of the coordination pattern as one activity or the other, that is, as a walk or a run.

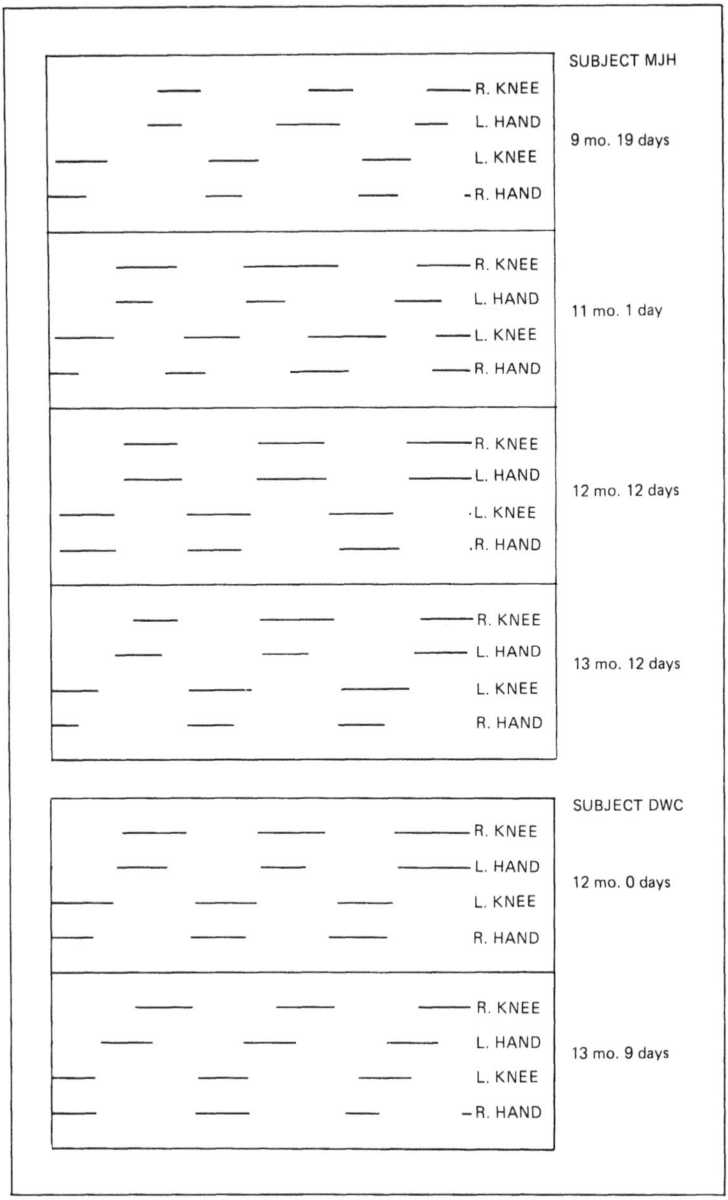

Figure 4. Pattern of swing and support for infants creeping on hands and knees. Solid lines represent the proportion of stride duration in support, the spaces represent swing duration. (From "Creeping patterns of human adults and infants" by Sparrow, W.A. (1989), *American Journal of Physical Anthropology*. Copyright 1988 by Alan R. Liss Inc. Reprinted by permission).

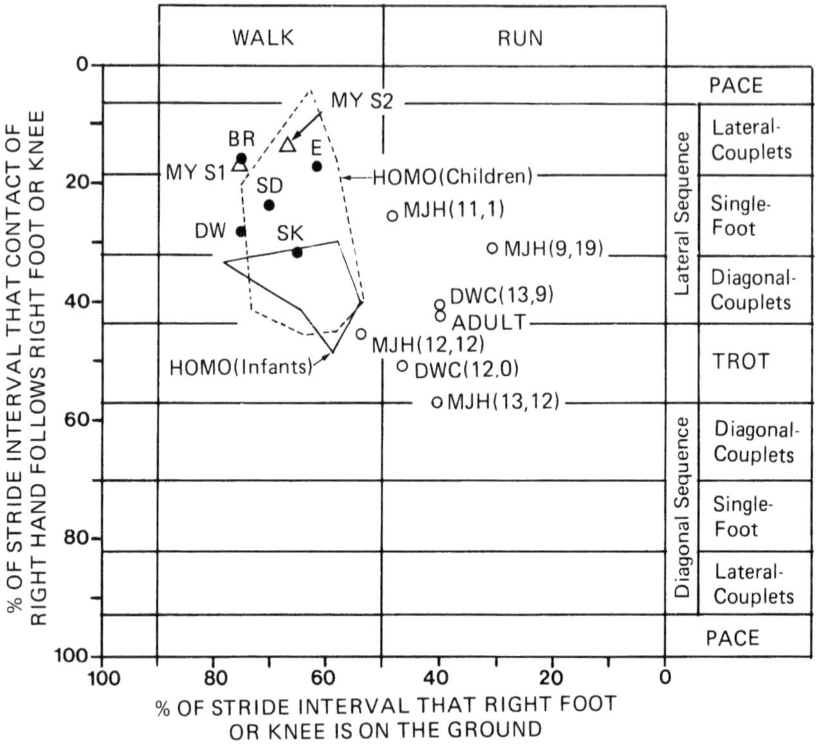

Figure 5. Support graph adapted from Hildebrand (1967) showing adult and infant creeping patterns. (From "Creeping patterns of human adults and infants" by Sparrow, W.A. (1989), *American Journal of Physical Anthropology.* Copyright 1988 by Alan R. Liss Inc. Reprinted by permission).

There are other areas of motor behaviour research that have devised ways of measuring inter-limb coordination. Studies of bimanual coordination have presented the coordination pattern of the hands using either outcome scores or kinematic variables. In Figure 6 are the trajectories of the left hand and right hand in a bimanual aiming task. The figure presents a convenient description of the path of the two hands. Other kinematic descriptions of the movement of the hands could also serve as measures of inter-limb coordination. For example, it would have been possible to plot vertical and horizontal displacement over time for the two hands. As with the angle-angle diagram in Figure 1, a trajectory diagram or a displacement-time graph only provide a qualitative description of the coordination pattern. In the next section consideration is given to how coordination patterns can be assessed

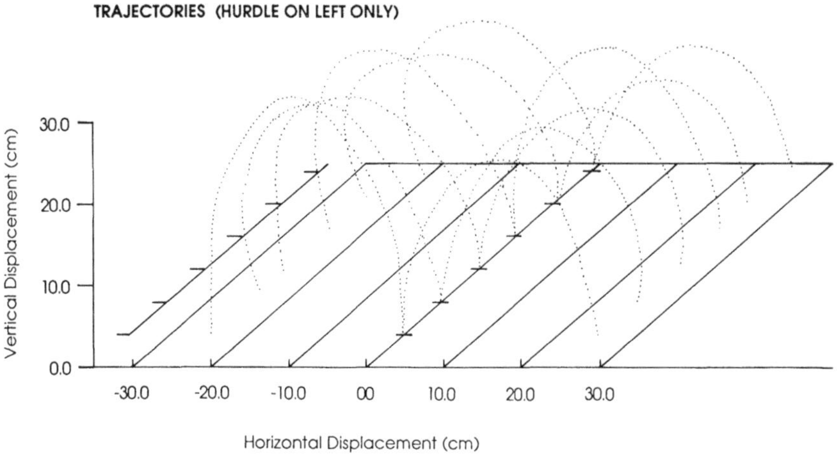

Figure 6. Trajectories for the left hand and right hand in a two-handed aiming movement. The left hand moves over a barrier and the right hand describes a similar trajectory even though no barrier is present. (From "On the space-time structure of human inter-limb co-ordination" by Kelso, J.A.S., Goodman, D., & Putnam, C.A. (1983), *Quarterly Journal of Experimental Psychology, 35A*, p. 366. Reprinted by permission).

quantitatively. Only by providing quantitative descriptions of the movement pattern can changes in coordination be reliably identified.

Measuring Changes in Coordination

Many avenues of motor behaviour research require measures of change in coordination. Enduring changes in coordination can be produced by learning, development, and recovery from trauma. Only recently, however, have the problems associated with measuring such changes in intra-limb and inter-limb coordination been addressed. Newell (1985), for example, refers to the fact that "eyeballing" figures to determine changes in movement topology has been the usual method of analysis. In response to this problem Sparrow, Donovan, van Emmerik, and Barry (1987) reviewed a number of quantitative methods for determining changes in relative motion plots. A formula was derived to measure the cross-correlation between the angles used to draw the angle-angle plots. An important feature of their cross-correlation formula was its ability to distinguish any differences in shape, size, and orientation, such that identical

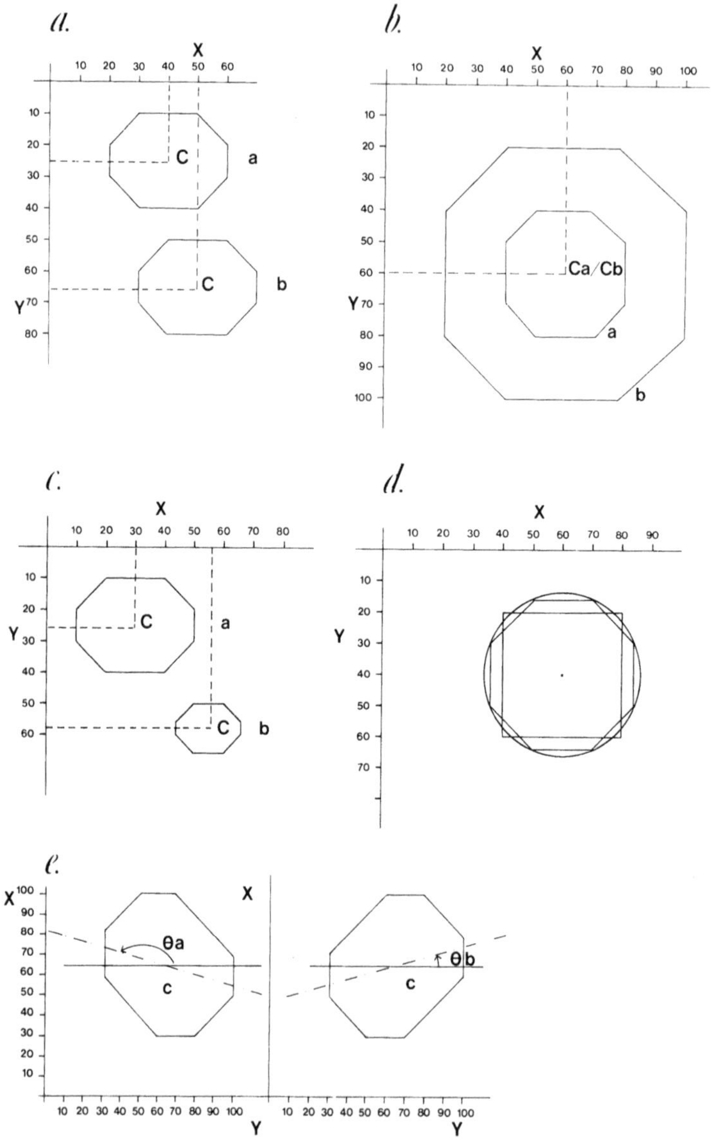

Figure 7. Hypothetical angle-angle diagrams showing the relationship between various pattern parameters. (a) Centroids changed. (b) Perimeter and area changed. (c) Area, perimeter and centroid changed. (d) Area, perimeter √area, and R Changed. (e) Orientation changed. (From "Using relative motion plots to measure changes in intra-limb and inter-limb coordination", by Sparrow, W.A. et al. (1987). *Journal of Motor Behavior, 19*, p. 121. Reprinted with permission of the Helen Dwight Reid Educational Foundation. Published by Heldref Publications, 4000 Albemarle St., Washington D.C. 20016. Copyright (c), 1987).

plots would give a maximum cross-correlation function of unity and less than identical plots would produce progressively smaller cross-correlation values. The importance of having a cross-correlation formula that is sensitive to such differences in the relative motion plots is illustrated below in Figure 7.

The diagrams show how size, shape, orientation, and pattern centroid can vary independently. Change in any one of these parameters introduces a degree of dissimilarity into the coordination patterns being compared. In diagram (b) of Figure 7, for example, the angle-angle plots **a** and **b** are the same shape but the maximum value of the cross-correlation coefficient R would not equal unity because of the difference in side length. Changes in any of the other pattern parameters, except the centroid, would also lead to comparisons between the plots with an R value of less than unity. Cross-correlation procedures similar to that presented by Sparrow et al., (1987) have been used to assess changes in relative motions due to practice (Sparrow & Zrizarry-Lopez, 1987), changes in walking speed (Shapiro, Zernicke, Gregor, & Diestel, 1981), and also to show refinements in time-varying kinematic data with practice (Den Brinker & Van Hekken, 1982).

It is important to note that the cross-correlation procedures described above can be used to assess changes in both intra-limb coordination and inter-limb coordination. The angle-angle data or kinematic time-varying data could be derived either from the same limb or from different limbs of the same subject. Most studies of inter-limb coordination simply use outcome scores to show differences in relative position or timing. It is anticipated that as motor behaviour research progresses attention will be focused on inter-limb differences in the movement pattern. It will be interesting to see if the expertise in measuring movement drives such experimentation or, on the other hand, some principles by which to explain such changes are put to test.

EXPERIMENTAL DESIGN

Traditionally motor skill learning experiments have employed between-subjects designs, with the effect of the independent variable(s) being confidently identified by comparing the experimental group with a control group. Such experiments also tend to require fairly large groups of subjects in order to obtain a sufficiently powerful test of the difference between treatments. When movement outcome measures alone are the values of the dependent variable such designs are practicable. When using coordination and control variables derived from an analysis of the movement pattern, however, such designs present a serious problem. All movement analysis systems have a common feature in that they are designed to accurately measure the position of body parts at fixed time intervals. The problem with this type of analysis is that it produces so much data that it is impractical to employ large-sample between-subjects designs. The alternative is to use some kind of single-subject design.

Single-Subject Designs

Single-subject designs have the advantage of requiring only one or a few subjects. The most basic type of single-subject design is the A-B-A design. The A condition is the baseline condition in which the subject performs the task prior to the introduction of the independent variable. This is equivalent in a way to the control condition of a true research design. In the B phase the treatment is introduced and its effect over trials is observed. In the second A condition the treatment is withdrawn, as in the more familiar "withdrawal" or "retention" phases of traditional motor learning experiments. If the effect of the independent variable is transient there will be a return to the original pre-treatment baseline. If, however, some relatively permanent change in behaviour has occurred there will not be a return to the performance level of the first baseline condition. Figure 8 shows a basic single-subject design.

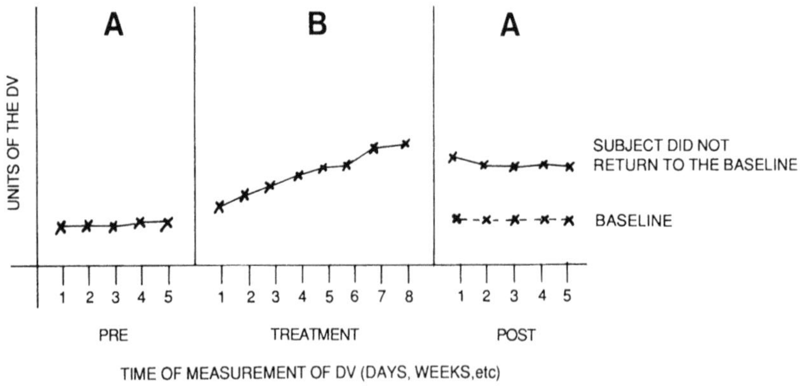

Figure 8. Basic single-subject design, the A-B-A design. First A is the baseline prior to treatment, B. Second A is the baseline following withdrawal of the treatment.

There are certain limitations, however, to the basic A-B-A design. (For a detailed discussion of single-subject designs and their limitations see Christensen, 1985.) One limitation is that behaviour might not return to baseline when the treatment is withdrawn. This being the case we cannot be absolutely sure that the treatment caused the change or whether some extraneous

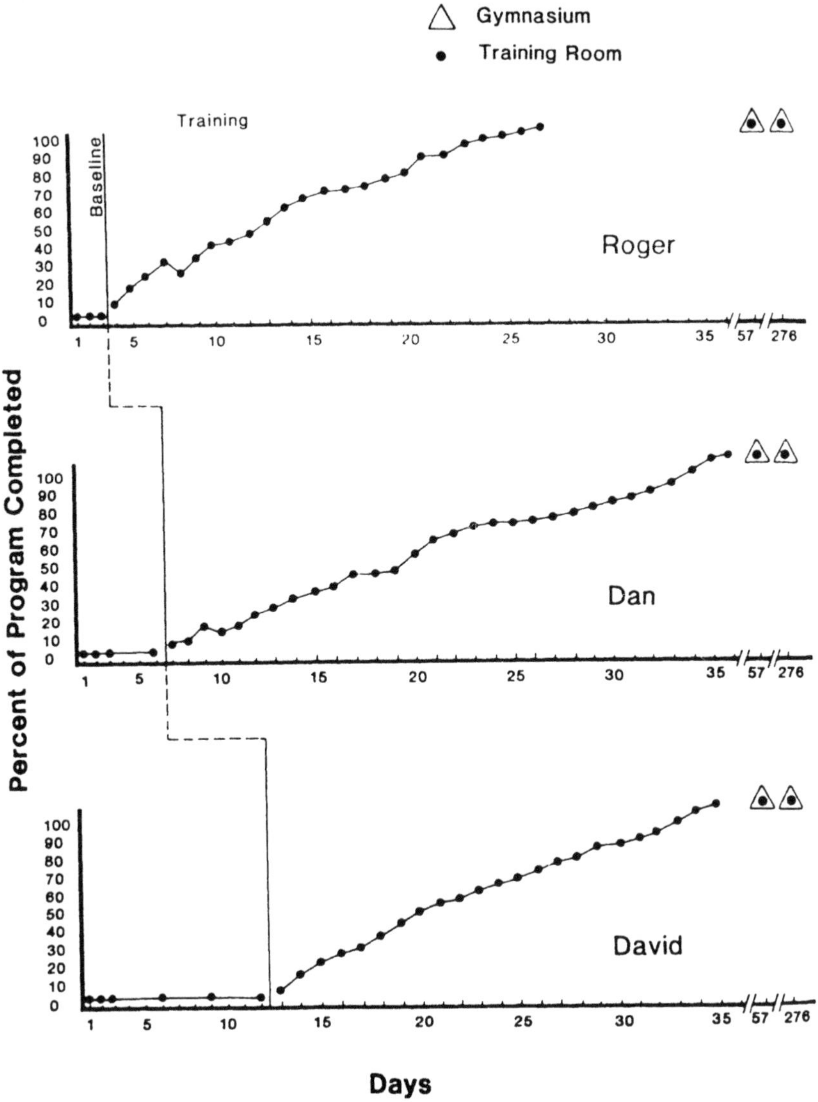

Figure 9. A multiple-baseline single-subject design showing the effectiveness of a behavioral program to teach a side-of-the-foot soccer pass. The Gymnasium and Training Room are the follow-up or "retention" trials to show the long-term effectiveness of the treatment. (From "Team sports for the severely retarded: training a side-of-the-foot soccer pass using a maximum-to-minimum prompt reduction strategy", Luyben, P.O. et al., (1986) *Journal of Applied Behavior in Analysis, 19*, 431-436. Reprinted by permission).

variable was responsible. One way to overcome this difficulty is to employ a design which does not rely on a return to baseline following the treatment. The multiple-baseline design illustrated in Figure 9 shows how the baseline performance of each subject acts as a control for the effectiveness of the treatment on the other subjects.

The soccer study by Luyben, Funk, Morgan, Clark, and Delulio (1986) shown in Figure 9 has a baseline in which the subjects were instructed to "Pass the ball". Under these conditions none of the subjects performed any of the nine "response components" (progressive parts of the task). Notice that the training procedure was introduced progressively later for Roger, Dan and David. The fact that the performance of Dan and David remained at baseline at the time Roger began the training program gives greater assurance that the change occurred due to training and not because of the influence of some extraneous variable. Following successful acquisition of the task there was a follow-up as indicated by the Gymnasium and Training Room data.

The major limitation to such designs is that the influence of the independent variable must be sufficiently powerful to show a clear effect with one or a few subjects. Such a requirement might not, however, prove to be an impediment to motor behaviour research if it forced researchers to focus on those variables that produce significant changes in behaviour. The major advantage of these designs is that the effect of an independent variable on the learning or control of movement can be evaluated with few subjects. This is of great importance when dealing with the large quantities of kinematic data needed to reliably describe changes in coordination and control.

A further consideration in favour of single-case designs is that they force attention on the individual's history of learning, relearning or developing a motor skill. That is not to say that data for the single case cannot be extracted from pooled group data but that a single case design demands a regard for individual differences and avoids information being lost in group summary statistics.

CONCLUSION

Despite their increasing facility with movement analysis techniques, motor behaviour researchers appear to be reluctant to focus their attention on the traditional issues of motor learning and motor development. The fields of motor learning, motor development, and rehabilitation, are all concerned with changes in movement pattern over time. Nevertheless, they are topics that appear to be underrepresented in mainstream motor behaviour research with respect to both empirical and theoretical study. It is possible that lack of theorising about learning and development is hindering work in these areas. Alternatively, it is possible that appropriate research designs and movement measurement procedures are impediments to progress. If such is the case, it is hoped that this paper might be of assistance in suggesting ways of overcoming problems associated with measuring changes in movement pattern over time.

REFERENCES

Burnside, L.H. (1927). Coordination in the locomotion of infants. *Genetic Psychology Monographs, 2*, 284-372.

Christensen, L. (1985). *Experimental Methodology.* London: Allyn and Bacon, Inc.

Den Brinker, B.P.L.M., & Van Hekken, M.F. (1982). The analysis of slalom-ski type movements using a ski-simulator apparatus. *Human Movement Science, 1*, 91-108.

Hildebrand (1967). Symmetrical gaits of primates. *American Journal of Physical Anthropology, 26*, 119-130.

Hoenkamp, E. (1978). Perceptual cues that determine the labelling of human gait. *Journal of Human Movement Studies, 4*, 59-69.

Kelso, J.A.S. Goodman, D., & Putman, C.A. (1983). On the space-time structure of human inter-limb co-ordination. *Quarterly Journal of Experimental Psychology, 35A*, 347-375.

Kugler, P.N., Kelso, J.A.S., & Turvey, M.T. (1980). On the concept of coordinative structures as dissipative structures. 1 Theoretical lines of convergence. In J.E. Stelmach & J. Requin (Eds.), *Tutorials in motor behavior* (pp. 3-47). Amsterdam: North-Holland.

Luyben, P.D., Funk, D.M., Morgan, J.K., Clark, K.A., & Delulio, D.W. (1986). Team sports for the severely retarded: training a side-of-the-foot soccer pass using a maximum-to-minimum prompt reduction strategy. *Journal of Applied Behavior Analysis, 19*, 431-436.

McIntyre, D.R., & Pfautsch, E.W. (1982). A kinematic analysis of the baseball batting swing involved in opposite-field and same-field hitting. *Research Quarterly for Exercise and Sport, 53*, 206-213.

Newell, K.M. (1985). Coordination, control and skill. In D. Goodman, R.B. Wilberg, & I.M. Franks (Eds.), *Differing perspectives in motor learning, memory, and control* (pp. 295-317). Amsterdam: North-Holland.

Schmidt, R.A., Zelaznik, H.N., Hawkins, B., Frank, J.S., & Quinn, J.T. Jr. (1979). Motor-output variability: A theory for the accuracy of rapid motor acts. *Psychological Review, 86*, 415-451.

Shapiro, D.C., Zernicke, R.F., Gregor, R.J., & Diestel, J.D. (1981). Evidence for generalized motor programs using gait patterns analysis. *Journal of Motor Behavior, 13*, 33-47.

Snyder, C.W. Jr., & Abernethy, B. (in press). *Understanding human action through experimentation.* Champaign, Illinois: Human Kinetics.

Sparrow, W.A. (1989). Creeping patterns of human adults and infants. *American Journal of Physical Anthropology, 78,* 387-401.

Sparrow, W.A., Donovan, E., van Emmerik, R., & Barry, E.B. (1987). Using relative motion plots to measure changes in intra-limb and inter-limb coordination. *Journal of Motor Behavior, 19*, 115-129.

Sparrow, W.A., & Zrizarry-Lopez, V.M. (1987). Mechanical efficiency and metabolic cost as measures of learning a novel gross motor task. *Journal of Motor Behavior, 19*, 240-264.

Winter, D.A., (1987). Are hypotheses really necessary in motor control research? *Journal of Motor Behavior, 19*, 276-279.

Approaches to the Study of Motor Control and Learning
J.J. Summers (Editor)

Chapter 6

CHILDREN'S MOTOR RHYTHM AND TIMING: A DYNAMICAL APPROACH

Helen Parker
University of Western Australia

Despite the complexity of the neuromotor system, highly patterned behaviours may be seen in rhythmic performances. By studying the development of motor rhythms in children, we may gain insight into the processes which coordinate and control action. In the development of movement skill, the rhythmic and timing characteristics of the motor performance undergo systematic, progressive changes. From early stereotyped rhythmic movements in infant movements (serial actions such as kicking, waving, shaking a rattle) we see the development of locomotor actions which, by their very nature, are serial actions and therefore rhythmic. The temporal characteristics of these gross rhythmic actions show firstly a narrow span of temporal control. That is, the young child's performances appear mainly one-paced. Older children are able to match the temporal demands of the environment much better. In adults, temporal synchronisation to a pace-maker becomes increasingly more accurate and stability of dynamical control at a wide tempo range is characteristic. This chapter reviews the literature on infant and children's motor rhythm and timing; provides an account of how the system's dynamics approach may be successfully used to investigate motor rhythms; and provides experimental data from the author's and published research as exemplars of this approach.

In coordinated rhythmic action, separate limbs are constrained to move together in relatively fixed phase relations. The resulting movement has fluency and temporal patterning. "Stated very generally, rhythmic movement is an instance of the formation of simplicity from complexity" (Kugler & Turvey, 1986, p.

408). How does such rhythmic fluency in action develop? Does the phasing between limbs change with development? How stable is the phasing in rhythmic action when performed at different speeds? The way coordinated rhythmic movement patterns emerge from the complex neuro-motor system and the nature of the constraint process are fundamental issues of interest to both motor development and motor control researchers.

To develop an empirical approach to these questions of rhythmic motor control this chapter reviews a wide range of developmental literature. Evidence for naturally occurring rhythmic movements in infants is reviewed. Speculation about the potential value of these movements to later developing control is presented as a precursor to the research on the temporal characteristics of children's rhythmic performance. Historical changes in rhythmic motor control theory is presented next to give the context for many of these developmental studies of motor rhythms. The relatively recent move to employ the approach and methods of complex systems dynamics to motor development, in general, and to interlimb coordination, in particular, is then reviewed in detail. Application of this research perspective in the author's own study of the development of multi-limbed rhythmic action supports the efficacy of the systems dynamics approach for understanding the nature of the control processes in motor rhythms.

MOTOR RHYTHMS IN INFANTS

Research on infants' motor behaviour has shown that stereotyped rhythmic movement, as well as reflexive movement, plays a significant part in normal motor behaviour from the early weeks of life (Kravitz & Boehm, 1971; Thelen, 1979, 1981; Wolff, 1967, 1968). These movements were called rhythmic stereotypies because they were distinctive, repeatable and performed apparently for their own sake without continual sensory regulation (Thelen, 1979). Since the regular temporal patterning in the infants' early actions does not appear to be merely stimulus driven, these movements provide interesting clues about the nature of the internal generation of timing of action. Wolff (1968) favoured innate oscillating control processes.

Both Kravitz and Boehm (1971) and Thelen (1979) conducted one-year longitudinal investigations, the former investigators relied on monthly parent report of 200 infants' rhythmic movements, whereas the latter used ethological methods in fortnightly observations of 20 infant's in their home settings. For Thelen's (1979) study, a bout of rhythmic stereotypy was defined as "a movement of parts of the body or the whole body that was repeated in the same form at least three times at regular short intervals of about a second or less" (p. 700). These studies confirmed Wolff's (1968) findings that rhythmic, stereotyped movements were a significant part of normal infants' developing movement repertoire and that each motor rhythm showed a clear developmental pattern.

From Thelen's (1979) data, up to 47 different rhythmic stereotypies were found in a typical infants' movement repertoire during the first year. These different rhythmic movements showed distinctive developmental patterns, as well as quite consistent onset ages in infants. For example, rhythmic actions of the legs gradually increased in frequency to a peak between 14 and 32 weeks, followed by a gradual decline in frequency to the end of the first year. Hands-and-knees rocking showed a sharper and shorter developmental history, with a burst of behaviours at 24 to 32 weeks, and very few bouts either before or afterwards. Within rhythmic categories, component behaviours showed a maturational trend. Whereas kicking movements began around 10 weeks of age, movements of the foot alone, such as ankle rotations, did not begin until much later, at around 34 weeks. Interestingly, the infant's sex was not a significant factor in any rhythmic category, except for earlier appearance of hands-and-knees rocking in girls (onset at 23.8 weeks) compared to boys (onset at 31.1 weeks).

Importantly, Thelen (1979) also found that the age of onset of rhythmic stereotypies was significantly related to the infant's neuromuscular maturation, as measured by the Bayley Infant Development Scale. The appearance of the stereotyped movements was closely associated (in all but very few cases) with the infant having just assumed that new posture. Thelen (1979) speculated that perhaps these stereotypies were manifestations of immature sensorimotor integration of inherent motor patterns. Perhaps this is an example of Bruner's (1968) notion of motor inflexibility preceding flexibility of action.

Since rhythmic stereotypes in infants often appeared when neural processing capacity became overloaded, Thelen (1979, 1981) also considered whether the rhythmic stereotypies were less demanding on sensory regulation by higher centres compared to more complex movements. Earlier Bruner (1968) and Fentress (1976) had also proposed this idea. Bruner (1968) had described the automatic rhythmic behaviours of breathing, swallowing, and "initial sucking" as systems involving relatively little information processing. These subcortical rhythmic motor patterns appeared in the absence of yet-to-be developed, appropriate goal-directed and corrected behaviour. "As maturation enlarges processing capacity, stereotyped behaviour is replaced by more variable and goal-corrected activity" (Thelen, 1979, p. 713).

Pathological conditions have been associated with both delayed appearance of rhythmic movement as well as abnormally long persistence and delay for re-incorporation of the rhythmic movements into instrumental actions. For example, Down syndrome infants, in contrast to normally developing infants, showed very late onset times into the second year, for behaviour that normally appears in the early months of the first year (Kravitz & Boehm, 1971; Wolff, 1967). Kravitz and Boehm (1971) had suggested that the onset timetable of common rhythmic motor patterns might be valuable indicators of early diagnosis of developmental retardation. This suggestion has merit in light of Thelen's (1979) finding that the timetable of rhythmic stereotypies is significantly related to neuro-developmental status.

From these findings, it is interesting to speculate how the rhythmic stereotypes might become incorporated into, or be related to, later developing serial actions. Wolff (1967, 1968) proposed that rhythmic stereotypies become incorporated into more complex activity through entrainment of their separate rhythms, a model of entrainment similar to that promoted by von Holst (1973). Wolff (1967, 1968) also proposed that rhythmical behaviours of infancy might be manifestations of an "intrinsic neural clock" which became the substrate of later serial order in behaviour.

> Motor development may then be viewed as the transformation of simple rhythmical repetitions or "circular reaction" into integrated actions, whose rhythmical origins are no longer apparent exactly because the component motor parts have been integrated and the associated rhythms have been submerged in complex phase sequences (Wolff, 1967, p. 215).

In summary, stereotyped, rhythmical movements are very much a normal part of human infants' motor development. These movements were shown to systematically change in quantity, quality, and duration throughout the first year. However, the significance of infant rhythmic stereotypies to later motor development and rhythmicity has not conclusively been determined and several hypotheses were advanced by the investigators:

(a) Rhythmic movements were precursors to more complex movements yet to develop (Bruner, 1968; Thelen, 1979);
(b) Phase interactions between the oscillations cause the emergence of new movements with qualitatively different timing (Wolff, 1968);
(c) Rhythmic stereotypies are immature patterns of behaviour requiring less processing capacity for control (Bruner, 1968; Fentress, 1976);
(d) These movements provided a "release" of neural tension appropriate to the level of development (Thelen, 1979; Wolff, 1967); and finally that
(e) The temporal mechanisms underlying the rhythmic stereotypes are used later in development to serially order cognitive behaviour, as well as mature motor behaviour (Wolff, 1967, 1968).

MOTOR RHYTHMS IN CHILDREN

In normal children, motor rhythms are manifest in voluntary actions such as unimanual, bimanual, or single limb movements, or in dancing and musical pursuits. Published studies of children's rhythmic performance are mainly descriptive in nature and rarely theory-based, which reflects the lack of a definitive theory of motor rhythms at the time the studies were conducted. Rhythmic movement control in children has been mainly studied using relatively simple tasks performed in time with some criterion rhythm. Rhythmic matching, or the ability to synchronise action with a beat, is one type of the class of movements named "synkinesis" (Prinz, 1987, p. 50) and requires the actor to generate an internal representation of the temporal pattern of the perceived event.

Rhythmic Single Limb Movements.

For example, a series of studies by Smoll (1974a, 1974b, 1974c, 1975a, 1975b, 1975c, 1975d) described various aspects of motor rhythm in children and adults performing a single limb, shoulder flexion-extension movement on a swinging lever apparatus. He measured timing and spatial errors in reaching the forward, outstretched position for both self-chosen and imposed movement tempos. Subjects studied were adults (aged 18 to 31 years) and children (aged 5 to 11 years).

From these studies, Smoll reported that adults and children had a reliable, preferred movement tempo. However, when the task required synchrony to "timing" beats, a metronome or flashing light, the error variance of performance depended on the subject's age. Young children were unable to accurately maintain the imposed tempo, whereas older subjects were more accurate and less variable in performance. Therefore, the ability to match a rhythm was found to be both age- and tempo-related.

Thomas and Moon (1976), using Smoll's (1974a) apparatus, investigated how well 5-year-old children performed at preferred and imposed tempos. The imposed tempo was at 0.55 Hz, with 0.9 second flexion and 0.9 second extension durations for the action. The children were required to keep time with either an auditory, visual, or visual-auditory signal. For children as young as this, both preferred and imposed conditions proved very difficult. The individual variant scores (VE) were equally high for all conditions - preferred, imposed auditory, imposed visual, and imposed visual-auditory. However, analysis of synchrony accuracy (absolute error of timing and spatial accuracy) showed that the children performed best under the auditory condition. Like Smoll (1975c), Thomas and Moon (1976) found there were no significant differences between 5-year-old girls and boys in all conditions.

More recently, Smoll and Schutz (1982) investigated the ability of adult subjects to match the beats of imposed tempos, both faster (+0.4, and +0.6 of a second) and slower (-0.4, and -0.6 of a second), than their preferred average tempo of arm swing. The results showed that "faster than" preferred tempo conditions led to greatest spatial errors in achieving the positional target. It was, however, the "slower than" condition which led to greatest timing errors.

Recently Geuze and Kalverboer (1987) studied timing inconsistency of serial, elbow flexion and extension movements in a group of normal children and a matched group of clumsy children for self-paced and externally paced conditions (at 0.5 Hz, 0.7 Hz, and 0.9 Hz). Neither a sex difference nor a consistent hand difference in the mean and standard deviation of the movement's contact or flight time was found. Multiple comparisons between the speed conditions showed that each comparison recorded significantly different duration variability. Of interest was the finding that, independent of clumsiness and age, external pacing showed improved consistency compared to the self-paced performance. It seemed that, in these children, the introduction of external pacing facilitated rhythmic timing consistency.

In the self-paced condition, clumsy children showed greater timing inconsistencies for the cycle time, contact time, and flight time compared to the control group. In the externally-paced condition, clumsy children as well as the younger controls (7 and 8 years of age) had greatest difficulty keeping synchrony with the "fast" pace condition. The authors also reported that these children seemed unperturbed by their inability to keep pace and that they tapped away at their own "normal" pace. This evidence suggested that for single limb, serial movements temporal difficulties arose from "fast" tempo rather than "slow" tempo synchrony conditions, although Thomas and Moon (1976) had found in 5-year-olds that both fast and slow tempos were equally difficult.

Rhythmic Tapping.

Other studies examining children's movement rhythms have used tapping tasks (e.g., Gardner, 1971; Thackray, 1969, 1972). Thackray (1969, 1972) evaluated the rhythmic ability of a large number of children (aged 8 to 15 years) on several rhythmic tasks which were scored on a points scale by a panel of expert judges. Results revealed, like other later studies, that there were no differences between the boys' (n = 545) and girls' (n = 556) rhythmic ability. However, some rhythmic abilities were shown to develop later than others. For example, phasing seemed to reach its peak accuracy last of all, whereas accent seemed to develop earlier than did timing and duration control. Thackray (1969) also found that the ability to maintain a steady tempo showed least improvement with increased age, but also points out that even many experienced musicians may be unreliable and erratic in this aspect. Rhythmic synchronisation and imitation were performed equally well by the 8-to 9-year-olds and the 11-year-olds. However, the youngest subjects had great difficulty in performing rhythmic pattern duplication. This result was also found by Gardner (1971), for his 6-year-old subjects. Interestingly, Thackray (1972) believed that overt movement was the foundation of rhythmic experience, a conclusion which concurred with the early published research on motor rhythms (Bolton, 1894;

Isaacs, 1920; Miner, 1903). He recommended that for children with rhythmic difficulties, motor rhythm training is of primary importance, whereas auditory rhythm training is of secondary importance.

Gardner's (1971) investigation of 6-, 8-, and 11-year-old children's rhythmic duplication ability, tested by tapping the pattern with a pencil, showed that when scored on a pass-fail criteria, no sex differences in rhythmic tapping performance existed. However, there were noticeable individual differences at each age level. By 11 years a ceiling effect was found in task difficulty. Although longer patterns showed more errors, a practice effect was noted in children's responses. Since performances were scored either pass or fail, Gardner's (1971) data did not reveal what aspect of rhythmic ability was improving as age increased.

In summary, motor rhythms and synchronisation ability in children has been assessed by a variety of tapping tasks or simple limb movements. These studies showed:

(a) Children were less consistent than adults in preferred rhythmic performance (Smoll, 1974b, 1974c, 1975c, 1975d);
(b) Rhythmic performance was not gender-related (Gardner, 1971; Smoll, 1975d; Thackray, 1969, 1972; Thomas & Moon, 1976);
(c) The accuracy of tempo matching depended on the age, and the speed compared to preferred speed (Geuze & Kalverboer,1987; Thomas & Moon, 1976); and finally
(d) Developmental disability was associated with greater variability during preferred tempo and rhythmic matching tasks (Geuze & Kalverboer, 1987).

Although these studies provided descriptive data of developing motor rhythms, a feature common among them was the lack of any explicit theoretical explanation for developing motor rhythms. In the next section, discussion turns to the evolution of rhythmic movement control theory.

HISTORY OF MOTOR RHYTHM THEORY

The dominant topic of early rhythm research was rhythmic perception rather than motor rhythms although, in 1903, Miner published a comprehensive study of motor rhythms. The earliest control notion was that rhythmic movements were serially chained together by rhythmic afference of the preceding movement (Isaacs, 1920; Miner, 1903; Stetson, 1905). Later, however, evidence from neuro-biological studies pointed to central control of rhythmic movement by neural networks called central pattern generators (von Holst, 1973). This work showed that rhythmic interactions between moving fins occurred independently of rhythmic, external stimulation. The notion of central pattern generators is still a widely accepted explanation of rhythmic movement control. Rhythmic stereotyped movements in infants were explained by internal oscillating processes (Wolff, 1967, 1968). In 1980, Kristan published a review of the different types of hard-wired neural pattern generators which have been identified by neuro-biological investigations. However, he cautioned that some rhythmic behaviour might not be predicted from such a reductionist approach to rhythmic control because of unknown behavioural effects resulting from interactions among particular neural pattern generators.

Cognitive and Systems Dynamics Approaches

Cognitive-based theories of motor control (Schmidt, 1982), and timing (Schmidt, 1982; Shaffer, 1982; Tyldesley & Whiting, 1975; Wing, 1980) have been advanced. Schmidt's (1982) motor control theory, hypothesised a generalised motor program which contained instructions for relative phasing and impulse timing for rhythmic performance. This motor program approach assumed that it is the cognitive processes which specify the temporal and force patterns of action, a so-called "top-down" control strategy. Several other cognitive timing models were based on the notion of internal "clocks", which either triggered movement (Wing, 1980), or provided temporal targets for movement (Shaffer, 1982), or drew timing from the duration of the movement itself (Tyldesley & Whiting, 1975).

From the late 1970's, a new direction for theorising about movement control, the systems dynamical approach, has appeared. The systems dynamics approach, in contrast to the cognitive motor program approach, assumes a predominant role of the system's underlying dynamics to self-organise movement patterns, a "bottom-up" control strategy. The systems dynamics strategy involves identifying low-dimensional variables which describe the behavioural patterning in complex systems and, from analysing the dynamics of these variables (that is, how they change over time), predict the future behaviour of the system (Kelso, 1988). In this view rhythmic movement control is self-organising and can be modelled by the principles of non-linear, limit cycle oscillators (Kugler & Turvey, 1987).

The cognitive and systems dynamical approaches offer contrasting explanations for the achievement of interlimb coordination and rhythmic timing. For interlimb coordination, the cognitive approach invokes the concept of the motor program, with explicitly generated timing and force parameters that determine the action topology. To control rhythmic timing, the relative timing of impulses of an action is stored as an immutable feature of the program. To increase or decrease the overall speed of rhythmic performance, an overall rate parameter is merely applied to the motor program (Schmidt, 1982).

By way of contrast, to account for interlimb coordination the dynamical approach invokes the notion of interacting coordinative structures. The coordinative structure is conceived as a functional synergy of neuro-muscular components. It is assembled to perform that particular task, but unlike the central pattern generator of neuro-biological studies, the coordinative structure is not conceived as a "hard-wired" neuromotor entity. Coordinative structures have been modelled as oscillating, energy-dissipating, self-organising assemblies with three limit cycle features: (1) preferred phasing and amplitude (attractor states), (2) frequency entrainment of oscillators, and (3) relative stability to perturbing influences such as scaled-up performance speed. In this theoretical approach, rhythmic timing is argued to be an emergent property of the coordinative structures' dynamical state. In other words, there is no explicit timing parameter controlling rhythmic movement (Kelso & Tuller, 1985).

MOTOR RHYTHM DEVELOPMENT AND SYSTEMS DYNAMICS

In the development of motor control, the attainment of stability in rhythmic coordination has yet to be fully explained. Since rhythmic movement is highly patterned temporally, it provides a window by which pattern formation in movement may be better examined and understood. The principles of systems dynamics has been recently employed to research the development of coordination in movement patterns (for example, Clark, Whitall, & Phillips, 1988; Roberton & Halverson, 1988; Thelen, 1985, 1986, 1988).

Thelen's (1988, 1989) recent synthesis of systems dynamics concepts with data from her research, provided a theoretical framework to explain how motor development might occur. She used systems dynamics' concepts of attractor states; stability and fluctuation; emergent pattern formation and coordinative structures; and order and control parameters to provide a principled account of motor development.

Longitudinal investigations of motor development have clearly identified that different coordination stages emerge (for example, Halverson, Roberton, & Langendorfer [1982] in overarm throwing; and Halverson & Williams [1986], Roberton & Halverson [1984, 1988] in hopping). From the systems dynamics approach, the development of greater movement diversity and complexity are explained by bifurcation processes. When a control parameter is scaled up, the relative stability of the system is disrupted. If these system fluctuations are large enough, due to a critical point in the scaling of the control parameter being reached, the system is driven to a new, more stable, solution. This process is called the bifurcation or phase shift. By such repeated bifurcations, movement complexity increases, resulting in multistabilities. In Thelen's (1988) view, "...development must be viewed as a series of more-or-less stable attractors that are task assembled,..." (p. 365).

Underlying any new stable attractor state is the formation of a new ensemble of components, called the coordinative structure. Practice, maturation, and social facilitation, Thelen (1988) speculated, stabilised the components within this new attractor state until some different scaling of a control parameter caused a new phase shift and further bifurcation.

According to systems dynamics, although multiple causes invoke change, the different control parameters which emerge to drive phase shifts do not themselves specify the nature of the change (Jeka & Kelso, 1989). This notion is supported by Thelen's developmental research. For example, her investigations of the changes in 2- to 4-month-old infants' stepping patterns, during a period of rapidly increasing fat deposition, identified body build as the control parameter in the first few months of an infant's first year (Thelen & Fisher, 1982; Thelen, Fisher, & Ridley-Johnson, 1984). In the second half of an infant's first year, however, Thelen found that other control parameters became predominant - extensor muscle strength for single leg support and neuro-motor maturation for upright stability. Giving assistance to balance enhanced the stepping performance of 10- and 11-month-old infants. However, assisted balance had little effect as a control parameter on either younger, pre-stepping infants or on older toddlers in whom upright stepping had become well established (Thelen, 1988). Thelen's synthesis of systems dynamics' principles with coordination development has provided a theoretical framework for new research paradigms for investigating the development of motor control. In the following section, two examples of how this approach was employed in investigations of children's gait coordination are discussed.

THE DEVELOPMENT OF COORDINATION

The focus for the majority of this work has been the development of intra- and interlimb coordination in locomotion. These studies have relevance to this discussion of motor rhythms because locomotion, as a serial action, is also rhythmic by nature. Their common theoretical approach was to view the development of interlimb coordination as the result of phase entrainment by self-sustaining, nonlinear oscillatory processes within the system (Clark et al., 1988; Clark & Whitall, 1989; Thelen, Kelso, & Fogel, 1987; Whitall, 1989). Phase entrainment of oscillating coordinative structures constrained the system complexity and resulted in different locomotor gaits. To test the stability of the particular interlimb coordination (phasing), the action is perturbed in some relevant way, such as by altering the inertia of the limbs (e.g., Whitall., 1989).

Children's Locomotion.

The first example chosen to illustrate the application of these systems dynamics principles is Whitall's (1989) study of children's running and galloping. She hypothesised that interlimb coordination was achieved by the phasing, entrainment, and structural stability characteristics of coupled, nonlinear, limit cycle oscillators. From a developmental perspective, it was assumed that alternate phasing of limbs in running was more efficient than the asymmetric phasing in galloping, and predicted that running would show greater phasing stability and entrainment at an earlier age than would galloping. In order that children should achieve the less efficient asymmetric phasing of galloping, Whitall (1989) argued that they would need to uncouple the symmetric pattern of running.

Forty females, eight children in each of the age groups 3, 4, 6, and 9 years plus an adult group, were studied. From the high speed film (64 fps) of the sagittal view of the subject's running and galloping at preferred speed, measures of interlimb phasing were made. The phasing pattern between limbs was measured as that proportion of the limb cycle (either in units of time or distance) when footstrike occurred on the contralateral limb for each successive pair of footstrikes. The dynamical constructs of phase locking and entrainment were quantified by measuring the consistency of the step timing phasing and distance phasing for consecutive contralateral footstrikes in each trial. To test the structural stability of the interlimb coordination, Whitall (1989) perturbed the limb's inertia by strapped a weight equivalent to 4% of body mass to one of the limbs and measuring the difference in mean phasing between the nonperturbed and perturbed conditions.

Results for the preferred speed condition showed that the phasing modes were distinctive between the two gaits in each age group. Running showed interlimb phasings of 50:50 for both timing and step distance measures, that is, the contralateral footstrike occurred at the 50% point of the other limb's step cycle. However, galloping showed an uneven timing phasing of 69:31 and an interlimb step distance phasing of 40:60. Since the variability of temporal and amplitude phasing measures was small, both between subjects and within gaits in the preferred tempo condition, it was concluded that the two gaits demonstrated phase locking. However, the unique gait phasings for running compared to galloping were interpreted to indicate significant entrainment differences between them.

Under weight perturbation, running showed no significant change in the mean temporal phasing of limbs. However in galloping, weight perturbation caused significant changes in temporal and amplitude phasing in the children. As predicted by Whitall (1989), structural stability in the gallop was developmentally related, with adults recording significantly lower perturbation effects compared to all other groups. Nine-year-olds were not different from 6-year-olds, who in turn, were not different from 4-year-olds. Whereas running showed equally stable temporal and amplitude stability, galloping showed greater temporal stability than amplitude stability. Amplitude instability in galloping was manifest in a change in the length of the next step after the weighted limb's swing and footstrike. However, amplitude readjustment to the altered limb inertias occurred within the first few of four galloping steps that were recorded.

From these findings, Whitall (1989) concluded that running showed the characteristics of nonlinear, limit cycle oscillator control at earlier ages compared to galloping. The systems dynamical approach appeared to be a useful approach for investigating developing gait coordination.

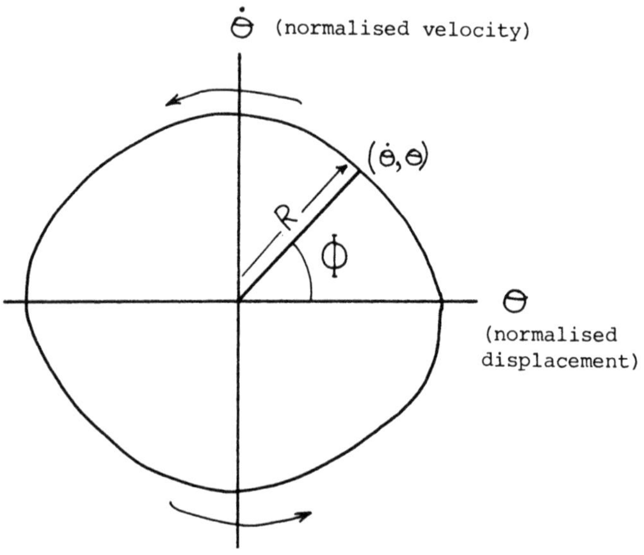

Figure 1. Stylised phase portrait with phase angle (Φ) and radial amplitude (R) marked.

Phase Portrait Analysis of Children's Interlimb Coordination.

The second example of a developmental study which was conducted from a systems dynamics approach is that of Roberton and Halverson (1988). They used the methodology of phase portraits to quantify interlimb phasing in dynamical terms.

Phase portrait analysis allows the quantification of the underlying dynamics and interactions of oscillating systems (Abraham & Shaw, 1982). For rhythmic joint movements, phase portraits are the cross-plots of range normalised joint velocity and displacement. Such plots may be quantified by two polar variables, phase angle, and radial amplitude (see Figure 1).

When phase portraits are constructed for repeated cycles of rhythmic joint action, one notes the relative "fuzziness" of the band of cycles (see Figure 2). This is an indication of the degrees of freedom encompassed in the coordinative structure. Tightly constrained, coordinated, one-degree of freedom motion in the phase plane would result in stable and consistent phase angles from cycle to cycle, a near-perfect circle and the band of "fuzziness" would be narrow.

Qualitative analysis of the shapes of trajectory segments of phase portraits is possible (Winstein & Garfinkel, 1989). This qualitative analysis relies on comparing the shape of segments of the phase portrait with trajectories produced by a known dynamical system. From this comparison one may infer the type of control underlying the dynamical system. According to Winstein and Garfinkel (1989) bursting-type control at the end of a trajectory produces a square shape, interrupted control produces cusps, and a smooth restoring force produces rounded segments at the extreme of the movement range. It appears from the literature that qualitative analysis of this type has not yet been used with developmental movement patterns.

For developmental studies, a number of questions arise regarding qualitative analysis. In what ways do the shapes of the phase portrait change with performers of different ages, with variations in performance tempos, and with limb preference? If phase portraits show systematic, age-related and tempo-related changes in topology then the underlying dynamics of the system are also changing (Roberton & Halverson, 1988).

Quantitative analysis of phase portraits is relatively more common. Consistent phase angle measures indicate that the underlying dynamics of the action are controlled by low-dimensional dynamic equations - that the system is coordinated. For example, at the initiation of upright independent gait, infants showed intralimb coordinative structures similar to adults (Truly, Clark, Phillips, & Caldwell, 1989). The phase angle of the thigh's reversal of direction on the shank's phase portrait for new walkers was not statistically different to that measured in adults. Although the infant's control of shank movement was more variable than adults to begin with, Truly et al., (1989) found that this difference had disappeared by 3 months of walking experience. They concluded that the combination of task and human anatomical constraints in independent upright walking "afforded" a single intralimb coordination, which was present at the beginning of independent walking. To test this notion further, future studies should measure thigh-shank coordination in infants' pre-walking stages, such as the "cruising" gait and supported walking.

In Roberton and Halverson's (1988) study of hopping development, changing leg action dynamics were explored in both the swing and the hopping limbs. This study is unique, at present, among the published developmental literature adopting the systems dynamical approach because of the longitudinal nature of the data. Hopping development was studied from film records in 7 children, each studied from 3 years of age for a minimum of 15 years. Kinematic data (angular displacement, velocity) were calculated from the film records sampled at 64 fps. Roberton and Halverson (1988) aimed to identify the emergence of relative interlimb phasing indicative of mature hopping.

Their data revealed timing invariances in the action of the support leg across developmental levels. From the earliest developmental stage of hopping through to the most advanced stage, the proportion of time of the total hop cycle from foot contact with the ground to deepest knee bend in hopping was constant. This early timing invariance compares with Truly et al's (1989) findings of timing invariances in the early stages of independent walking. During hopping development, the other three limbs gradually become entrained to this support limb, however Roberton and Halverson (1988) showed that the entrainment proceeded differently in different children. Some children started swinging the swing limb before pumping their arms bilaterally, while other children did the reverse.

Differences were revealed in the phase portraits of the support knee action. The phase portraits illustrated clear shape differences between the developmental levels described for hopping. The pattern changed from a spiral, to a top-loop, and then to a bottom-loop pattern with increased hopping skill. In Winstein and Garfinkel's (1989) analysis, such loops show the influence of position-dependent forces that oppose motion such as in pendular and spring-like systems.

Interlimb coordination in hopping was measured from the phase angles in the contralateral limb's phase portrait at (a) the initiation of the swing limb's forward movement, and (b) the beginning of the support limb's extension. Roberton and Halverson (1988) predicted that interlimb coordination would be quantified by consistent phase angles at each of the four developmental levels seen in hopping. Briefly, these levels showed the following characteristics. In Level 1, children show one or two rudimentary hops with only momentary flight achieved through a "pull-up" action in the support leg. In Level 2, the action has advanced to a "fall and catch" style which is achieved by combining a forward body lean with a minimal amount of knee and ankle extension to push against the ground. By Level 3 hopping is performed with a projected takeoff, which also shows a short delay between the flexion motions of the ankle and knee at landing and their extension motions at takeoff. In this stage the swing leg begins to assist the production of force by swinging forwards during the supporting leg's extension action. The fourth level is the most advanced, with well-timed actions to absorb the landing forces and to roll forward to the ball of the foot prior to the extension of the ankle and knee joints. Roberton and Halverson (1988) predicted that Level 4 phase angle values would be different because of new coordination relationships at this higher skill level and also that the phase angle variability for developmental Level 4 would be less. The developmental levels in hopping were based on behavioural description of the lower limb movements. Level 3 children attempt to pump the swing leg whereas in Level 4 children, the range of the swing leg forward-backward motion is increased.

Results for the support leg showed that this leg's phase angle was significantly different at Level 3 (0.66 radians) compared to Level 4 (0.98 radians) at the initiation of the forward swing of the swing limb. However, no significant developmental difference was apparent in the swing limb's phase angles at the initiation of support knee extension. Further, timing of the occurrence of peak forward velocity of the swing leg with the occurrence of the beginning of support knee extension showed no significant difference between Level 3 and Level 4 children.

On the basis of two further results that related interlimb coordination to the velocity of limbs, Roberton and Halverson (1988) speculated that velocity per se, rather than phase angle, was the coordinating variable used in the hop. The first of these two results was the simultaneous initiation of forward movement of the swing leg with the landing (within 15 ms of landing). The second result showed that peak forward swing velocity of the swing knee was almost simultaneous with the beginning of support knee extension (30 ms after peak swing velocity). Phase angles of these same features, by contrast, showed high intra-subject variability and thus it was concluded that hopping coordination did not rely on position-velocity, or phase angle, states.

Overall, Roberton and Halverson (1988) concluded that the findings supported a systems dynamical interpretation. They viewed the support limb to be like a "forcing oscillator" (Abraham & Shaw, 1982; von Holst, 1973), to which the swing limb gradually became entrained. The timing of swing leg forward movement showed developmental changes, whereas the timing of peak velocity of the swing leg with respect to the support knee's extension showed no developmental changes. The swing leg motion was entrained to the oscillation pattern of the already occurring (in a developmental sense) support knee extension. Results did not point to the reverse process of the support limb entraining to the swinging limb. The developmental difference apparent between Levels 3 and 4 was shown to be due to earlier initiation of the forward movement in the swinging limb. This occurred, it was proposed, to fit the on-going dynamics of the support limb, as well as to accommodate the longer swing duration evident at Level 4 hopping.

Four-Limbed Rhythmic Coordination

In order to understand the process of development of stable, four-limbed coordination there is a need to investigate the control of multi-limbed rhythmicity and its temporal flexibility in a setting as natural and unconstrained as possible. Investigating natural actions, rather than contrived ones, retains ecological validity in such studies.

To date, no published studies have been found on a dynamical analysis of four-limbed rhythmic coordinated action in children, although Jeka and Kelso (1988) reported the relative stability of different coordination modes for hand and feet tapping movements in adults under the stress of external pacing. To fill this gap, the systems dynamics approach was applied to the development of a four-limbed rhythmic movements in a rhythmic matching paradigm. The task chosen for analysis was the starjump (or jumping jacks) (Parker, 1990a).

In starjumping, contralateral limbs are abducted and adducted in mirror-image, with repetitive astride jumps. Since this skill is not typically classified as a fundamental motor skill of childhood, little information exists in the literature about its developmental timetable (Keogh, 1968, 1969; Magalhaes, Koomar, & Cermak, 1989). Nevertheless, the skill is one encountered by children during physical education classes, fitness exercises and playground games.

Keogh's (1968, 1969) survey of the mastery of starjumping, as part of a larger study of the development of limb control in normal children, showed age-related improvements and sex differences in performance at volitional cadence. For 570 children the passing percentage of boys was 8% (at 5 years of age), 42% (at 6 years), and 62% (at 7 years), while for girls the corresponding percentages were 30% (5 years), 55% (6 years), and 97% (7 years). At combined ages of 8 and 9 years, 85% of a sample of 60 boys compared to 97% of 60 girls passed the assessment. Keogh (1968) suggested that females' advanced physiological maturity might explain this result (see also Greulich & Pyle, 1959). However, there is also strong evidence for gender differences in children's play (for example, Sutton-Smith, Rosenberg, & Morgan, 1963), which could contribute to the earlier acquisition of rhythmic coordination by girls compared to boys.

Recently, Magalhaes et al., (1989) reported developmental changes in starjumping of 5 to 9 year old boys and girls. They reported that starjumps were performed quite skilfully above the age of 7 years (with a performance score of 92% and better), however below this age consistent and correct performance was not the norm (63% and 74% performance scores for 5- and 6-year-olds respectively). These age differences were statistically significant, however in contrast to Keogh's findings, starjumping performance was not sex-related in any of the measures. Because starjumping showed reliable differences among young children, Magalhaes et al. (1989) recommended that their starjump scale might be a useful screening tool to assess the level of bilateral motor coordination in young children.

Two aspects require particular attention in the investigation of the development of children's multi-limbed rhythmic movements. The first relates to the dynamical investigation of the development of entrainment among all limbs in the action. Upper limb action, and its incorporation into hopping, was evaluated only descriptively in Roberton and Halverson's (1988) developmental levels. However, phase portrait methods allow a quantitative approach to describing the development of multi-limbed coordination. The second aspect relates to measuring the internal consistency of the dynamic variables during repeated cycles of action by children. Developmental data published so far, has focused on dynamic descriptions from the phase portrait of either a single cycle of the action (for example, Roberton & Halverson, 1988) or of very few steps in locomotion (for example, Clarke, Clark, Phillips, & Caldwell, 1989; Truly et al., 1989; Whitall, 1989). These two aspects were focused on in Parker's (1990a) study of starjumping.

Three groups of 11 males aged 7, 9, and 18+ years were asked to perform starjumps at their preferred tempo and at metronome-paced trials slower and faster than this. The subjects aimed to keep in time with the metronome beat as accurately as possible. In all, six trials were performed at the following paces - PR, the self-paced preferred tempo; S2, 125% of preferred tempo interjump interval (IJI, slowest); S1, 120% of preferred IJI (slow); PM, 100% of preferred IJI (preferred tempo, metronome-paced); F1, 90% of preferred IJI (fast); and F2, 80% of preferred IJI (fastest). An electronic metronome presented the pacing beat for starjumping. Since the pacing tempo was set in relation to each individual's preferred tempo the relative "difficulty" of the pacing for each individual was controlled.

VICON motion analysis system was used to track the motions of reflective joint markers in the frontal plane at 60 Hz sampling frequency for 5 starjump cycles (that is, 11 repetitive astride-and-together jumps). FMAP software (Wood, 1985) smoothed the raw data with a Butterworth, second-order recursive, low pass, digital filter set to 8.5 Hz and calculated the angular displacement and angular velocity of each upper and lower limb. Footswitches recorded the timing of each successive ground contact. Timing and phase portrait variables were analysed by general linear models MANOVA for Age (3 groups) X Limb Type (arm or leg) X Tempo (6 levels, repeated), with post hoc Tukey comparisons ($p < 0.05$).

Rhythmic Timing Results

For rhythmic timing in starjumping, children's ability to match the pacing beat supported earlier findings of Smoll (1974b,c, 1975c,d) and Thomas and Moon (1976). Temporal synchrony was measured as the difference in time between the instance of each footfall and each metronome beat. The mean synchrony error (constant error, CE) and intra-subject variability (variable error, VE) were calculated and normalised to percentage of the interbeat duration. Statistically significant age, group, and tempo interactions were found in both the percentage accuracy and percentage variability data from the repeated measures MANOVA (Parker & Lockwood, 1988).

At tempos slower than preferred pace, the youngest children recorded significantly greater mean constant and variable errors of rhythmic synchrony. At the slowest, slow, and metronome-paced preferred tempos the 7-year-olds recorded the highest "lead" errors of all groups with mean values of 158.6%, 140.8%, and 125.1%, respectively (scores of 100% signify perfect synchrony; >100% signify a "lead" error). For these same tempos, 9-year-olds scored 125.4%, 115.4%, and 108.4%, and adults scored 111.5%, 109.9%, and 106.2%, respectively. For the fast and fastest tempos all groups scored within 4% of perfect synchrony and the differences between the aged groups failed to reach significance.

For percentage variability (%VE), 7-year-olds scored 11.5% (at the slowest tempo), 6.8% (slow tempo), 2.7% (metronome-paced preferred tempo), 2.0% (fast), and 2.4% (fastest), whereas adults scored less than 2% error across all tempos. Tukey post hoc comparisons showed the differences between adults and 7-year-olds were significant at each tempo. The respective comparative scores for 9-year-olds were 5.7%, 3.5%, 1.9%, 1.7%, and 1.1%.

In summary, results showed that the ability to synchronise starjumps with the pacing beat was both age- and tempo-related. For the slow tempos, the youngest subjects were unable to slow their performances enough to match the beat, however they were able to speed up to match the faster tempos. At the faster tempos they were not significantly different to older children and adults. The variability with which the 7-year-olds matched the beat also reduced as the tempo increased, although they were significantly more variable than adults at all tempos.

Phase Portrait Results

Phase portraits of the right shoulder at each tempo for an Adult, a 9-year-old, and 7-year-old are shown in Figure 2. From these illustrations it can be seen that the adult shows greater consistency (the trajectories are less "fuzzy") compared to the children at any tempo. It can also be seen that the shape and size of the portraits change as the performance tempo increases. Both qualitative and quantitative methods were employed to analyse the phase portraits.

Qualitative analysis of phase portrait shapes revealed age- and tempo-related changes in the nature of the underlying dynamical control. For the shoulder joint, adults showed smooth, oval-shaped portraits which became increasingly square as tempo increased. Oval shapes at the extreme range of movement are characteristic of smooth restoring forces, as in "elastic-type" control. However, square profiles indicate a change to a "bursting-type" control. In contrast, 7-year-olds show less squareness at fast tempos and more cusps at slow tempos in the phase portraits. Cusps, according to Winstein and Garfinkel (1989) are

RIGHT SHOULDER PHASE PORTRAITS IN STARJUMPING

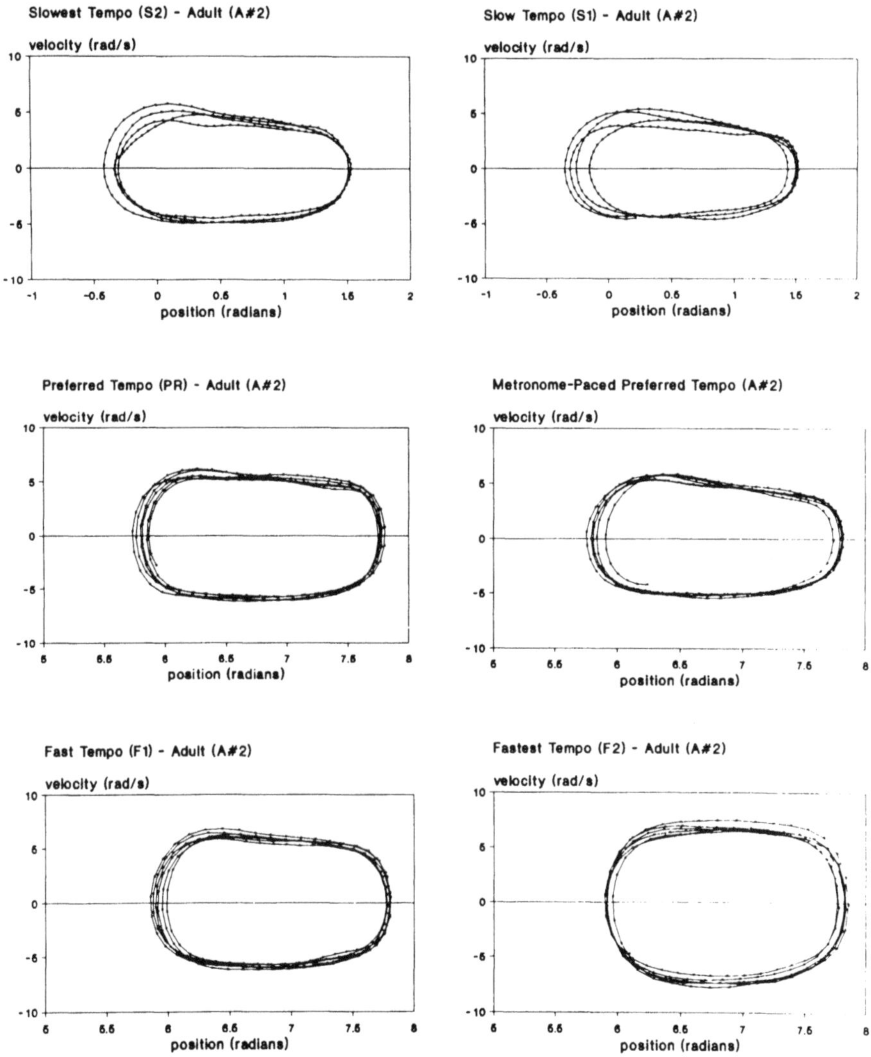

Figure 2(a). Phase portraits of the right shoulder of an adult starjumping at different tempos.

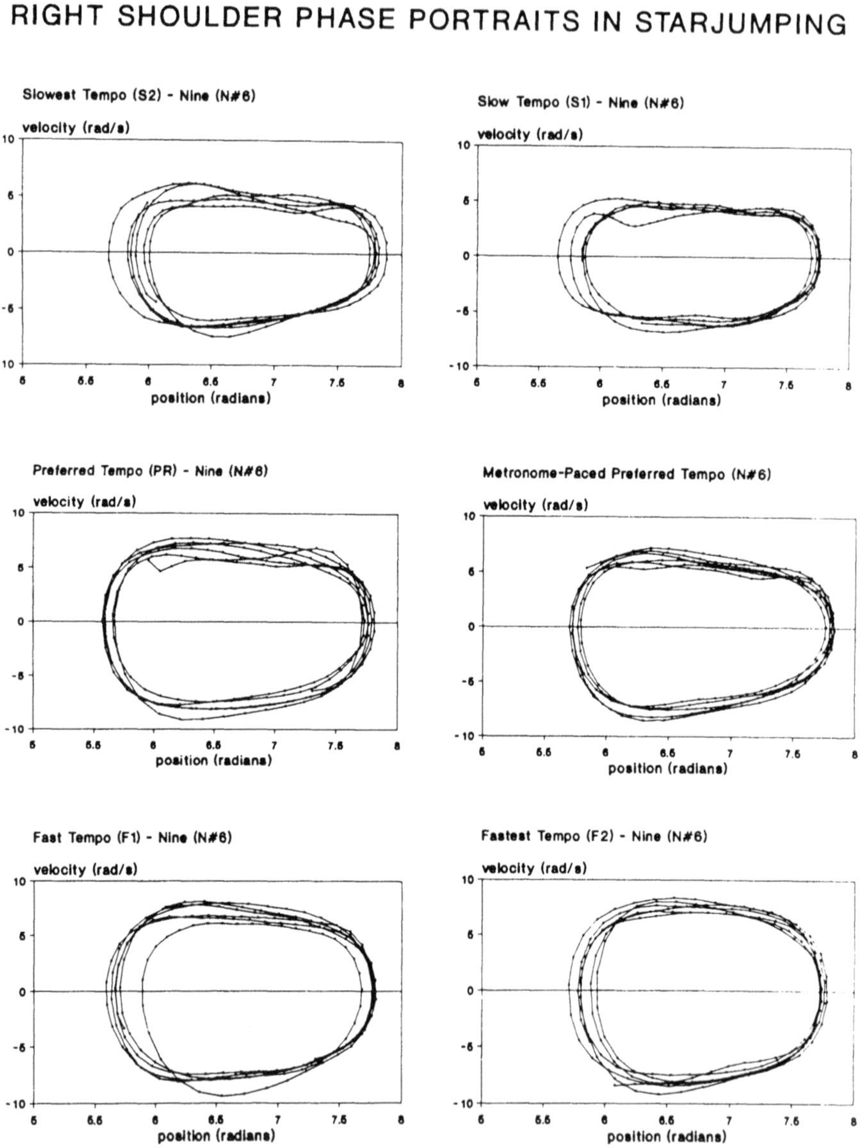

Figure 2(b). Phase portraits of the right shoulder of a 9-year-old starjumping at different tempos.

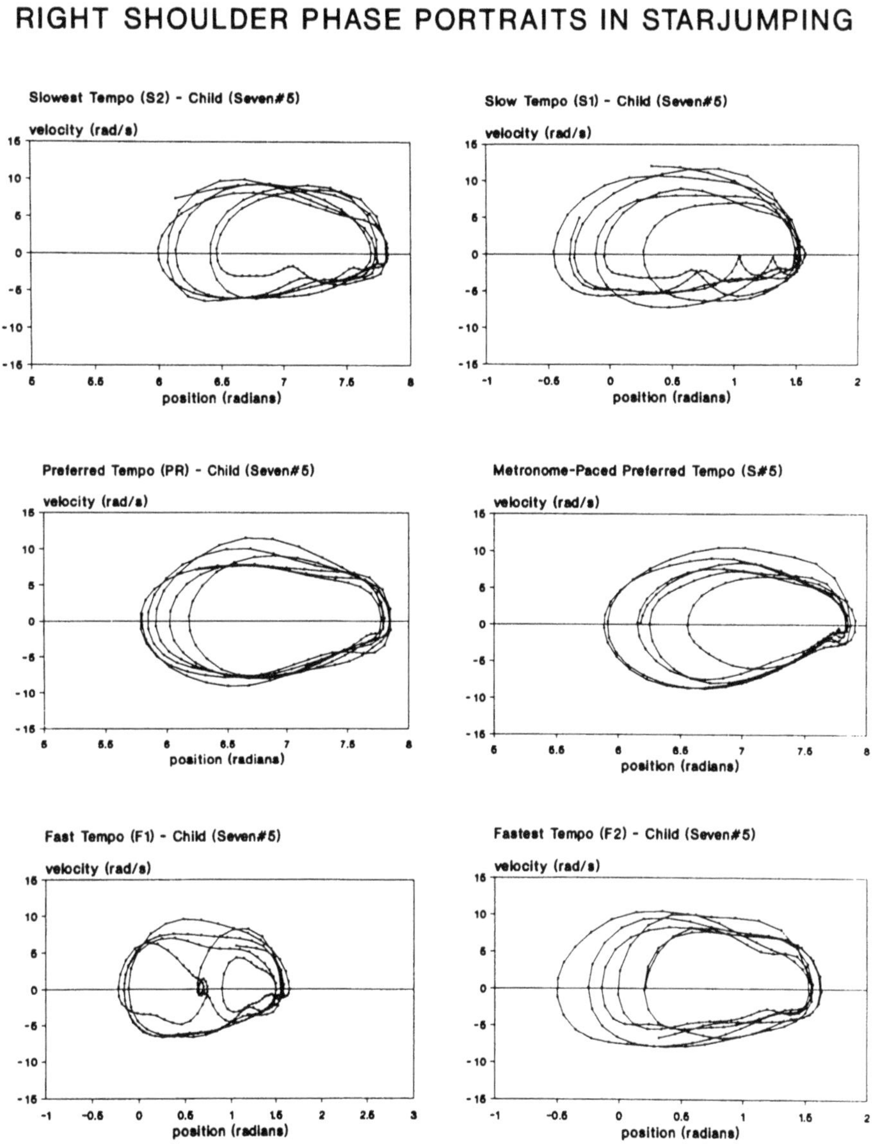

Figure 2(c). Phase portraits of the right shoulder of a seven-year-old starjumping at different tempos.

indicative of interrupted or perturbed dynamical control. The 9-year-old has phase portraits with adult-like characteristics.

Quantitative analyses of the phase portraits were made by measuring the phase angle and radial amplitude for range normalised plots at the instance of each successive foot contact in each trial (see Figure 1). From these raw measures, three dependent variables were extracted as descriptors of the hypothesised limit cycle behaviour:

(a) Phase preference - mean contact phase angle;
(b) Interlimb entrainment - standard deviation of contact phase angle; and
(c) Dynamic stability - standard deviation of radial amplitude.

Overall, it was expected that preferred tempo performance would be the most stable at each age, but as tempos deviated from this tempo it was predicted that stability would deteriorate in young children but remain relatively unchanged for adults. Thus, adult performers were expected to maintain phase preference, interlimb entrainment, and stability across all the performance tempos.

Analysis of the data showed significant interactions between age, group, and performance tempo in phase preference (Figure 3), entrainment (Figure 4), and dynamic stability (Figure 5).

Phase preference data revealed that the mean phase angles of 7-year-olds were significantly lower than 9-year-olds and adults at the two faster than preferred tempos for "in" contact data, and for both slow and fast tempos for "out" contact data. The two older groups did not show significant changes in mean phase angles for hips or shoulders across tempo. Therefore, phase preference was characteristic of the starjumping in adults and older children, but not in young children.

Interlimb entrainment data (the variability of phase angles), showed adults had significantly lower standard deviations across all tempos compared to either the 9- or 7-year-olds for "in" cycle data. In turn, 9-year-olds recorded significantly lower standard deviations than 7-year-olds at the two preferred pace trials. For the "out" cycle the 7-year-olds were significantly more variable than the Adults across all tempos. Interestingly, 9-year-olds performed with greater variability than Adults at the extreme tempos only. Thus dynamic fluctuation in interlimb coordination was revealed in children at the most extreme tempos in the range. Within the children's groups, the 7-year-olds' interlimb entrainment was much poorer than that of 9-year-olds at the two preferred tempos and the fast tempo. In Figure 4b, both Adults and 9-year-olds show little difference between arm or leg phase angle variability across tempos. However, the 7-year-olds show an interaction between limb phase angle variability and the two fast tempos. As tempo quickened, the phase angle variability for their legs increased, while the phase angle variability of their arms decreased.

In summary, the phase angle variability data showed that in adults, interlimb entrainment was consistently strong regardless of the performance tempo.

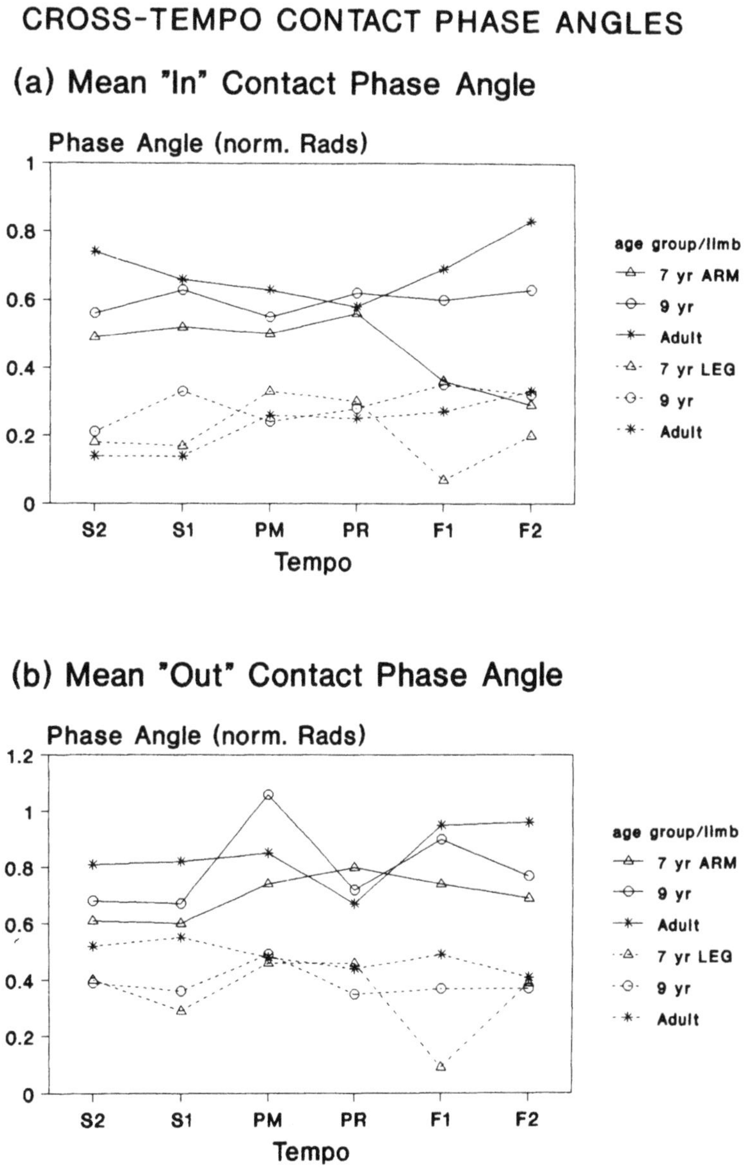

Figure 3. Phase preference as indicated by mean phase angles of children and adults starjumping at different tempos. "In" and "Out" refer to the together and astride feet contact positions respectively. "In" denotes phase angle at "in" contact position. "Out" denotes phase angle at "out" contact position. Refer to text for tempo categories.

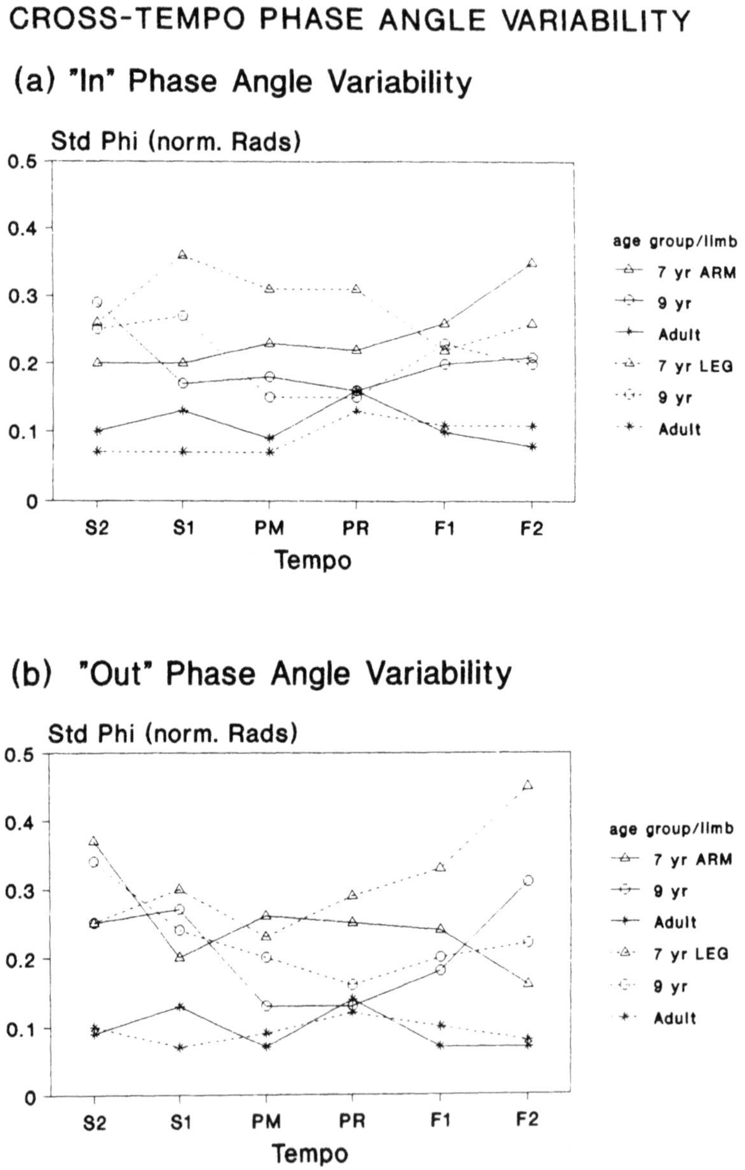

Figure 4. Entrainment strength as indicated by phase angle variability of children and adults starjumping at different tempos. "In" and "Out" refer to the together and astride feet contact positions respectively. "In" denotes phase angle at "in" contact position. "Out" denotes phase angle at "out" contact position. Refer to text for tempo categories.

However, in children once performance tempos shifted away from preferred tempos interlimb entrainment became more variable, particularly for the 7-year-olds.

Stability in the system dynamics ("fuzziness" of phase plots) to perturbing effects of tempo was quantified by the variability of the radial amplitude of the phase portraits (see Figure 5). Results showed that adults had significantly lower phase portrait variability than both children's groups at all performance tempos, except at the preferred tempo for 9-year-olds. At this tempo, the variability of radial amplitude for adults and 9 year old children was equivalent. The 9-year-olds had significantly lower variability than the 7-year-olds for all tempos but the metronome-paced preferred tempo. Data also revealed that for children the arms recorded significantly lower radial amplitude standard deviations than the legs at all performance tempos, but for adults the difference between the arms and legs was small and not statistically significant. Therefore, the overall stability or "fuzziness" of the limb's phase portrait revealed developmental differences.

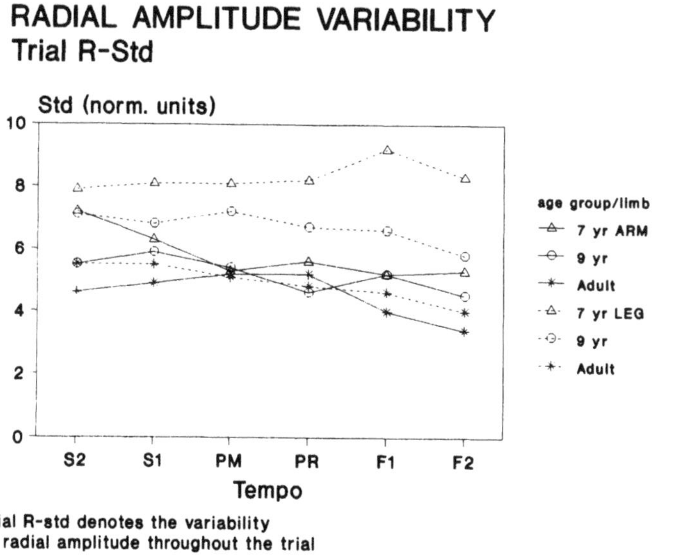

Figure 5. Dynamic stability as indicated by radial amplitude variability of children and adults starjumping at different tempos. "In" and "Out" refer to the together and astride feet contact positions respectively. Refer to text for tempo categories.

Discussion

In summary, rhythmic timing and phase portrait variables in starjumping were affected by age and performance tempos. The temporal data showed that both mean error (%CE) and synchrony variability (%VE) were significantly greater for 7-year-olds compared to 9-year-olds and adults. However, slow tempos were the most difficult for the youngest children to match, with characteristically high "lead" errors. For the faster tempos, however, their synchrony errors were not significantly different to older children and adults. The variability with which the 7-year-olds matched the beat also reduced as the tempo increased, although they were significantly more variable than adults at all tempos (Parker, 1990a; Parker & Lockwood, 1988).

Taken as a whole, phase portrait analysis revealed that starjumping control was like coupled, nonlinear oscillators with limit cycle properties. Importantly, however, the evidence showed that each predicted characteristic of limit cycle oscillation was age-related and tempo-related. Phase preference was evident in adults across all tempos, but only at faster than preferred tempos for young children. Interlimb entrainment for adults was tightly coupled at all tempos but for children performing at other than preferred tempos, the interlimb entrainment became less tightly coupled. Finally, dynamic stability was evident in adults at all tempos, in contrast to children who showed stability only at preferred tempos. When required to perform at tempos slower and faster than the preferred tempos, instability or fuzziness was greater in children (Parker, 1990a, 1990b, in preparation). This concurs with Thelen's (1988, 1989) notion that development consists of a series of relatively stable phase attractor states, and that these fluctuate under the influence of particular control parameters.

Therefore, immature, developing control systems show motor rhythm instability in the face of changed performance tempos. Youngest children showed an inability, as yet, to slow down enough to synchronise starjumps with slower than preferred tempos while the dynamical data revealed a stronger phase preference, at these same slower tempos. Regardless of the actual tempo of the slow beat, it appeared that the youngest children performed closer to their own preferred pace. A similar finding was reported by Geuze and Kalverboer (1987). They reported that in rhythmic synchronisation of a forearm movement, the tempo of clumsy and young children's movement was irrespective of the pacing beat. For the young starjumping children, scaling the gain in the system's oscillator control downwards appeared not yet achievable. However, increasing the gain was achievable, as shown in children's accurate temporal synchrony for the faster beat trials. One consequence of achieving this was a change in phase preference and weaker interlimb entrainment in the limb dynamics. Such a change was not seen in the data of older children and adults - phase preference was maintained across the different tempo conditions as was temporal synchronicity. Whitall (1989) showed a similar stronger phase locking and structural stability in adults than in young children for the galloping gait, although this was tested by weight perturbation not tempo perturbation.

The children's starjumping data revealed that the features of the nonlinear, limit cycle oscillator model are evident at self-selected performance tempos but become less apparent at other pacing tempos. Further, the ability to increase the frequency gain by these young children was not necessarily concomitant with improved dynamical stability.

Self-paced multi-limbed, rhythmic coordination develops with increased stability in phase preference and entrainment features of self-organised limit cycle dynamics. However, to perform rhythmic matching tasks also demands some level of cognitive constraint over the self-organising system dynamics with regard to correcting the temporal mismatch between the beat and the response.

When a child successfully performs a rhythmic matching task, we observe that the child's motor performance speed is adjusted to match the external beat. To achieve control of a multi-limbed skill and perform it synchronously with a beat, the dynamics of the neuromotor system need to be constrained at least at two levels - the cognitive and dynamical. At the cognitive level, the child must firstly perceive the tempo of beats and their own tempo. Secondly, kinaesthetic-auditory cross-modal matching must occur to detect any temporal mismatch, and then the lead or lag errors be corrected by setting the system to drive the action at a faster or slower pace. If the action is to remain topologically the same, then at the dynamical level, the strength and mode of interlimb coordination should be maintained. However, in order to scale-up or scale-down the tempo, an internal forcing oscillator's gain is increased or reduced, in some way, to produce faster or slower frequencies respectively. In a tightly coupled system, other oscillator frequencies are autonomously entrained to match this frequency - multiple limbs remain coordinated with the beat.

By way of conclusion, quantitative modelling of motor development from the systems dynamic approach is in its infancy. There is much work still to be done to understand the nature of the constraint process that produces stable, coordinated, rhythmic movement. The empirical and theoretical challenge presented by the dynamical perspective is to determine which control variable(s) operate to promote stability or fluctuations in motor development. As stated above, the effects of any particular control variable would vary and different variables have potency over developmental time (Thelen, 1988). To identify control variables, increased variability and vulnerability of system stability to perturbations is mooted as a tool by which to investigate developmental transitions to new and relatively stable phase states.

REFERENCES

Abraham, R.H., & Shaw, C.D. (1982). *Dynamics - The geometry of behaviour, Part I: Periodic behavior*. Santa Cruz, CA: Aerial Press.

Bolton, T.L. (1894). Rhythm. *Journal of Psychology*, *6*, 145-238.

Bruner, J. (1968). On voluntary action and its hierarchical structure. In A. Koestler & J.R. Smythies (Eds.), *Beyond reductionism. New perspectives in the life sciences* (pp. 161-179). New York: Macmillan.

Clarke, L.C., Clark, J.E., Phillips, S.J. & Caldwell, G. (1989). Intralimb coordination in walking: Does the lower extremity act as coupled non-linear limit-cycle oscillator [Abstract]. *Proceedings of the Annual Conference of NASPSPA Psychology of Motor Behavior and Sport*. Kent State University, Kent, OH, June 1-4.

Clark, J.E., & Whitall, J. (1989). Changing patterns of locomotion: From walking to skipping. In Woollacott, M., & Shumway-Cook, A. (Eds). *Development of posture and gait across the lifespan*. Columbia, SC: University of South Carolina Press.

Clark, J.E., Whitall, J., & Phillips, S.J. (1988). Human interlimb coordination: The first 6 months of independent walking. *Developmental Psychobiology*, *21*, 445-456.

Connolly, K. (1980). The development of competence in motor skills. In C.H. Nadeau, W.R. Halliwell, K. Newell & G.C. Roberts (Eds). *Psychology of motor behavior and sport - 1979* (pp. 229-252). Champaign, Ill: Human Kinetics.

Fentress, J.C. (1976). Dynamic boundaries or patterned behaviour: Interactions and self-organization. In P.P.G. Bateson & R.A. Hindle (Eds.), *Growing Points in Ethology* (pp. 135-170). Cambridge: Cambridge University Press.

Gardner, H. (1971). Children's duplication of rhythmic patterns. *Journal of Research in Music Education*, *19*, 355-360.

Geuze, R.H., & Kalverboer, A.F. (1987). Inconsistency and adaptation in timing of clumsy children. *Journal of Human Movement Studies*, *13*, 421-432.

Greulich, W.W., & Pyle, S.I. (1959). *Radiographic atlas of skeletal development of the hand and wrist* (2nd ed.). London: Oxford Press.

Halverson, L.E., Roberton, M.A., & Langendorfer, S. (1982). Development of the overarm throw: Movement and ball velocity changes by the seventh grade. *Research Quarterly for Exercise and Sport*, *53*, 198-201.

Halverson, L., & Williams, K. (1986). Developmental sequences for hopping over distance: A pre-longitudinal screening. *Research Quarterly for Exercise and Sport*, *56*, 37-44.

Isaacs, E. (1920). The nature of the rhythm experience. *Psychological Review*, *27*, 270-297.

Jeka, J.J., & Kelso, J.A.S. (1988, Abstract). Dynamic patterns of multi-limb coordination. In J.A.S. Kelso, A.J. Mansell, & M.F. Shlesinger (Eds.),

Dynamic patterns in complex systems (p. 403). Singapore: World Scientific Publishers.

Jeka, J.J., & Kelso, J.A.S. (1989). The dynamic pattern approach to coordinated behavior: A tutorial review. In S.A. Wallace (Ed.), *Perspectives on the coordination and regulation of movement* (pp. 1-47). Amsterdam: North-Holland.

Kelso, J.A.S. (1988). Introductory remarks: Dynamic patterns. In J.A.S. Kelso, A.J. Mandell; & M.F. Shlesinger (Eds.), *Dynamic patterns in complex systems* (pp. 1-5). Singapore: World Scientific.

Kelso, J.A.S., & Tuller, B. (1985). Intrinsic time in speech production: Theory, methodology , and preliminary observations. *Haskins Laboratories Status Report on Speech Research* SR-81 (pp. 23-39). New Haven, CT.

Keogh, J.F. (1968). *Developmental evaluation of limb movement tasks, Technical Report 1-68*. Department of Physical Education, University of California, Los Angeles.

Keogh, J.F. (1969). *Analysis of limb and body control tasks. Technical Report 1-69.* Department of Physical Education, University of California, Los Angeles.

Kravitz, H., & Boehm, J. (1971). Rhythmic habit patterns in infancy: Their sequence, age of onset, and frequency. *Child Development*, *42*, 399-413.

Kristan, W.B. (1980). Generation of rhythmic motor patterns. In H.M. Pinkster & W.D. Willis (Eds.), *Information processing in the nervous system* (pp. 241-263). New York: Raven Press.

Kugler, P.N. and Turvey, M.T. (1986). *Information, natural law, and the self-assembly of rhythmic movement*. Hillsdale, NJ: Lawrence Erlbaum Associates.

Magalhaes, L.C., Koomar, J.A., & Cermak, S.A. (1989). Bilateral motor coordination in 5- to 9-year-old children: A pilot study. *The American Journal of Occupational Therapy*, *43*, 437-443.

Miner, J.B. (1903). Motor, visual and applied rhythms [Monographs]. *Psychological Review*, *5*, 1-106.

Parker, H.E. (1990a). *The development of coordination and timing in a rhythmic multi-limbed task*. Unpublished doctoral thesis, University of Western Australia, Perth.

Parker, H.E. (1990b, July). *The development of multi-limbed coordination in rhythmic movement. The systems dynamic approach*. Paper presented at the VIth National Developmental Conference, Perth, Australia.

Parker, H.E. (in preparation). *Rhythmic multi-limbed coordination in children*.

Parker, H.E., & Lockwood, R. J. (1988, August). Temporal stability in rhythmic jumping. *Abstract on Proceedings of XXIVth International Congress of Psychology*, Sydney, Australia.

Prinz, W. (1987). Ideo-motor action. In H. Heuer & A.F. Sanders (Eds.), *Perspectives on perception and action* (pp. 47-76). Hillsdale, NJ: Lawrence Erlbaum Associates.

Roberton, M.A. & Halverson, L.E. (1984). *Developing children - Their changing movement: A guide for teachers*. Philadelphia: Lea & Febiger.

Roberton, M.A., & Halverson, L.E. (1988). The development of locomotor coordination: Longitudinal change and invariance. *Journal of Motor Behavior*, *20*, 197-241.

Schmidt, R.A. (1982). *Motor control and learning*. Champaign, Ill: Human Kinetics.

Shaffer, L.H. (1982). Rhythm and timing in motor skill, *Psychological Review*, *89*, 109-122.

Smoll, F.L. (1974a). Assessment of spatial and temporal elements of rhythmic ability. In M. Wade & R. Martens (Eds.), *Psychology of motor behavior and sport* (pp. 314-320). Champaign, Ill: Human Kinetics.

Smoll, F.L. (1974b). Development of rhythmic ability in response to selected tempos. *Perceptual and Motor Skills*, *39*, 767-772.

Smoll, F.L. (1974c). Development of spatial and temporal elements of rhythmic ability. *Journal of Motor Behavior*, *6*, 53-58.

Smoll, F.L. (1975a). Preferred tempo in performance of repetitive movements. *Perceptual and Motor Skills*, *40*, 439-442.

Smoll, F.L. (1975b). Between-days consistency in personal tempo. *Perceptual and Motor Skills*, *41*, 731-734.

Smoll, F.L. (1975c). Preferred tempo of motor performance: Individual differences in within-individual variability. *Journal of Motor Behavior*, *7*, 259-263.

Smoll, F.L. (1975d). Variability in the development of spatial and temporal elements of rhythmic ability. *Perceptual and Motor Skills*, *40*, 140.

Smoll, F.L., & Schutz, R.W. (1982). Accuracy of rhythmic motor behavior in response to preferred and nonpreferred tempos. *Journal of Human Movement Studies*, *8*, 123-138.

Stetson, R.H. (1905). A motor theory of rhythm and discrete sensation. *Psychological Review*, *12*, 250-270.

Sutton-Smith, B., Rosenberg, B.G., & Morgan, E.F. (1963). Development of sex differences in play choices during pre-adolescence. *Child Development*, *34*, 119-126.

Thackray, R. (1969). *Rhythmic abilities and their measurement*. Unpublished Ph.D. Thesis, University of London, London.

Thackray, R. (1972). Rhythmic abilities in children: *Music Education Research Papers* (No.5). London: Novello.

Thelen, E. (1979). Rhythmical stereotypies in normal human infants. *Animal Behaviour*, *27*, 699-715.

Thelen, E. (1981). Kicking, rocking and waving: Contextual analysis of rhythmical stereotypies in normal human infants. *Animal Behaviour*, *29*, 3-11.

Thelen, E. (1985). Developmental origins of motor coordination: Leg movements in human infants. *Developmental Psychobiology*, *18*, 1-22.

Thelen, E. (1986). Treadmill-elicited stepping in seven-month-old infants. *Child Development*, *57*, 1498-1506.

Thelen, E. (1988). Dynamical approaches to the development of behavior. In J.A.S. Kelso, A.J. Mandell & M.F. Shlesinger (Eds.), *Dynamic patterns in complex systems* (pp. 348-367). Singapore: World Scientific Publishing Co.

Thelen, E. (1989). Self-organization in the developmental process: Can systems approaches work? In M.R. Gunnar (Ed.), *Systems and development: The 22nd Minnesota Symposium on Child Development* (pp. 77-117). Hillsdale, NJ: Lawrence Erlbaum Associates.

Thelen, E., & Fisher, D.M. (1982). Newborn stepping: an explanation for a "disappearing" reflex, *Developmental Psychology*, *18*, 760-775.

Thelen, E., Fisher, D.M., & Ridley-Johnson, R. (1984). The relationship between physical growth and a newborn reflex. *Infant Behavior and Development*, 7, 479-493.

Thelen, E., Kelso, J.A.S., & Fogel, A. (1987). Self-organizing systems and infant motor development. *Developmental Review*, 7, 39-65.

Thomas, J.R., & Moon, D.H. (1976). Measuring motor rhythmic ability in children. *Research Quarterly*, *47*, 20-32.

Truly, T.L., Clark, J.E., Phillips, S.J., & Caldwell, G.E. (1989). Getting the system started: Intralimb coordination for gait initiation in newly walking infants [Abstract]. *Proceedings of the North American Society of the Psychology of Sport and Physical Activity*, (p. 10). Kent State University, Kent, OH.

Tyldesley, D.A., & Whiting, H.T.A. (1975). Operational timing. *Journal of Human Movement Studies*, *1*, 172-177.

Von Holst, F. (1973). *The behavioural physiology of animals and man: The collected papers of Erich von Holst*. Coral Gables, Fl: University of Miami Press.

Whitall, J. (1989). A developmental study of the interlimb coordination in running and galloping. *Journal of Motor Behavior*, *21*, 409–428.

Wing, A.M. (1980). The long and short of timing in response sequences. In G.E. Stelmach & J. Requin (Eds.), *Tutorials in motor behavior* (pp. 469-486). Amsterdam: North-Holland.

Winstein, C.J., & Garfinkel, A. (1989). Qualitative dynamics of disordered human locomotion: A preliminary investigation. *Journal of Motor Behavior*, *21*, 373-391.

Wolff, P.H. (1967). The role of biological rhythms in early psychological development. *Bulletin of the Menninger Clinic*, *3*, 197-218.

Wolff, P.H. (1968). Stereotypic behaviour and development. *The Canadian Psychologist*, *9*, 474-483.

Wood, G.A. (1985). *Film motion analysis system users manual*. Perth, Australia: Department of Human Movement and Recreation Studies, University of Western Australia.

Approaches to the Study of Motor Control and Learning
J.J. Summers (Editor)

Chapter 7

MULTI-SENSORY CONTROL OF COORDINATED MOVEMENT

Patrick Haggard
Medical Research Council
Applied Psychology Unit, Cambridge

...Sense sure you have,
Else could you not have motion.

Hamlet.

This paper discusses how information from many sensory sources might contribute to coordinated movements of a limb involving many muscles and joints.

WHAT IS COORDINATION?

Few natural movements involve activity at a single joint only. Even everyday reaching movements typically use at least the shoulder and elbow joints (Morasso, 1981; Soechting & Lacquaniti, 1981), while maintaining balance may involve ten or more joints distributed throughout the body (Nashner & McCollum, 1985).

Multi-effector[1] movements are more flexible than single-effector movements, but place a greater computational load on the motor control system. Even a simple "kinematic chain", consisting of three effectors and two planar joints,

---

[1] The term 'effector' is used to mean a component unit of the motor system which is involved in performing a movement. An effector is thus a muscle-joint system.

allows the endpoint (e.g., the hand) of the chain to move freely within a plane. However, the movement trajectories that humans actually produce are not randomly distributed over the whole of the available range of configurations of the chain. Not all possible endpoint paths are observed, indicating that movements of the participating effectors are systematically related. That is, effectors which could move independently, in fact move together as a group. Sometimes a single property of one effector's movement, such as its timing or its amplitude will constrain the timing or amplitude of another effector (e.g., Yamanishi, Kawato, & Suzuki, 1980). In other cases, there will be a systematic relationship between the kinematics of one effector and a second throughout a movement (Turvey, Rosenblum, Schmidt, & Kugler, 1986). In both cases, the effectors are said to be *coordinated*.

THE APPROACH

This paper approaches this problem of coordination from an information-processing standpoint. Sensory information from many sources forms the input to the system controlling coordinated movement, and the movements of multiple effectors form the output. This problem is characteristic of all information-processing problems: in sensing stimuli relevant to movement, considerable integration or data reduction is necessary to extract the key patterns of an unfolding movement from thousands of individual receptors in many sensory modalities. The Central Nervous System (CNS) then faces the inverse problem of specifying appropriate responses and of coordinating the movement, of computing the contribution of individual effectors to the response, and of distributing the computed instructions to muscles in the periphery. This combination of data reduction and expansion makes the use of sensory information for coordinated movement fruitful territory for the models of the information-processing psychologist. Despite this, there is rather little discussion in the literature of how and why coordination of effectors is achieved (Haggard & Wing, unpublished research). While the physiological literature contains many studies of the mechanisms of movement control, few discuss coordination between multiple effectors. Psychological studies, by contrast, have often focused on bilateral coordination, comparing the simultaneous performance of two tasks, which are often fairly similar, performed with the left and right hands (Kelso, Southard, & Goodman, 1979; Turvey et al., 1986). However, the computational problems of coordination are perhaps clearer when multiple joints are coordinated in the control of a single limb. In this latter case, there are no obvious similarities between the effectors involved, and the contribution of each effector to the task is more easily expressed than in the bilateral case. For this reason, the rest of this paper will focus primarily on movements of a single limb.

The approach of this paper also draws on two decades of research on the control of multi-joint robotic manipulators (Whitney, 1969, 1972). Despite considerable research, most robots still do not coordinate movements of their effectors. Sometimes only one joint moves at a time. In other cases, the contributions of the various joints are determined using fixed rules, which do not attempt to relate the activity at one joint to the activity at another. This paper borrows some of the methods of robotics, and uses them to model coordination in biological movement. The approach may help to make more explicit how many sensory inputs help to produce coordination of many effectors in human movement. This may in turn point the way to more sophisticated robotic movement.

THE NEED FOR COORDINATION

There are two distinct reasons why the motor control system might favour such coordinated relationships between effectors: a decision problem when selecting limb configurations, and an implementation problem in simultaneously controlling multiple effectors.

A limb with three or more joints can achieve a given position of the hand or endpoint with an infinite number of joint configurations, and can produce a given endpoint trajectory with an infinite set of joint trajectories. The motor control system, therefore, faces a decision problem in selecting one set of joint configurations and joint trajectories from the infinite number available. Roboticists have given this problem of kinematic redundancy a more precise definition: Whenever the number of controllable joints of a multi-effector limb exceeds the number actually needed to perform a given task, the limb is said to be redundant for that task (Wolovich, 1987). This discrepancy between the number of effectors available and the minimum number required clearly increases with the anatomical complexity of the limb, making the decision problem faced by the motor control system more severe.

Once appropriate joint configurations and trajectories have been chosen, actually implementing them introduces a further challenge for the motor control system. The Soviet physiologist Bernstein (1967) appreciated that the control of all the effectors in a complex kinematic chain demands considerable information processing by the CNS. Neural commands must be sent to every muscle, and the movement of every effector must be monitored. Both the amount of information and the transmission rates required seemed unfeasible. This lead Bernstein to investigate methods which the CNS might exploit to make the control of multi-effector movement more tractable. Bernstein showed how a hierarchical organisation comprising several levels of simple, specialised modules, each dedicated to a particular function, and each receiving inputs from and passing inputs to other modules at other levels offered an informationally economical approach. Harnessing groups of effectors to work together could solve the problem of the limited capacity of the motor control system. When effectors are coordinated, high-level control of an action need not make reference to individual effectors, but can address groups of effectors as a single unit.

ACHIEVING COORDINATION

Coordination between distinct effectors can be achieved in at least three distinct ways. These are mechanical, pre-planned, and sensor-driven coordination, which are now considered in turn.

The mechanical configuration of anatomical structures may encourage particular relationships between effectors. In the lower limb, for example, the gastrocnemius muscle crosses the knee and ankle joints at each end of the tibia. This arrangement ensures that the knee and ankle joints flex and extend together. This produces a fixed pattern of coordination between knee and ankle, useful in locomotion and jumping (van Ingen Schenau, 1989). Mechanical linkages of this kind have also proved valuable in a number of robotic devices (Raibert, 1986).

While such mechanisms give a clear example of coordination, they are inflexible. Their fixed configuration means that the selective use of just one of the effectors in the limb is not possible unless other muscles are also activated. Therefore, simple mechanical linkages cannot make a general contribution to coordination.

Coordination could result from the nervous system computing and prescribing in advance a relationship between all the effectors involved in a movement. The primary motor cortex, the premotor area, and the supplementary motor area have long been assigned precisely this role (Penfield & Rasmussen, 1950). Single neurones in the motor cortex appear to facilitate multiple effectors involved in a task as a group (Cheney & Fetz, 1985; Muir & Lemon, 1983). While prior computation and storage of movement plans clearly do occur (Day et al., 1989, Monsell, 1984), some researchers have suggested that prior computation alone is not a practicable means of achieving coordinated movement (Kelso, 1982; Kugler & Turvey, 1986). For example, the computations involved in specifying the time-course of activation for all the muscles contributing to a multi-effector movement are complex, because of task constraints and dynamical interactions between effectors (Hollerbach & Flash, 1982). The complexity of these calculations increases rapidly with the number of effectors involved. The computations may also be inaccurate, perhaps due to poor representation of the initial configurations of effectors. Unexpected perturbations occurring during the movement may also cause difficulties. While a purely open-loop strategy of this kind clearly has limitations, it can be combined very successfully with sensory knowledge of results. A variety of sensors can provide information each time the movement is performed, and this can be used to update the initial conditions for subsequent performance.

In addition to knowledge of results, sensory systems can also play a role in coordinating effectors during the course of the movement itself through feedback control. A feedback system allows the desired relationships between effectors to be implemented more reliably than pre-planned coordination, since spatio-temporal uncertainty can be eliminated by sensing the current state of the effectors and adjusting command signals accordingly, providing the update rate for the commands is adequate.

Sensory-driven coordination could produce *rapid, remote, flexible* adjustments to multi-effector movements. A coordinated response is *remote* when it involves activity of one or more effectors that can nevertheless function independently of the site where the driving sensory input occurred (Marsden, Merton, & Morton, 1981). On this definition, any peripheral response to a central sensory source, such as vision, qualifies as remote. Note that the physical distance between a sensory source and the responding effector does not have to exceed a fixed threshold for the response to be remote: functional independence of stimulus and the responding effector(s) are more important than their separation in centimetres. The *speed* of sensorimotor networks has been widely studied, and the latencies of various kinds of stimulus-response mappings are known. Physiologically "hardwired" responses such as the stretch reflex have latencies as low as 20 ms, while voluntary movements have a latency of 120 ms or more. The latency of sensor-driven responses can offer important clues about the neural structures involved in the organisation of movement. Thus, Marsden, Merton, and Morton, (1976) noted that the latency of stabilising "tulip" responses by the flexor pollucis longus muscle was around 40-50 ms when a brief perturbation was delivered to the thumb, while the latency of responses in the flexor hallucis longus muscle was 75-90 ms when the perturbation was delivered to the big toe. This pattern of latencies is consistent with both responses involving cortical loops. Finally, a coordinated response is *flexible* if the relation between the effectors can be modulated as appropriate: rather than being a fixed consequence of the sensory input, the pattern of coordination between effectors depends on the current task demands.

Rapid, remote, flexible activity are the key properties of multiple effectors working together as a group. Sensory-driven coordination can provide greater flexibility than pre-planned and mechanical coordination, and can provide faster responses than pre-planned coordination. Therefore, sensors must play a major role in coordinating multi-effector movements.

RELEVANCE OF EXISTING MODELS OF SENSING TO COORDINATION

Sherrington's (1947) classic model of the sensorimotor reflex arc underlies much modern thinking about the role of sensing in movement control. But most movements can use sensory information from a large number of different sensory sources to monitor and adjust the patterns of muscle activation in many effectors. Therefore, only the very simplest of motor behaviours can successfully be analysed using the reflex model's association of a single sensory message with a single, local, stereotyped motor response. Sherrington was, of course, very aware of this complexity, and stressed that "integration" was a crucial feature of the nervous system. However, his descriptions of integration are qualitative rather than quantitative, and the sensorimotor reflex arc remains his most explicit model. Unfortunately, the simple reflex model does not generalise well to such cases of multiple sensory input being used to coordinate multiple motor outputs: the mapping of many sensors onto many effectors cannot be achieved by many mappings of a single sensor onto a single effector along the lines of the the reflex arc. In particular, the Sherringtonian model cannot suggest which particular sensory input variables are specifically assigned to which motor output variables, nor how such assignment might occur.

Perhaps the clearest demonstration that there are multiple sensory inputs to the motor control system comes from considering the different sensory modalities and receptors that can contribute. These include joint receptors, tendon organs, muscle spindles, and four classes of cutaneous sensor, and the vestibular system. Vision characterises the organism's movement relative to environmental surfaces (Lee & Lishman, 1975), and can also be used for proprioception of any effector (Wing & Fraser, 1983). These many sensory sources are discussed at greater length later.

Using the Inputs

How are the afferent messages from these multiple sensory sources used to coordinate the states of multiple effectors? Unfortunately, this complex mapping has not been adequately considered in the literature, though a number of separate approaches are discernible.

Often, the control of a single effector or of a set of effectors uses a combination of sensory signals from different sensors. For example, fusimotor control of a muscle uses information from both the primary and secondary receptors in the muscle spindle which code rate of change of muscle length and muscle length respectively. Again, position information from muscle spindles and tension information from Golgi tendon organs may be used in the compliance control of a muscle (Houk, 1979).

On the other hand, a single sensory source can be used in the control of multiple effectors. This possibility was recognised by Sherrington, and expanded by his successors. The suggestion of "principles of combination" for reflexes - the reflex inhibition of antagonists and reflex facilitation of synergists in the spinal stretch reflex, for example - still plays a major part in some theories of action (Gallistel, 1980). However, these principles of combination are mainly concerned with the coordination of many muscles moving one effector, rather than the coordination of many independent effectors.

A second tradition, found primarily in the psychological literature, has used higher-level concepts such as kinaesthesis, proprioception and somatosensation (e.g., Laszlo & Bairstow, 1983), which describe what the sensory information is about, rather than relating to any particular sensory sources or model of sensorimotor function. Recently, psychologists have concentrated on whether sensory information is used during the course of a movement (Keele, 1982). By contrast, rather little work has studied *how* any sensory information might be used.

Roboticists have perhaps confronted the computational difficulties associated with using many sensory inputs to control many effectors more directly, because of their applied perspective. Early in the development of robotics, researchers realised that robots equipped with sensors would prove more useful than robots simply following feedforward commands, since they could interact more successfully with their environment. However, research in sensor-based robotics was delayed due to difficulties with the motoric side of robot control (Lumelsky & Brooks, 1989). Two, rather different strands of research emerged. One approach, motivated by the need for engineering solutions, fitted existing sensor technologies to existing robots, particularly in assembly tasks, only to discover that the provision of sensory capability did not of itself guarantee better performance. Sometimes the design of the robotic manipulator made it clear how sensory information should be related to motor commands. For example, tension sensors in the tendons of the JPL hand (Salisbury, 1985) can be directly related to joint torques. In tactile sensing, by contrast, it is often not clear how to relate the sensory information to the control of the robot's motors.

A second approach drew inspiration from Artificial Intelligence. This research sought to process and analyse sensory signals to build up a "world model" of the robot's environment. Once an accurate world model was obtained, it could be used to guide action. However, this approach has perhaps not fulfilled its promise: first generating useful models of the world has proved surprisingly difficult. Second, notions of world models have been derived largely from vision (Marr, 1982), and may not generalise easily to other sensory modalities. Finally, the notion of a world model implies considering perception independently of action, and may not make the control of movement any easier. Replacing low-level perceptual representations with higher-level ones may not solve the fundamental problem of how to use sensory information in goal-directed action (Turvey, 1977).

A MODEL OF SENSING FOR COORDINATION

Drawing on these contributions from psychology, physiology, and robotics, one can model the use of sensing for the coordination of a multi-effector limb using the following flow-diagram. The model aims to describe how sensory information is used in biological motor control, but could also suggest how sensory information might be used in the control of a robot manipulator. The account of sensing presented in the model is not new, but it does relate sensing to coordinated movement more explicitly than traditional models. The boxes in the diagram represent the various stages of processing in the use of sensory information to coordinate multiple effectors. Later, these stages of processing will be presented more quantitatively using a set of four matrix operations, which are also marked in the figure.

Starting at the top of Figure 1, environmental events provide stimuli for the available receptors. Since many sensors detect movements of the effectors rather than, or in addition to, events in the external world, the activation of an effector is itself considered an environmental event.

The availability of sensory receptors is the next consideration. Many sensory receptors provide information simultaneously about the state of a limb. For example, a soleus muscle may contain many hundreds of muscle spindles, and around sixty Golgi tendon organs. Visual information comes from a single location in the body, but often dominates in the control of action (Lee & Aronson, 1974). Work in robotics shows that the availability of sensors is not a trivial issue: the choice of which sensors are used, and where they are placed on the robot arm is crucial to robot performance (Cheung & Lumelsky, 1989).

Which physical dimensions does a particular sensor transduce, and how does it transduce them? In the last hundred years, the physiology of many receptors has been established. However, debate continues on a number of issues, such as the precise role of muscle spindles (Matthews, 1981), and the ways in which joint capsule receptors measure joint angles (Grigg, 1975). Evolution has produced very specialized receptor cells, which are remarkably efficient at transducing particular stimuli. Robot sensors, by contrast, are often fairly poor, and inefficient at transducing a single physical dimension, particularly in the case of tactile sensing. Poor sensing often leads to inappropriate robot motion, and thus poor overall performance. On the other hand, roboticists have sometimes invented new transducers not available to biological systems, such as proximity sensors (Cheung & Lumelsky, 1989).

Sensory integration, the next stage in the model, is perhaps the least understood, although its importance has been recognised since the work of

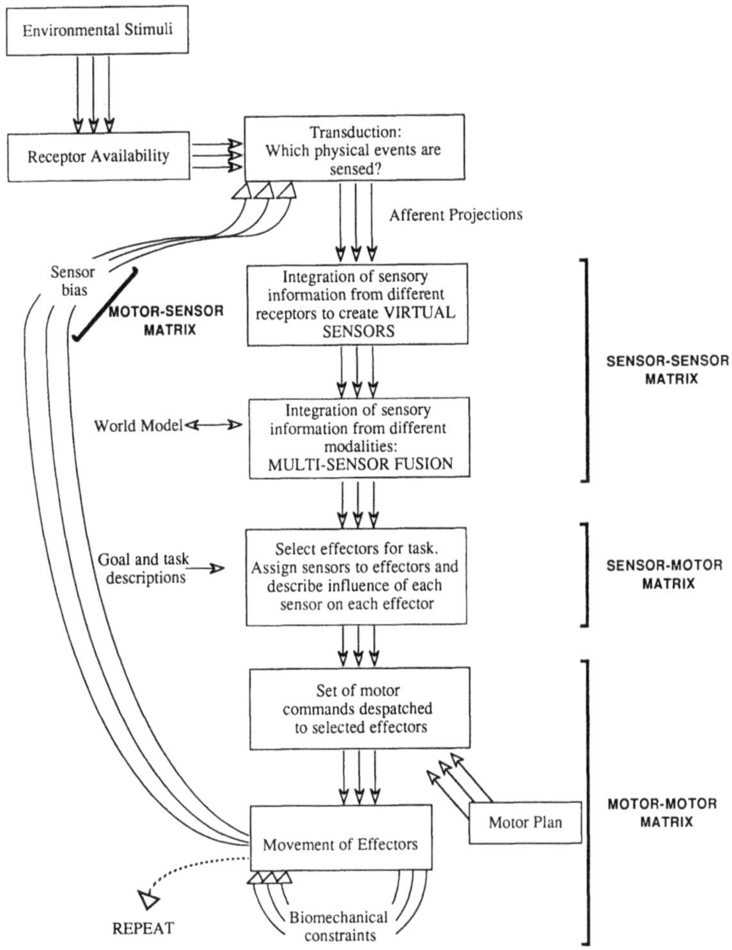

Figure 1. An information processing model of using many sensory sources to coordinate many effectors.

Sherrington (1947). Integration seems to be of two forms. Both have the common goal of grouping together sensory signals carrying information about related features of the stimulus.

First, information from adjacent receptors within a single sensory modality must be processed in parallel, since the information is about spatially adjacent portions of the stimulus. For example, information from many tactile receptors in adjacent areas of glabrous skin must be pooled to create a representation of the extended surface of an object, rather than just a set of local deformations. Similarly, signals from the three orthogonal semicircular canals must be integrated to create a full 3-dimensional description of the head's movement. This level of integration achieves data reduction: a plethora of raw sensory information from many sensors is reduced to a more coherent representation of environmental events. The outputs of this stage are the readings of a set of *virtual sensors*, or higher-level sensory channels offering reduced but more useful representations.

The second stage of sensory integration is more sophisticated: information from distinct sensory modalities, which transduce very different physical properties of the stimulus, must be combined to create an objective representation of the state of the organism, its own effectors and other objects in the environment. For example, information from the semicircular canals and the otoliths is combined at a very early stage of processing, perhaps to allow combination of information about rotatations and translations of the head relative to the gravitational vertical. Also, tactile sensors in the skin may be used to sense contact forces, but the contribution of active muscle contraction to these contact forces will need to be removed at higher levels of processing, if tactile information about environmental surfaces is required. This second kind of integration is a crucial feature of mammalian cortex: many neurons have been found to respond to combinations of a number of sensory inputs such as muscle position and muscle force (Jennings, Lamour, Soli, & Fromi, 1983) or a tactile stimulus on a particular part of the body and a visual stimulus from a corresponding point in space (Sparks & Nelson, 1985).

Psychological studies of this kind of sensory integration have often used postural tasks, since many sensory systems, including vision, the vestibular system, and tactile sensing, all contribute to the control of posture. These different sensory sources can be traded off against each other (Lee & Lishman, 1975) to discover how this information is integrated into a single, coherent representation (Droulez & Dorlot, 1988).

This second form of integration has also been a major issue in robotics, where it is often known as "multi-sensor fusion" (Durrant-Whyte, in press), a usage followed in this paper. Traditionally, roboticists' interest in multi-sensor fusion has been in creating more reliable world models by using many sensory sources in collaboration. However, multi-sensor fusion is important even if an explicit world model is not required. This alternative possibility of using sensory information directly in the control of action, without world models as an intermediary, has received rather little attention, although "behaviour-based control" (Brooks, 1986; Connell, 1989) has pointed towards its potential.

Interestingly, the roboticists' focus on the need for a high-level stage between sensing and action parallels a continuing debate in psychology. Some researchers, first behaviourists, and later perception-action theorists (Turvey, 1977), saw a direct connection between environmental stimuli and motor responses. Others, (e.g., Hebb, 1949) argued that some higher level intermediary was required: behaviour was too sophisticated and organised to result from simple links between sensing and action. The debate continues.

The goal of both kinds of sensory integration is to bring together sensory signals into coherent groups. All the sensory information within such a group is directed at a particular physical feature of the environment or of the body, despite the information's disparate origins. By this means, the vast barrage of afferent information is translated into a form which is useful for action. The outputs of the sensory integration stage, together with some specification of the movement's goals can then be used to choose *which* effectors will be used during the task, and what movement each effector will make. Determining how the multiple sensory signals contribute to the control of the multiple effectors is the key problem at this stage.

Finally, once the assignment of sensory sources to effectors has been made, the appropriate commands must be dispatched to each effector at the appropriate time.

The resulting movements of each effector will be monitored by the available sensors, and the cycle leading from sensing to movement will repeat. In biological systems, the processes represented by the model seem to occur continuously: sensory information about the environment is taken in all the time, and appropriate motor responses can be made at any time. Thus, the model is not serial and discrete, but parallel and continuous: the arrows of Figure 1, therefore, indicate only the flow of information, and not a hierarchy of control or a temporal sequence of processing stages. Most robotic implementations, by contrast, are serial and discrete: sensors are polled in strict rotation once in each cycle, the relevant calculations are performed, and the commands sent to the motors are updated in strict rotation, again only once in each cycle. Delays inevitably occur between sensing an environmental event and a motor response to that event. In biological systems, these delays are due to the limited speed of neural conduction and central processing. In robots, by contrast, these operations are often virtually instantaneous, but delays arise because sensors are polled and motor commands updated only periodically. Clearly, a higher update rate involves shorter delays, and thus better performance.

Because of sensorimotor delays, coordinated movement can never be driven instantaneously by sensory information. If the sensorimotor delays become too great, the system becomes unstable and uncontrollable (Poulton, 1974). Some researchers have used the difficulties posed by sensorimotor delays to argue against the importance of sensor-driven coordination (Abbs & Winstein, 1988), while others have commented that sensor-driven responses are remarkably rapid (Marsden et al., 1981), and have accordingly given them an important function in motor control.

THE MATRIX APPROACH

Sensory information must go through many stages of processing before it becomes useful for coordinated movement. Multi-sensor fusion, the assignment of sensors to effectors and mechanical interactions between effectors all introduce complexities which make local computational models inadequate. Further, the use of many sensors in coordinated control of many effectors cannot be modelled as a set of many independent local feedback systems, since many *remote* mappings, in which a sensory source is used to control a remote effector, may occur. The remote effector may, in turn, cause movements of other effectors, due to the biomechanics of the limb, perhaps altering the reading of a remote sensor. All these mutual interactions will be occurring simultaneously. Therefore, any model of sensing for coordinated multi-effector movement must be distributed and parallel. Independent, local circuits cannot do the job.

A set of matrices offers a convenient way of modelling these effects of many sensory inputs on many effectors. The matrix representation is intended as a characterisation of the information-processing involved in coordination, rather than as a detailed description of neural control. The use of matrix representations is consistent with current modelling techniques in robotics.[2]

Sensor-Motor Matrix

The sensor-motor matrix forms the major component of the matrix representation of coordination. It specifies how information from each sensor influences the activity of each effector. Each row of this matrix represents one effector, and each column of the matrix represents one sensor. Each cell in the matrix contains a gain factor for the relation between the particular sensory input and the particular motor output represented by that cell. The actual motor output of a particular effector depends on the sensor inputs and the gain values in the cells in the relevant row of the matrix, by matrix multiplication. Multiple sensory inputs are thus mapped onto multiple motor outputs. A further vector of DC offsets can be added if required. These offsets could be used to represent background levels of activity in the effectors, such as muscle tone, which occur even in the absence of a functional sensory input. These operations can be expressed in the following equation:

---

[2] E.g., GEC-Marconi's MICCON robot control system, which prompted some of the thoughts in this paper. Reference: Techbrief MS19, available from GEC-Marconi Research Centre, West Hanningfield Road, Great Baddow, Chelmsford CM2 8HN.

Vector of Motor Outputs	=	Sensor-Motor Matrix	*	Vector of sensor inputs	+	Vector of offsets

This matrix represents the computations involved in selection and assignment of sensory signals to effectors. An entry of zero in a particular cell of the sensor-motor matrix implies that that particular sensor has no influence on the activity of that particular effector. Non-zero entries in a cell indicate that the sensor is assigned some influence over the effector. The sensor-motor matrix is likely to express the influence of virtual sensors rather than individual receptors, for reasons of economy of information. A representation of the goal of the movement, in addition to a representation of the current state of the limb as provided by the sensor readings, will generally be required to specify the cell entries in the matrix. Some motor learning theories (Schmidt, 1982) suggest a convenient way of representing a movement's goal as a set of sensor readings which would be obtained on successful completion of the task, and with which current sensor readings can be compared. This suggests one way of allowing the goal of a movement to affect the cell entries in the sensor-motor matrix. Because of sensorimotor delays, the motor outputs of each effector will be responses to recent, rather than instantaneous sensory signals.

Temporal Implications of the Matrix Representation

The contents of the sensor-motor matrix need not be fixed throughout the course of an action, but may be updated as the action progresses. Incoming sensory information may be used to guide the adjustment of the contents of the matrix. Some successful robotic implementations have used a finite number of discrete mappings of motors to sensors corresponding to independent stages of an action (Connell, 1989; Raibert, 1986). This would correspond to updating the contents of the matrix only periodically. A biological system could, on the other hand, adjust the contents of the matrix continuously. The contents of the sensor-motor matrix could be considered as a time series (Box & Jenkins, 1970), with the current contents of the matrix being a function of its contents at earlier times. Note that the proposal of a matrix representation for sensor-driven coordination does not imply *how* the contents of the sensor-motor matrix are updated. However, a combination of the specification of the goal and incoming sensory information are probably involved.

Finally, the matrix representation itself is not temporal: rather it relates the *states* of sensory sources (i.e., sensor readings) to the *states* of the effectors. Temporal characteristics of movement are supplied by the time-varying nature of the sensor-motor matrix, and of the sensory input itself, as action develops.

A large part of motor control research has focused on the processes expressed by this matrix. However, for a complete understanding of how sensory information contributes to coordinating many effectors, three further relations must be considered. These relations are expressed by a motor-sensor matrix, a motor-motor matrix, and a sensor-sensor matrix. Many features of the sensor-motor matrix discussed above, such as temporal delays and adjustments to the contents of the matrix during the course of an action, clearly apply to the other three matrices as well.

The Motor-Sensor Matrix

This matrix captures the way that the state of an effector can influence sensors. Obviously, many peripheral receptors sense the physical properties of effectors: e.g., the length of a muscle affects muscle spindles since it provides their primary stimulus. This "raw" response of receptors to their immediate stimulus is a result of peripheral anatomy, rather than a computational element of the motor control system. It is, therefore, included in the input vector of sensor readings, rather than in the motor-sensor matrix itself.

Rather, the motor-sensor matrix expresses how movement of an effector can influence sensors by modulating the sensors' gain, rather than by an actual change in the physical dimension that the sensor monitors. The motive for such motor-sensor influences may be informational economy: moving an effector inevitably has effects on the readings of its associated sensors, such as joint receptors, muscle spindles, and Golgi tendon organs. If the movement is a voluntary, controlled response, the barrage of sensory feedback associated with it may produce an overload of redundant and unhelpful information, since the sensory consequences of the movement would have been anticipated at the time the movement was commanded, and might arrive too late to be useful anyway, if the movement were purely ballistic. Therefore, the gain on particular sensors may be turned down when an effector is active. The sensors so affected will include those local to the moving effector, but may also include remote sensors as well. For example, movement of the shoulder and/or elbow could transport the hand over a highly textured surface, where suppression of superfluous cutaneous input from the hand might be desirable.

Under other circumstances such as fine manipulation, an increased feedback gain may improve movement accuracy. Further, movements of effectors may form part of a sensory strategy, as when saccades are used to foveate a new and salient stimulus, or when the hand explores an object's surface to gain tactile information. In such cases, the movements made by the effectors may suggest an important role for some sensory sources, and disregard of other sources. Both possibilities can be expressed in the matrix.

A number of neurophysiological studies have found evidence for motoric influences on the gain of a sensor, typically by observing modulated activity in cortical neurons which is attributable to an impending movement rather than to any actual change in stimulation (see Prochazka, 1989 for a review). The motor-sensor matrix captures such influences occurring in the model between the stages of movement and sensory transduction.

The Motor-Motor Matrix

The motor-motor matrix captures the results of the movement of each effector on other effectors, due to the biomechanical linkages between degrees of freedom. The motor control system often takes advantage of the biomechanical properties of an effector to coordinate movements. Therefore, the distinction between the control of movement and the physics of movement is somewhat artificial, as many researchers have emphasised (Kugler & Turvey, 1986; Mussa-Ivaldi, Morasso, & Zaccaria, 1988). For example, the bi-articular gastrocnemius muscle in the leg ensures that rotations of the knee and ankle joints are coordinated in a way which provides efficient timing and force production for jumping and locomotion (van Ingen Schenau, 1989). This linkage could be expressed by a gain factor in the cell relating knee and ankle joints in the motor-motor matrix.

Branching axons in the descending motor pathways are another source of motor-motor interaction. Around 30% of motor cortex neurons branch out to innervate more than one muscle (Sears & Stagg, 1976). Taken by itself, a branching axon provides the same, rather inflexible variety of coordination as a fixed mechanical linkage between effectors. However, additional muscles may be used as antagonists to vary the precise relationship between the movements of the effectors involved.

Motor-motor influences will not always be so constructive. Interaction torques are present whenever a multi-joint limb is moved. Exerting a torque at the shoulder joint, for example, results in coriolis and centripetal torques around the elbow joint which are a nonlinear function of the torque at the shoulder. These interaction torques are not negligible (Hollerbach & Flash, 1982) and must be included in the computations of the motor control system.

Finally, many studies have shown that deafferented humans can produce learned coordinated movements, even without visual feedback (Rothwell et al., 1982; Sanes, Mauritz, Dalakas, & Evarts, 1985). In such cases, coordination is often attributed to a pre-arranged plan to maintain a particular relationship between the movement of each of a set of effectors. Since sensory information is absent, the coordination observed cannot be due to the sensor-sensor, sensor-motor, or motor-sensor matrices. However, if a planned pattern of coordination is treated as a kind of influence of one effector on another, a motor plan could be included in the motor-motor matrix. Planned relationships between effectors would be at a higher level than direct biomechanical interactions. They might, for example, involve duplicating the abstract neural representation of one effector's movement, and applying it to another. Both the motor plan, and biomechanical interactions, then, make the movements of effectors interdependent, without the mediation of sensing, and both can be included in the motor-motor matrix.

The Sensor-Sensor Matrix

Sensory receptors do not interact directly. However, the interpretative nature of higher sensing processing involves combining information from one sensory source with information from another. For example, the overall activity of one set of virtual sensors often partially determines the nature of the stimulus, and thereby makes a particular pattern of activation of additional virtual sensors more probable than any alternative patterns (e.g., Droulez & Darlot, 1988). Thus, the sensor-sensor matrix specifies a gain factor for relating the levels of activation of each virtual sensor to every other virtual sensor involved in a task. A further vector of DC offsets can be added if required.

The readings of two sensors may be systematically related because of an underlying relationship between the physical dimensions that each measures. For example, muscle spindle and Golgi tendon organ activity are related because the spring-like qualities of muscle ensure that muscle tension depends on muscle length (Rack & Westbury, 1969). In this case, the one sensor does not *cause* the activation of the other directly, but rather both are effects of the muscle's actual and preferred lengths. Interactions of this kind, therefore, do not belong in the sensor-sensor matrix.

The traditional laboratory demonstration of the "polystyrene brick effect" offers a good example of these interpretative, heuristic processes at work by illustrating the dramatic effects of their failure. In the demonstration, a student prepares to catch a brick thrown to him by the demonstrator. The student has used visual information to infer that the object she will catch will be heavy and rigid, and therefore prepares an appropriate two-handed catch and braced stance. The student has expectations of the tactile sensory experiences that will be associated with catching the brick. When the brick turns out to be made of polystyrene, the student's heuristics are foiled, often producing a fumble, over and above general bewilderment and peer ridicule. The student's anticipation could be characterised within the matrix system for the task by placing a high gain factor in the cell relating a visual input to a tactile input.

This adjustment of sensor-sensor relations is, of course, a major element of many pattern recognition systems based on neural networks. A neural network "learns" to produce characteristic patterns of activation in response to characteristic stimuli. When a novel stimulus with only some of the attributes of previous stimuli is encountered, the pattern of activation elicited will depend on the test stimulus' *degree* of similarity with the previous stimuli.[3]

The representation provided by the sensor-sensor matrix is a pattern of sensory activity reflecting the sensed attributes of the stimulus, and also the system's previous experience of such stimuli. The output could be considered as a world-model, and could be included in a library of stimulus descriptions. This library in turn provides the influence of past experiences on present stimulation.

Since the four processes represented by these four matrices operate in parallel, they can be incorporated into a single, large sensorimotor matrix [S]. This larger matrix is a mapping from a set of sensor readings and effector states to a new set of sensor readings and effector states. As an example, Figure 2 below shows how [S] might be constructed for a limb, similar to the human forearm, which contains two effectors (e.g., the shoulder and elbow) and two virtual sensors. The vector of DC offsets is a combination of the four vectors of DC offsets occurring with each component matrix. For simplicity, each sensor is considered to be attached to an effector, and reports the joint angle of its effector, although the matrix representation could clearly apply to other forms of sensor also.

While all of the four matrices will contribute to the mapping, the sensor-motor matrix will typically have the dominant say. The sensor-sensor matrix will be more important in tasks with a distinct perceptual component, such as those involving discriminative stimuli. The motor-motor matrix is likely to become more important as the mechanical connections between effectors become more numerous and more complex.

---

[3] Consider a network which has experienced previous stimuli possessing attributes A1, A2, and A3, detected respectively by three sensors S1, S2, and S3. A novel stimulus possesses A1 and A2, but has not yet been observed to possess A3. Nonetheless, the novel stimulus is likely to be quite similar to the previous stimuli, since they share some attributes. The pattern of activation that would be associated with A3 if it were present will thus be supplied by the network itself. Thus, the sensors S1 and S2 which detected A1 and A2 could simulate the effect of A3 on S3, even in the absence of appropriate activity in S3. Alternatively, heuristic modification of peripheral activity could actually occur: the threshold for a sensor involved in detecting A3 may be lowered, or its level of activity increased to reflect the probability that A3 is present. If the heuristic value turns out to be incorrect, future uses of the network will use a revised value for the probability of A3 given A1 and A2. This ability to respond appropriately to partial input is an intrinsic consequence of the way that the system learns, and is a major attraction of neural network models (McLelland & Rumelhart, 1987).

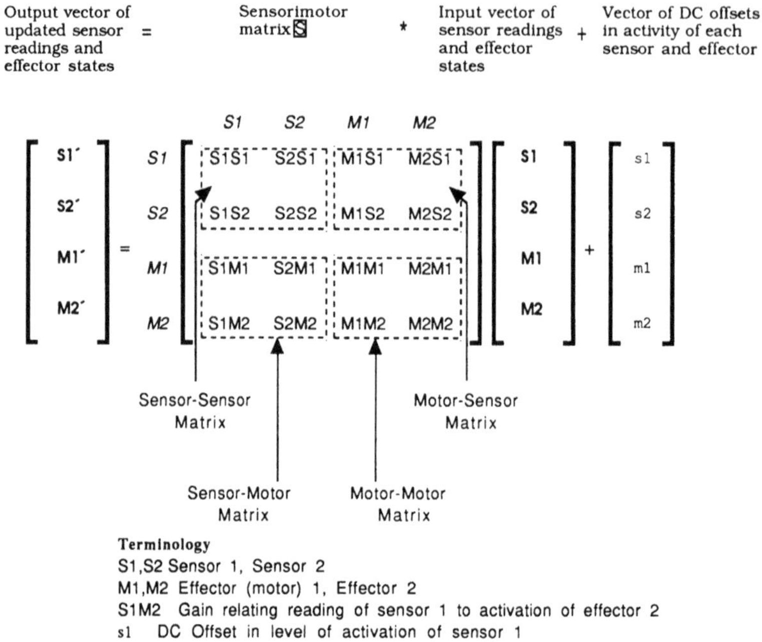

Figure 2. A matrix representation of using many sensory sources to coordinate many effectors.

Limitations of the Matrix Representation

The matrix representation is, of course, linear. That is, a given change in the input values will produce the same change in the output values whatever the existing input values are. Can a linear mapping from sensors to motors really capture the full range of coordinated movement? This question is best tackled by distinguishing two different senses in which sensorimotor systems may be nonlinear.

First, the relation between one particular sensory input variable and one particular output variable, considered alone, is unlikely to be linear. This is because each motor output variable is determined by many sensory inputs: a motor output may depend not only on an immediate sensory source, but also on suppression and enhancement from other sensory sources, as stressed earlier. These phenomena are conveniently expressed by the matrix representation. Although the matrix representation does model the output as a linear function of the whole input, the representation can nonetheless be rich, because it is parallel and distributed over many inputs and outputs. Nonlinearity in the sense of distributedness is therefore, not problematic.

The second aspect of nonlinearity in sensorimotor systems includes dynamic responses (the system's behaviour depends on the rate of change of the input), saturation effects (the system's behaviour changes at extremes of the range on inputs), and adaptation (changes in the system as inputs change). Nonlinear dynamics present particular difficulties for the matrix approach. The matrices relate the *state* of a set of inputs to the *state* of a set of outputs, whereas phenomena such as coarticulation of movement (Kelso, Salzman, & Tuller, 1986), and dynamic interactions between limb segments (Hollerbach & Flash, 1982) suggest that the motor outputs depend on higher order derivatives of state information (i.e., velocity, acceleration etc.) rather than on state information alone. Further, most sensory systems respond to transients, as well as to steady-state inputs (as Table 1 will later show).

Should the matrix representation be expanded to include these higher derivatives in the control scheme? If nonlinearities appear crucial to coordinated movement, the original equation relating a vector of outputs to a vector of inputs *via* the sensorimotor matrix could be expanded: the vector of outputs would also depend on the rate of change of input states *via* an additional differential matrix. However, the computations required to produce a coordinated movement of a limb increase each time a higher order of control is included.

Model-referenced adaptive controllers (MRACs) suggest an alternative way of understanding nonlinearities in the sensorimotor system (Åström, 1983). Where a control system's output is a nonlinear function of its input, the system can sometimes be linearized by including an MRAC in the control loop. The MRAC adaptively modulates the closed loop gain and phase so as to compensate for the system's nonlinearities, producing a linear relation between input and output. The MRAC thus "cancels out" for the nonlinearities inherent in the system, so that overall behaviour of the system is linear. Extending these concepts to motor control, the matrix representation might offer a good overall description of coordinated movement, although the behaviour of individual neural structures might be nonlinear. The cerebellum seems a plausible candidate for the role of compensatory gain modulation (Stein, 1986).

Thus, nonlinear dynamical influences constitute a more fundamental problem for the matrix approach than distributedness. Which of these features contributes most to the complexity of coordinated movement remains an empirical question.

Local vs Remote Effects

The matrix representation usefully expresses the distinction between local and remote use of sensory information. According to our definition, coordinated multi-effector movement depends on controlling an effector using information from other, remote effectors within the limb. These remote influences are overlaid upon a basic system of local, regulatory control which provides essential characteristics of the effectors such as muscle tone and compliance. For example, the muscle spindles provide a servo-assisted control system for the local muscle, but can also have remote coordinating effects, due to reflex inhibition of antagonist muscles, and reflex excitation of synergists.

The matrix representation conveniently captures this difference between local and remote control. The local, regulatory control is represented by the diagonal terms in the four matrices above, while the remote, coordinating control is represented by the off-diagonal terms. Thus, an uncoordinated motor control system could have a number of effectors each of which was appropriately regulated by an associated sensor, with each sensor-effector pair being independent of each other pair.

The mathematical expression of these local, regulatory influences is not the same for each matrix. In the sensor-motor matrix, the diagonal terms would be nonzero and the off-diagonal terms would be zero. In the motor-motor matrix, by contrast, the diagonal terms would presumably be zero, since the activation or movement of an effector would neither inhibit nor excite further activation of that effector. In many cases, such as saccadic eye movements (Matin, 1974) and tactile sensing (Angel & Malenka, 1982), movement of an effector inhibits the associated sensor, suggesting negative diagonal terms in the motor-sensor matrix. By contrast, positive feedback is an important feature of neural networks for pattern recognition (McClelland & Rumelhart, 1987), suggesting positive diagonal terms in the sensor-sensor matrix. Despite these differences, the diagonal terms in each matrix capture local effects distinct from the coordination captured by the off-diagonal terms.

The differing roles of peripheral and central sensory sources in motor control may be related to the local/remote distinction. Physiologists have traditionally thought of the sensory systems located in the limb itself as local regulatory systems for maintaining muscle tone and preventing injury, while the central senses, such as vision, specified the goal of a movement independently of particular effectors. However, the notion that peripheral systems are purely regulatory now seems less sustainable. Cutaneous signals are strongly represented in somatosensory cortex, and it seems as though even muscle spindles may have a considerable cortical projection (Gandevia & Burke, 1988). More directly, Cordo (1988) has shown that "kinaesthetic" information, probably originating from many peripheral sources, about one effector can be used to coordinate a second, remote effector. The further problem, of how an object-centred visual representation maps onto a set of effector movements, remains. These difficulties are postponed in this paper, and it is assumed that the matrix representation can map both peripheral and central sensory information onto appropriate effector movements. Nevertheless, the transformation of visual information about the environment into motor commands remains a major problem in motor control.

Relating Sensory Function to the Matrix Representation of Coordination

The psychological study of sensing has traditionally focused on psychophysics rather than on the role of sensing in the control of action. Some researchers have argued that this is misguided (Bootsma, 1988). Perhaps because of this traditional emphasis, the ways in which different sensory sources may contribute to coordinated movement are not adequately understood.

The matrix representation proposed above helps in understanding the role of sensing in coordination by distinguishing three distinct components: the sensor-motor, motor-sensor and sensor-sensor matrices. Accordingly, Table 1 characterises the principal sensory systems in terms of the operations represented by the matrices.

The first column describes the number, location, and distribution of receptors each sensory system, while the second column describes the physical dimensions which each class of receptor transduces. Column 3, describing the contribution of each class of sensor to motor control, corresponds to the function of the sensor-motor matrix. Integration with other sensory systems, corresponding with the sensor-sensor matrix, is described in column 4, while column 5 describes motoric contributions to sensing, and thus corresponds to the motor-sensor matrix. The table as a whole aims to show how existing knowledge of sensory systems can be related to the matrix representation of coordination.

MANIPULATION: AN EXAMPLE OF COORDINATION WITH MANY INPUTS AND MANY OUTPUTS.

Manipulating a grasped object provides a good example of the problems of using multiple sensory inputs in the control of multiple effectors. Consider a task which involves picking up a peg from a tray, transporting it to a target location, and inserting it into a hole. Typically, at least two effectors, the shoulder and elbow joints, will be used to position the hand. A number of fingers, each with three joints, may then be used to grip the peg. Such tasks could involve many sensory sources, including muscle spindles, Golgi tendon organs, joint receptors, cutaneous receptors and vision. Interestingly, the

Table 1: Summary of functions of sensory systems

Sensor	**1. Distribution of receptors**	**2. Physical events signalled**	**3. Uses of signals in motor control**
Vision	o Rod and Cone receptors densely packed on retinae. o High spatial acuity.	o Activity within a portion of electromagnetic spectrum reaching the eye.	o Judging environmental features relevant to movement, e.g., distances and time to connect (Gibson, 1950), and location of targets (Poulton, 1974). o Representation of effectors, and particularly of end-effector (Jeannerod, 1988). This becomes vital in deafferented patients (Rothwell et al., 1982; Sanes et al., 1985).
Joint receptors	o A small number are found distributed through joint capsules and ligaments (Freeman & Wyke, 1967). The cat knee joint has been the focus of most studies.	o Deformations of joint capsule caused by changes in the joint angle between two adjacent effectors. o Slowly adapting (Ruffini) and rapidly adapting (Pacinian) receptors and fibres code joint position and joint movement respectively (Skolgund, 1956). Many afferent fibres are directionally sensitive, showing best response for either flexion or extension of the joint.	o Respond best at extreme joint-angles, but poorly in mid-range o Possible importance as end stops, coding extreme joint angles (Skoglund, 1973; Grigg, 1975), and thus preventing anatomically damaging hyperextension of joints. o Now thought to contribute little to normal movement control (Lee & Kelso, 1979).
Golgi Tendon Organs	o A small number are found in most tendons. o Located in series with muscle, at the musculo-tendinous junction, serving as the serial head of parallel muscle fibres.	o Muscle tension. Almost no response related to muscle length due to low compliance of tendons.	o Estimating muscular forces. o May contribute to the protective "clasp-knife reflex", causing muscle collapse at extreme tension (Prochazka & Ward, 1980). o Tension feedback from GTOs may combine with length feedback from muscle spindles to implement compliance control (Houk, 1979).
Muscle spindle receptors	o Muscle length (static response), and rate of change of muscle length (dynamic response). o Information about many muscles around a joint specifies the position and movement of the joint and related effectors generally (Clark & Horch, 1986).	o Slowly adapting and rapidly adapting receptors and fibres code tension and rate of change of tension respectively (Prochazka & Ward, 1980).	o Spindles provide the afferent information used in the rapid monosynaptic stretch reflex, and probably also in the long loop reflex, which act to maintain a muscle at a specified length. o Provide a servo-assisted control loop for controlling muscle length. Thus spindles, may be thought of as " the first line of defense against perturbations" (Stein, 1982, p. 221).

Vestibular system	o 3 fluid-filled semicircular canals in orthogonal planes positioned adjacent to each middle ear. The end-organs are hair cells which detect movement of the fluid in the canals. o 2 otolith organs, the utricle and saccule, are located on each side of the head, adjacent to the canals. The end-organs are hair cells suspending the otoliths themselves from membranes fixed in the chamber walls (Hardy, 1934).	o Canals: transduce rotational accelerations of the head. Accelerations cause relative motion between the canals and the fluid they contain. However, the "leaky integrator" dynamics of the canals ensure that the signal in the afferent fibres represents head angular velocity as well as acceleration. Both rapidly and slowly adapting afferent fibres are found. o Otoliths: transduce linear accelerations of the head. State response of otolith organs may indicate the gravitational vertical. Both rapidly and slowly adapting fibres are found.	o The vestibular system plays a key role in postural responses and control of locomotion. o Vestibular system has an important role in two important reflexes. The vestibulo-ocular reflex (Robinson, 1981) allows the eyes to fixate while the head moves. The vestibulo-collic reflex allows the head to remain correctly oriented with respect to the environment while the rest of the body moves (Outerbridge & Melvill Jones, 1976). In both cases, the vestibular system detects motion in the head, and commands are sent to the eye and neck muscles which are proportional and opposite to the head movement which occured.
Cutaneous receptors	o Found in varying densities throughout the skin. o Density of receptors is higher in glabrous (i.e., hairless, ridged) skin, in vulnerable zones (e.g., eyelids) and in erogenous zones. Receptors are particularly dense in the hands and fingertips (Valbo & Johansson, 1978). o The four major types of receptor (Pacinian corpuscle, Meissner corpuscle, Merkel cell and Ruffini ending) have different anatomical structure, and are distributed differently within the skin.	All the cutaneous receptors respond to deformations of the skin. o Different receptor types respond to different types of deformation, thus sensing many different types of physical event (Petit & Galifret, 1978). Some classes of receptor respond to sustained deformations and others to transient deformations. The latter respond optimally to vibratory stimuli of characteristic frequencies, and their discharge is phase-locked to a stimulus event. o Each receptor has a receptive field. The receptive field structure is preserved at higher levels of processing.	Cutaneous receptors have two clear functions in movement control: o description of contacts with objects in the outside world or with other effectors. This is particularly important in manipulation (Valbo & Johansson, 1978). o description of effector position and movement. Almost any movement causes stretching and compression of the skin over the joints and related effectors. This may be particularly important in the fingers of man and higher primates, and may be less relevant for the position sense of other, more proximal joints.

Table 1 (continued): Summary of sensory systems

Sensor	4. Integration with other sensory signals	5. Motoric contribution to sensory processes
Vision	o considerable integration with other modalities such as touch, sound, vestibular senses and somatosensation in mammalian superior colliculus (Sparks & Nelson, 1985). o Vision has long been thought to collaborate with other senses in adaptive learning during early childhood (Morgan, 1977).	A number of low-level motor-sensor relationships allow maximum exchange of information between animal and environment: o Eye movements, such as vergence, accommodation, smooth pursuit and saccades, allow more and better information about stimuli to be transduced. o low-level reflex orienting responses involving eye and neck musculature, to allow rapid orientation responses (Carpenter, 1977; Robinson, 1981). o The processing of visual information is suppressed during saccades (Matin, 1974).
Joint receptors	Special role in sensing extreme range of joint movement suggests functional separation of joint receptor signals from other sensory signals. So, while joint receptors may code the same dimension as muscle spindles, they appear to do so for a separate purpose.	Response of joint receptors is affected by muscle activity (Clark & Burgess, 1975).
Golgi Tendon Organs	GTO coding of muscle tension may be integrated with spindle coding of muscle length, at least at cortical levels (Jennings et al., 1983) to provide compliance control strategies (Houk, 1979), which may be particularly valuable during contact movements.	Not known.
Muscle spindle receptors	Spindle coding of muscle length may be integrated with GTO coding of muscle tension, at least at cortical levels (Jennings et al., 1983), to provide compliance control strategies (Houk, 1979).	The motoric aspect of spindle activity is crucial to their function: o g efferents projecting to interfusal muscle fibres cause contraction of fibres within the spindle itself. This contraction determines the afferent responses of the spindle. o The g activation was thought to be a motor command signifying desired length, detected by spindle receptors as part of a length servo (Merton, 1953). However, g activation does not precede the major extrafusal a activation (Valbo, 1971).

Vestibular system	o Vestibular information is integrated with vision, cutaneous information from the soles of the feet, and information about the position of effectors, to specify posture. o Second-order neurones combine information from all the ipsilateral semicircular canals and the otoliths at a fairly low level (Baker et al., 1984), perhaps to produce a complete geometrical description of head kinematics (Droulez & Dorlot, 1988).	Not known.
Cutaneous receptors	o Cutaneous sensing is integrated with pain and temperature sensing from the receptor level right up to somatosensory cortex (e.g., Boring, 1942, p. 466). o Sakata and Iwamura (1978) found somatosensory cortex neurones tuned to a combination of elbow-joint flexion and tactile stimuli. At a more abstract level, the same authors report "grasp neurones" which are tuned to a given hand configuration and a given pattern of skin contact.	"Active touch" has long been recognised as an important phenomenon by psychologists (Gibson, 1966). Haptic examination of objects invariably involves active exploration, i.e., moving either the object or the hand so as to maximise the useful information about the object that is gained. This technique also discloses the object dynamically, which may be useful given the many rapidly adapting cutaneous receptors. Manipulation is a motoric component of haptic perception aimed at improving information exchange: it is therefore analogous to foveation in vision. o There is also evidence for the suppression of cutaneous sensing during movements (Angel & Malenka, 1982).

peg-in-hole task, as it is called, has been unofficially adopted by roboticists as a criterion for dexterity in robot control systems.

First, we consider those aspects of the peg-in-hole task which are expressed by the sensor-motor matrix. In the approach phase of the task, the preshaping of the hand to grasp the peg must be coordinated with the transport of the hand towards the target (Jeannerod, 1981; Wallace & Weeks, 1988). In normal prehension, the hand aperture increases gradually to a maximum as the hand approaches the target, and then closes more abruptly in the final few centimetres. Recent research has shown that the regular pattern of coordination of preshaping and hand transport can be rapidly modified when a change in conditions is sensed. Paulignan, MacKenzie, Marteniuk, and Jeannerod (1990), for example, asked subjects to reach for an object indicated by a target light. During the course of the approach phase, the original target light was switched off, and a new object to be grasped was indicated by a second target light coming on. Paulignan et al., observed changes in hand transport within 100 ms of the change in targets. Thus, visual information about the target position appears to be available during the movement. Interestingly, compensation for the change in targets was not restricted to hand transport. The hand preshaping component of the movement was adjusted in a way which depended on the adjustment of hand transport, ensuring a successful grasp of the object. The adjustments of hand preshaping typically involved substantial wrist rotation to orient the hand towards the new target. Further, whereas closing the grasp to obtain the object usually involves finger movements only (Wing, Turton, & Fraser, 1986), some changes in target position resulted in an increased contribution by the thumb, and a decreased contribution by the index finger. Thus, visual sensory information is used continually to produce rapid responses by many effectors. The responses are flexible, in the sense of being context-dependent, and they are coordinated, since the response of one effector is not independent of the response of the others, but rather the responses of all the effectors together help to achieve the changed goals of the task.

Haggard and Wing (1990) found evidence of coordination of hand preshaping with hand transport which was less likely to depend on vision. If hand transport was perturbed by an unexpected pull on the subjects' arm from an electric actuator, a rapid compensatory adjustment of hand aperture was also observed: hand aperture continued to increase for a short period after the onset of the perturbation, and then began to close slightly before resuming normal preshaping. The adjustment of hand aperture was consistent with subjects attempting to maintain a fixed relationship between the two effector variables of hand transport and hand aperture. While subjects could have used vision to detect the onset of the perturbation, it seems more plausible that sensory receptors in the arm detected the sudden pull by the actuator, leading to a remote adjustment by effectors involved in controlling hand preshaping.

Compensatory adjustment also occurs among the fingers of the hand. In isotonic pincer grip, for example, Cole and Abbs (1986) observed a reciprocal relationship between the contributions of the Metacarpophalangeal and Proximal Interphalangeal joints. There was considerable variability from trial to trial in the distance travelled by each joint, but a smaller than normal displacement of one joint was accompanied by a larger than normal displacement of the other joint, thus ensuring that the fingertip always met the thumb to form the pincer grip at the same point in Cartesian space. Since the two joints can be moved independently, the coordinated relationship could be due to a sensor-motor mapping between the sensors in one segment of the finger and the muscles controlling the other.

Finally, Cordo (1988) has recently offered clear evidence for the use of kinaesthetic information about the state of one effector at an independent remote effector. In a task similar to frisbee throwing, his subjects could time opening of the hand to occur when elbow rotation reached a target value, even when the arm could not be seen, and the course of elbow rotation was unpredictable due to a randomised motor load. However, it is not clear which sensory sources Cordo's subjects used to coordinate the two movements.

Returning to the peg-in-hole task, when the fingers actually contact and grasp the object, the nature of the task, and thus the cell entries in the sensor-motor matrix, suddenly change. Cutaneous sensors detecting the first contact with the object could cause this switch. During the contact phase, cutaneous sensing yields important information about the movement and stability of the object within the hand's grip. A number of studies have observed rapid, coordinated grip responses based on cutaneous information. Cole and Abbs (1989), for example, found that an unexpected downward pull on a grasped object elicited a rapid increase in the grip force exerted by the finger and thumb. Since this response did not occur if the hand itself was tugged downwards with the same force, the modulation of grip force was a flexible, task-dependent response to the object slipping, rather than a generalised "startle" response to the perturbation.

Research by Johansson and colleagues confirms that the sensorimotor mappings involved in grasping are distributed and flexible. Johansson and colleagues found that, when subjects lifted small objects with a precision grip, the grip force used showed a margin of error over and above the force required to prevent the object slipping (Westling & Johansson, 1984). Further, the grip force was increased between trials where the object's surface was changed from rough to smooth. In cases where the object did begin to slip, grip force began to increase on average after 74 ms, and continued to increase until the slipping stopped. Microelectrode recordings from single fibres in the median nerve during these tasks showed that cutaneous sensory information was associated with the object slipping (Johansson & Westling, 1987). Since the compensatory adjustment of grip force disappeared under conditions of cutaneous anaesthesia, cutaneous sensing appears to play a key role in the coordination of grip.

The way in which cutaneous information influences the various effectors involved in grip has not been fully understood. However, increases in grip force cannot be achieved by one effector alone: if just the finger muscles contracted during precision grip and the thumb muscles were not activated, the net force would produce a displacement of the object rather than an increase in grip force. So, when the task requires keeping the object stationary, the thumb muscles must also be activated: coordination of many independent effectors seems to be necessary.

When the grasped object must be moved or regrasped, the sensor-motor mapping is likely to be even more distributed and complex. More distal effectors, such as the extrinsic and forearm muscles, function as fixators during manipulation, and must adjust during regrasping to ensure accurate and stable hand positioning. Simultaneous recording from a number of muscles during grasping operations could elucidate the nature of the sensor-motor mapping involved.

Further evidence for the importance of a number of sensory sources in manipulation comes both from studies of surgically deafferented animals (Munk, 1909) and from clincal studies of patients with peripheral sensory neuropathy (Rothwell et al., 1982; Sanes et al., 1985). Typically, while these studies have reported rather little impairment in gross movement of proximal effectors, both animal and human studies have observed considerable deficits in fine manipulation (Fromm & Evarts, 1978). These deficits include an inability to maintain a constant grip force, difficulty in maintaining finger positions providing appropriate grip configuration in the absence of vision, and inability to detect and respond to unexpected displacements of the effectors, or of the object being grasped.

The existing physiological literature offers rather few clues about sensor-sensor mappings in manipulation. A number of psychophysical studies have evaluated the relative contributions of joints, muscles, tendons, and skin sensors to the sense of finger position and finger movement, typically by anaesthetising or otherwise disabling all but one of these sensory sources (see Clark & Horch, 1986, for a review). Much less is known about the way these sensory sources combine in normal movement. However, some sensor-sensor mappings have been found, notably for cutaneous sensing. For example, the receptive fields of cutaneous afferents from Meissner corpuscles and Merkel cells exhibit edge enhancement effects akin to those in the visual system (Johansson & Vallbo, 1983). This is an instance of the integration of many receptors into "virtual sensors", and serves to enhance the representation of edges in the stimulus.

Evidence for multi-sensor fusion comes largely from the discovery of single units in specialised areas of cortex, such as superior colliculus or optic tectum, which respond to particular stimuli in more than one modality (Sparks & Nelson, 1987). For example, some units respond optimally to a combination of a visual stimulus in a particular location on the retina, and a tactile stimulus on a particular part of the body. Typically, these units detect novel and salient stimuli. They often interface with motor pathways to produce a rapid, appropriate orienting response. Thus, while these units do integrate sensory information, they do so for a purpose that is computationally much simpler than world-modelling. The location, and even the existence of the world-model in the cortex remains obscure. However, all these varieties of sensor-sensor mapping could be included together in the sensor-sensor matrix.

Because of the complexity of the kinematic chain during grasping, movement of just one effector in the chain will cause a barrage of new afferent information from many sensory sources. Therefore, suppression of sensory information during movement may be important. While Angel and Malenka (1982) have reported such suppression for electrical stimuli, suppression has yet to be demonstrated for more natural tactile stimuli.

In contrast to the apparent need for sensory suppression, there is considerable physiological evidence for the *facilitation* of sensors by voluntary movements likely to involve those sensors. For example, neurons in somatosensory area 1 which receive cutaneous input become active before voluntary movement. This biasing behaviour ensures that subsequent stimulation produces greater neural activity than would otherwise occur. Prochazka (1989) concludes "cutaneous sensory transmision tends to be reduced during stereotyped motor tasks, but is elevated above resting levels in novel situations or during exploratory tasks" (p. 294).

Psychologists have also recognized active elements of cutaneous sensing, for example when the hands explore an object to gain more information during haptic object recognition (Klatzky, Lederman, & Reed, 1987). The exploratory movements observed are directed at salient perceptual features. These active, strategic aspects of sensing may be connected with the physiological process of sensory bias.

The motor-motor mappings in manipulation are probably extremely complex, as already noted. If the grasped object is rigid, as in the peg-in-hole task, then isolated movement of a joint in any one finger will cause movement of the other joints in that finger, resulting in movement of the grasped object, and thus movement of the other fingers. The consequences will be a highly nonlinear function of the original movement. The anatomy of the primate hand, particularly the large number of biarticular muscles, ensures that movements of many of the joints in the fingers are interdependent. For example, the proximal interphalangeal joint cannot be flexed without also flexing the distal interphalangeal joint. The two joints can be moved independently, however, when the fingertip is in contact with a rigid surface. The motor-motor mappings in the fingers, then, may depend critically on how each finger is involved in the grasp.

Despite their complexity, the biomechanical characteristics of the effectors are not just a nuisance, and may themselves help in the control of stable grasps. Recent robotic models have suggested that stable grasps could be assembled by taking advantage of the biomechanics of the hand itself. Each finger would act as a spring, whose preferred state would bring the finger tip to a point at the centre of the ellipse defined by all the finger's contacts on the object. The force that the finger exerts on the grasped object depends on the finger's departure from the preferred state, and on a term characterising the Cartesian compliance of the finger, which in turn depends on the compliance of the individual muscles and joints. This technique, known as *remote centre compliance* (Cutkosky, 1985) guarantees that small perturbations to the grasped object or to an individual finger will not affect the stability of the grasp. Hanafusa and Asada (1977) demonstrated the practical advantages of this approach by building a robot hand with elastic fingers.

Thus, the biomechanical relationships provided by the compliant hand-object system, and captured in the motor-motor matrix, can substantially ease the computational load in control of grasping. Indeed, Cutkosky and Kao (1989) showed that, even when biomechanical linkages between joints were not part of the design of a robot hand, they would still form a valuable part of the robot's control scheme, since coupled fingers can produce any required stiffness of the grasped object, in any arbitrary direction, whereas uncoupled fingers cannot produce some stiffnesses in some directions. They, therefore, concluded that "coupling terms among the joints on different fingers... (of a robot hand) provides... considerably more control. than we could obtain from independently servoed fingers" (p. 159). With further research, compliance control is likely to make robot hands considerably more dextrous than was possible with traditional position control schemes.

Since human prehension is normally stable and successful, the motor control system can clearly cope with these interactions between effectors, despite the computational complexity that seems to be involved.

CONCLUSION

A coordinated movement involves many effectors working together towards a goal. Sensory information from a large number of sources is often used to coordinate effectors. Representing the mutual influences of sensors and effectors via a matrix of weights offers a useful way to capture this complexity and distributedness.

ACKNOWLEDGEMENTS

I am grateful to the Wellcome trust for a Prize Studentship which made this research possible. I am also grateful to Alan Wing, Paul Cordo and Roger Lemon for comments and advice. Some earlier stages of this research were supported by a contract awarded to Alan Wing and Patrick Haggard by the Office of Naval Research.

REFERENCES

Abbs, J.H. & Winstein, C.J. (1988). Functional contributions of rapid and automatic sensory-based adjustments to motor output. In M. Jeannerod (Ed.) *Attention and Performance XIII* (pp. 627-652). Hillsdale, NJ: Lawrence Erlbaum Associates.

Angel, R.W. & Malenka, R.C. (1982). Velocity-dependent suppression of cutaneous sensitivity during movement. *Experimental Neurology, 77,* 266-274.

Åström, K.J. (1983). Theory and applications of adaptive control a survey. *Automatica, 19,* 471-486.

Bernstein, N. (1967). *The coordination and regulation of movement.* London: Pergamon.

Bootsma, R.J. (1988). *The timing of rapid interceptive actions.* Amsterdam: Free University Press.

Boring, E.G. (1942). *Sensation and perception in the history of experimental psychology.* New York: Appleton-Century.

Box, G.E.P. & Jenkins G.M. (1970). *Time Series Analysis: Forecasting and control.* San Francisco: Holden-Day.

Brooks, R.A. (1986). A layered intelligent control system for a mobile robot. *IEEE Journal of Robotics and Automation, RA-2,* 14-23.

Carpenter, R.H.S. (1977). *Movements of the eyes.* London: Pion.

Cheney, P.D. & Fetz, E.E. (1985). Comparable patterns of muscle facilitation evoked by individual corticomotoneuronal (CM) cells and by single intracortical microstimuli in primates: Evidence for functional groups of CM cells. *Journal of Neurophysiology, 53,* 784-786.

Cheung, E. & Lumelsky, V.J. (1989). Proximity sensing in robot manipulator motion planning: System and implementation issues. *IEEE Transactions on Robotics and Automation, 5,* 740-751.

Clark, F.J., & Horch, K.W. (1986). Kinaesthesia. In K. Boff (Ed.) *Handbook of Perception and Performance, Volume 1* (pp. 13/1-13/62). New York: Wiley Interscience.

Cole, K.J. & Abbs, J.H. (1986). Coordination of three-joint digit movements for rapid finger-thumb grasp. *Journal of Neurophysiology, 55,* 1407-1423.

Cole, K.J. & Abbs, J.H. (1989). Grip force adjustments evoked by load force perturbation of a grasped object. *Journal of Neurophysiology, 60,* 1513-1522.

Connell, J.H. (1989). A behaviour-based arm controller. *IEEE Transactions on Robotics and Automation, 5,* 784-791.

Cordo, P.J. (1988). Kinesthetic coordination of a movement sequence in humans. *Neuroscience Letters, 92,* 40-45.

Cutkosky, M.R. & Kao, I. (1989). Computing and controlling the compliance of a robotic hand. *IEEE Transactions on Robotics and Automation, 5,* 151-165.

Cutkosky, M.R. (1985). *Robotic grasping and fine manipulation.* Boston: Kluwer Academic.

Day, B.L., Rothwell, J.C., Thompson, P.E.D., Maertens de Nordhout, A., Nakashima, K., Shannon, K. & Marsden, C.D. (1989). Delay in the execution of voluntary movement by electrical or magnetic stimulation in intact man: Evidence for the storage of motor programm in the brain. *Brain, 112,* 643-649.

Droulez, J. & Dorlot, C. (1988). The geometric and dynamic implications of the coherence constraints in three-dimensional sensor-motor interactions. In M. Jeannerod (Ed.) *Attention and Performance XIII* (pp. 495-526). Hillsdale, NJ: Lawrence Erlbaum Associates.

Durrant-Whyte, H. (in press). Geometric sensor fusion in robotics. In T.C Henderson & E. Grant (Eds.). *Traditional and non-traditional robotic sensors.* Berlin: Springer-Verlag.

Freeman, M.A.R., & Wyke, B. (1967). The innervation of the knee joint: an anatomical and histological study in the cat. *Journal of Anatomy, 101,* 505-532.

Fromm, C. & Evarts, E.V. (1978). Motor cortex responses to kinaesthetic inputs during postural stability, precise fine movements and ballistic movement in the conscious monkey. In G. Gordon (Ed.) *Active touch* (pp. 105-117). Oxford: Pergamon.

Gallistel, C.R. (1980). *The organization of action: A new synthesis.* Hillsdale, NJ: Lawrence Erlbaum Associates.

Gandevia, S.C. & Burke, D. (1988). Projection to the cerebral cortex from proximal and distal muscles in the human upper limb. *Brain, 111,* 389-403.

Gibson, J.J. (1950). *The perception of the visual world.* Boston: Houghton Mifflin.

Gibson, J.J. (1966). *The senses considered as perceptual systems.* Boston: Houghton Mifflin.

Grigg, P. (1975). Mechanical factors influencing response of joint afferent neurones from cat knee. *Journal of Neurophysiology, 38,* 1473-1484.

Haggard, P.N. & Wing, A.M. *Multi-sensory control of coordinated robotic and biological movement.* Unpublished report prepared for the Office of Naval Research.

Haggard, P.N. & Wing, A.M. (1990). Remote responses to perturbation in human prehension. Manuscript submitted for publication.

Hanafusa, H. & Asada, H. (1977). Stable prehension by a robot hand with elastic fingers. *Proc. 7th International Symposium on Industrial Robots*, (pp. 361-368) Tokyo.

Hardy, M. (1934). Observations on the innervation of the macula sacculi in man. *Anatomical Record, 59*, 403-478.

Hebb, D.O. (1949). *The organization of behaviour.* New York: Macmillan.

Hollerbach, J.M. & Flash, T. (1982). Dynamic interactions between limb segments during planar arm movement. *Biological Cybernetics, 44,* 67-77.

Houk, J.C. (1979). Regulation of stiffness by skeleto-motor reflexes. *Annual Review of Physiology, 41,* 99-114.

Jeannerod, M. (1981). Intersegmental coordination during reaching at natural objects. In J. Long & A.D Baddeley (Eds.). *Attention and Performance, IX* (pp. 153-169). Hillsdale, NJ: Lawrence Erlbaum Associates.

Jeannerod, M. (1988). *The neural and behavioural organization of goal-directed movements.* Oxford: Oxford University Press.

Jennings, V.A., Lamour, Y., Soli, H. & Fromm, C. (1983). Somatosensory cortex activity related to position and force. *Journal of Neurophysiology, 49,* 1216-1229.

Johansson, R.S. & Vallbo, A.B. (1983). Tactile sensory coding in the glabrous skin of the human hand. *Trends in Neurosciences, 6,* 27-32.

Johansson, R.S. & Westling, G. (1987). Signals in tactile afferents from the fingers eliciting adaptive motor responses during precision grip. *Experimental Brain Research, 66,* 141-154

Keele, S.W. (1982). Learning and control of coordinated motor patterns: The programming perspective. In J.A.S. Kelso (Ed.) *Human motor behavior: An introduction* (pp. 143-160). Hillsdale, NJ: Lawrence Erlbaum Associates.

Kelso, J.A.S. (1982). Two strategies for investigating action. In J.A.S.Kelso (Ed.). *Human motor behavior: An introduction* (pp. 283-287). Hillsdale, NJ: Lawrence Erlbaum Associates.

Kelso, J.A.S., Salzman, E., & Tuller, B. (1986). A dynamical perspective on speech production, *Journal of Phonetics, 14,* 29-61.

Kelso, J.A.S., Southard, D.L. & Goodman, D. (1979). On the coordination of two-handed movements. *Journal of Experimental Psychology: Human Perception and Performance, 5,* 229-238.

Klatzky, R.L., Lederman, S.T. & Reed, C. (1987). There's more to touch than meets the eye: The salience of object attributes for haptics with and without vision. *Journal of Experimental Psychology: General, 116,* 356-369.

Kugler, P.N. & Turvey, M.T. (1986). *Information, natural law, and the self-assembly of rhythmic movement.* Hillsdale, NJ: Lawrence Erlbaum Associates.

Laszlo, J.I. & Bairstow, E.J. (1983). Kinaesthesia: Its measurement, training and relationship to motor control. *Quarterly Journal of Experimental Psychology, 35A,* 411-422.

Lee, D.N. & Aronson, E. (1974). Visual proprioceptive control of standing in human infants. *Perception & Psychophysics, 15,* 529-532.

Lee, D.N. & Lishman, J.R. (1975). Visual proprioceptive control of stance. *Journal of Human Movement Studies, 1,* 87-95.

Lee, W.A., & Kelso, J.A.S. (1979). Properties of slowly adapting joint receptors do not readily predict perception of limb position. *Journal of Human Movement Studies, 5,* 171-181.

Lumelsky, V.J., & Brooks, R.A. (1989). Sensor-based planning and control in robotics. *IEEE Transactions on Robotics and Automation, 5,* 713-715.

Marr, D.M. (1982). *Vision.* San Francisco: Freeman.

Marsden, C.D., Merton, P.A. & Morton, H.B. (1976). Stretch reflex and servo-action in a variety of human muscles. *Journal of Physiology, 259,* 531-560.

Marsden, C.D., Merton, P.A. & Morton, H.B. (1981). Human postural responses. *Brain, 104,* 513-534.

Matin, E. (1974). Saccadic supression: A review and an analysis. *Psychological Bulletin, 81,* 899-917.

Matthews, P.D.C. (1981). Muscle spindles: Their messages and their fusimotor supply. In V.B. Brooks (Ed.) *Handbook of Physiology, Section 1: The Nervous System* (Volume 2 pp. 189-228). Bethesda: American Physiological Association.

McClelland, J.L. & Rumelhart, D.E. (1987). *Parallel distributed processing. Volume 2: Psychological and biological models.* Cambridge, MA: MIT Press.

Merton, P.A. (1953). Speculations on the servo-control of movement. In J.L. Malcolm & J.A.B. Gray (Eds.), *The spinal cord* (pp. 247-255). London: Churchill.

Monsell, S. (1984). Programming of complex sequences: Evidence from the timing of rapid speech and other productions. In H. Heuer & C. Fromm (Eds.), *The generation and modulation of action patterns* (pp. 72-86). Berlin: Springer Verlag.

Morasso, P. (1981). Spatial control of arm movements. *Experimental Brain Research, 42,* 223-227.

Morgan, M.J. (1977). *Molyneux's Question.* Cambridge: Cambridge University Press.

Muir, R.B. & Lemon, R.N. (1983). Cortico-spinal neurons with a special role in precision grip. *Brain Research, 261,* 312-316.

Munk, H. (1909). Über die Folgen des Sensibilitätsverlustes der Extremität für deren Motilität. Kap XIII. In: *Über die Funktionen von Hirn und Rückenmark,* Gesamelte Mitteilungen, (pp. 247-285). Hirschwald, Berlin.

Mussa-Ivaldi, F.A., Morasso, P. & Zaccaria, R. (1988). Kinematic networks: A distributed model for representing and regularizing motor redundancy. *Biological Cybernetics, 60,* 1-16.

Nashner, L.M., & McCollum, D. (1985). The organization of human postural movements: A formal basis and experimental synthesis. *Behavioral and Brain Sciences, 8,* 135-172.

Outerbridge, J.S., & Melville-Jones, G. (1976). Reflex vestibular control of head movements in man. *Aerospace Medicine, 42,* 935-940.

Paulignan, Y., MacKenzie, C., Marteniuk, R. & Jeannerod, M. (1990). The coupling of arm and finger movements during prehension. *Experimental Brain Research, 79,* 431-435.

Penfield, W. & Rasmussen, T. (1950). *The cerebral cortex of man.* New York: Macmillan.

Petit, J., & Gallifret, Y. (1978). Sensory coupling function and the mechanical properties of the skin. In G. Gordon (Ed), *Active touch* (pp. 19-27). Oxford: Pergamon.

Poulton, E.C. (1974). *Tracking and manual control.* London: Academic Press.

Prochazka, A. (1989). Sensory motor gain control: A basic strategy of motor systems? *Progress in Neurobiology, 33,* 281-307.

Prochazka, A. & Ward, P. (1980). Tendon organ discharge during voluntary movement in cats. *Journal of Physiology, 303,* 385-390.

Rack, P.M.H. & Westbury, D.R. (1969). The effects of length and stimulus rate on tension in the isometrice cat soleus muscle. *Journal of Physiology, 204,* 443-460.

Raibert, M.H. (1986). *Legged robots that balance.* Boston: MIT Press.

Robinson, D.A. (1981). Control of eye movements. In V.B. Brooks (Ed) *Handbook of Physiology* (Vol 2, Part 2, pp. 1275-132). Bethesda: American Physiological Association.

Rothwell, J.C., Traub, M.M., Day, B.L., Obeso, J.A., Thomas, P.K. & Marsden, C.D. (1982). Manual motor performance in a deafferented man. *Brain, 105,* 515-542.

Sakata, H., & Iwamura, Y. (1978). Cortical processing of tactile information in the first somato-sensory and parietal association areas in the monkey. In G. Gordon (Ed.) *Active touch* (pp. 54-72). Oxford: Pergamon.

Salisbury, J.K. (1985). Design and control of an articulated hand. In M.T. Mason & J.K. Salisbury (Eds). *Robot hands and the mechanics of manipulation* (pp. 151-167). Cambridge, MA: MIT Press.

Sanes, J.N., Mauritz, K-H., Dalakas, M.C. & Evarts, E.V. (1985). Motor control in humans with large-fibre sensory neuropathy. *Human Neurobiology, 4,* 101-114.

Schmidt, R.A. (1982). The schema concept. In J.A. S. Kelso (Ed.) *Human motor behavior: An introduction* (pp. 219-238). Hillsdale, NJ: Lawrence Erlbaum Associates.

Sears, T.A. & Stagg, D. (1976). Short-term synchronisation of intercostal motor neurone acitivity. *Journal of Physiology, 263,* 357-381.

Sherrington, C.S. (1947). *The integrative action of the nervous system.* Cambridge: Cambridge University Press.

Skoglund, S. (1956). Anatomical and physiological studies of knee joint innervation in the cat. *Acta Physiologica Scandinavica, 36,* supplement 24, 1-101.

Skoglund, S. (1973). Joint receptors and kinaesthesia. In A. Iggo (Ed.) *Handbook of Sensory Physiology, Vol 2: Somatosensory System* (pp. 111-136). New York: Springer-Verlag.

Soechting, J.F. & Lacquaniti, F. (1981). Invariant characteristics of a pointing movement in man. *Journal of Neuroscience, 1,* 710-720.

Sparks, D.L. & Nelson, J.S. (1987). Sensory and motor maps in the mammalian superior colliculus. *Trends in Neurosciences, 10,* 312-317.

Stein, J.F. (1982). *An introduction to neurophysiology.* Oxford: Blackwell Scientific.

Stein, J.F. (1986). The role of the cerebellum in the visual guidance of movement. *Nature, 323,* 217-221.

Turvey, M.T. (1977). Preliminaries to a theory of action with reference to vision. In R. Shaw & G. Bransford (Eds.) *Perceiving, acting and knowing: Toward an ecological psychology* (pp. 211-265). Hillsdale, NJ: Lawrence Erlbaum Associates.

Turvey, M.T., Rosenblum, L.D., Schmidt, R.C. & Kugler, P.N. (1986). Fluctuations and phase symmetry in coordinated rhythmic movements. *Journal of Experimental Psychology: Human Perception and Performance, 12,* 564-583.

Vallbo, A.B. (1971). Muscle spindle response at the onset of isometric voluntary contractions in man. Time difference between fusi-motor and skeleto-motor effects. *Journal of Physiology, 318,* 405-443.

Vallbo, A.B., & Johansson, R.S. (1978). The tactile sensory innervation of the glabrous skin of the human hand. In G. Gordon (Ed.). *Active touch* (pp. 29-54). Oxford: Pergamon.

van Ingen Schenau, G.J. (1989). From rotation to translation: Constraints on multi-joint movements and the unique action of bi-articular muscles. *Human Movement Science, 8,* 301-337.

Wallace, S.A. & Weeks, D.L. (1988). Temporal constraints in the control of prehensile movement. *Journal of Motor Behavior, 20,* 81-105.

Westling, G. & Johansson, R.S. (1984). Factors influencing the force control during precision grip. *Experimental Brain Research, 53,* 277-284.

Whitney, D.E. (1969). Resolved motion rate control of manipulators and human prostheses. *IEEE Transactions on Man-Machine Systems, 10,* 47-53.

Whitney, D.E. (1972). The mathematics of coordinated control of prosthetic arms and manipulators. *ASME Journal of Dynamic Systems, Measurement and Control, 94,* 303-309.

Wing, A.M. & Fraser, C. (1983). The contribution of the thumb to reaching movements. *Quarterly Journal of Experimental Psychology, 35A,* 297-309.

Wing, A.M., Turton, A. & Fraser, C. (1986). Grasp size and accuracy of approach in reaching. *Journal of Motor Behavior, 18,* 245-260.

Wolovich, W.A. (1987). *Robotics: Basic analysis and design.* New York: Holt, Rinehart and Winston.

Yamanashi, J., Kawato, M., & Suzuki, R. (1980). Two coupled oscillators as a model for the coordinated finger tapping by both hands. *Biological Cybernetics, 37,* 219-225.

Approaches to the Study of Motor Control and Learning
J.J. Summers (Editor)

Chapter 8

CONTROL OF RAPID ARM MOVEMENT

L.R.T. Williams
University of Otago

The interest in control mechanisms underlying rapid arm swings is followed from early work with refractoriness of movement to current concern with anticipatory activity of so-called "postural" muscles. A tentative model is presented as a framework that highlights the combination of percept and action and the interaction of subject and surround. The results of experimental work confirm the Anticipatory Postural Activity (APA) effect in terms of reliability, consistency and coherency; and in particular the role of APA in the construction and implementation of actions is highlighted. Of fundamental importance is the nature of the force field and the perception of the future state of the subject and the surround. In addition to a closer investigation of dynamical relationships, future experiments should involve manipulation of behavioural conditions. As understanding develops it should continue to be applied to therapeutic and rehabilitation settings.

This chapter is concerned with the control mechanisms underlying the production and amendment of rapid arm movements. It begins with a brief outline of earlier studies of the phenomenon known as the "Psychological Refractory Period" (PRP) and leads into more recent work where the theoretical perspective is developed further. This perspective combines percept and action into a general model that outlines major features of a theory of emergent action. It also provides a framework for the laboratory's research in this area. The third section focuses on the relationship of leg muscle action to the production of rapid arm swings and presents some recent experimental findings. The final section provides a brief summary along with a discussion of future research directions.

REFRACTORINESS OF ARM SWINGS

One of the prime areas of interest for our laboratory has always been with questions to do with the learning and control of large body movements. In the early 1970s, we carried out several studies of the phenomenon known as the "psychological refractory period" (e.g., Williams, 1971a, 1971b, 1973). This "PRP" effect was demonstrated as a delay in reaction to the second of a pair of closely-spaced stimuli (RT2). Prior to that time, the PRP effect was usually examined with small movements such as the pressing or releasing of keys or the tracking of a target with and hand-held stylus and the theoretical framework was characterised by models of information processing such as the "Single-Channel" concept advanced by Welford (1952). An important study, however, was that conducted by Henry and Harrison (1961) who found that if the second stimulus (S2) arrived after approximately halfway through the reaction time (RT1) to the first stimulus (S1), subjects could not reverse the first movement before it was completed.

It was notable that in contrast to most other studies in the area, Henry and Harrison used a moderately large arm swing for the primary movement and it's reversal for the second response. Their work led to our concern with investigating two kinds of refractoriness. One was termed "temporal refractoriness" where the emphasis was on changes in RT2, while the other was called "movement refractoriness" where the focus was more directly on the inability to modify the primary movement (Williams, 1971a). The series of experiments continued to use extended arm swings and studied variables such as the type, complexity, and speed of the second movement (Williams, 1973, 1974, 1975, 1978), and evidence was found to support a programming explanation of refractoriness, that was characterised by adaptability of the controlling processes. It was also noted that two components of responding were important. One was the intentional command and the other was the reflex contribution that accompanied movement at high frequencies.

As the series developed, kinematic and neuromuscular variables were investigated; and Bernstein's (1967) influence became more apparent with consequent emphasis on muscle synergies, structural prescriptions, and the indication that force and muscle sequencing were independent properties of the arm swing and its modification.

> The PRP phenomenon, therefore, is seen not as a program disorder but as a particular context where the emergent properties of movement have a special influence on the achievement of intentional amendment (Williams, Sullivan, & Kerr, 1985, p. 227).

A MODEL FOR EMERGENT ACTION

More recently, we have made a start on studying the actions of leg muscles and their role in controlling rapid arm swings. One of the aims is to gain further understanding of the supportive role of the legs and how this integrates with the actions of the upper limbs. The perspective taken is guided by the model of how movement solutions may be achieved (Figure 1).

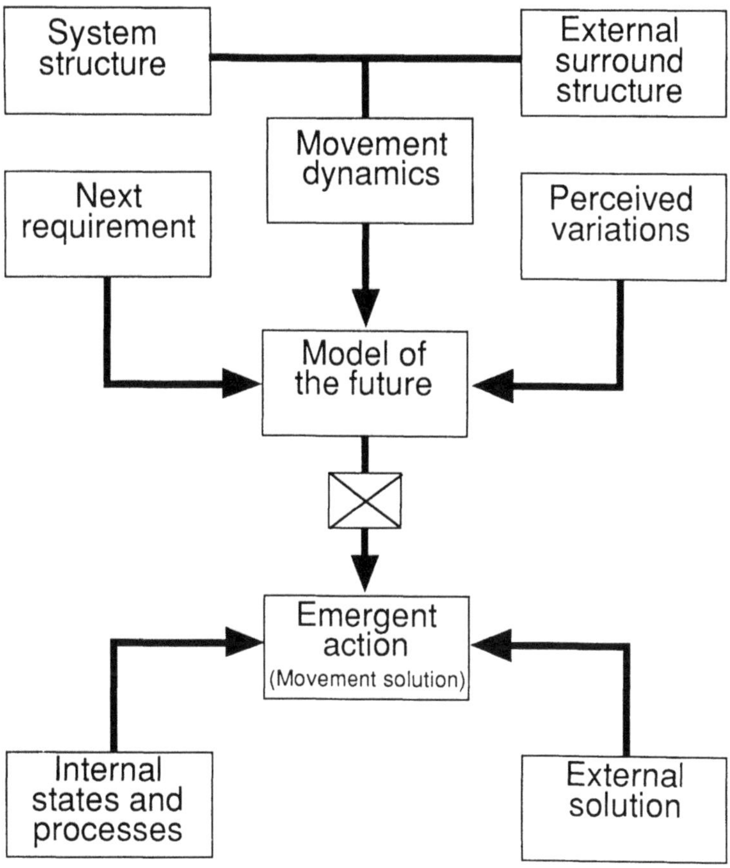

Figure 1. A model for the solution of movement problems.

Figure 1 presents a tentative model of how movement solutions may be achieved. It is a general representation that incorporates ideas from Bernstein (1967), Gahery and Massion (1981), Higgins (1980), and Lee, Buchanan, and

Rogers (1987) in an attempt to synthesise the major processes involved in producing solutions to motor problems.

A striking feature about producing movements such as rapid arm swings, is that the future state of the organism needs to be accounted for rather well if the system is to remain relatively stable. As suggested by Bernstein (1967) the first step is to formulate the motor problem in terms of a model of the future. This requirement is central to ideas represented in Figure 1. It is to be noted that the model of the future is formed not only from extrapolating the perceived variations in the surrounding environment, but also from the future requirements of the system.

More recent statements of this theme have come from Susan Higgins (1985) who describes goal-directed movement as an emergent property of a system interacting with its surround. Moreover, she emphasises the unified nature of the system's structure, the dynamics of the movement and the external surround. These perspectives are incorporated into Figure 1. The line linking "system structure" with "external surround structure" represents this interaction which relates to the force field and the perception of the future state. The result is a prescription of the essential dynamical aspects which becomes part of the model of the future. The upper half of the model emphasises the higher level cognitive processes which are concerned with programming and planning.

Once the model of the future is formed, the command string with feedforward and feedback loops produce the emergent action. A challenge for motor control theorists is to understand how an individual integrates internal states and processes with external demands to produce movement solutions. The efficacy of these solutions will be reflected by skilled coordination, reduced entropy, and minimal disturbance to system stability.

The laboratory's program of research is concerned with the theoretical perspective outlined in the present model. Since this perspective combines percept and action, several movement situations and experimental paradigms are being employed. The present program of work includes for example, studies of serial movement, cyclical movement, multilimb movement, simple reaction time (RT), choice RT, and coincident timing. The remainder of this chapter, however, will be restricted to the presentation of some recent work that focuses specifically on the interaction of posture and voluntary upper limb movement. This will be followed by a consideration of future directions.

THE ROLE OF LEG MUSCLES IN THE PRODUCTION OF RAPID ARM SWINGS

While there is a great deal known about reflex mechanisms for regulating posture, there has been less systematic investigation of the extent to which anticipatory postural components are related to voluntary limb action.

Although several studies support the view that postural adjustments can interact closely with voluntary response components (e.g., Belen'kii, Gurfinkel, & Pal'tsev, 1967; Bouisset & Zattara, 1987; El'ner, 1973; Fukuda, 1961; Jones, 1965; Lee, 1980), there is a lack of clearly quantified evidence to support the view that anticipatory postural activity (APA) is a part of programmed voluntary movement. One exception is Lee (1980) who reported robust correlations between electromyographical (EMG) activity of postural muscles and initiation of arm movement; another is the study by Bouisset and Zattara (1987) which showed that APA is especially sensitive to biomechanical variables.

Recent work from our laboratory is in accordance with previous EMG studies showing reliable APA, and robust time-locking of APA with RT. Additional evidence has suggested that such interactions may hold for different classes of upper limb movement (Williams, 1987).

The present section reports on a study that was designed to extend previous work (Bel'enkii et al., 1967; Lee, 1980; Williams, 1987) first, by increasing the number of muscles simultaneously recorded and second, by studying further several types of arm swing. The major questions addressed are as follows:

1. In the latent period of voluntary upper limb movement, is anticipatory activation of lower limb muscles confirmed?
2. Are muscle activation patterns similar over repeated trials?
3. Is the temporal sequence of muscle activity consistent over repeated observations?
4. Is preparatory activation coupled to the initiation of voluntary movement?
5. To what extent are the findings influenced by different types of voluntary movement?

Answers to the questions about consistency and coupling should help clarify the extent to which preparatory activity may be regarded as a valid part of the processes controlling voluntary limb action. For example, a high degree of sequential and temporal invariance would support the view of centrally preprogrammed control. The presence of strong coupling between preparatory changes and initiation of the voluntary movement would emphasise the integral nature of these two elements of control.

Comparison of different types of arm swing should reveal specific functional synergies, and support the view that they form the basis for reliable and efficient interaction between the movement system and the surround (Gelfand, Gurfinkel, Tsetlin, & Shik, 1971).

Method

Subjects stood in a comfortable position with the right hand resting against a microswitch. The task was a simple RT one where the period between the warning light (W) and the signal to move (S) was randomly varied between 2, 3, and 4 sec. In response to S, the subject swung the right arm in a predetermined manner to a position designated by a strip of soft cardboard. Instructions emphasised remaining relaxed while waiting for the signal lights and moving the arm (which is kept straight throughout) in a fast but controlled speed to finish at the defined end-point.

An acceleration signal was provided by an accelerometer attached to the subject's right wrist, and EMG data were provided by pairs of electrodes (2.5 cm apart) on nine muscles. For all swing conditions, the ipsilateral and contralateral pairs for biceps femoris, rectus femoris, gastrocnemius, and tibialis anterior of the legs were monitored, along with the shoulder muscle appropriate to the direction of the arm movement (either the anterior or posterior deltoid). The ground electrode was placed on the subject's forehead. Skin resistance of less than 10 K ohms was required for each electrode pair. The signal from the RT key was used only as a trigger channel. An APC IV microcomputer with the Computerscope Phi package was used for data acquisition and analysis. All data were captured directly on to hard disk at a frequency of 500Hz and simultaneously recorded on a 14-channel FM tape for backup.

Five right-handed males were the subjects. Testing was carried out in a single session where 30-32 trials for each swing condition were administered. Four swing types were used with the order balanced over subjects who had a 3 min rest (seated) while the RT key and cardboard target were re-sited. The swing conditions were:

Sagittal - Forward (SF): From a standing position with arms at the side, the direction was forward-upward in the sagittal plane to finish with the arm in the vertical position.

Sagittal - Backward (SB): The starting position was with the arm horizontal and directly in front of the right shoulder. The swing direction was downward-backward in the sagittal plane to pass through the vertical and end just behind the line of the body.

Horizontal - Backward (HB): Starting from a similar position to SB (except that the hand was opposite the left shoulder with the palm faced down) the direction was horizontal and backward to end at a comfortable position just behind the line of the shoulders.

Horizontal - Forward (HF): A horizontal swing as in HB except that the starting position was directly in line with the shoulders and the end-point was just past the medial line with the hand in line with the left shoulder.

The major steps in data processing consisted of trial-by-trial examination of all channels, rectification and integration of EMG, measurement of onset latencies for every trial, and subsequent signal averaging over trials.

Results

Figure 2 shows the conditioned EMG signals and acceleration profiles for the first 10 trials for one of the subjects under the SF condition. Apart from the relatively diffuse activity of the ipsilateral gastrocnemius muscle and to a lesser extent the contralateral gastrocnemius, each muscle shows a high degree of profile similarity from trial to trial; and viewing across muscles suggests sequential coherence. Close inspection revealed that such consistency was characteristic over all trials - which was verified by comparing the results of averaging different numbers of trials (Williams, 1988). The results for the other four subjects were also consistent and coherent with the only anomaly being the inability to determine clear onset times for the gastrocnemius muscles for one of the subjects.

Table 1. Mean Latencies (ms) of Pooled Data in Ascending Order [a]

SB		SF		HB		HF	
BFC	166	BFI	134	BFC	131	BFI	141
RFI	173	TAI	174	RFI	150	RFC	158
PD	181	AD	212	PD	163	TAI	165
RT	214	TAC	215	GC	168	TAC	206
RFC	272	RFC	223	RT	219	GI	212
TAI	290	GI	234	TAC	239	AD	212
BFI	294	RFI	241	TAI	267	RT	215
GI	320	BFC	263	GI	286	GC	299
TAC	323	GC	265	BFI	295	BFC	309
VEL	410	RT	269	RFC	297	RFI	327
GC	445	VEL	591	VEL	440	VEL	501

[a] RT = reaction time, VEL = velocity, AD = anterior deltoid, PD = posterior deltoid, BF = biceps femoris, RF = rectus femoris, TA = tibialis anterior, G = gastrocnemius. Abbreviations ending in C and I refer to contralateral and ipsilateral respectively.

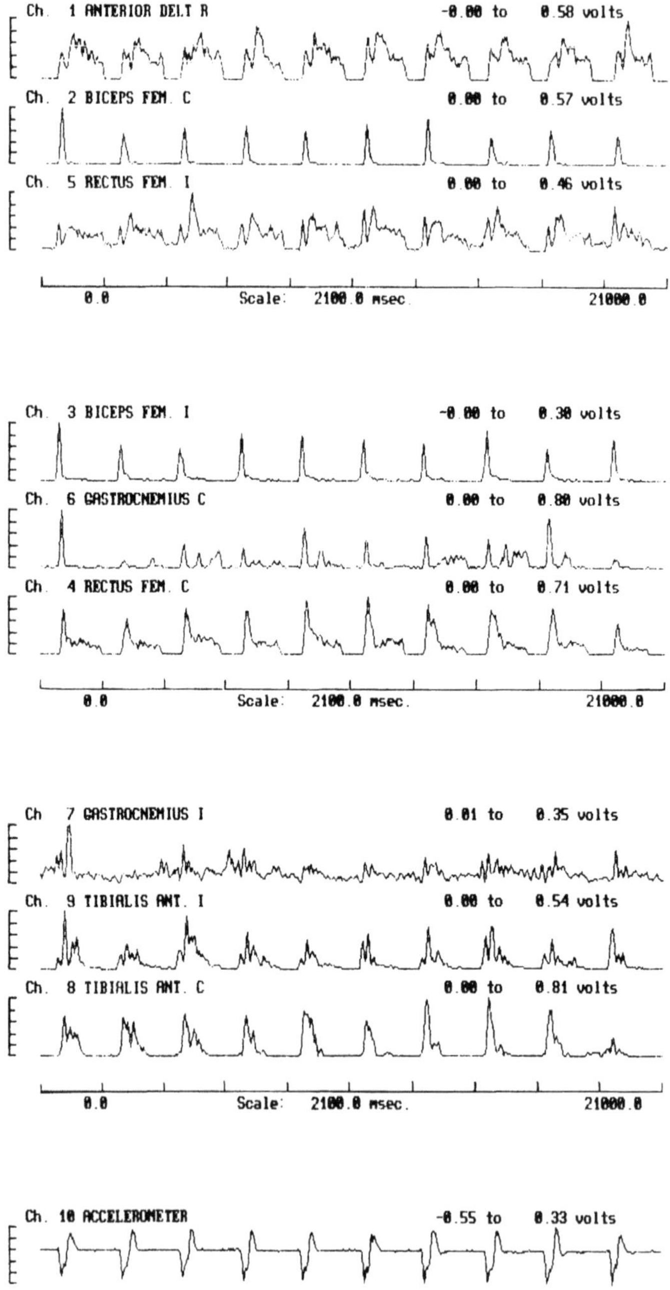

Figure 2. Electromyographic responses for the first 10 trials of the sagittal forward (SF) swing for one subject. The acceleration signal is the bottom trace.

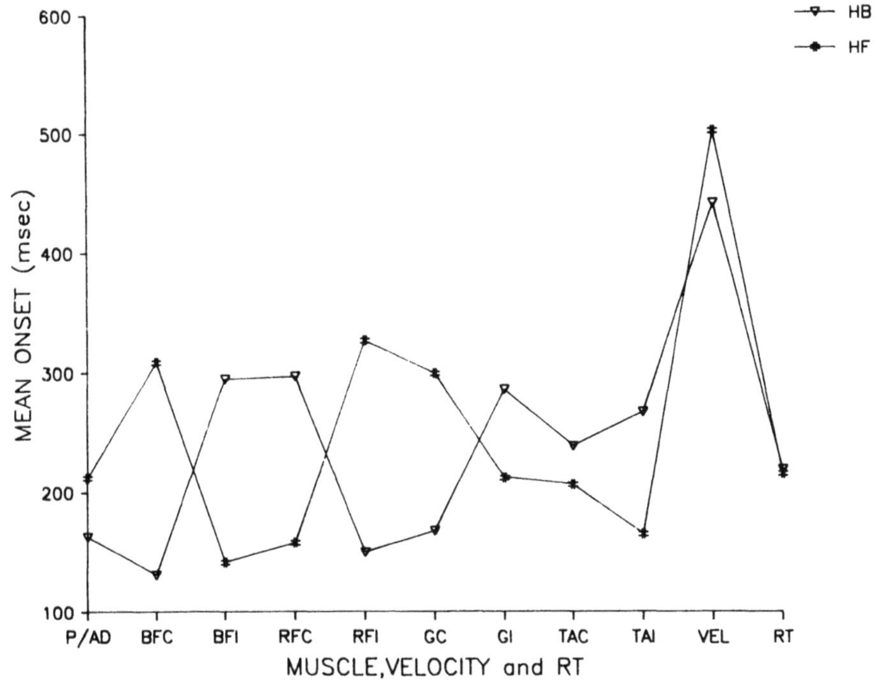

Figure 3. Mean onset times for HF. RT = reaction time, VEL = peak velocity, AD = anterior deltoid, BF = biceps femoris, RF = rectus femoris, TA = tibialis anterior, G = gastrocnemius. Abbreviations ending with C and I refer to contralateral and ipsilateral, respectively.

With regard to the SB, HF, and HB swings, although there were expected changes in muscle sequence, the data demonstrated the same level of consistency.

Onset latencies were measured for every trial for each swing condition; and while differences between subjects were maintained, there was a marked similarity of the onset profiles within each swing type. Figure 3 presents these results for HF as an example. Included in the figure is RT, which was measured as the first point of excursion of the acceleration signal, and peak velocity (VEL) which was found by integrating acceleration. The graph shows that for every subject, certain muscles became active prior to RT.

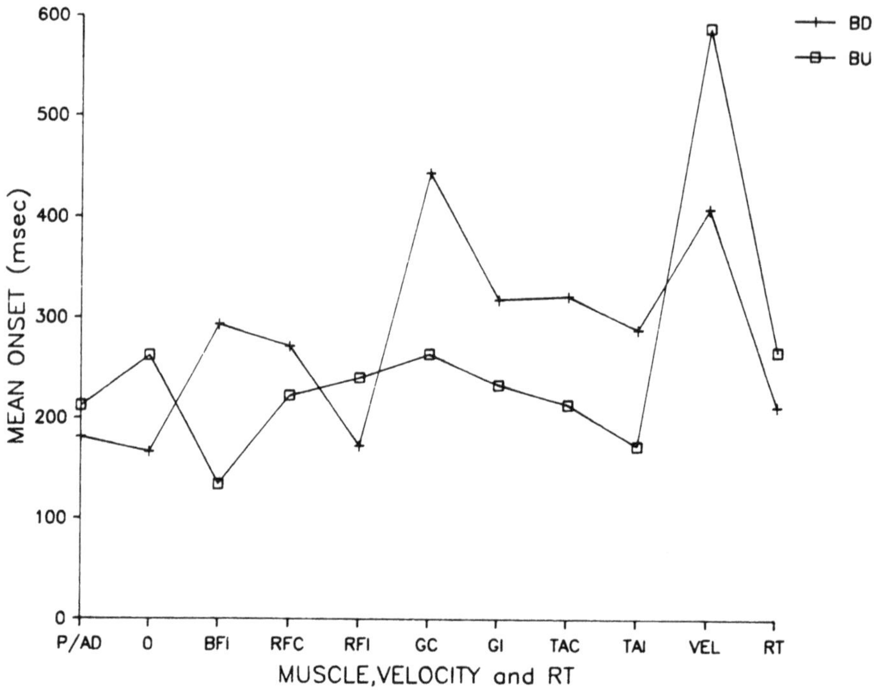

Figure 4. Onset times averaged over subjects for the two sagittal swing conditions. RT = reaction time, VEL = peak velocity, P/AD = posterior/anterior deltoid, BF = biceps femoris, RF = rectus femoris, TA = tibialis anterior, G = gastrocnemius. Abbreviations ending with C and I refer to contralateral and ipsilateral, respectively.

In order to characterise these findings further, onset times were pooled for all trials over all subjects and then averaged. Figure 4 compares the two sagittal swings and illustrates the finding that the synergistic relationship among the muscles varies accordingly with the class of movement. Moreover, as seen in Table 1, this variation includes different amounts of APA. With the SF swing for example, most of the muscles led by BFI are activated prior to movement onset since there is a great deal of work against gravity; while in contrast, the SB swing which is assisted by gravity is led by BFC and has much less APA. Comparison of the two swings in the horizontal plane (HF and HB in Figure 5) confirms further such specificity. These findings are in close agreement with the hypothesis that the solution to motor problems involve highly specific functional synergies. In testing coherence more formally, different kinds of correlational analysis were used. The first type was a within - subject correlation between all latencies (including RT and VEL) carried out over all available trials. The results for the different swings are summarised in

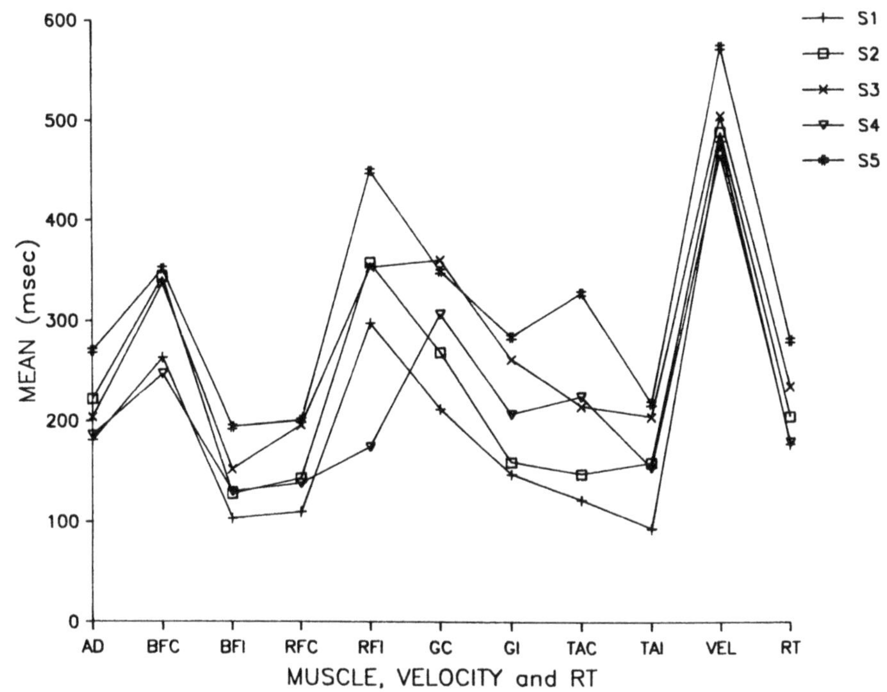

Figure 5. Onset times averaged over subjects for the two horizontal swing conditions. RT = reaction time, VEL = peak velocity, P/AD = posterior/anterior deltoid, BF = biceps femoris, RF = rectus femoris, TA = tibialis anterior, G = gastrocnemius. Abbreviations ending with C and I refer to contralateral and ipsilateral, respectively.

Table 2 in the rows designated "w/s #" and "w/s %". For SF, 92% of the within-subject inter-muscle correlations (EMG) were significant; as were 93% of the EMG-RT correlations and 91% of those for EMG-velocity. SB has corresponding figures of 66, 78, and 83% and the HB figures are less than those for HF.

The second analysis simply pooled all the data over subjects before correlating within swing type. These results, which are also summarised in Table 2, generally show higher percentages of statistically significant correlations and emphasise the robustness of the inter-relationships within swing type. The third correlational analysis was conducted within subjects. However, in this case the variables were trials and the profile made up by the EMG, RT, and VEL latencies for a given trial was correlated with that of another trial. All pairs of trials were correlated. The results are summarised

Table 2. Summary of Significant Correlations ($p<.05$)[a]

SWING TYPE	EMG	EMG - RT	EMG - VEL	EMG - PROFILE
SF w/s #	152/165	40/43	39/43	2151/2151
w/s %	92	93	91	100
pooled #	32/36	9/9	9/9	--
pooled %	89	100	100	--
SB w/s #	95/144	28/36	30/36	1399/1415
w/s %	66	78	83	99
pooled #	30/36	8/9	9/9	--
pooled %	83	89	100	--
HF w/s #	157/180	42/45	40/45	2064/2064
w/s %	87	93	89	100
pooled #	36/36	9/9	40/45	--
pooled %	100	100	89	--
HB w/s #	96/180	31/45	34/45	2140/2158
w/s %	53	69	76	99
pooled #	36/36	9/9	9/9	--
pooled %	100	100	100	--

[a] w/s # refers to the number of significant within-subject correlations expressed in relation to the total number available, and w/s % expresses the ratio as a percentage. The pooled data are for correlations calculated across subjects.

in the right column of Table 2 where it is seen that practically every profile correlation was significant.

Discussion

The results of this experiment have shown that muscle activity in the preparation phase of voluntary movement is consistent and coherent in terms of sequential and temporal features. It is also evident that considerable coupling of such activity occurs; and that it ranges over both preparatory and execution phases of the voluntary response. In addition, there is strong evidence indicating that anticipatory postural muscle activity is time-locked to the initiation of voluntary movement.

These findings support the view that postural activity prior to onset of voluntary movement is an important component of the planned response. While this role may be described in terms of "pre-tuning" the motor apparatus, close coupling of this pre-movement activity with parameters of the voluntary action emphasises the highly integrated nature of the complex kinematic chain. The early onset of postural activity that is coupled with the main "task" muscles fits in well with the view that the central program controlling the action prepares for system stabilisation as well as the voluntary limb movement (Gahery & Massion, 1981; Gelfand et al., 1971). The findings are also in accordance with the present model of the control of emergent action based on modelling the future state of the organism and its relation to the surround.

However, such results can pose a problem for information processing models and the measurement of central processing time. While RT and fractionated RT have been widely used as measures of processing time, it appears that if the planned movement will affect stability of the system, then the overt action that first emerges as part of the response may result not from "task" muscles but from muscles directly concerned with stability.

GENERAL DISCUSSION

The present findings illustrate the flexible, adaptable, and coherent manner in which action plans are formulated to solve movement problems. Moreover, it is becoming increasingly clear that to achieve a greater understanding of the interaction of living systems and their surrounds, more attention needs to be devoted to the dynamics of systems as they relate to force characteristics of the motor field and as they relate to the organism's perception of the future state.

In considering force characteristics surrounding rapid limb movements, there seem to be two complimentary features. One is the generation of a flow of force that moves mechanically through the system. The requirement here is to generate momentum through a chain of linked segments so that the target segment (or segments) move appropriately. The emphasis here is on the *construction* of the primary movement sequence.

The second feature is the need for the *maintenance* of system stability. However, it does not seem reasonable to suppose that APA is part of a program just to preserve stability. It can also be part of the desired action and have a role in the necessary generation of the flow of force through the system. These two features therefore, need to be interactive since it seems unlikely that the system can organise one in the absence of the other. The processes of construction and maintenance are thus complimentary, parallel, and interactive.

The experiment presented here illustrates how different classes of movement require functional synergies that are specific to task requirements. As emphasised by Bouisset and Zattara (1987), this specificity is largely dependent on the resultant force flow as it relates to the centre of gravity of the system. In the sagittal swings for example, the resultant force flow can be described as being essentially linear where the primary movement action does not cross the line of gravity. In contrast, the horizontal class of movements have a strong rotational component where the action does cross the line of gravity. The central nervous system is clearly sensitive to these important biomechanical factors and is able to produce the emergent action using specific synergies that are appropriate for the system's future force field as it interacts with the environmental force field.

DIRECTIONS FOR FUTURE RESEARCH

The work presented here is incomplete. So far it has concentrated on the reliability of relationships between timing parameters and has investigated the characteristics of different movement classes. Current work involves several areas. One is studying the relationship between EMG amplitudes and acceleration parameters as a function of different force fields. The strategy employed so far is to have subjects forcefully halt the primary arm swing (SF) at a designated position. The results indicate that in comparison to "non-halt" conditions, certain muscles are activated even sooner. In addition muscles involved in halting the movement become activated earlier in a manner that resembles the SB primary swing (Williams, 1988).

Other experiments use a serial arm movement task that has three directional changes (in the horizontal plane) to study the effects of response uncertainty. In comparing simple and choice RT conditions, preliminary findings indicate that while the muscles primarily involved in initiating arm movement are activated earlier for the simple situation, certain upper leg muscles are activated slightly earlier under the choice condition. Moreover, these leg muscles are those that are expected to be closely involved in producing the appropriate force flow between the leg columns (Williams & Morrison, 1990).

Studies of the effects of physical fatigue on APA are in progress and preliminary findings for onset latency confirm robust inter-muscle relationships and strong correlations between the major upper leg muscles and the onset of the primary upper arm movement. It also appears, however, that while APA is still apparent for specific leg muscles when they are fatigued, amplitude of their response is reduced. As our understanding of this area develops we also need to continue seeking to make contributions to the applied problems faced by workers in the field of physical therapy and rehabilitation of movement coordination. Examples of such work are given by Lee (1989) with broad perspectives well set out in the recent book by Carr and colleagues (Carr, Shepherd, Gordon, Gentile, & Held, 1987).

ACKNOWLEDGMENTS

This work was supported by the University Grants Committee (grant numbers 32-566, 32-586, and 32-610); and the University of Otago Research Committee (DHA-805, DHA-813 and DHA-817). Appreciation is also expressed to Miss K. Fleming for assistance with data capture.

REFERENCES

Belen'kii, V.Y., Gurfinkel, V.S.,& Pal'tsev, Y.I. (1967). Elements of control of voluntary movements. *Biofizika, 12*, 135-141.

Bernstein, N. (1967). *The co-ordination and regulation of movements.* New York: Pergamon.

Bouisset, S., & Zattara, M. (1987). Biomechanical study of the programming of anticipatory postural adjustments associated with voluntary movement. *Journal of Biomechanics, 20*, 735-742.

Carr, J.H., Shepherd, R.B., Gordon, J., Gentile, A.M., & Held, J.M. (1987). *Movement Science: Foundations for physical therapy in rehabilitation.* Rockville, Maryland, Aspen.

El'ner, A.N. (1973). Possibilites of correcting the urgent voluntary movements and the associated postural activity of human muscles. *Biofizika, 18*, 907-911.

Fukuda, T. (1961). Studies in human dynamic postures from the viewpoint of postural reflexes. *Acta Oto-laryngologica Supplementum, 161,* 1-52.

Gahery, Y., & Massion, J. (1981). Coordination between posture and movement. *Trends in Neuroscience, 81*, 199-202.

Gelfand, I.M.,Gurfinkel, V. S., Tsetlin, M.L., & Shik, M.L. (1971). Some problems in the analysis of movements. In I.M. Gelfand, V.S. Gurfinkel, S.V.

Fomin, & M.L. Tsetlin (Eds.), *Models of the structural-functional organization of certain biological systems* (pp. 329-345). Cambridge, Mass: MIT Press.

Henry, F.M., & Harrison, J.S. (1961). Refractoriness of a fast movement. *Perceptual and Motor Skills, 13,* 351-354.

Higgins, S. (1985). Movement as an emergent form: Its structural limits. *Human Movement Science, 4,* 119-148.

Jones, F.P. (1965). Method for changing stereotyped response patterns by the inhibition of certain response sets. *Psychological Review, 72,* 196-214.

Lee, W.A. (1980). Anticipatory control of postural and task muscles during rapid arm flexion. *Journal of Motor Behavior, 12,* 185-196.

Lee, W.A. (1989). A control systems framework for understanding normal and abnormal posture. *American Journal of Occupational Therapy, 43,* 291-301.

Lee, W.A., Buchanan, T.S., & Rogers, M.W. (1987). Effects of arm acceleration and behavioral conditions on the organization of postural adjustments during arm flexion. *Experimental Brain Research, 66,* 257-270.

Welford, A.T. (1952). The 'psychological refractory period' and the timing of high-speed performance - a review and theory. *British Journal of Psychology, 43,* 2-19.

Williams, L.R.T. (1971a). Refractoriness of a long movement. *Research Quarterly, 42,* 212-219.

Williams, L.R.T. (1971b). Refractoriness of an extended movement to directional change. *Journal of Motor Behavior, 3,* 289-300.

Williams, L.R.T. (1973). Psychological refractoriness of two serial motor responses. *Research Quarterly, 44,* 24-33.

Williams, L.R.T. (1974). Effects of number of alternatives on the psychological refractoriness of an extended movement. *Journal of Motor Behavior, 6,* 227-234.

Williams, L.R.T. (1975). Effects of complexity on movement refractoriness. *Research Quarterly, 46,* 177-183.

Williams, L.R.T. (1987). Control of rapid arm movement and anticipatory postural activity. Paper presented at the *Fifth International Australasian Winter Conference on Brain Research*, Queenstown, New Zealand.

Williams, L.R.T. (1988). The role of anticipatory activity of postural muscles in the control of arm movements. Paper presented at the *XXIV International Congress of Psychology*, Sydney, Australia.

Williams, L.R.T., & Morrison, S. (1990). Preparation and programming for a movement series. Paper presented at the *Commonwealth and International Conference on Physical Education, Sport, Health, Dance, Recreation and Leisure,* Auckland, Australia.

Williams, L.R.T., & Sullivan, S.J. (1978). Effects of movement speed on the refractoriness of an extended movement to reversal. *Journal of Human Movement Studies, 4,* 70-84.

Williams, L.R.T., Sullivan, S.J., & Kerr, G.K. (1985). Movement refractoriness: The influence of response structure and speed. *Human Movement Science, 4*, 203-228.

PART III

VISUO-MOTOR PROCESSES

Approaches to the Study of Motor Control and Learning
J.J. Summers (Editor)

Chapter 9

VISUOMOTOR CONTROL IN GOAL-DIRECTED MOVEMENTS

Graham K. Kerr
Oxford University

The intention of this chapter is to outline some of the experimental approaches I have undertaken in attempting to understand the mechanisms involved in visuomotor control. This research has primarily been directed at understanding the time course of the processes that occur between the reception of visual information and the issuing of a motor command. In the first part of the chapter an outline of some of the complexities involved in the production of visually guided movements is described. Secondly, an experiment is presented in which the temporal and spatial relationship between eye and arm movements was examined in a simple motor task, both at an unskilled and skilled level of performance. This experiment serves to describe characteristics typical of actual eye and arm movements and to outline some control processes that have been inferred from different levels of analysis. In the third part of the chapter the summary of an experiment is presented which was designed to ascertain the temporal constraints governing the utilisation of visual information prior to and during a movement. This experiment has been able to illustrate both the parallel and serial processing capacities of the visuomotor control system.

COMPLEXITIES OF VISUOMOTOR CONTROL

In performing goal-directed movements within our environment we constantly acquire and process a rich variety of visual information. This information is used both to locate objects in peripersonal and extrapersonal space and to plan and guide appropriate motor actions. But this is no easy feat given that visual information is primarily specified within a coordinate system that is relative to the external world (extrinsic coordinates) and motor information is specified within a coordinate system that is relative to the body (intrinsic coordinates). Each of these coordinate systems may also have a number of possible representations (e.g., Cartesian, polar, muscle length, joint angle). Thus in order for these different sources of motor and sensory information to be integrated, the diverse neural signals and their respective coordinate domains must be combined within a common representational base (Knudsen, DuLac, & Esterly, 1987; Lacquaniti, 1989; Stein, 1989).

In both neurophysiological and cognitive terms, the processing of afferent and efferent information arising from the visual and motor systems appears immensely difficult. The complexity involved in these processes is manifest in the large number of intermediate connections that exist between the visual and motor cortices. Thus visual control of movement is not the result of direct cortico-cortico connections but involves the linking of visual, motor, and parietal cortices via subcortical pathways including the basal ganglia and the cerebellum (Stein, 1986). Cognitive approaches towards understanding visuomotor control have recognised this inherent complexity by proposing that control processes are distributed (Arbib, 1981) according to a heterarchical organisation (Turvey, Shaw, & Mace, 1978), and that they are reliant on different levels of sensorimotor representation (Saltzman, 1979).

Understanding the processes and variables essential to the representation and control of movement has been a major challenge for motor control researchers. That these are able to be inferred from events and regularities in the kinematic profile of movement is a major assumption underlying the study of movement behaviour (Bernstein, 1967). What has been observed at a behavioural level is that movements appear to display both continuous and intermittent control (Craik, 1947; Miall, Weir, & Stein, 1986; Neilson, Neilson, & O'Dwyer, 1988; Stein, Miall, & Weir, 1987). This may in part be due to the nature of the visual information and the mechanisms involved in its acquisition. Certainly, predictable visual information appears to involve different control mechanisms in the production of movement than unpredictable information (Miall et al., 1986; Stein et al., 1987). Examination of saccadic eye movement and manual responses has implicated several control mechanisms that appear to be involved in visuomotor control and which have a corollary with neurophysiological processes. These include mechanisms involved in the preparation of movement based on the predictability of the visual stimulus, feedforward or efference copy mechanisms for the early control of movement, and mechanisms involved in feedback control (Becker & Jurgens, 1979; Cordo, 1987; Jeannerod & Prablanc, 1983).

That the performance of goal-directed movements is highly dependent on the processing of visual information has been emphasised by the degradation in performance that occurs when visual information is altered or removed. When limited visual information is available, such as when targets are briefly presented or vision of the limb is partly or wholly excluded, there is an increase in spatial error of both saccadic eye and arm movements (Jeannerod, 1988; Mather, 1985). There are considerable deviations from normal trajectories when visual information is delayed (Smith & Bowen, 1980) or prismatically altered (e.g., Held, 1965; Held & Freedman, 1963). Movements to intercept moving objects are also dependent on the amount of time that visual information is available (e.g., Whiting, Gill, & Stephenson, 1970).

The visual properties of a target have also been shown to exert a profound influence on the movement trajectory. Smaller targets, which may be equated with a higher index of difficulty, generally result in slower movements and more corrections during the terminal phase of the movement. These discrete corrections have been considered to be mediated by closed-loop visual feedback (e.g., Crossman & Goodeve, 1983; Fitts, 1954). But there may also be an overall slowing down of the whole movement trajectory (e.g., Marteniuk, MacKenzie, Jeannerod, Athenes, & Dugas, 1987), and more constrained terminal trajectories may also occur (Soechting, 1984). Grasp size during reaching has also been found to be adjusted in accordance with the perceived size of an object although independent of the transport component of the movement (Jeannerod, 1981; cf. Wing, Turton, & Fraser, 1986).

Controlling visually guided movements can, therefore, be seen to be a very complex process. The transition from the reception of afferent visual information to the efferent motor commands entails transformations of the neural signals. Moreover, how the involved control processes govern these input/output relationships is very much dependent on the nature of the task and the environment within which it is performed. Still we have been able to identify some of the control mechanisms and the manner in which they exert their influence. In the following sections of the chapter some of these processes will be presented in conjunction with experiments that I have undertaken that have examined the relationship between concurrent eye and arm movements.

LEARNING AND PERFORMANCE OF A STEP TRACKING TASK

In this section of the chapter I will present some of the findings of an experiment in which subjects were required to perform a simple step tracking task. The purpose of this experiment was to examine the temporal and spatial relationships between the eye and the arm and to ascertain whether these relationships changed with practice. Subjects were required to track targets displayed on an oscilloscope screen by moving a manipulandum, the angular position of which was monitored as a cursor on the screen (Fig. 1). The discrete elbow extension movements, which were performed as fast and accurately as possible, were practised by seven subjects for 80 trials a day over

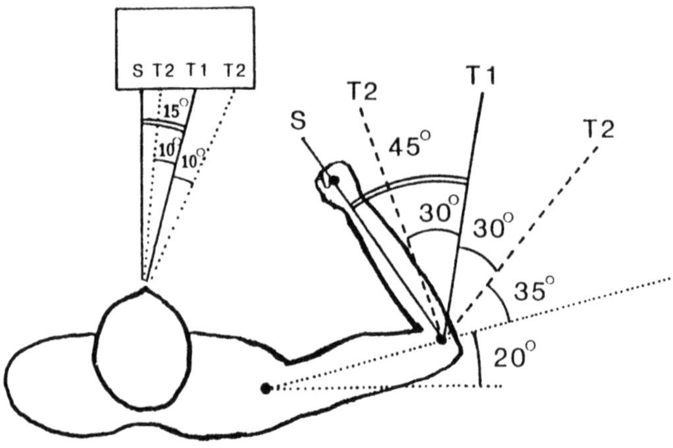

Figure 1. Experimental arrangement illustrating target angles and locations for eye and arm movements. Eye movements were recorded by the electro-oculographic (EOG) method (Shackel, 1967). Arm movements were performed with a manipulandum which constrained subject's actions to the horizontal plane. Electromyographic (EMG) activity was recorded from the lateral head of triceps (agonist) and the biceps brachii (antagonist). A reaction time paradigm was used for the presentation of the targets. Prior to each trial subjects were given a verbal "ready" signal upon which they fixated the start target and aligned the manipulandum cursor with the start position. A warning light was then illuminated and was followed, after a variable delay (1.5s, 2s, 2.5s), by a horizontal pulse-step of the target to the right (T1). This target step corresponded to a visual angle of 15° and an elbow extension angle of 45°.

a three day period. An example of the changes that occurred with practice for one subject have been illustrated in Figure 2.

Eye Movements

The visual information that is available for the production and execution of goal-directed movements is highly dependent on retinal sensitivity to different visual stimuli, where the eye is directed, and whether it is moving or not. The eye movements that were associated with the present experiment are known as saccades. They primarily serve to direct visual information onto the fovea and are considered to be the only eye movements that can be voluntarily produced (Carpenter, 1988).

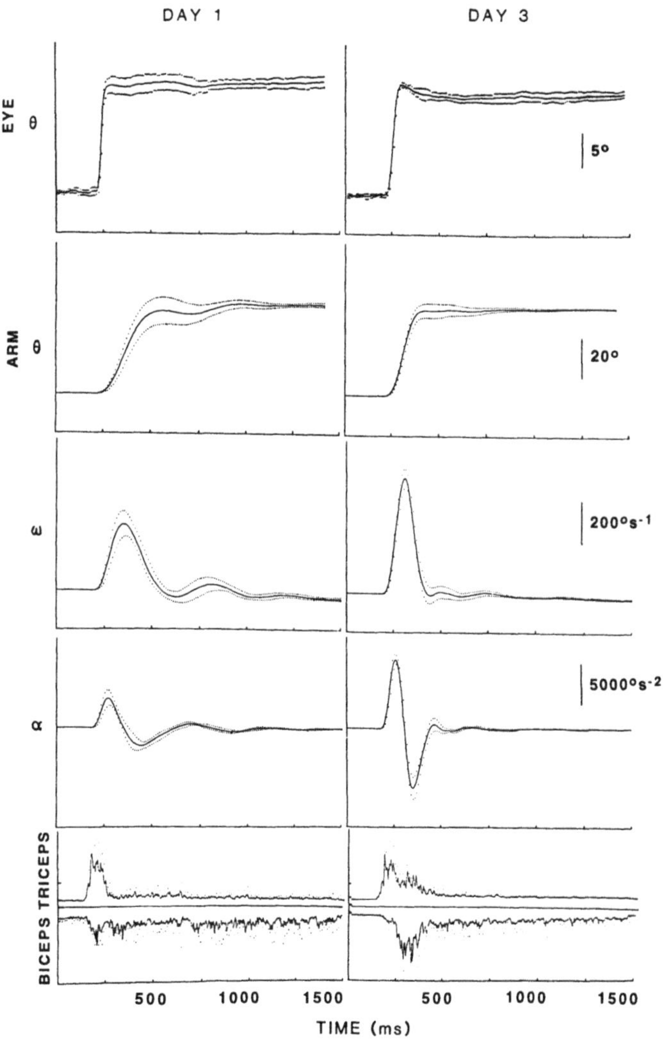

Figure 2. Performance of one subject at the start and finish of practice. These data represent the mean (±1SD) performance of the first block of eight trials on day one and the last block of eight trials on day three. The figure contains, from top to bottom, eye displacement averaged to onset of the eye movement, and arm displacement, velocity, acceleration and triceps and biceps EMG averaged to onset of the arm movement.

Saccade Initiation. Three important properties of these saccades are apparent when the displacement record of the eye, depicted at the top of Figure 2, is considered. First there was an average delay of 287 ms in initiating the movement. This delay reflects the time taken to detect the target and to compute and initiate the required motor command. It can be influenced by a number of factors including target luminance (Wheeless, Cohen, & Boynton, 1967), target predictability (e.g., Fuchs, 1967; Stark, Vossius, & Young, 1962), movement amplitude (e.g., Bartz, 1962; White, Eason, & Bartlett, 1962), and attention (Fischer, 1986, 1987). Decreases in saccadic reaction time with increased practice have been reported (Fischer, Boch, & Ramsperger, 1984; Fischer & Ramsperger, 1986), although no such changes were obtained in the present experiment.

Saccade Duration. Secondly, once commenced, the eye moved very rapidly to the target. The brief duration of the saccade (83 ms) emphasised its ballistic nature. However, despite the rapidity of saccades, their kinematic profiles are able to be influenced by the required task and instructional set (Crawford, 1984; Viviani & Berthoz, 1977), and are also dependent on the direction of the movement (Collewijn, Erkelens, & Steinman, 1988; Pelisson & Prablanc, 1988).

Spatial Accuracy. Finally, at the start of practice, the initial saccade undershot the target by up to 1.25° on 39% of trials and a corrective saccade was required to attain the target. Saccades to suddenly presented targets have been reported to fall short of the target by about 10% (Becker & Fuchs, 1969; Pelisson & Prablanc, 1988; Prablanc, Masse, & Echallier, 1978). The frequency (Prablanc et al., 1978) and the magnitude of this undershoot have been found to increase with the amplitude of the required movement (Vivianni & Swensson, 1982). One possible reason for this undershoot is that it is due to the incomplete or faulty computation of the saccade amplitude (Fischer, 1987). A rapidly initiated saccade may, therefore, undershoot the target because of the greater uncertainty of the targets position (Collewijn et al., 1988). This hypothesis is supported by the present experimental results when it is considered that, by the end of practice, saccades were more accurate (14.8°) and required fewer corrections (21%). Presumably subjects produced more accurate saccades in this instance because they were able to learn the position of the target, which always appeared at the same location. Saccadic accuracy is also increased when targets are continuously visible (Collewijn et al., 1988).

Processing Visual Information During Eye Movements. The ballistic properties of saccades present a potential problem to the visual system. Because of their rapidity the image that is projected onto the retina is likely to be blurred. And because the eye is directed at a new spatial location the visual world may appear to have abruptly shifted. However, certain mechanisms exist that prevent the perception of motion during saccades and also ensure the perception of a stable external visual world. This appears to be accomplished by the inactivation of motion-dependent mechanisms which are sensitive to stimuli of high temporal and low spatial frequency (Burr, Holt, Johnston, & Ross, 1982; Burr & Ross, 1986). Some 40 ms before the eye moves there is an increase in the visual threshold which lasts up to 100 ms after the commencement of the saccade (Latour, 1962). Consequently, the saccade itself has often been considered to be a period of inactive information processing (e.g., Matin, 1974).

Control Processes Inferred from Corrective Saccades. However, investigations of corrective saccades have indicated that visual information may not necessarily be totally excluded during a saccade. Corrective saccades have been considered to be calculated during the fixation period following the primary saccade and, therefore, to be based on an estimate of visual error derived from reafferent information (Carpenter, 1988; Salthouse & Ellis, 1980). However, the observation that corrective saccades follow saccades performed in the dark has indicated that this does not appear to be the only source of error information (Becker & Fuchs, 1969). This hypothesis has been further supported by the observation that errors in directions of primary saccades are corrected with very short latencies in the order of 5 ms to 80 ms (Vivianni & Swensson, 1982). In addition, saccades have been reported to be voluntarily amended with a very short intervening fixation period and sometimes with no fixation period at all (Becker et al., 1981; Viviani & Berthoz, 1977). These observations indicate that the retinal information that signals the position of the actual target may be combined with extraretinal information that signals the position of the eye (Vivianni & Swensson, 1982). Thus visual information may be obtained prior to and during a saccade. Even the brief presentation of a target during a saccade has been found to provide sufficient information to enable accurate corrective saccades to be produced (Hallett & Lightstone, 1976a,b).

Arm Movements

There are a number of levels at which we can examine the performance of a goal-directed arm movement. An appreciation of these different levels of analysis may be gleaned from an examination of the descriptors of the arm movement depicted in Figure 2. These include the angular displacement, velocity, and acceleration of the arm and, at the bottom of the figure, the electromyographic (EMG) activity from representative agonist (lateral head of triceps) and antagonist (biceps brachii) muscles. From this figure it can be seen that, for all of these movement descriptors, there are some obvious differences between the start and end of practice. Each of these adds to our understanding as to how movements are controlled and will be addressed in turn.

Movement Initiation. I would first like to consider some factors involved in the initiation of the arm movement following the presentation of the target. Many authors have considered rapid limb movements to be fully programmed prior to their initiation and for alterations in this motor program to be reflected in the latency of a movement (e.g., Anson, 1982; Glencross, 1972, 1973; Henry & Rogers, 1960). Reaction time has been found to be influenced by properties that are intrinsic to a visual stimulus such as intensity (Niemi & Lehtonen, 1982) and target size (Glencross, 1976; Klapp & Greim, 1979; Siegel, 1977). These properties contribute to the perceptual attributes of a stimulus and its detectability from other objects and environmental stimuli. Factors related to the type of response have also been shown to be influential. These include movement duration (Klapp & Erwin, 1976; Klapp, Wyatt, & Lingo, 1974), movement amplitude (Glencross, 1973; Williams, 1971a; cf Lagasse & Hayes, 1973), and the number of movement sequences in a response (e.g., Anson, 1982; Glencross, 1972; Henry & Rogers, 1960; Norrie, 1974; cf Klapp, 1981). Other factors such as temporal uncertainty of target presentation (Welford, 1968), the number of stimulus alternatives (Hick, 1952; Hyman, 1953), and stimulus-response compatibility (Marteniuk, 1976; Welford, 1968) may also influence reaction time.

Many of the above results have used the onset of an overt movement as a measure of reaction time. But this measure does not allow a complete assessment of central or peripheral contributions. This limitation can be overcome to some extent by recording the EMG activity of the agonist muscles which allows the reaction time to be fractionated into premotor time and motor time components (Weiss, 1965). Premotor time represents central nervous system processing and constitutes the interval between the stimulus and EMG onset. Motor time, or electromechanical delay, constitutes the interval between EMG onset and the overt movement. Further division of the reaction time may also be undertaken if electroencephalographic activity from areas of the visual and motor cortex is recorded. This method enables periods of visual reception time, opto-motor integration time, central motor outflow time, and peripheral motor time to be distinguished (Wood, 1977).

The reaction times obtained in the present experiment indicated that there was a refinement of the motor processes used in the preparation and production of the arm movement. The latency of the arm movement decreased from 281 ms at the start of the first days practice to a latency of 260 ms by the end of the final day. This reduction appeared to be within the movement preparatory stages as indicated by the decrease in onset of the triceps EMG activity from 248 ms to 226 ms. That some improvement should occur is not surprising given the spatial predictability of the target. Reductions with practice have previously been reported for reaction times and their premotor component (Clarkson & Kroll, 1978; Morris, 1977), although decreases in the motor time component have also been found (Lofthus & Hanson, 1981).

Movement Kinematics. An obvious feature of the arm movement records obtained during the first days practice (Fig. 2) was that they consisted of an initial distance covering phase, which fell short of the target, followed by a terminal corrective phase. The initial phase was characterised by a single velocity peak, and a single acceleration and deceleration peak; features which have often been described as characteristic of rapid movements. The initial phase has been considered to be preprogrammed and performed open loop whereas closed loop visual feedback has been thought to regulate the terminal phase (e.g., Crossman & Goodeve, 1983; Vince, 1948; Woodworth, 1899).

One model for the control of rapid arm movements that has stemmed from observations of the initial consistency in kinematics has been that of 'impulse variability'. This model proposes that the information contained within the initial command controls the magnitude of scalable acceleration (Schmidt, Zelaznik, Hawkins, Frank, & Quinn, 1979) or acceleration and deceleration phases (Meyer, Smith, & Wright, 1982) which determine the final limb position. However, except for some limited experimental situations, these models do not adequately account for observable movement behaviour. The pattern of accelerative and decelerative forces is largely asymmetrical, and there is large variability in the decelerative portion of movement (Marteniuk et al., 1987; Soechting, 1984; Zelaznik, Schmidt, & Gielen, 1986).

The discrete corrections observed during the terminal phase of the movement have been the basis for iterative correction models of control. These models postulate that each correction is based on visual feedback obtained from previous submovements (Craik, 1947; Crossman & Goodeve, 1983; Keele, 1968; Vince, 1948). In correspondence with Fitts' law (1954), the corrections are predicted to increase with the difficulty of the movement and to determine the total movement time. However, the analyses of movement trajectories has not revealed a consistent relationship between either the duration or number of submovements and movement time as predicted by these models (Jagacinski, Repperger, Moran, Ward, & Glass, 1980). In addition these discrete corrections have been observed during movements performed without visual feedback (Jeannerod, 1984).

The occurrence, duration, and magnitude of these kinematic features are influenced by task constraints, movement strategy, and skill level (Brooks, 1981; Hoffman & Strick, 1986; Marteniuk et al., 1987; Moore & Marteniuk, 1986; Soechting, 1984). Thus, in the present experiment on the last day of practice the initial limb movement was performed faster, for a shorter duration, over a greater distance, and with fewer terminal corrections. The velocity profile and the acceleration and deceleration phases were also more symmetrical and there was a noticeable decrease in their variability (Fig. 2). Such changes with practice are in agreement with those previously reported in the literature (Beggs & Howarth, 1972; Brooks, Kennedy, & Ross, 1983; Darling & Cooke, 1987a; Georgopoulos, Kalaska, & Massey, 1981; Moore & Marteniuk, 1986).

Electromyographic Activity. Underlying the kinematic features of movement are the patterns of EMG activity from the agonist and antagonist muscles. Certain EMG patterns have been identified which provide some insight as to how arm movements are organised and controlled. These patterns have been found to be dependent on the task required (Person, 1958), the strategy adopted by the subject (Mustard & Lee, 1987), and on the direction (Wadman, Boerhout, & Denier van der Gon, 1980), and speed of movement (Hallett, Shahani, & Young, 1975; Lestienne, 1979; Maton, LeBozec, & Cnockaert, 1980).

The pattern of EMG activity at the start of practice consisted of a burst of activity in the triceps in conjunction with continuous activation of the biceps. By the end of practice the biceps activity had become more burstlike and there was evidence of an extension of the initial triceps burst which at times appeared as a second distinct burst. These latter patterns of EMG activity are characteristic of those found in rapid arm movements (e.g., Benecke, Meinck, & Conrad, 1985; Brown & Cooke, 1984; Hallett et al., 1975; Lestienne, 1979; Marsden, Obeso, & Rothwell, 1983; Maton et al., 1980). The changes also appeared to represent a decrease in cocontraction of the agonist and antagonist muscles, particularly during the terminal phase of the movement. The phasing of EMG activity has previously been reported to become less variable and more synchronised with practice as the mode of control shifts from one of cocontraction of opposing muscle groups to one of reciprocal activation (Ludwig, 1982; Moore & Marteniuk, 1986; Payton & Kelly, 1972; Person, 1958; cf. Darling & Cooke, 1987b). Reported changes in the magnitude of EMG activity with practice, however, have been inconsistent both within and between studies (Moore & Marteniuk, 1986).

It is from such regular patterns of EMG activity that hypotheses of central controlling mechanisms have originated. Stable patterns of EMG activity have been recorded between component muscles within flexor and extensor muscle groups during both agonist and antagonist roles (Bouisset, 1983) and appear to be independent of differences in the fibre types of component muscles (Bejaoui, LeBozec, & Maton, 1987; LeBozec & Maton, 1987). Some form of central control has been further suggested by the observation that at least the initial agonist burst and part of the antagonist burst are completed before movement onset (Hallett et al., 1975; Wadman, Denier van der Gon, Geuze, & Mol, 1979), and that these temporal sequences persist in the absence of afferent information (e.g., Forget & Lamarre, 1987; Rothwell et al., 1982). Afferent input has also been found not to affect the initial burst of agonist EMG activity for a period of at least 100 ms (e.g., Garland & Angel, 1971; Hallett et al., 1975; Wadman et al., 1979).

Central control of movements has also been suggested from experiments in both humans (Kelso & Holt, 1980) and monkeys (Bizzi, Polit, & Morasso, 1976; Polit & Bizzi, 1978, 1979), in which the final position of a previously learned movement was reached in the absence of normal afferent information. In these latter experiments final position was accomplished despite physical perturbations. This equifinality has been considered to be achieved by the setting of a tonic level of EMG activity in agonist and antagonist muscles (Lestienne, Polit, & Bizzi, 1981), although this view has been disputed (Matheson, Hallett, Berardelli, Weinhaus, & Inzucchi, 1985).

The 'mass-spring' model is an attempt to explain movement control based on the consideration that muscles possess spring-like properties. In this muscle-level model limb trajectory and final position are determined by the stiffness which is dictated by the ratio of activation levels in opposing muscle groups. It allows for the production of movements from a large range of initial conditions, and for the control of movement dynamics by the adjustment of stiffness and dampening parameters (Kelso, Holt, Kugler, & Turvey, 1980; Kelso, Tuller, & Harris, 1983). However, criticisms have been made of both the deafferentation studies and the behavioural experiments which support this model (Fel'dman & Latash, 1982; Hasan & Enoka, 1985; Matheson et al., 1985; Vincken, Gielen, & Denier van der Gon, 1983).

In this vein it is worthwhile remembering that EMG activity reflects the activity of motor units in response to activation of motoneurone pools by central commands (Mustard & Lee, 1987). These motoneurone pools are also influenced monosynaptically or via interneurones by proprioceptive information arising from muscle spindles and other peripheral sensory receptors (Desmedt & Godaux, 1978; Fel'dman, 1986; Fel'dman & Latash, 1982; Hasan & Enoka, 1985). As the movement progresses the segmental afferent input increases its influence, according to the adjusted reflex gain (Angel, 1977; Hallett et al., 1975; Wadman et al., 1980). At least part of the control during the latter part of the movement may be achieved by the interaction of reflexes with the mechanical properties of the muscles (Cooke, 1979, 1980a,b; Nichols & Houk, 1976). Afferent dependent reflex mechanisms are, therefore, able to influence the patterns of EMG activity observed during movement (Ghez & Martin, 1982; Gordon & Ghez, 1984, 1987a; Soechting, 1973; Soechting, Ranish, Palminteri, & Terzuolo, 1976; Viviani & Terzuolo, 1973). Variations in the moment-arms of muscles during the course of a movement may also affect this relationship (Hasan & Enoka, 1985). Thus, because the relationship between the movement and the sources of the observed EMG is complex (Ghez & Vicario, 1978; Sittig et al., 1985, 1987) explanations of control based primarily on muscle properties are likely to be an oversimplification (Darling & Cooke, 1987c, Fel'dman, 1986).

EYE AND ARM MOVEMENTS

Temporal Relationship

Initiation. Some measure of the temporal interdependence of the eye and arm movement control systems may be provided by a comparison of the lag between the onset of the saccadic eye movement and the arm movement. The typical sequence of events reported by previous authors has been that the initiation of a saccadic eye movement is followed by movement of the arm. This lag of the arm movement has been reported as 20 ms (Megaw & Armstrong, 1973), 60 ms (Angel, Alston, & Garland, 1970), and 100 ms or more (Herman, Herman, & Maulucci, 1981; Prablanc, Echallier, Komilis, & Jeannerod, 1979). These results indicate that the eye moves first in order that the target may be accurately located.

In the present experiment, however, only 41% of the saccadic eye movements at the start of day one were initiated earlier than the arm movement. In fact the eye lagged the arm by an average 5 ms, although there was considerable variability in this measure (SD = 40 ms). But by the end of the final day's practice, the decrease in reaction time of the arm movement had resulted in 82% of the saccades lagging behind the arm movement by an average 29 ms (SD = 35 ms). This lag in initiation of the saccadic eye movement was even greater if the onset of the arm movement was taken as the onset of the triceps EMG activity. Figure 3 illustrates this relationship as a linear regression of eye versus arm reaction time. In this figure the broken line represents the line along which the data would lie if saccadic reaction time was equal to arm reaction time. Points above the line therefore represent responses where the saccade was initiated after movement of the arm. Some previous reports have found that initiation of EMG activity in neck and arm muscles was coincident with the initiation of the saccade (Biguer, Jeannerod, & Prablanc, 1982, 1985). Thus, the lag in arm movement has primarily appeared to be due to the electromechanical delay (or motor time component) of the musculoskeletal apparatus.

The strength of the relationship between the eye and arm has been inferred from the correlation between their respective reaction times. High correlations have been interpreted as implicative of some interdependence between visual and motor processes during early stages of movement preparation and that information from these sources are processed in parallel (Biguer et al., 1982, 1985; Gielen, van den Heuvel, & van Gisbergen, 1984; Prablanc et al., 1979). The regression illustrated in Figure 3 showed that with practice there was a slight increase in the correlation from .60 to .70 between the respective reaction times. Correlations in the order of .50 (Gielen et al., 1984; Prablanc et al., 1979) and as high as .80 and .93 (Herman et al., 1981; Fischer & Rogal,

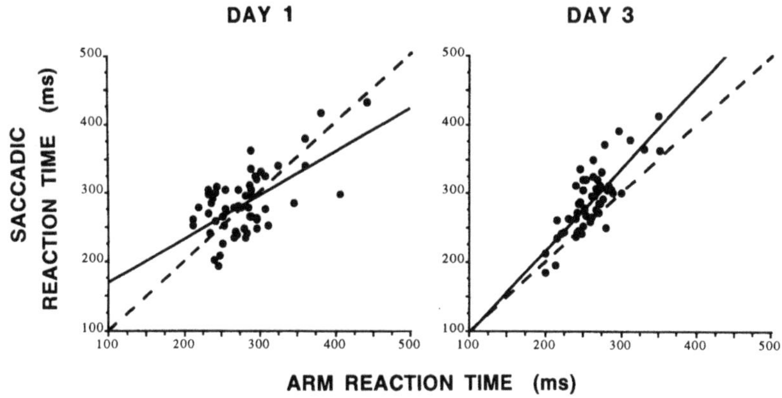

Figure 3. Linear regression of eye versus arm reaction time (solid line) for all subjects on the first and last eight trials of practice. The broken line represents the line along which the data would lie if saccadic reaction time was equal to arm reaction time.

1986) have previously been obtained. Fischer and Rogal (1986) have reported these correlations to decrease when the initial fixation point was turned off prior to movement onset (.50), when there was decreased attention to the initial fixation point (.78), and after extended practice (.73). However, in the latter case high correlations were restored by instructing subjects to pay greater attention to the initial fixation point. These results have been interpreted by Fischer and Rogal (1986) as suggestive of an attentional influence on the preparation of eye and arm movements. In fact it may be that the switching on and off of these attentional mechanisms explains some of the delays in movement initiation that were observed between the eye and the arm in the present study. In this experiment the target and manipulandum cursors were superimposed and, although the target had been presented, the cursor representing the arm position remained in the same location as the start target. This may have continued to act as a fixation point and inhibited the disengagement of attention and, therefore, the initiation of the saccade.

But it is also possible that, within this stable experimental environment, the strategy adopted by subjects enabled them to use earlier cues originating from the arm movement so that appropriate motor corrections could be initiated more rapidly. Delaying execution of the saccade until after commencement of the arm movement may have allowed earlier processing of visual information about the performance of the arm movement, even before the arm reached the target. The early portion of the arm movement would contain information of the higher derivatives of position which have been postulated to be essential control parameters (Fuchs, 1962; Gordon & Ghez, 1987b; Hoffman & Strick, 1986). Thus, with practice, subjects may have progressed from a mode of movement control based on positional information of target and arm to one centered on the refinement of movement kinematics and kinetics. Such transitions have been reported to occur during the practice of reaching movements in the sagittal plane (Schneider, Zernicke, Schmidt, & Hart, 1986) and in the performance of continuous tracking tasks (Fuchs, 1962; Marteniuk & Romanow, 1983). However, the onset of the eye movement, although it lagged behind the arm, still occurred prior to peak jerk (third derivative of position). Even after extended practice, the eye was moving when the higher kinematic features of the arm movement, such as peak acceleration and jerk, were most prominent. This would imply that there was a reduction in the available visual information pertaining to these kinematic features because of the elevation in the visual threshold prior to a saccadic eye movement. Although some visual information may still be accessed by visuomotor control processes because visual information is not totally excluded during a saccadic eye movement (Burr et al., 1982; Hallett & Lightstone, 1976a,b).

Duration. It is also important to know whether the eye arrives at the target before the arm. If this was not the case it would imply that foveation of the target was not essential for successful achievement of the movement goal. In fact, because of the saccades relatively brief duration, the eye always did arrive at the target prior to the arm. At the start of practice arrival of the eye was coincident with peak acceleration of the arm. By the end of practice the time of arrival of the eye was between peak acceleration and peak velocity of the arm. This indicates that some form of spatial information obtained from the newly foveated image was available for the successful completion of the movement. However, this is only a partial description of the changes that occurred in the eye and the arm with practice. One of the reasons for the differences in arrival time of the eye at the target relative to the arm movement was because the duration of the arm movement had decreased. Thus, at the start of practice visual information of the initial motion of the arm was available for a longer duration than at the end of practice. This suggests that early in practice the strategy unconsciously adopted by subjects placed greater reliance on visual feedback. But as subjects became more skilful they were able to refine their internal representation of the movement and their strategy shifted to one in which the initial movement was performed predominantly in an open-loop mode of control.

Spatial Relationship. Another means of examining the relationship between the eye and the arm has been to assess whether there was any correlation between measures of their respective spatial errors. If during later stages of preparation and execution the eye and the hand were not so tightly coupled, then lower correlations in their spatial accuracies would be expected. In the present experiment a comparison of amplitude errors for the eye and the arm revealed no significant correlation for either the first (r = .046) or last (r = -.055) day of practice. These results, therefore, suggested some independence of the control mechanisms governing the actual execution of the eye and arm movements. Some independence of control has also been suggested by the different directional errors that have been reported for the eye and arm (Megaw & Armstrong, 1973), and by uncorrelated errors of gaze and hand in open-loop pointing movements (Prablanc et al., 1979).

INFERRING CONTROL PROCESSES FROM MOVEMENT CORRECTIONS

One of my initial interests was in establishing whether visual information was able to be processed in parallel with motor information or whether these processes were subject to serial delays. The results of the above experiment had suggested that there was some interaction between visual and motor processes during movement preparation but that during movement execution these processes were essentially independent. If visual information was denied to the motor system during movement execution then correcting a movement error based on visual information would incur a delay in the order of the movement's duration. Although many studies have reported visual feedback delays that support this notion there is some contention as to how long the actual delays are. Estimates have ranged from 400 ms (Vince, 1948; Woodworth, 1899), to 260 ms (Cordo, 1987; Keel & Posner, 1968), and to 100 ms (Carlton, 1981; Cordo, 1987; Smith & Bowen, 1980; Zelaznik, Hawkins, & Kisselburgh, 1983). However, it is unlikely that movement corrections are based solely on a simple servo-like mechanism with a fixed time delay, simply because such a mechanism would not be able to respond rapidly enough to changes in the environment. And even if this were the sole error-correcting mechanism it is difficult to explain why there should be such a wide range of reported visual feedback times. One possibility for this range of processing times is that more than one mechanism is involved in the error correction process. And this, in fact, seems to be the case. Several experiments have indicated that limb movements are not performed in a completely preprogrammed manner, but are subject to continuous visually mediated regulation. Thus, when more information about the target or the response is available movements are performed more accurately (Cordo, 1987; Gordon & Ghez, 1987b; Henning, Favilla, & Ghez, 1988; Prablanc et al., 1979). Even if vision of the limb is not available during movement, accuracy is improved if the target is continuously visible (Prablanc et al., 1979). Such results imply

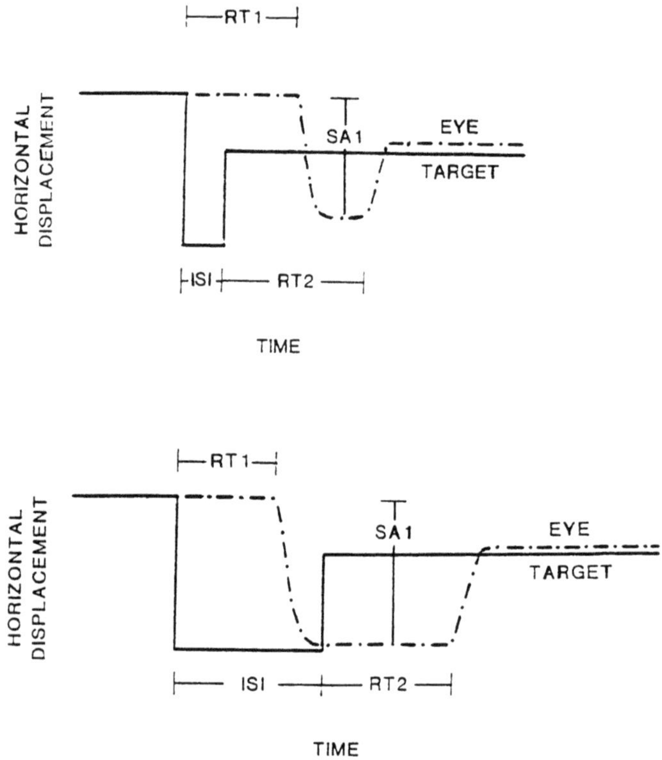

Figure 4. Experimental paradigm illustrating typical saccadic responses to two successive step movements of the target. The first and second step corresponded respectively to visual angles of 15° and ±10°, and elbow angles of 45° and ±30°. Only one amendment direction was presented on each day of testing. The second target step occurred at one of ten stimulus intervals. Five of these were timed from the presentation of the first target (40, 80, 120, 160, 200 ms) and five from the onset of the elbow extension movement (0, 50, 100, 150, 200 ms). The reaction times to the first and second target step have been respectively labelled RT1 and RT2, and the amplitude of the first saccade SA1. Top: the second step of the target occurs prior to onset of the first movement. Bottom: the second step of the target occurs after onset of the first movement.

that movements are subject to some form of feedforward modulation and control. It has been hypothesised that this feedforward control is achieved via a corollary discharge mechanism and is responsible for the movement corrections that have been observed at 100 ms (Cordo, 1987). Abbs (1982) has termed this an afferent-dependent feedforward process, and Jeannerod (1988) has termed it proactive control.

Many of the above results have been obtained from experiments in which vision of the target or the hand was either removed or reinstated at some time during the preparation or performance of the movement. An alternative method of investigating eye and arm movement control processes, and one which I have employed, has involved shifting the location of a visual target at some time prior to or during a movement. In such an experiment subjects are required to amend their initial movement and to achieve the new target location as fast as possible. In this second study subjects were required to amend their initial movement by either reversing or continuing to a new target location. The change in target location occurred on 40% of trials at random inter-stimulus intervals (ISI) (see Fig. 4 for details of experimental paradigm). A typical trial for a reversal and continuation response at an ISI of 160 ms is displayed in Figure 5. At the top of the figure the eye movement displacement shows the saccadic responses to the two target steps. Underneath are the angular displacement, velocity, and acceleration for the arm movement and the EMG activity of representative agonist and antagonist muscles.

Temporal Delays

The data for this experiment were quantified in terms of the reaction times to the first (RT1) and second target steps (RT2), and the amplitude traversed at the end of the first and second movement. These data for one subject have been illustrated in Figure 6 for saccadic eye movements and in Figure 7 for arm movements. In these figures the data have been expressed as a function of the time at which the target location changed relative to the onset of the first arm movement. Thus all negative values on the ordinate represent the time when the initial target shifted to a new location prior to onset of the subject's first arm movement. All positive values represent a change in target location that occurred after the onset of the subject's first arm movement.

Two types of responses were obtained in this experiment. The first type consisted of movements that were directed straight to the second target. They occurred more frequently the earlier the second target step occurred relative to onset of the first movement; that is, when the ISI was short and when the reaction time for the first movement was sufficiently long. These have been called final angle responses (Becker & Jurgens, 1979) and have been depicted as solid circles for the reaction time data (Figs. 6 & 7, top) and the amplitude data (Figs. 6 & 7, bottom). An obvious feature of this response type for saccades was that they occurred more frequently when a reversal amendment was required. In fact the subject whose data is depicted in Figure 6 performed all of their saccades directly to the second target if the second target step

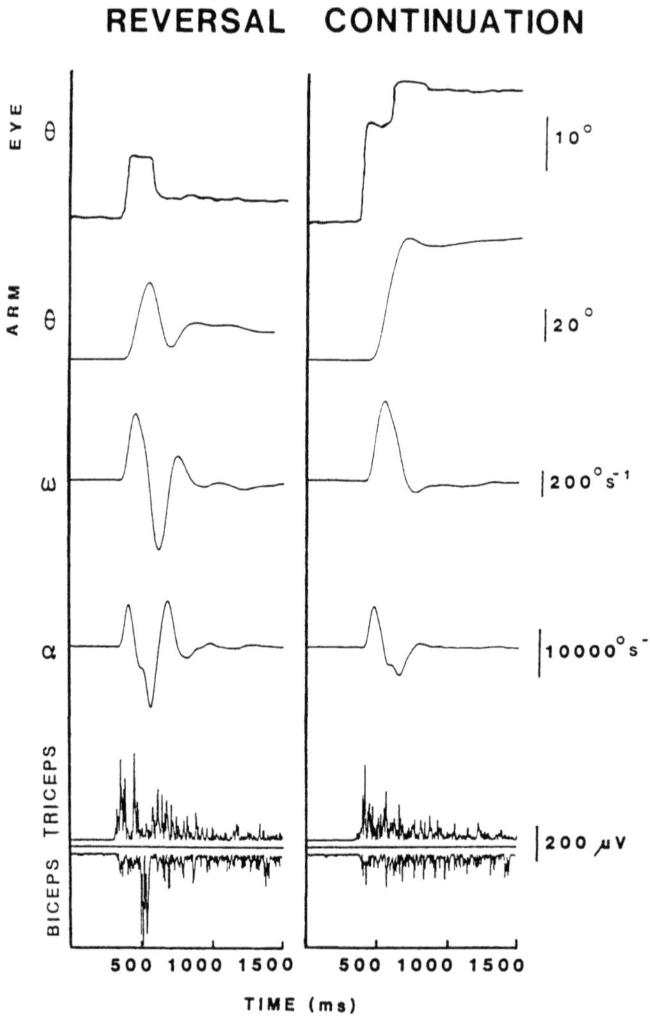

Figure 5. Typical trial for a reversal and continuation amendment when the second target step occurred at an inter-stimulus interval of 160 ms. The figure contains, from top to bottom, eye displacement, arm displacement, velocity, acceleration and triceps and biceps EMG.

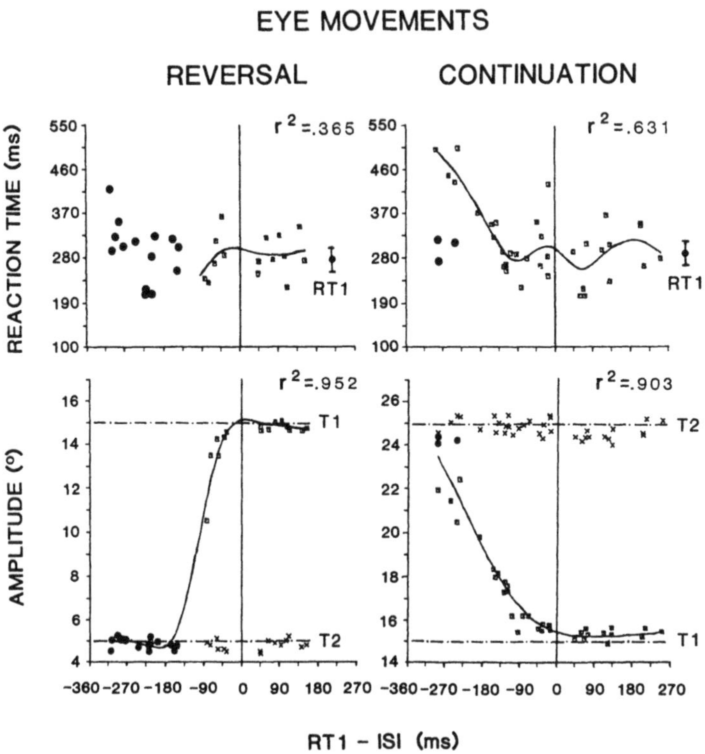

Figure 6. Saccadic reversal and continuation responses for one subject expressed as the interval between the change in target location and initiation of the first movement (ISI-RT1). Curves were fitted with a cubic spline function (Woltring, 1986). Top: Average reaction time (±1SD) to the first target step (RT1); reaction time to the second target step (□); reaction time of responses directly to the second target (●). Bottom: Amplitude of first saccade (□) and final eye position (x); amplitude of responses directly to the second target (●).

occurred earlier than 100 ms prior to the onset of the first movement. For the arm movements, by contrast, there were more final angle responses when the movement amendment required continuation of the initial response.

The second type of response consisted of movements that were performed in two steps, the first to the initial target location and the second to the new target location. These responses occurred more frequently the later the change in target location occurred and have been called initial angle responses (Becker & Jurgens, 1979). For both the eye and arm movements in the present

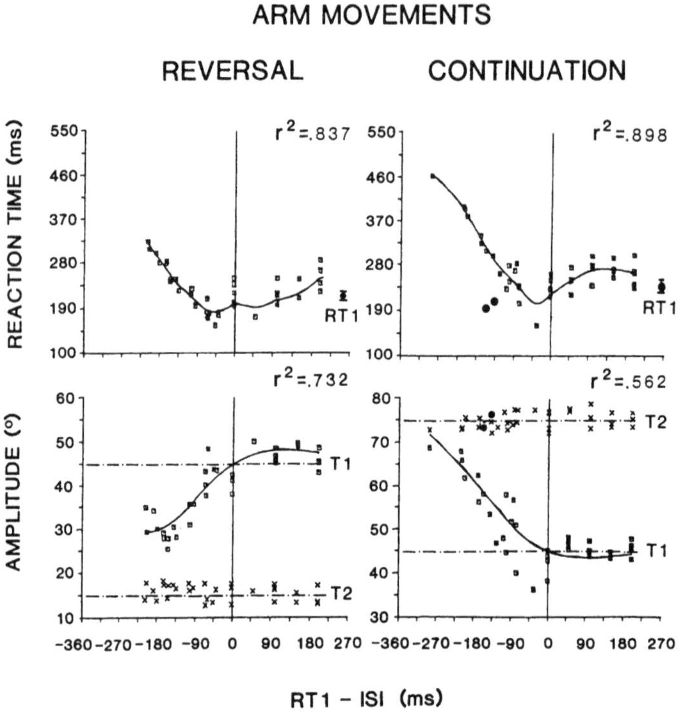

Figure 7. Arm reversal and continuation responses for one subject expressed as the interval between the change in target location and initiation of the first movement. Top: Average reaction time (±1SD) to the first target step (RT1); reaction time to the second target step (□); reaction time of responses directly to the second target (●). Bottom: Amplitude of first arm movement (□) and final arm position (x); amplitude of responses directly to the second target (●).

experiment, when the target location change occurred sufficiently early relative to movement onset, the reaction time to this target change was lengthened. However, this reaction time decreased as the second target step occurred closer to movement onset, until a minimum was reached. This minimum occurred at about 90-100 ms prior to movement onset for the eye movements and at about 50 ms for the arm movements. The curves that represent these trends, which were obtained using a cubic spline method (Woltring, 1986), have been depicted at the top of Figures 6 and 7. The only exception to these trends in RT2 was for reversal amendments in which many of the responses to early changes in target location were mainly directed straight to the second target (e.g., Fig. 6, top left). Similar trends in RT2 have previously been obtained for both saccadic eye movements (e.g., Bartlett, Eason, & White, 1961; Kerr & Lockwood, 1987, 1988; Megaw, 1975; Wheeless, Boynton, & Cohen, 1966), and arm movements in the sagittal plane (e.g., Henry & Harrison, 1961; Welford, 1959; Williams, 1971b; Williams & Sullivan, 1978; Williams, Sullivan, & Kerr, 1985) and horizontal plane (Kerr, 1984, 1989). This trend, of an increased delay followed by a decrease, was originally thought to be due to limitations in the capacity of central mechanisms to process more than one stimulus at a time. According to "single-channel" theory there was a "bottleneck" at some point in the processing in which a second stimulus had to await until the processing of the first stimulus had been completed (Welford, 1968). In a similar manner Henry and Roger's (1960) "memory drum" theory considered that responses were resistant to modification while the motor program was being discharged to the muscles. More recent examinations of the refractory period phenomena in rapid arm movements have indicated that there are two sources of delay: one concerned with the processing of the two stimuli (central refractoriness) and one arising from the movement (movement refractoriness) (Williams & Sullivan, 1978; Williams et al., 1985).

A prediction that arose from single channel theory was that the production of a second response would incur an additional delay which was proportional to the time remaining between the second target step and the onset of the first movement. Thus, as the available shared processing time for the two target steps decreased, the reaction time to the second target step (RT2) would decrease with a constant slope of -1 until a minimum delay, equivalent to a normal reaction time, was reached at movement onset. But deviations in this trend, in which a minimum was not reached until some time after movement onset, have been reported (Williams, 1971b). This continued elevation in RT2 has been attributed to influences arising from the initial response and supports the notion of "movement refractoriness" proposed by Williams and Sullivan (1978) and Williams et al. (1985).

However, an unexpected finding of the second experiment was that the initial minimum in RT2 occurred earlier than predicted. Moreover, there was a second increase in RT2 up until movement onset, which was followed by a decrease, often until a second minimum was reached. This trend was most pronounced for the eye movements, although it must be noted that there was considerable variability in subjects responses at longer amendment intervals. This period between the first and second minimum coincides with the reported time course of saccadic suppression during which the visual threshold is elevated (Carpenter, 1988). Thus, one reason for this second increase in delay may be because the second target was harder to detect. But it is also possible that there was insufficient time to complete certain computational processes associated with the second response prior to the initiation of the first movement. Presumably these take a certain length of time and if there was insufficient time for their completion prior to initiation of the first response then an additional delay would be incurred. This argument presumes though that such initial computational processes can proceed concurrently and at the same speed as those for the first movement.

Amplitude Alterations

Another noticeable result was that the amplitude of the initial movement was adjusted towards the second target. Thus, when the second target step occurred sufficiently early, relative to the onset of the first movement, the first movement was able to be amended such that the final target was immediately achieved. But the later the target was presented the less the amplitude of the initial movement was able to be adjusted. The movement, therefore, ended at an intermediate position between the first and second targets. For saccades this amplitude transition was observed provided the second target was presented 100 ms or more prior to movement onset. For arm movements, in which subjects had to increase the amplitude of their initial movement, the amplitude alteration was possible if the second target step occurred 135 ms prior to movement onset. But for reversal amendments only two subjects showed a large adjustment of the initial movement towards the second target; this occurred provided the target was presented 67 ms or more prior to movement onset, and only a small alteration was obtained for three other subjects.

Amplitude adjustments have previously been obtained for both saccadic eye movements (e.g., Aslin & Shea, 1987; Becker & Jurgens, 1979; van Asten, Gielen, & de Winkel, 1988) and arm movements (Barrett & Glencross, 1988a,b; Georgopoulos et al., 1981; Gottsdanker, 1966; Vince, 1948). These results suggest that early in movement preparation visual information is continuously processed and can be integrated into the intended movement with minimal delay. Furthermore, the proportional alteration in amplitude indicates that some form of averaging buffer may be utilised in the involved computational processes (Becker & Jurgens, 1979).

Because the amplitude alterations were manifest in both eye and arm movements there is an implication that both control systems had access to some form of shared spatial representation. Presumably this shared access occurred prior to movement onset because when the movement was initiated it already contained the appropriate stimulus amplitude information. But further analysis of movement amplitudes indicated that there was some evidence of interdependence between visual and motor control processes during early stages of response execution. This was manifest as a slight but significant correlation between the amplitudes traversed by the eye and the arm at the end of their respective primary movements (reversals, $r = .229$ $p = .002$; continuation, $r = .658$ $p = .0001$). In contrast, there was no significant correlation between eye arm movement amplitude for single step control trials (reversal control, $r =$

-.029; continuation control, r = -.06). One possibility for this result is that during this period of the movement there is a greater reliance on movement amplitude information derived from a shared spatial representation. Indeed, if corollary discharge mechanisms were exerting a controlling influence during the early period of movement execution then some relationship between the amplitudes would be expected because their "open-loop" regulation is based on the latest available visual information of the target location. This lends some support to Cordo's (1987) hypothesis that movement corrections observed within the first 100 ms of a response are independent of visual feedback and involve the incorporation of stimulus amplitude information into the response via a corollary discharge process.

Mechanisms of Visuomotor Control

The experimental observations that the amplitudes of movements were able to be altered have previously been interpreted as indicative of 'real time' control of movement with few response delays. But the results of the present experiment also indicate that both eye and arm movement responses may exhibit increased temporal delays. These results are apparently mutually exclusive. On the one hand they imply that there are serial limitations on processing more than one stimulus at the same time. But on the other hand they indicate that there is a continuous monitoring of visual afferent information with concomitant adjustments of the initial response. However, this apparent discrepancy may be explained if the relationship between the temporal delays and alterations in movement amplitude is considered. Provided that the new visual information arrives 100 ms or more before the start of a movement it may be incorporated into the intended movement with minimal delay. But this early processing is at the expense of extra delays in producing a second corrective movement. Presumably these delays arise because a new movement cannot proceed until the amplitude computations for producing the first movement have been completed. Thus, although visual information appears to be subject to parallel processing during early stages of response preparation, as evidenced by alterations in the initial movement amplitude, there is a serial 'bottleneck' in the processing of visuomotor information which results in a refractory period between two motor responses.

FUTURE DIRECTIONS

The present chapter has touched briefly on some of the issues facing those attempting to understand how we use visual information in the guidance of movement. The experiments I have described have been concerned with discrete movements about a single joint. They are very much 'laboratory type' tasks in that constraints are placed on both the visual environment and the required motor task. Such controlled experimentation is important in learning how visual and other sensory information are able to be utilised in the control of movements. In the present experiments this approach has provided an understanding of how eye and arm movements are coordinated and how this relationship changes with skill level. It has also enabled an assessment of the processing constraints that govern visually guided movements. A future challenge, however, lies in identifying the neural correlates of these processes and in determining whether such processes are generalised to movements more typical of everyday actions.

ACKNOWLEDGEMENTS

The experiments described in this chapter were conducted at the Department of Human Movement and Recreation Studies, The University of Western Australia, as part of the authors Ph.D. studies. Gratitude is expressed to Dr. R. Lockwood, Dr. D. Larkin, Associate Professor G. Wood, Associate Professor B. Blanksby and to Professor J. Ross for their advice and support. Appreciation is also expressed to Dr. R.C. Miall, Oxford University, Dr. D. Larkin, The University of Western Australia, and to Dr. J. Summers, University of Melbourne for their comments on this manuscript.

REFERENCES

Abbs, J.H. (1982). A speech-motor-system perspective on nervous-system-control variables. *Behavioral and Brain Sciences, 5*, 541-542.

Angel, R.W. (1977). Antagonist muscle activity during rapid arm movements: central versus proprioceptive influences. *Journal of Neurology, Neurosurgery, and Psychiatry, 40*, 683-686.

Angel, R.W., Alston, W. & Garland, H. (1970). Functional relations between the manual and oculomotor control signals. *Experimental Neurology, 27*, 248-257.

Anson, J.G. (1982). Memory drum theory: Alternative tests and explanations for the complexity effects on simple reaction time. *Journal of Motor Behavior, 14*, 228-246.

Arbib, M.A. (1981). Perceptual structures and distributed motor control. In V.E. Brooks (Ed.) *Handbook of physiology. Section I: The nervous system. Vol. 2: Motor control (pp. 1449-1480). Part* 2. Baltimore: Williams & Wilkins.

Aslin, R.N. & Shea, S.L. (1987). The amplitude and angle of saccades to double-step target displacements. *Vision Research*, 27, 1925-1942.

Barrett, N.C. & Glencross, D.J. (1988a). The double-step analysis of rapid manual aiming movements. *Quarterly Journal of Experimental Psychology, 40*, 299-322.

Barrett, N.C. & Glencross, D.J. (1988b). The amplitude transition function and the manual and oculomotor control systems. *Psychological Bulletin, 104*, 363-372.

Bartlett, N.R., Eason, R.G., & White, C.T. (1961). Latency of ocular fixation upon the second of two successive stimuli. *Perceptual and Motor Skills, 13*, 259-268.

Bartz, A. (1962). Eye movement latency, duration and response time as a function of angular displacement. *Journal of Experimental Psychology, 64*, 318-324.

Becker, W. & Fuchs, A.F. (1969). Further properties of the human saccadic system: Eye movements and correction saccades with and without visual fixation points. *Vision Research, 9*, 1247-1258.

Becker, W. & Jurgens, R. (1979). An analysis of the saccadic system by means of double step stimuli. *Vision Research, 19*, 967-983.

Becker, W., King, W.M., Fuchs, A.F., Jurgens, R., Johanson, G., & Kornhuber, H.H. (1981). Accuracy of goal-directed saccades and mechanisms of error correction. In A.F. Fuchs & W. Becker (Eds.). *Progress in oculomotor research* (pp. 29-37). Amsterdam: Elsevier, North-Holland.

Beggs, W.D.A. & Howarth, C.I. (1972). The movement of the hand towards a target. *Quarterly Journal of Experimental Psychology, 24*, 448-453.

Bejaoui, K., LeBozec, S., & Maton, B. (1987). Modulation of slow and fast elbow extensor EMG tonic activity by stretch reflexes in man. *European Journal of Applied Physiology, 56*, 97-104.

Benecke, R., Meinck, H.M., & Conrad, B. (1985). Rapid goal-directed elbow flexion movements: Limitations of the speed control system due to neural constraints. *Experimental Brain Research, 59*, 470-477.

Bernstein, N. (1967). *The co-ordination and regulation of movements*. Oxford: Pergamon Press.

Biguer, B., Jeannerod, M., & Prablanc, C. (1982). The coordination of eye, head, and arm movements during reaching at a single visual target. *Experimental Brain Research, 46*, 301-304.

Biguer, B., Jeannerod, M., & Prablanc, C. (1985). The role of position of gaze in movement accuracy. In M.I. Posner & O.S.M. Marin (Eds.) *Mechanisms of attention. Attention and performance XI* (pp. 407-424). Hillsdale, N.J.: Lawrence Erlbaum Associates.

Bizzi, E., Polit, A., & Morasso, P. (1976). Mechanisms underlying achievement of final head position. *Journal of Neurophysiology, 39*, 435-444.

Bouisset, S. (1983). Fundamental motor patterns in simple voluntary movements. In H. Matsui & K. Kobayashi (Eds.), *Biomechanics VIII-B* (pp. 615-625). Champaign, IL: Human Kinetics.

Brooks, V.B. (1981). Task related cell assemblies. In O. Pompeiano & C. Ajmone Marsan (Eds.), *Brain mechanisms and perceptual awareness* (pp. 295-309). New York: Raven Press.

Brooks, V.B., Kennedy, P.R., & Ross, H.G. (1983). Movement programming depends on understanding of behavioral requirements. *Physiology & Behavior, 31*, 561-563.

Brown, S.H. & Cooke, J.D. (1984). Initial agonist burst duration depends on movement amplitude. *Experimental Brain Research, 55*, 523-527.

Burr, D.C., Holt, J., Johnston, J.R., & Ross, J. (1982). Selective depression of motion sensitivity during saccades. *Journal of Physiology (London), 333*, 1-15.

Burr, D.C. & Ross, J. (1986). Visual processing of motion. *Trends in Neurosciences, 9*, 304-307.

Carlton, L.G. (1981). Visual information: The control of aiming movements. *Quarterly Journal of Experimental Psychology, 33A*, 87-93.

Carpenter, R.H.S. (1988). *Movements of the eyes*. London: Pion.

Clarkson, P.M. & Kroll, W. (1978). Practice effects on fractionated response time related to age and activity level. *Journal of Motor Behavior, 10*, 275-286.

Collewijn, H., Erkelens, C.J., & Steinman, R.M. (1988). Binocular co-ordination of human horizontal saccadic eye movements. *Journal of Physiology, 404*, 157-182.

Cooke, J.D. (1979). Dependence of human arm movements on limb mechanical properties. *Brain Research, 181*, 493-497.

Cooke, J.D. (1980a). The organization of simple skilled movements. In G.E. Stelmach & J. Requin (Eds.), *Tutorials in motor behavior* (pp. 199-212). Amsterdam: North-Holland.

Cooke, J.D. (1980b). The role of stretch reflexes during active movements. *Brain Research, 181*, 493-497.

Cordo, P.J. (1987). Mechanisms controlling accurate changes in elbow torque in humans. *Journal of Neuroscience, 7*, 432-442.

Craik, K.J.W. (1947). Theory of the human operator in control systems. I. The operator as an engineering system. *British Journal of Psychology, 38*, 56-61.

Crawford, T.J. (1984). The modification of saccadic trajectories. In A.G. Gale & F. Johnson (Eds.), *Theoretical and applied aspects of eye movement research* (pp. 95-102). Amsterdam: North-Holland.

Crossman, E.R.F.W. & Goodeve, P.J. (1983). Feedback control of hand-movement and Fitts' law. Paper presented at the meeting of the Experimental Psychology Society, Oxford, England, July, 1963. Reprinted in *Quarterly Journal of Experimental Psychology, 35A*, 251-278.

Darling, W.G. & Cooke, J.D. (1987a). Changes in the variability of movement trajectories with practice. *Journal of Motor Behavior, 16*, 348-363.

Darling, W.G. & Cooke, J.D. (1987b). Movement related EMGs become more variable during learning of fast accurate movements. *Journal of Motor Behavior, 19*, 311-331.

Darling, W.G. & Cooke, J.D. (1987c). A linked muscular activation model for movement generation and control. *Journal of Motor Behavior, 19*, 333-354.

Desmedt, J.E. & Godaux, E. (1978). Ballistic skilled movements: Load compensation and patterning of the motor commands. In J.E. Desmedt (Ed.), *Cerebral motor control in man: Long loop mechanisms. Progress in Clinical Neurophysiology, Vol 4* (pp. 21-55). Basel: S. Karger.

Fel'dman, A.G. (1986). Once more on the equilibrium-point hypothesis (λ model) for motor control. *Journal of Motor Behavior, 18*, 17-54.

Fel'dman, A.G., & Latash, M.L. (1982). Interaction of afferent and efferent signals underlying joint position sense: Empirical and theoretical approaches. *Journal of Motor Behavior, 14*, 174-193.

Fischer, B. (1986). The role of attention in the preparation of visually guided eye movements in monkey and man. *Psychological Research, 48*, 252-257.

Fischer, B. (1987). The preparation of visually guided saccades. *Reviews in Physiology, Biochemistry & Pharmacology, 106*, 1-35.

Fischer, B., Boch, R., & Ramsperger, E. (1984). Express-saccades of the monkey: Effect of daily training on probability of occurrence and reaction time. *Experimental Brain Research, 55*, 232-242.

Fischer, B. & Ramsperger, E. (1986). Human express saccades: effects of randomization and daily practice. *Experimental Brain Research, 64*, 569-578.

Fischer, B. & Rogal, L. (1986). Eye-hand coordination in man: a reaction time study. *Biological Cybernetics, 55*, 253-261.

Fitts, P.M. (1954). The information capacity of the human motor system in controlling the amplitude of movement. *Journal of Experimental Psychology, 47*, 381-391.

Forget, R. & Lamarre, Y. (1987). Rapid elbow flexion in the absence of proprioceptive and cutaneous feedback. *Human Neurobiology, 6*, 27-37.

Fuchs, A.F. (1967). Periodic eye tracking in the monkey. *Journal of Physiology (London), 193*, 161-171.

Fuchs, A.F. (1962). The progression-regression hypotheses in perceptual-motor skill learning. *Journal of Experimental Psychology, 63*, 177-182.

Garland, H. & Angel, R.W. (1971). Spinal and supraspinal factors in voluntary movement. *Experimental Neurology, 33*, 343-350.

Georgopoulos, A.P., Kalaska, J.F., & Massey, J.T. (1981). Spatial trajectories and reaction times of aimed movements: Effects of practice, uncertainty, and change in target location. *Journal of Neurophysiology, 48*, 725-743.

Ghez, C. & Martin, J.H. (1982). The control of rapid limb movement in the cat. III. Agonist-antagonist coupling. *Experimental Brain Research, 31*, 1-12.

Ghez, C. & Vicario, D.S. (1978). The control of rapid limb movement in the cat. II. Scaling of isometric force adjustments. *Experimental Brain Research, 33*, 191-203.

Gielen, S.C.A.M., van den Heuvel, P.J.M., & van Gisbergen, J.A.M. (1984). Coordination of fast eye and arm movements in a tracking task. *Experimental Brain Research, 56*, 154-161.

Glencross, D.J. (1972). Latency and response complexity. *Journal of Motor Behavior, 4*, 251-256.

Glencross, D.J. (1973). Response complexity and the latency of different movement patterns. *Journal of Motor Behavior, 5*, 95-104.

Glencross, D.J. (1976). The latency of aiming movements. *Journal of Motor Behavior, 8*, 27-34.

Gordon, J. & Ghez, C. (1984). EMG patterns in antagonist muscles during isometric contraction in man: relations to response dynamics. *Experimental Brain Research, 55*, 167-171.

Gordon, J. & Ghez, C. (1987a). Trajectory control in targeted force impulses. II. Pulse height control. *Experimental Brain Research, 67*, 241-252.

Gordon, J. & Ghez, C. (1987b). Trajectory control in targeted force impulses. III. Compensatory adjustments for initial errors. *Experimental Brain Research, 67*, 253-269.

Gottsdanker, R. (1966). The effect of superseding signals. *Quarterly Journal of Experimental Psychology, 18*, 236-249.

Hallett, M., Shahani, B.T., & Young, R.R. (1975). EMG analysis of stereotyped voluntary movements in man. *Journal of Neurology, Neurosurgery, and Psychiatry, 38*, 1154-1162.

Hallett, P.E. & Lightstone, A.D. (1976a). Saccadic eye movements towards stimuli triggered by prior saccades. *Vision Research, 16*, 99-106.

Hallett, P.E. & Lightstone, A.D. (1976b). Saccadic eye movements to flashed targets. *Vision Research, 16*, 107-114.

Hasan, Z. & Enoka, R.M. (1985). Isometric torque-angle relationship and movement-related activity of human elbow flexors: implications for the equilibrium point hypothesis. *Experimental Brain Research, 59*, 441-450.

Held, R. (1965). Plasticity in sensorimotor systems. *Scientific American, 213*, 84-94.

Held, R. & Freedman, S. (1963). Plasticity in human sensorimotor control. *Science, 142*, 455-462.

Henning, W., Favilla, M., & Ghez, C. (1988). Trajectory control in targeted force impulses: V. Gradual specification of response amplitude. *Experimental Brain Research, 71*, 116-128.

Henry, F.M. & Harrison, J.S. (1961). Refractoriness of a fast movement. *Perceptual and Motor Skills, 31*, 351-354.

Henry, F.M. & Rogers, D.E. (1960). Increased response latency for complicated movements and a "memory drum" theory of neuromotor reaction. *Research Quarterly, 31*, 448-458.

Herman, R., Herman, R., & Maulucci, R. (1981). Visually triggered eye-arm movements in man. *Experimental Brain Research, 42*, 392-398.

Hick, W.E. (1952). On the rate of gain of information. *Quarterly Journal of Experimental Psychology, 4*, 11-26.

Hoffman, D.S. & Strick, P. (1986). Step-tracking movements of the wrist in humans. I. Kinematic analysis. *The Journal of Neuroscience, 6*, 3309-3318.

Hyman, R. (1953). Stimulus information as a determinant of reaction time. *Journal of Experimental Psychology, 45*, 188-196.

Jagacinski, R.J., Repperger, D.W., Moran, M.S., Ward, S.L., & Glass, B. (1980). Fitts' law and the microstructure of rapid discrete movements. *Journal of Experimental Psychology: Human Perception and Performance, 6*, 309-320.

Jeannerod, M. (1981). Intersegmental coordination during reaching at natural visual objects. In J. Long & A. Baddeley (Eds.), *Attention and performance IX* (pp. 153-169). Hillsdale, NJ.: Lawrence Erlbaum Associates.

Jeannerod, M. (1984). The timing of natural prehension movements. *Journal of Motor Behavior, 16*, 235-254.

Jeannerod, M. (1988). *The neural and behavioural organization of goal-directed movements*. Oxford: Clarendon Press.

Jeannerod, M. & Prablanc, C. (1983). The visual control of reaching movements. In J. Desmedt (Ed.), *Motor control mechanisms in health and disease* (pp. 13-29). New York: Raven Press.

Keele, S. W. (1968). Movement control in skilled motor performance. *Psychological Bulletin, 70*, 387-403.

Keele, S.W. & Posner, M. (1968). Processing of visual feedback in rapid movements. *Journal of Experimental Psychology, 77*, 155-158.

Kelso, J.A.S. & Holt, K.G. (1980). Exploring a vibratory systems analysis of human movement production. *Journal of Neurophysiology, 43*, 1183-1196.

Kelso, J.A.S., Holt, K.G., Kugler, P.N., & Turvey, M.T. (1980). On the concept of coordinative structures as dissipative structures: II. Empirical lines of convergence. In G.E. Stelmach & J. Requin (Eds.), *Tutorials in motor behavior* (pp. 49-70). Amsterdam: North-Holland.

Kelso, J.A.S., Tuller, B., & Harris, K.S. (1983). A "dynamic pattern" perspective on the control and coordination of movement. In P.F. MacNeilage (Ed.), *The production of speech* (pp. 138-173). New York: Springer-Verlag.

Kerr, G.K. (1984). *Refractoriness and control of arm movements with one and two degrees of freedom.* Masters Thesis, Faculty of Physical Education, University of Otago, Dunedin, New Zealand.

Kerr, G.K. (1989). Saccadic eye movements and rapid arm movements in a double-step tracking task. *Society for Neuroscience Abstracts, 15*, 785.

Kerr, G.K. & Lockwood, R.J. (1987). Saccadic reactions to double-step stimuli: the influence of movement amendment direction. *Society for Neuroscience Abstracts, 13*, 1090.

Kerr, G.K. & Lockwood, R.J. (1988). Refractoriness of saccadic eye movements to a two-choice movement amendment. *International Journal of Neuroscience, 40*, 59-60.

Klapp, S.T. (1981). Motor programming is not the only process which can influence RT: some thoughts on the Marteniuk and MacKenzie analysis. *Journal of Motor Behavior, 13*, 320-328.

Klapp, S.T. & Erwin, C.I. (1976). Relation between programming time and duration of the response being programmed. *Journal of Experimental Psychology, 100*, 368-374.

Klapp, S.T. & Greim, D.M. (1979). Program control of aimed movements revisited: The role of target visibility and symmetry. *Journal of Experimental Psychology: Human Perception and Performance, 5*, 509-521.

Klapp, S.T., Wyatt, E.P., & Lingo, W.M. (1974). Response programming in simple and choice reactions. *Journal of Motor Behavior, 6*, 263-271.

Knudsen, E.I., DuLac, S., & Esterly, S. (1987). Computational maps in the brain. *Annual Review of Neuroscience, 10*, 41-65.

Lacquaniti, F. (1989). Central representations of human limb movement as revealed by studies of drawing and handwriting. *Trends in Neurosciences, 12*, 287-291.

Lagasse, P.P. & Hayes, K.C. (1973). Premotor and motor reaction time as a function of movement extent. *Journal of Motor Behavior, 5*, 25-32.

Latour, P.L. (1962). Visual thresholds during eye movements. *Vision Research,* 2, 261-262.

LeBozec, S. & Maton, B. (1987). Differences between motor unit firing rate, twitch characteristics and fiber type composition in an agonistic muscle group in man. *European Journal of Applied Psychology, 56*, 350-355.

Lestienne, F. (1979). Effects of inertial load and velocity on the braking process of voluntary limb movements. *Experimental Brain Research, 35*, 407-418.

Lestienne, F., Polit, A., & Bizzi, E. (1981). Functional organization of the motor process underlying the transition from movement to posture. *Brain Research, 230*, 121-131.

Lofthus, G.K. & Hanson, C.J. (1981). Fractionated reaction times and performance times as a function of practice. *American Journal of Physical Medicine, 60*, 190-197.

Ludwig, D.A. (1982). EMG changes during acquisition of a motor skill. *American Journal of Physical Medicine, 61*, 229-243.

Marsden, C.D., Obeso, J.A., & Rothwell, J.C. (1983). The function of the antagonistic muscle during fast limb movements in man. *Journal of Physiology, 335*, 1-13.

Marteniuk, R.G. (1976). *Information processing and motor skills*. New York: Holt, Rinehart, & Winston.

Marteniuk, R.G., Mackenzie, C.L., Jeannerod, M., Athenes, S., & Dugas, C. (1987). Constraints on human arm movements trajectories. *Canadian Journal of Psychology, 41*, 365-378.

Marteniuk, R.G. & Romanow, S.K.E. (1983). Human movement organization and learning as revealed by variability of movement, use of kinematic information, and Fourier analysis. In R.A.Magill (Ed.), *Memory and control of action* (pp. 167-197). Amsterdam: North-Holland.

Mather, J.A. (1985). Some aspects of the motor organization of the oculomotor system. *Journal of Motor Behavior, 17*, 373-383.

Matheson, J., Hallett, M., Berardelli, A., Weinhaus, R., & Inzucchi, S. (1985). Failure to confirm a correlation between electromyogram and final position. *Human Neurobiology, 4*, 257-260.

Matin, E. (1974). Saccadic suppression: A review and an analysis. *Psychological Bulletin, 81*, 899-916.

Maton, B., LeBozec, S., & Cnockaert, J.C. (1980). The synergy of elbow extensor muscles during dynamic work in man. II. Braking of elbow flexion. *Journal of Applied Physiology, 44*, 271-178.

Megaw, E.D. (1975). Saccadic eye-movements and the refractory period. In P.M.A. Rabbitt & S. Dornic (Eds.), *Attention and performance V* (pp. 383-394). London: Academic Press.

Megaw, E.D. & Armstrong, W. (1973). Individual and simultaneous tracking of a step input by the horizontal saccadic eye movement and manual control system. *Journal of Experimental Psychology, 100*, 18-28.

Meyer, D.E., Smith, J.E.K., & Wright, C.E. (1982). Models for the speed and accuracy of aimed movements. *Psychological Review, 89*, 449-482.

Miall, R.C., Weir, D.J., & Stein, J.F. (1986). Manual tracking of visual targets by trained monkeys. *Behavioral Brain Research, 20*, 185-201.

Moore, S.P. & Marteniuk, R.G. (1986). Kinematic and electromyographic changes that occur as a function of learning a time-constrained aiming task. *Journal of Motor Behavior, 18*, 397-426.

Morris, H.H. (1977). Effects of practice and set upon reaction time and its fractionated components. In D.M. Landers & R.W.Christina (Eds.), *Psychology of motor behavior and sport* (pp. 259-268). Champaign, IL: Human Kinetics.

Mustard, B.E. & Lee, R.G. (1987). Relationship between EMG patterns and kinematic properties for flexion movements at the human wrist. *Experimental Brain Research, 66*, 247-256.

Neilson, P.D., Neilson, M.D., & O'Dwyer, N.J. (1988). Internal models and intermittency: A theoretical account of human tracking behavior. *Biological Cybernetics, 58*, 101-112.

Nichols, T.R. & Houk, J.C. (1976). Improvement in linearity and regulation of stiffness that results from actions of stretch reflex. *Journal of Neurophysiology, 39*, 119-142.

Niemi, P. & Lehtonen, E. (1982). Foreperiod and visual stimulus intensity: a reappraisal. *Acta Psychologica, 50*, 73-82.

Norrie, M.L. (1974). Effects of movement complexity on choice reaction and movement times. *Research Quarterly, 45*, 154-161.

Payton, O.D. & Kelley, D.L. (1972). Electromyographic evidence of the acquisition of a motor skill. A pilot study. *Physical Therapy, 52*, 261-266.

Pelisson, D. & Prablanc, C. (1988). Kinematics of centrifugal and centripetal saccadic eye movements in man. *Vision Research, 28*, 87-94.

Person, R.S. (1958). An electromyographic investigation on co-ordination of the activity of antagonist muscles in man during the development of a motor habit. *Pavlovian Journal of Higher Nervous Activity, 8*, 13-23.

Polit, A. & Bizzi, E. (1978). Processes controlling arm movements in monkeys. *Science, 201*, 1235-1237.

Polit, A. & Bizzi, E. (1979). Characteristics of motor programs underlying arm movements in monkeys. *Journal of Neurophysiology, 42*, 183-194.

Prablanc, C., Echallier, J.F., Komilis, E., & Jeannerod, M. (1979). Optimal response of eye and hand motor systems in pointing at a visual target. I. Spatio-temporal characteristics of eye and hand movements and their relationships when varying the amount of visual information. *Biological Cybernetics, 35*, 113-124.

Prablanc, C., Masse, D., & Echallier, J.F. (1978). Error correcting mechanisms in large saccades. *Vision Research, 18*, 557-560.

Rothwell, J.C., Traub, M.M., Day, B.L., Obeso, J.A., Thomas, P.K., & Marsden, C.D. (1982). Manual motor performance in a deafferented man. *Brain, 105*, 515-542.

Salthouse, T.A. & Ellis, C.L. (1980). Determinants of eye-fixation duration. *American Journal of Psychology, 93*, 207-234.

Saltzman, E. (1979). Levels of sensorimotor representation. *Journal of Mathematical Psychology, 20*, 91-163.

Schmidt, R.A., Zelaznik, H., Hawkins, B., Frank, J.S., & Quinn, J.T. (1979). Motor-output variability: A theory for the accuracy of rapid motor acts. *Psychological Review, 86*, 415-451.

Schneider, K., Zernicke, R.F., Schmidt, R.A., & Hart, T.J. (1986). Modulation of limb dynamics during the learning of rapid arm movements. *Proceedings of the North American Congress on Biomechanics* (pp. 77-78), Montreal (Quebec), Canada, 25-27 August, 1986.

Shackel, B. (1967). Eye movement recording by electro-oculography. In P.H. Venables & I. Martin (Eds.), *A manual of psychophysiological methods* (pp. 301-334). Amsterdam: North-Holland.

Siegel, D.S. (1977). The effect of movement amplitude and target diameter on reaction time. *Journal of Motor Behavior, 9*, 257-265.

Sittig, A.C., Denier van der Gon, J.J., & Geilen, S.C.A.M. (1987). The contribution of afferent information on position and velocity to the control of slow and fast human forearm movements. *Experimental Brain Research, 67*, 33-40.

Sittig, A.C., Denier van der Gon, J.J., Geilen, S.C.A.M., & van Wijk, A.J.M. (1985). The attainment of target position during step-tracking movements despite a shift of initial position. *Experimental Brain Research, 60*, 407-410.

Smith, W.M. & Bowen, K.F. (1980). The effects of delayed and displaced visual feedback on motor control. *Journal of Motor Behavior, 12*, 91-101.

Soechting, J.F. (1973). Modelling of a simple motor task in man: Motor output dependence on sensory input. *Kybernetic, 14*, 25-34.

Soechting, J.F. (1984). Effect of target size on spatial and temporal characteristics of a pointing movement in man. *Experimental Brain Research, 54*, 121-132.

Soechting, J.F., Ranish, N.A., Palminteri, R., & Terzuolo, C.A. (1976). *Brain Research, 105*, 21-44.

Stark, L., Vossius, G., & Young, L.R. (1962). Predictive control of eye tracking movements. *IRE Transactions on Human Factors Electronics, HFE-3*, 52-57.

Stein, J.F. (1986). Role of the cerebellum in the visual guidance of movement. *Nature, 323*, 217-221.

Stein, J.F. (1989). Representation of egocentric space in the posterior parietal cortex. *Quarterly Journal of Experimental Physiology, 74*, 583-706.

Stein, J.F., Miall, C., & Weir, D. (1987). The role of the cerebellum in the visual guidance of movement. In M. Glickstein, C. Yeo, & J. Stein (Eds.), *Cerebellum and neuronal plasticity* (pp. 175-191). Plenum Publishing.

Turvey, M.T., Shaw, R.E., & Mace, W. (1978). Issues in the theory of action: Degrees of freedom, coordinative structures and coalitions. In J. Requin (Ed.), *Attention and performance VII* (pp. 557-595). Hillsdale, NJ.: Lawrence Erlbaum Associates.

van Asten, W.N.J.C., Gielen, S.C.A.M., & de Winkel, M.E.M. (1988). The effect of isoluminant and isochromatic stimuli on latency and amplitude of saccades. *Vision Research, 28*, 827-840.

Vince, M.A. (1948). Corrective movements in a pursuit task. *Quarterly Journal of Experimental Psychology, 1*, 85-103.

Vincken, M.H., Gielen, S.C.A.M., & Denier van der Gon, J.J. (1983). Intrinsic and afferent components in apparent muscle stiffness in man. *Neuroscience, 9*, 529-534.

Viviani, P. & Berthoz, A. (1977). Voluntary deceleration and perceptual activity during oblique saccades. In R. Baker & A. Berthoz (Eds.), *The control of gaze by brainstem neurons* (pp. 23-28). New York: Elsevier.

Viviani, P. & Swensson, R.G. (1982). Saccadic eye movements to peripherally discriminated visual targets. *Journal of Experimental Psychology: Human Perception and Performance, 8*, 113-126.

Viviani, P. & Terzuolo, C.A. (1973). Modelling of a simple motor task in man: Intentional arrest of an ongoing movement. *Kybernetic, 14*, 35-62.

Wadman, W.J., Boerhout, W., & Denier van der Gon, J.J. (1980). Responses of the arm movement control system to force impulses. *Journal of Human Movement Studies, 6*, 280-302.

Wadman, W.J., Denier van der Gon, J.J., Geuze, R.H., & Mol, C.R. (1979). Control of fast goal-directed arm-movements. *Journal of Human Movement Studies, 5*, 3-17.

Weiss, A.D. (1965). The locus of reaction time changes with set, motivation and age. *Journal of Gerontology, 20*, 60-64.

Welford, A.T. (1959). Evidence of a single channel mechanism limiting performance in a serial reaction task. *Quarterly Journal of Experimental Psychology, 11*, 193-210.

Welford, A.T. (1968). *Fundamentals of skill*. London: Methuen.

Wheeless, L.L., Boynton, R.E., & Cohen, G.H. (1966). Eye-movement responses to step and pulse-step stimuli. *Journal of the Optical Society of America, 56*, 956-960.

Wheeless L.L., Cohen, G.H., & Boynton, R.E. (1967). Luminance as a parameter of the eye-movement control system. *Journal of the Optical Society of America, 57*, 394-400.

White, C.T., Eason, R.G., & Bartlett, N.R. (1962). Latency and duration of eye movements in the horizontal plane. *Journal of the Optical Society of America, 52*, 210-213.

Whiting, H.T.A., Gill, E.B., & Stephenson, J.M. (1970). Critical time intervals for taking in flight information in a ball-catching task. *Ergonomics, 13*, 265-272.

Williams, L.R.T. (1971a). Reaction time and large response units. *New Zealand Journal of Health, Physical Education and Recreation, 4*, 46-52.

Williams, L.R.T. (1971b). Refractoriness of an extended movement to directional change. *Journal of Motor Behavior, 3*, 289-300.

Williams, L.R.T. & Sullivan, S.J. (1978). Effects of movement speed on the refractoriness of an extended movement to reversal. *Journal of Human Movement Studies, 4*, 70-84.

Williams, L.R.T., Sullivan, S.J., & Kerr, G.K. (1985). Movement refractoriness: The influence of response structure and speed. *Human Movement Science, 4*, 203-228.

Wing, A.M., Turton, A. & Fraser, C. (1986). Grasp size and accuracy of approach in reaching. *Journal of Motor Behavior, 18*, 245-260.

Woltring, H.J. (1986). A fortran package for generalized, cross-validatory spline smoothing and differentiation. *Advances in Engineering Software*, *8*, 104-113.

Wood, G.A. (1977). An electrophysiological model of human visual reaction time. *Journal of Motor Behavior, 9*, 267-274.

Woodworth, R.S. (1899). The accuracy of voluntary movement. *Psychological Monographs, 3(2, Whole No. 13).*

Zelaznik, H.N., Hawkins, B., & Kisselburgh, L. (1983). Rapid visual feedback processing in single-aiming movements. *Journal of Motor Behavior, 15*, 217-236.

Zelaznik, H.N., Schmidt, R.A., & Gielen, S.C.A.M. (1986). Kinematic properties of rapid aimed hand movements. *Journal of Motor Behavior, 15*, 217-236.

Approaches to the Study of Motor Control and Learning
J.J. Summers (Editor)

Chapter 10

THE PROCESSING OF VISUAL FEEDBACK IN RAPID MOVEMENTS: REVISITED

Denis Glencross and Nicholas Barrett
Curtin University

Keele and Posner (1968) claimed to have estimated the minimum processing time for visual information (e.g., 190 - 260 msec). This chapter examines the evidence for visually based amendments during very rapid movements and questions whether, indeed, it is even possible to establish an absolute processing time for visual error information. Two visually based error correction mechanisms are proposed. For precision movements, displaying an initial impulse followed by a visual correction, processing time is related to the magnitude of error. Small errors are thought to require a normal reaction time in accord with Keele and Posner's (1968) estimate. Intermediate magnitude errors allow the subject to prepare the correction in advance and await visual confirmation at the end of the initial impulse. Visual processing here may be as rapid as 130 msec. Large magnitude error corrections do not await any visual confirmation. A qualitatively different and very rapid loop may also serve to constrain response variability even for movements as fast as 80 msec. It is questioned whether these processes may be fully understood in isolation from other sources of ocular information. In particular, future research must address the close interaction between retinal and extraretinal information.

In 1968, Steven Keele and Michael Posner published a paper in the *Journal of Experimental Psychology* entitled 'Processing of Visual Feedback in Rapid Movements'. This seminal paper, at the time, had a major influence on both the theoretical modelling of human motor control and the paradigms subsequently adopted. In their paper, Keele and Posner argued that there was a minimum amount of time necessary for the processing of visual information associated with a movement. "If a movement is made quite slowly, visual feedback may be used in guiding it to an accurate termination. However, visual feedback may not influence the accuracy of very rapid movements" (Keele & Posner, 1968, p. 155).

In the present chapter we review the original study in the light of research into the question of visual information processing and motor control over the past twenty years. In particular, we question the validity of the basic assumption that there exists some absolute amount of time necessary to process visual feedback from a movement.

KEELE AND POSNER'S (1968) ORIGINAL STUDY

The Original Experiment

In the original experiment, subjects made discrete movements to small circular targets (0.25 in. diameter) over a distance of 6 in. from the starting position. There were two such targets each side of the starting position on the 45°-225° axis. The trials were conducted in the dark, except that a circle of light surrounded the circumference of the target. The whole experimental area (the targets to start position) was illuminated (this was referred to as the feedback light) and enabled the subject to see the hand (and stylus) and targets. The feedback light was programmed to turn off immediately on leaving the starting position and when this occurred the whole room was in the dark. The procedure involved the subjects making paced movements, which they had previously practiced, with duration of 150, 250, 350, or 450 msec. Subjects were required to make the movements as spatially accurate as possible and to keep the movement duration within ± 10% of the specified duration. The other important procedural manipulation was that randomly, on half the trials, the feedback light was turned off at the start of the movement and remained off until the target was hit (or missed).

The predictions were quite straightforward. If there was time to process and use the visual information, during a particular movement duration, then the 'lights-on' trials should be more accurate than the 'lights-off' trials. However, if there was not sufficient time, the 'lights-on' and 'lights-off' trials should be equally accurate (or inaccurate), in terms of hitting or missing the target.

The Original Results

The findings indicated that accuracy, as measured by the proportion of target misses, was closely related to the movement duration; the longer the duration, the more accurate the movement when the lights remained on. The important result was that when the lights were turned off at the start of the movement, the proportion of misses increased significantly for the 250, 350, and 450 msec duration movements (0.58, 0.52, 0.47 respectively), compared with the 'lights-on' condition (0.47, 0.28, 0.15 respectively). However, at the 150 msec duration condition, the proportion of misses were equivalent for the 'lights-on' and 'lights-off' conditions, 0.68 and 0.69 respectively. These results are summarised in Figure 1.

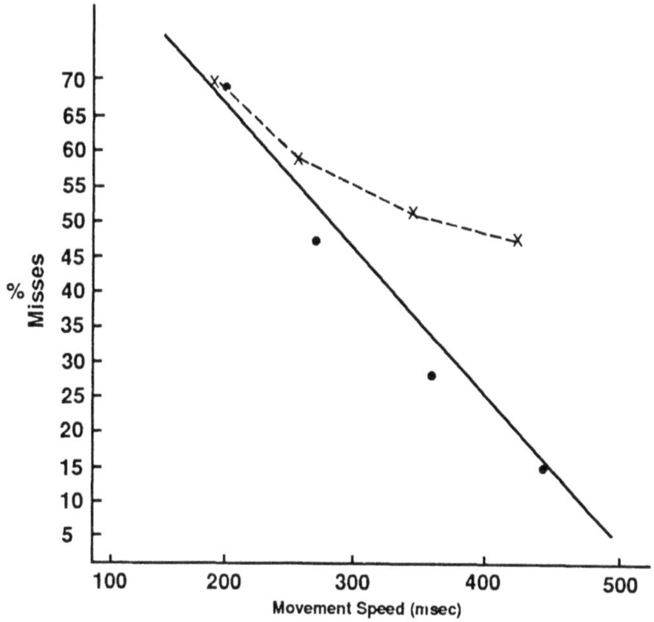

Figure 1. Keele & Posner's (1968) data illustrating percentage misses as a function of movement speed and the illumination condition (Dashed lines = OFF condition; solid lines = ON condition).

Let us state Keele and Posner's (1968) conclusion; "...the minimum duration for processing visual feedback from a movement appears to be between 190 and 260 msec" (p. 157). This estimate is derived from the actual movement times for the shortest duration movement (190/185 msec instead of 150 msec) and the next shortest duration (267/254 msec instead of 250 msec). This visual processing time is somewhat less than previous estimates. Vince (1948) and Woodworth (1899), for example, observed that reciprocal tapping movements are not benefited by visual feedback for movement duration in the order of 450 msec. If we use this value of 450 msec as the visual processing time, however, we are including the time to reverse direction in any estimate based on reciprocal tapping. By using a discrete movement paradigm, Keele and Posner (1968) ensured that their own measurements for the visual processing time did not include the time taken to reverse directions. Slow processing times were also reported by Hick (1949) and Pew (1966). Hick (1949) tricked subjects into executing an incorrect movement during a step tracking task. A period of 300 msec elapsed prior to the detection of the error and the amendment of the movement. Similar results are reported in Pew (1966). He required subjects to maintain a target in the centre of an oscilloscope screen by means of two buttons causing target acceleration either to the left or to the right. When the oscilloscope display was blacked out for 410 msec following a response, the modal corrective reaction time before the next response was 300-350 msec after the end of the black-out. The rather high estimates of 300-350 msec reported by Hick (1949) and Pew (1966) may be due, as Christina (1970) has pointed out, to the added element of complete surprise to see the movement error occur.

Keele and Posner's (1968) results suggested that the more time there was available to process (use) the visual information, the greater was the accuracy, "...accuracy increased as movement time increased even when the feedback light was turned off, though not as much as when it remained on" (p. 157). The implication of the results taken as a whole is that accuracy is related to the time available to process visual information. However, this relationship ceases somewhere between 190 and 260 msec, because there is not sufficient time to use the visual information, even if it is available.

In summary, Keele and Posner (1968) reasoned that since visual information requires a specific time to be processed, then there should be a corresponding movement speed, faster than this processing time, at which visual feedback can no longer make a useful contribution to controlling the accuracy of an aimed movement. As we have seen, the visual processing time was thought to have been discovered at a movement speed of between 190 and 260 msec. In the next section we present supporting evidence for Keele and Posner's approach. In subsequent sections we address the weaknesses in their argument.

Supporting Evidence

A number of research findings appeared to bolster Keele and Posners' (1968) arguments. Sometimes, in a left-right choice step tracking situation, the subject will initiate a response in a direction opposite to that specified by the target light. Gibbs (1965), for example, noted that amendments to a step-tracking directional error response which were measured from response onset took in the order of 240 msec, at least during the early stages of practice. Note that this step-tracking directional error situation differs from Hicks' (1949) step tracking error situation since in the former situation the errors are subject generated rather than experimenter generated. Gibbs' (1965) conclusion that this time of 240 msec represented the processing time in the visual feedback loop concurs with Keele and Posner (1968). The time decreased with practice, however, and this was presumed to represent a shift towards proprioceptive control and even to control via an efference copy (e.g., Angel, 1976). It is not clear, however, whether the information for the error corrections in Gibbs (1965) is supplied at the initiation of the error response (see comments by Glencross & Barrett, 1989; Schmidt & Gordon, 1977). If we cannot be sure when the processing leading to the error correction commences then, clearly, we cannot be confident in our estimation of the error correction reaction time.

In an extension of Keele and Posner's paradigm, Beggs and Howarth (1970) investigated the effect of disrupting the visual feedback loop at the initiation of a movement, and also at different stages as the limb approached the target. An infrared beam was located at different distances between the homebase and target. As the tapping stylus passed through the beam, illumination of the target display and room was extinguished. When illumination was extinguished early in the trajectory, Beggs and Howarth (1970) reported more errors (measured in terms of the root mean square error) than if the illumination was extinguished towards the end of the trajectory. They argued that there should be no improvement in accuracy of an aiming movement for any additional illumination after a point corresponding to one corrective reaction time prior to target contact. That is, there should be a 'breakpoint' in the function relating errors to the distance of the infrared beam from the target and from this 'breakpoint' the corrective reaction time could be derived. Their estimate for the visual processing time was in the order of 290 msec which corresponds quite well with that of Keele and Posner (1968). It is possible the larger estimation by Beggs and Howarth (1970) reflects the study of a reciprocal tapping situation.

In a replication and extension of Keele and Posner's (1968) experiment, in our own laboratory, we required subjects to make discrete movements to a target in a fixed duration. However, during the course of the movement the illumination was switched off at randomly varying intervals, so that the final phase of the movement to the actual target was in the dark. This procedure is a variation of the ON-OFF procedure used by Beggs and Howarth (1970). In our experiment, subjects produced movements over a distance of 21 cms to a 1.4 cm diameter target. After leaving the starting position the illumination was turned off at 0, 100, 150, 200, 250, 300, 350, 400 and 500 msec, (Note at 0 msec the whole movement was made in the dark, at 500 msec the whole movement was made with the lights on). In addition, we employed an OFF-ON condition. For the OFF-ON condition illumination was always extinguished at the initiation of a response and, then, returned after various intervals (again

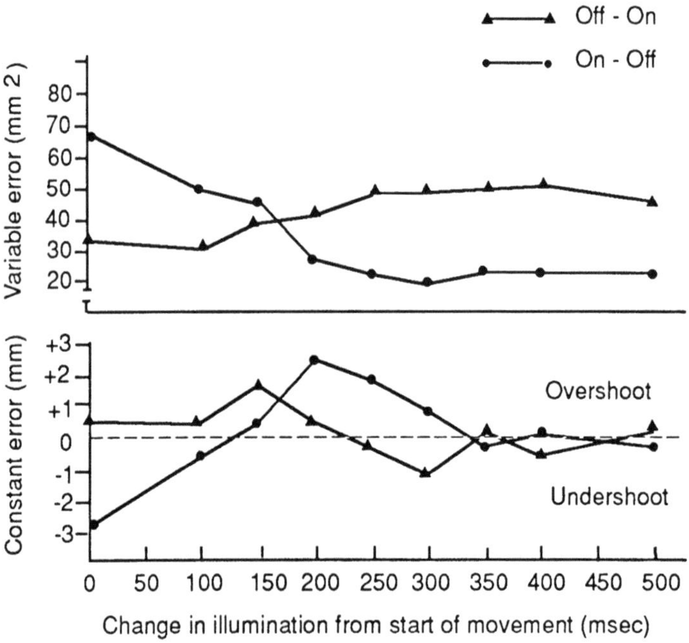

Figure 2. Variable and constant errors as a function of the change in illumination from the start of the movement. In the ON-OFF condition, the movement commenced with full vision and subsequently, the illumination was switched off. In the OFF-ON condition, the movement commenced without vision and subsequently, the illumination was switched on. Movement time was 450 ± 45 msec.

these intervals were 0, 100 msec and then at 50 msec increments through to 400 msec, and 500 msec). Subjects were instructed to produce movement times of 450 ± 45 msec, and trial by trial they were given feedback on their actual duration times. Target accuracy was expressed in terms of variable error and signed constant error. Variable error refers to the variation or dispersion of movement endpoints around the target, whereas constant error refers to the position of movement endpoints relative to the target. Thus, a negative constant error is registered if the subject undershoots the target. A positive constant error indicates a target overshoot. The results from this study are reported in Figure 2. In general, the variable error data replicates Keele and Posner and are in accord with the previous studies. For both the ON-OFF and OFF-ON plots of variable errors, there appears to be a 'breakpoint' representing a point at which either maximum accuracy or maximum variability is attained. For the

ON-OFF condition, a breakpoint occurs at 200 msec indicating that allowing any additional visual information beyond this point has no additional benefit for accuracy. For the OFF-ON condition, a 'breakpoint' occurs at 250 msec indicating that if visual feedback is presented beyond this point, it is of no value in the control of the trajectory of the movement. Since subjects produced movement times of 450 msec, the variable error data suggests a visual processing time in the order of 200-250 msec. The constant error data will be addressed later.

Wallace and Newell (1983) compared no vision and vision trials in a Fitts tapping task. Only at an index of difficulty (ID) corresponding to 4.58 BITS or more did they observe a lower error rate associated with the availability of vision. Since at ID 4.58 movement time was roughly 250 msec, these results also agree with those of Keele and Posner (1968). Similar results are also reported in Glencross and Barrett (1983).

Such findings fit well into a discrete error correction model (e.g., Craik, 1947; Crossman & Goodeve, 1963/1983; Keele, 1968; Howarth, Beggs, & Bowden, 1971). Here the subject selects a series of motor programs which eventually translate into a series of submovements. As Zelaznik, Hawkins, and Kisselburgh (1983) summarise:

> ...the previous movement produced error and the next motor program is selected to reduce the error. The reasons for the ...delays (of the magnitude reported in the above studies) in the processing of visual feedback could be the result of the delays in selecting new motor programs" (pp. 234-235).

If this is the mechanism by which visual feedback mediates in the accuracy of an aiming movement then a corollary assumption would indeed be that there is a specific processing time for visual information. Since, furthermore, the minimum reaction time to a visual stimulus is approximately 200 msec (e.g., Klemmer, 1957) it would be expected that the correction to visually based movement errors would also take a corresponding time.

The notion of a visually mediated discrete correction control process is borne out by an examination of movement patterns. Discrete corrections, indicated by a discontinuity in the movement pattern, are very clearly defined for very short microscopic movements (e.g., Langolf, Chaffin, & Foulke, 1976) but less so for larger amplitude movement trajectories. Using a sampling rate of 30 samples/second, Langolf et al. (1976) failed to observe similar breaks in large amplitude movement patterns. Carlton (1980), however, increased his sampling rate to 222 samples/second and readily observed discrete corrections even for large amplitude movements (see also Meyer, Abrams, Kornblum, Wright, & Smith, 1988). As Langolf et al. (1976) themselves point out, inertial damping of the arm may smooth out and mask the changes in control for large amplitude movements to some extent. What is interesting from Langolf et al's (1976) data for microscopic movements is that the discontinuities in their movement traces showed up some 200 msec after movement initiation. That is, the information for the error correction seemed to be processed in a time compatible, again, with Keele and Posner's (1968) estimate.

Of course, it could be argued that the discontinuities observed in the trajectories of aimed movements need not be a result of visually mediated feedback mechanisms. Meyer et al. (1988), for example, entertained the possibility that submovements could be programmed before response initiation as part of a "submovement series... [which] might then follow a predetermined course regardless of the outcomes achieved by primary submovements"(p. 364). Meyer et al. (1988), nevertheless, reported that removing the view of the response cursor in a rapid wrist rotation task increased error rates in terms of the percentage of submovement series that failed to terminate within the objective target region. It seems reasonable to conclude, therefore, that the generation of corrective submovements is visually mediated.

There was, therefore, emerging evidence from the analysis of movement patterns and the illumination manipulation paradigm that was interpreted in favour of Keele and Posner (1968). However, there were nuances in the data that questioned whether an absolute processing time for visual information would in fact be discovered. So influential had Keele and Posner's paper become that there was the danger that it might become a Procrustes bed. In the following sections we take issue with Keele and Posner's paper on two counts. Namely, (1) that there is a unitary mode for visual processing, and (2) that a minimum time for visual processing is in the order of 190-260 msec.

KEELE AND POSNER (1968) REAPPRAISED

Conflicting Evidence

Keele and Posner (1968) sought to establish a specific time for visual processing and this notion has also become the central tenet of iterative correction models of aimed movements (e.g., Crossman & Goodeve, 1963/1983; Keele, 1968; Howarth, et al., 1971). However, there is mounting evidence which questions both this notion of a constant time and, also, that Keele and Posner's estimate represents a minimum processing time.

Beggs and Howarth's (1970) estimate of a visual processing time of 290 msec was a mean corrective reaction time estimate derived from only three of their eight obtained functions (see their Figure 1). For a tapping speed of 85 strokes/minute they obtained, from the discontinuity in the respective line, a visual processing time of 165 msec; at 100 strokes/min. - 285 msec; at 125 strokes/min. - 290 msec; at 141 strokes/min. - 295 msec. The other lines showed no discontinuity. Beggs and Howarth (1970) discounted the corrective reaction time of 165 msec, presumably for being anomalous, and averaged the other three results to arrive at the processing time of 290 msec. Beggs and Howarth's results, however, suggest instead that the speed at which the subject was required to tap actually determined the corrective reaction time. Reinterpreted, the data tell us that slow tapping either showed a short corrective reaction time or at very slow speeds no breakpoint. As the tapping speed was increased, so too was the magnitude of the corrective reaction time until, for very fast movements, the actual time needed to initiate a correction was now longer than the movement itself. Movement time was a main determinant of corrective reaction time. Another concern with Beggs and Howarth's study is that their conclusions are based on variable errors. Conceivably, for example, the overall spread of movement endpoints may remain the same even though some shift in their mean location has changed. If we return to our data in Figure 2, we see that the variable error data does indeed support Beggs and Howarth (1970). The constant error data, however, suggests that visually based adjustments are still happening beyond the corresponding 'breakpoints' in the variable error plots.

Langolf et al's (1976) data also challenged the notion of a constant visual processing time from their analyses of breakpoint times for microscopic movements. The breakpoints, it will be recalled, reflect a discrete, visually mediated correction. The mean breakpoint time was Keele and Posnerian (e.g., 195 msec) but what is of interest is the considerable variability in the data. Even when we observe a series of corrections within the same movement it appears that successive corrections are accomplished in different times (e.g., Jagacinski, Repperger, Moran, Ward, & Glass, 1980). The first correction takes in excess of 290 msec whereas the final correction could be achieved in less than 190 msec. Intermediate corrections had intermediate durations.

Given the wide variability for breakpoints observed by Langolf et al. (1976), it might be reasonable to expect that visual feedback may have some limited benefit for movements of 190 msec or faster. This might be the case even if we allowed for a shift in the overall corrective reaction time distribution with movement time, as Beggs and Howarth's (1970) data indicated.

That visual information may have some benefit for very rapid movements was in fact suggested in a paper by Smith and Bowen using a visual delay paradigm. Smith and Bowen (1980) delayed view of the responding limb by 66 msec during target directed movements ranging in duration between 150 and 650 msec. Constant errors were reported to be different between delayed trials and undistorted trials even at movement times of 150 msec. Smith and Bowen (1980) drew the conclusion that since a movement of 150 msec duration can be affected by a visual delay of 66 msec then the processing time for the visual feedback underlying this effect must be somewhat less than 100 msec. In terms of the constant errors, aiming had shifted from undershooting (-1.50 mm) for undistorted trials to overshooting (+3.20 mm) when visual feedback was delayed. Though challenging, the data is not easy to interpret in view of the standard deviation data (e.g., Glencross & Barrett, 1989). There was a doubling of variability on delayed trials as compared to undistorted trials. As Beggs and Howarth (1988) have suggested, moreover, an anomaly may have occurred since even under undistorted vision, the distribution of errors for a movement time of 150 msec was low and also failed to follow the trend of increased error distribution with decreased movement time.

Smith and Bowen (1980) did not directly design their experiment in order to assess the effects of visual information on movement accuracy. However, in 1983, Zelaznik, Hawkins, and Kisselburgh published their reappraisal and refinement of Keele and Posner's (1968) study. The appearance of Smith and Bowen's (1980) data and other data (e.g., Carlton, 1981, to be discussed later) had by now questioned Keele and Posner's estimate of the visual processing time (190-260 msec) and raised doubts that a constant processing time might be found.

Zelaznik et al's (1983) Analysis of Rapid Movements

Zelaznik et al. (1983) argued that by randomly presenting the vision and no vision (0.5 probability) trials in Keele and Posner's (1968) original study, meant that subjects would have been uncertain as to whether an upcoming trial was to be completed with or without illumination. This may have encouraged the subjects to prepare to control all movements in the absence of vision. Should a trial with visual feedback available then occur, there would be added delays due to the cost of having prepared for a blind movement.

Zelaznik et al. (1983) further argued that Keele and Posner's (1968) measurement of error, in terms of hits and misses, itself would not be sensitive enough to detect all but the most gross of errors. Two conditions could have identical percent hits and yet have widely different dispersions of the movement endpoints. Zelaznik et al. based their results, therefore, on Henry's (1974) composite error score, E. Figure 3 plots the error data for Zelaznik et al's Experiment 3 in which the subjects performed the no-vision and vision trials in separate blocks.

As can be seen from Figure 3, more errors are produced when the trials are performed without illumination than with illumination at all movement speeds except for the very rapid 70 msec movements. There was a large error difference, particularly for errors measured in the dimension parallel to the horizontal trajectory (i.e., E-distance) even for a movement speed of 150 msec. These results are in stark contrast to those of Keele and Posner. In a previous experiment (Zelaznik et al., 1983, Experiment 1), furthermore, a similar advantage for vision had been reported for a movement time of 100 msec. This would set the visual processing time to be in the order of 70-100 msec. It is

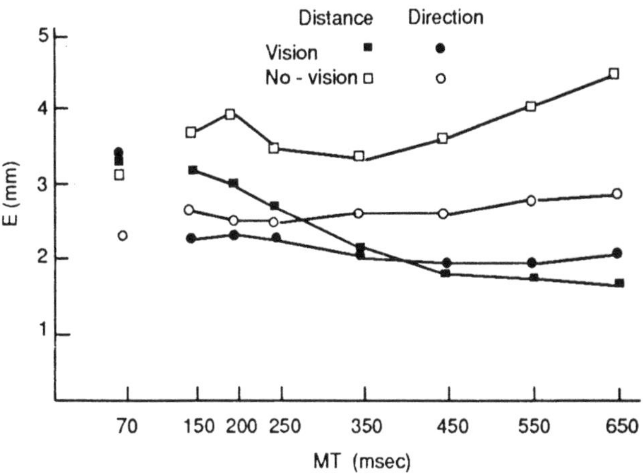

Figure 3. Target accuracy (E) as a function of movement time and illumination condition for errors measured in the dimensions parallel (i.e., E-distance) and perpendicular (i.e., E-direction) to the horizontal trajectory. From Zelaznik et al. (1983), Journal of Motor Behavior, 15, 217-236. Reprinted with permission of the Helen Dwight Reid Educational Foundation. Published by Heldref Publications, 4000 Albemarle St., N.W., Washington, D.C. 20016. Copyright 1983.

interesting to note that this time may be equivalent to the summed afferent and efferent delay times (see review by Barrett & Glencross, 1988a).

Although error differences were reported both when subjects were certain and also uncertain about the availability of visual feedback for movement speeds of as fast as 100 msec, the difference is larger for the certain condition. This is consistent with the notion that subjects prepare to receive visual information. A combination of an insensitive error measurement and randomly presenting vision and no vision trials in the same block may, therefore, have led Keele and Posner (1968) to overestimate the visual processing time.

In the absence of an alternative explanation, Zelaznik et al. (1983) provided convincing evidence for the very rapid processing of visual information. The results cannot be explained, for example, in terms of the environment remaining constant on visual trials but not so during no-vision trials. In their Experiment 2, Zelaznik et al. (1983) required subjects to begin their movements in the absence of visual feedback. Therefore, the environment remained constant for the no-vision trials only. Again, the error difference resulting from the availability of visual feedback showed up. Nor could the difference be attributed to the use of visual feedback to update the response on subsequent trials. Disrupting visual feedback was detrimental even when the vision and no-vision trials were alternated (Zelaznik et al., 1983, Experiment 4).

Zelaznik et al's (1983) data, nevertheless, confound the effects of constant and variable error by using a composite error score. Beggs and Howarth (1988) and Howarth and Beggs (1985) have clearly made the case for the theoretical and logical distinction between variable and constant error. Elliot and Allard (1985) have replicated Zelaznik et al's (1983) study using variable and constant error in addition to radial error which reflects the mean distance of movement endpoints relative to the target centres. For both variable and radial error the most errors were a result of performing blocked trials with the lights off. Only for radial errors was the greatest benefit derived from performing blocked trials with the lights on. The radial error data, therefore, supports Zelaznik et al's (1983) observation that visual information is used most efficiently if subjects are certain it will be available.

The constant error data reported in Elliot and Allard (1985) suggested a further factor that may have contributed to Keele and Posner's (1968) overestimation of the visual processing time. When the vision and no-vision trials were presented randomly, there was an increase in the magnitude of undershooting both when the lights were on and off. The constant errors may have thus contributed more to the hits and misses measure which in turn would have marred any effects detectable from the measurement of variable or radial errors.

Elliot and Allard (1985) also tried to shed some light on why, in both their study and also Zelaznik et al's (1983), subjects did not take advantage of the visual information present in the random condition. By measuring initial reaction time they proposed to show up any differences in strategy across conditions. However, no differences could be found. The reasons for superior processing of vision when the availability is certain remains a matter of speculation.

Zelaznik et al's (1983) results have important implications for Keele and Posner's (1968) earlier study. If vision can be shown to be of benefit to the accuracy of rapid movements in the order of 70-100 msec, then visual feedback can modulate the trajectory of a movement even when there is no evidence for any discontinuity of the movement pattern. Here again, the possibility is raised that not only is the visual processing time highly variable but that visual amendments may reflect qualitatively different processes. Indeed, if we return to Figure 2, we see that in our own replication of Beggs and Howarth's (1970) study, variable and constant error have been affected differently by changes in illumination. Examination of the constant error data suggests that visual information is being processed more rapidly than the variable error data suggests. Zelaznik et al. (1983) suggested that lengthy delays in the visual amendment process may indicate the selection of a new motor program. Conceivably, this underlies the discontinuities that are observed in movement patterns. On the other hand, the rapid processing suggested in their own study may reflect visually mediated corrections of the execution of a motor program rather than the selection of a new motor program.

For both Keele and Posner (1968) and Zelaznik et al. (1983), the basic approach was to find the fastest movement at which vision could still have some influence on response outcome and conclude that this must be the visual processing time. This research suggests a possible role for visual information in very rapid movements. Can we make conclusions, however, from the observations of visual information processing at fast movement times about visual processing in slower movements? If we look at Zelaznik et al's (1983) Figure 1, we note that for all movement times up to 300 msec, the difference in error between vision and no vision trials is equivalent. For slower movements, however, the difference (seen in Zelaznik et al., 1983, Figure 2) in error with and without vision increased with movement time. This different pattern of results suggests that visual feedback is being processed in different ways for the fast and slow movements. In the next section, then, we ask whether Keele and Posner's (1968) estimate may, nevertheless, apply to visual feedback processing as the limb approaches the target during an aimed movement of greater than 300 msec duration.

Carlton's (1981a) Analysis of Slower Precision Movements

Carlton (1981a) examined visually based amendments as the limb approached a target. He did this by blocking vision of the stylus by means of a metal shield placed in the subject's line of vision. Carlton demonstrated that withdrawing visual feedback about the hand from the initial portion of the aiming movement did not affect the movement outcome. However, if 75% or more of the distance from the homebase to the target remained unsighted then there was an increase in both movement times and also error rates (Carlton, 1981a, Experiment 1). In a subsequent experiment Carlton (1981a, Experiment 2) withdrew visual feedback from the initial 75% (and also 93%) of the movement amplitude and used high-speed cinematographic techniques to measure the time from when the stylus first became visible until the initiation of a corrective movement could be derived from the movement's kinematic profile. The mean visual processing time was estimated to be 135 msec. On average, individual trials differed quite markedly from this value by 21 msec. This estimated visual processing time is nevertheless much shorter than Keele and Posner's (1968) estimate.

Carlton's data, therefore suggested that the visually mediated reorganisation of the motor program as the limb approached the target could also be achieved quite rapidly. Interestingly, the visual corrective reaction time of 135 msec corresponds well with the intersaccadic pause during ocular responses to visual

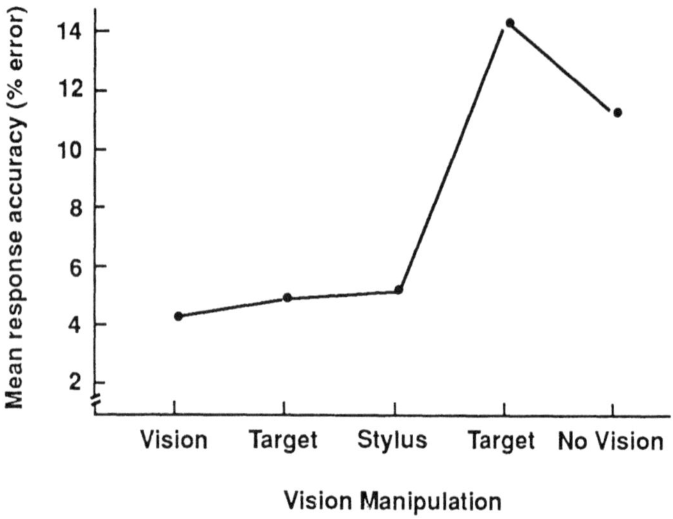

Figure 4. Mean response accuracy as a function of the vision manipulation condition. From Carlton (1981b). Reproduced with permission.

stimuli (e.g., Henson, 1978), and begs for a comparison of visual processing across control systems.

Beggs and Howarth (1988), however, have taken issue with Carlton's (1981a) conclusions. They draw particular attention to Carlton's assumption that the only source of information about hand position should come from visual feedback available as soon as the hand becomes visible. Beggs and Howarth (1988) argue that once the target has been fixated, visual hand position is not used for control. Instead, "kinaesthetic or proprioceptive information about the hand, and visual target position information, may be used to generate an intersensory error signal" (p. 52). Carlton (1981b) has, however, presented results that refute this position. Carlton (1981b) examined movement accuracy (hits and misses) in terms of complete vision; target plus stylus vision only, stylus vision only, target vision only, and no vision. If, as Beggs and Howarth (1988) argued, hand position is quite adequately derived from proprioceptive sources, then providing stylus information would only be redundant information. Consequently, the stylus vision only and no vision conditions would be expected to display equivalent error rates. Furthermore, the target vision only condition would be expected to be associated with a relatively low error rate. Carlton (1981b), however, reported quite the opposite findings. His data, reproduced in Figure 4, suggests that response accuracy is largely dependent on visual error information about hand position.

One way to interpret Carlton's (1981a) data is to say that the subject is not awaiting the completion of the initial submovement before selecting the new motor program for a secondary submovement. Instead, it is possible that the subject produces a deliberate error. In doing so, the motor system would know in advance the direction and approximate amplitude of the corrective response. These aspects of the corrective response could be programmed in parallel with the ongoing preparation and execution of the initial response. The final corrective motor program would await visual confirmation at the end of the initial impulse and these final specifications are completed within 135 msecs when the corrective response is initiated.

Barrett and Glencross (1989) argued that rather than selecting a new program, the system, instead, reorganises the already existing motor program. They provide evidence that amending an undershoot is achieved more readily than amending an overshoot. For such reasons, Prablanc, Pelisson, and Goodale (1986) have suggested that subjects initially undershoot (rather than overshoot) the target prior to making feedback-based adjustments. However, MacKenzie, Sivak, and Elliott (1988) make the point that in slower positioning movements, undershooting may reflect an intersensory positional judgment rather than a deliberate strategy.

Step analyses of the saccadic system suggest that the visual processing time in Carlton's (1981a) study may have depended on the magnitude of the error. Becker and Jürgens (1979) have proposed that if the magnitude of an upcoming error is small (<3 deg), as assessed via a predictive extraretinal feedback pathway, then the intersaccadic latency will equal a normal saccadic reaction time. However, for saccades with errors ranging in magnitude from 3-15 deg, preparation for the corrective saccade will begin at once but the final program will require some visual confirmation. The intersaccadic pause here would be in the order of 130 msec. As noted above, this is the processing time reported by Carlton (1981a) for manual aiming responses. Perhaps a processing time in the order of 190-260 msec would have been observed for manual aiming responses with smaller errors. The visual information in Carlton's (1981a) study may have served to confirm the suitability of an already programmed corrective response.

If the error is of a very large magnitude, the system initiates a corrective response without awaiting any visual confirmation. This has been observed for double step tracking responses in both the oculomotor (e.g., Becker & Jürgens, 1979; Deubel, Wolf, & Hauske, 1984) and manual (e.g., Barrett & Glencross, 1988b; Georgopoulos, Kalaska, & Massey, 1981; Gielen, van der Heuvel, & Dernier van der Gon, 1984) control systems. The relationship of this research to Carlton's may be seen if we realise that in the double step tracking task the superceding step stimulus serves as an artificially induced movement error signal.

Depending on the magnitude of the upcoming error, visual information may even form the basis for the complete reorganisation of the initial program. If the error is very large, however, the error correction is initiated without awaiting any visual confirmation. The measured time for visual processing under these different error situations will be quite different. In essence, we are arguing, along with Keele and Posner (1968), that a visually based amendment should take a normal reaction time. There are, however, strategies (for example, the generation of a deliberate error) that can substantially reduce the duration of the visual sampling period at the end of the initial aimed movement to a target. In addition, Zelaznik et al's (1983) data and our own constant error data (see Figure 2) suggest that vision may subserve a qualitatively different role in constraining the variability of even very rapid movements. If we abandon the search for an absolute processing time, what then are the implications for future research? In the next section, we examine a possible paradigm for future research.

FUTURE DIRECTIONS

Keele and Posner (1968) sought to establish some absolute value for the time to process visual information. Subsequent research, rather than simply refining their measurements, has suggested this notion be abandoned. Instead, there is a need now to specify the different modes of processing by which visual information may be used to control aiming movements. The very rapid adjustments noted by Zelaznik et al. (1983), for example, are qualitatively different from the visually based adjustments during slower precision movements.

The issue to which we wish to turn now is whether visual processes may be neatly dissected and studied in isolation. Rather than viewing visual processing from this simplistic perspective it is necessary to view retinal (visual feedback) information as an interacting component within a broader concept of "ocular" information. In the next section, we ask whether retinal information is the only source of information supplied by the eye. For any reaching task in which a target must be captured by the hand there is a concomitant capturing or foveation of the target by the oculomotor system. Could the movement of the eyes also contribute non-retinal information? What does this eye-hand coordination reveal about the processes underlying the accuracy of an aimed movement?

The Contribution of Extraretinal Information

Under conditions of target uncertainty and movement time constraints, a number of studies (e.g., Paillard, 1982; Prablanc, Echallier, Komilis, & Jeannerod, 1979a) have reported that the eyes move to the target before the hand does. Indeed, the target may be foveated before the limb movement is initiated. When the subjects are free to move their eyes and limb as they please, however, although the saccade remains closely time locked to the initiation of the limb movement, the order of occurrence is no longer important (e.g., Abrams, Meyer, & Kornblum, 1990). Limb movements are equivalent whether they follow or are preceded by the saccadic response. Nevertheless, the eye always arrives at the target well over 200 msec prior to the limb (see Abrams et al., 1990, Figure 1). This behaviour has led to speculation over the role of eye movements in the accuracy of limb movements. Since the eyes arrive first the target will be foveated as the limb homes in. Since detailed information about target position is provided by foveal vision, foveation may form the basis for the correction of the trajectory of the hand. Paillard (1980) makes a distinction between peripheral and central vision. He proposes that a limb movement is initially programmed on the basis of information derived from the peripheral retina concerning target position. Once the target is foveated, however, error corrections are then programmed on the basis of information this time derived from central vision and concerning the relative positions of the target and hand. This accords well with Carlton's (1981a) findings.

It must be asked, however, whether such retinal information relating to the positions of the hand and target is the only source of information provided by the ocular apparatus. After all, as the eyes move, there will be a corresponding proprioceptive trace of their behaviour (movement information). Furthermore, the efferent commands to the eyeballs could provide a source of information about eye position (position information). For the oculomotor system, as Guthrie, Porter, and Sparks (1983) point out, the eyes move under constant loads and, therefore, a copy of the ocular efferent commands would provide information regarding position of the eye. This information is referred to as extraretinal information and may underlie the control of aimed limb movements. Prablanc et al. (1979), for example, report that subjects who cannot see their hand produce less errors if the target remains visible than if it is extinguished once the limb has responded. Pelisson, Prablance, Goodale, and Jeannerod (1986) have shown, furthermore, that removing vision of the hand during an aiming movement does not prevent subjects from modifying their movement in response to a sudden shift in the target location. This will happen even if subjects do not realise a target step has occurred. Therefore, these amendments are not just predictive corrections made on the basis of an observed shift in target position. In the absence of vision, proprioceptive, limb information or extraretinal information may underly movement accuracy.

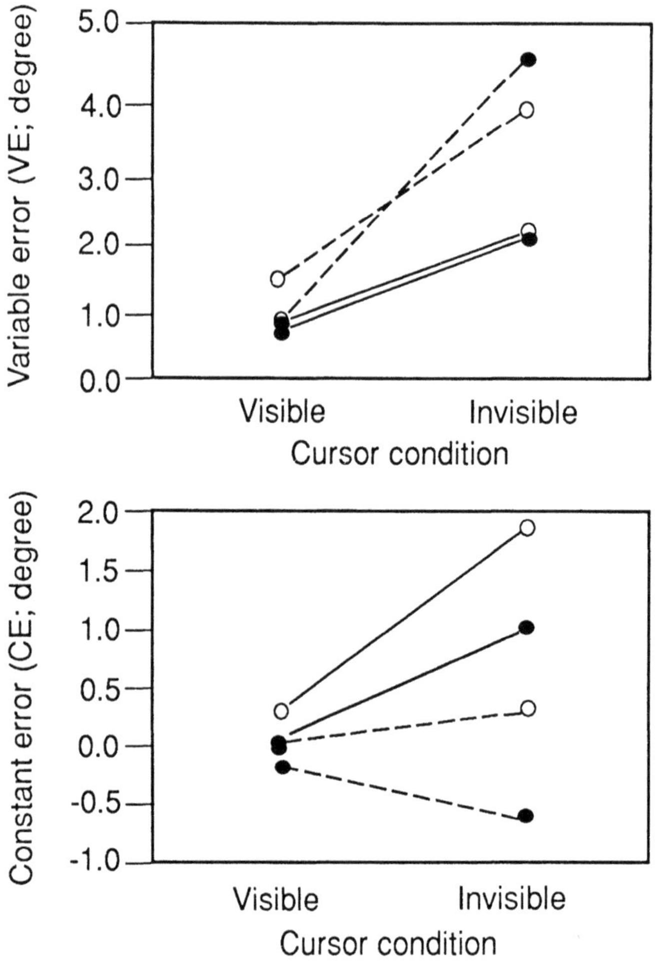

Figure 5. Upper panel: Mean variable error (VE, degrees) for wrist rotations. Lower panel: Mean constant error (CE, degrees) for wrist rotations. Positive values denote movements that overshoot the centre of the target; negative values denote movements that undershoot it. (Filled circles = saccade condition; open circles = control condition; solid lines = 10° targets; dashed lines = 39.5° targets.) Copyright (1990) by the American Psychological Association. Reprinted by permission.

A recent study by Abrams et al. (1990) has rigorously examined the role of eye movements in wrist rotations. In their Experiment 2, on half the trials subjects could move their eyes as they wished. On the other half of the trials, the subjects were required to keep their eyes fixated on the home position so that the wrist rotations were performed in the absence of any eye movements. For each condition the cursor either remained visible or disappeared at movement onset. Abrams et al. reasoned that if, for trials in which the cursor was not visible, there was no difference between the free eye movement and prohibited eye movement conditions, then it could be concluded that eye movements were of no importance in the accuracy of limb movements. Their results are illustrated in Figure 5.

Figure 5 indicates that prohibiting eye movements increases limb error even for blind movements. Constant error increased under eye movement prohibition for both cursor visibility conditions suggesting, furthermore, that eye movements, when permitted, do not simply provide retinal information about the responding limb. This finding suggests a role for ocular information in movement accuracy. Accuracy is an outcome of the intimate relationship between retinal and extraretinal information.

In a subsequent experiment, Abrams et al. (1990, Experiment 3) showed that the distance travelled by the initial impulse of a limb movement depended on whether the target was foveated following a smooth-pursuit eye movement or a saccade. Further differences were noted in the error correction phase. This suggests that having the eyes directed at the target is not all that matters as has been previously suggested (e.g., Hansen & Skavenski, 1977). A role for extraretinal information relating to eye movements (*movement* information) is thus implicated. There was, however, no difference in endpoint accuracy between the pursuit and saccade conditions which implicates a role for extraretinal *position* information. The results of Abrams et al. (1990), therefore, suggest that extraretinal information about both the movement and also the position of the eyes is useful in limb control. Movement and position of the eyes thus provide information which interacts with retinal information during limb control. So close is this relationship that if we are to understand the role played by visual feedback we must also understand the role played by extraretinal information. An important direction for future research is, therefore, to view and analyse visual processing within this overall context of ocular information.

CONCLUSION

Keele and Posner (1968) sought to elucidate the processing of visual feedback in rapid movement. Their results have formed the basis for much of our current thinking regarding the processes underlying limb accuracy. In the present chapter, we examined Keele and Posner's (1968) assumptions. In particular, we examined their claim to have measured the minimum visual processing time. On the basis of recent research questions, it is questioned whether: (1) the minimum visual processing time is within the order of 190-260 msec proposed by Keele and Posner (1968), (2) an absolute value for visual processing may be found, and (3) indeed there is even a unitary mode for visual processing. Processing time appears to be a function of movement time (e.g., Beggs & Howarth, 1970) and the particular task (e.g., Elliot & Allard, 1985). One approach to explaining the variability of processing times has been to propose different modes of processing. Barrett and Glencross (1989) proposed, for example, that the processing time for visual feedback as the limb approaches a target depends on the magnitude of the error. Only for very small unpredictable errors one might expect a visual processing time similar to that proposed by Keele and Posner (1968). Carlton's (1981a) results, however, suggest that subjects are able to reduce this time by generating a deliberate error and programming the correction in advance. Under these circumstances, visual processing represents either the confirmation of the already structured corrective program or the final refinement of the predicted error correction, and takes in the order of 130 msec. Zelaznik et al's (1983) data suggest an additional qualitatively different automatic mode of processing that may operate even for very rapid movements. If we are to understand the ability to produce accurate aimed movements, however, then it is crucial that we no longer treat information from the eye just as visual information but, instead, in terms of "ocular" information in which retinal and extraretinal information interact. From this perspective, the practice of treating visual feedback as if it may be dissected out and studied in isolation is questioned.

REFERENCES

Abrams, R.A., Meyer, D.E. & Kornblum, S. (1990). Eye-hand coordination: Oculomotor control in rapid aimed limb movements. *Journal of Experimental Psychology: Human Perception and Performance*, *16*, 248-267.

Angel, R.W. (1976). Efference copy in the control of movement. *Neurology*, *26*, 1164-1168.

Barrett, N.C. & Glencross, D.J. (1988a). The amplitude transition function and the manual and oculomotor control systems. *Psychological Bulletin*, *104*, 363-372.

Barrett, N.C. & Glencross, D.J. (1988b). Double-step analysis of rapid manual aiming movements. *Quarterly Journal of Experimental Psychology*, *40A*, 299-322.

Barrett, N.C. & Glencross, D.J. (1989). Response amendments during manual aiming movements to double-step targets. *Acta Psychologica*, *70*, 205-217.

Becker, W. & Jürgens, R. (1979). An analysis of the saccadic system by means of double-step stimuli. *Vision Research*, *19*, 964-983.

Beggs, W.D.A. & Howarth, C.I. (1970). Movement control in a repetitive motor task. *Nature*, *225*, 752-753.

Beggs, W.D.A. & Howarth, C.I. (1988). Unpaced aiming - a control theory explanation. In A.M. Colley and J.R. Beech (Eds.), *Cognition and Action in Skilled Behaviour* (pp 49-64). Amsterdam: North-Holland.

Carlton, L.G. (1980). Movement control characteristics of aiming responses. *Ergonomics*, *23*, 1019-1023.

Carlton, L.G. (1981a). Processing visual feedback information for movement control. *Journal of Experimental Psychology: Human Perception and Performance*, *1*, 1019-1030.

Carlton, L.G. (1981b). Visual information: The control of aiming movements. *Quarterly Journal of Experimental Psychology*, *33A*, 87-93.

Christina, R.W. (1970). Minimum visual feedback processing time for amendment of an incorrect movement. *Perceptual and Motor Skills*, *31*, 991-994.

Craik, K.J.W. (1947). Theory of the human operator in control systems 1. The operator as an engineering system. *British Journal of Psychology*, *38*, 56-61.

Crossman, E.R.F.W. & Goodeve, P.J. (1963). Feedback control of hand-movement and Fitts' Law. Unpublished communication to the Experimental Psychology Society, Oxford. Published in *Quarterly Journal of Experimental Psychology*, 1983, *35A*, 251-278.

Deubel, H., Wolf, W. & Hauske, G. (1984). The evaluation of the oculomotor error signal. In A.G. Gale and F. Johnson (Eds.), *Theoretical and Applied Aspects of Eye Movement Research* (pp. 55-62). Amsterdam: North-Holland.

Elliot, D. & Allard, F. (1985). The utilization of visual feedback information during rapid pointing movements. *Quarterly Journal of Experimental Psychology*, *37A*, 407-425.

Georgopoulos, A.P., Kalaska, J.F., & Massey, J.T. (1981). Spatial trajectories and reaction times of aimed movements: Effects of practice, uncertainty, and change in target location. *Journal of Neurophysiology*, *46*, 725-743.

Gibbs,C.B. (1965). Probability learning in step-input tracking. *British Journal of Psychology*, *56*, 233-242.

Gielen, C.C.A.M., van den Heuvel, P.J.M., & Dernier van der Gon, J.J. (1984). Modification of muscle activation patterns during fast goal-directed arm movements. *Journal of Motor Behavior*, *16*, 2-19.

Glencross, D.J. & Barrett, N.C. (1983). Programming precision in repetitive tapping. *Journal of Motor Behavior*, *15*, 191-200.

Glencross, D.J. & Barrett, N.C. (1989). Discrete aiming movements. In D. Holding (Ed.), *Human Skills* (pp. 107-146). New York: Wiley.

Guthrie, B.L., Porter,J.D., & Sparks, D.L. (1983). Corollary discharge provides accurate eye position information to the oculomotor system. *Science*, *221*, 1193-1195.

Hansen, R.M. & Skavenski, A.A. (1977). Accuracy of eye position information for motor control. *Vision Research*, *17*, 919-926.

Henry, F.M. (1974). Variable and constant performance error within a group of individuals. *Journal of Motor Behavior*, *6*, 149-154.

Henson, D.B. (1978). Corrective saccades: Effects of altering visual feedback. *Vision Research*, *18*, 63-67.

Hick, W.E. (1949). Reaction time for the amendment of a response. *Quarterly Journal of Experimental Psychology*, *77*, 155-158.

Howarth, C.I. Beggs, W.D.A., & Bowden, J. (1971). The relationship between speed and accuracy of movement aimed at a target. *Acta Psychologica*, *35*, 207-218.

Howarth, C.I. & Beggs, W.D.A. (1985). The control of movements by multisensory information. In Heuer, H.,Kleinbeck, U., & Schmidt, K.H. (Eds), *Motor behaviour: Programming, control and acquisition* (pp. 125-151). Berlin: Springer-Verlag.

Jagacinski, R.J., Repperger, D.W., Moran, M.S., Ward, S.L., & Glass, B. (1980). Fitts' Law and the microstructure of rapid discrete movements. *Journal of Experimental Psychology: Human Perception and Performance*, *6*, 309-320.

Keele, S.W. (1968). Movement control in skilled motor performance. *Psychological Bulletin*, *70*, 387-403.

Keele, S.W. & Posner, M.I. (1968). Processing of visual feedback in rapid movements. *Journal of Experimental Psychology*, *77*, 155-158.

Klemmer, E.T. (1957). Simple reaction time as a function of time uncertainty. *Journal of Experimental Psychology*, *54*, 195-200.

Langolf, G.D., Chaffin, D.B. & Foulke, J.A. (1976). An investigation of Fitts' Law using a wide range of movement amplitudes, *Journal of Motor Behavior*, *8*, 113-128.

MacKenzie, C.L., Sivak, B., & Elliott, D. (1988). Manual localization of lateralized visual targets. *Journal of Motor Behavior*, *20*, 443-457.

Meyer, D.E., Abrams, R.A., Kornblum, S., Wright, C.E., & Smith, J.E.K. (1988). Optimality in human motor performance: Ideal control of rapid aimed movements. *Psychological Review*, *95*, 340-370.

Paillard, J. (1980). The multichanneling of visual cues and the organization of a visually guided response. In G.E. Stelmach & J. Requin (Eds.), *Tutorials in motor behavior* (pp. 259-278). Amsterdam: North-Holland.

Paillard, J. (1982). The contribution of peripheral and central vision to visually guided reaching. In D. Ingle, M. Goodale., & R. Mansfield (Eds.), *Analysis of visual behaviour* (pp. 367-385). Cambridge: MIT Press.

Pelisson, D., Prablanc, C., Goodale, M.A., & Jeannerod, M. (1986). Visual control of reaching movements without vision of the limb: II Evidence of fast unconscious processes correcting the trajectory of the hand to the final position of a double-step stimulus. *Experimental Brain Research*, *62*, 303-311.

Pew, R.W. (1966). Performance of human operators in three-state relay control system with velocity-augmented displays. *Journal of Experimental Psychology*, *71*, 764-771.

Prablanc, C., Echallier, J.F., Komilis, E., & Jeannerod, M. (1979). Optimal response of eye and hand motor systems in pointing at a visual target : 1. Spatio-temporal characteristics of eye and hand movements and their relationships when varying the amount of visual information. *Biological Cybernetics*, 35, 113-124.

Prablanc, C., Pelisson, D., & Goodale, M.A. (1986). Visual control of reaching movements without vision of limb. 1. Role of retinal feedback of target position in guiding the hand. *Experimental Brain Research*, *62*, 293-302.

Schmidt, R.A. & Gordon, G.B. (1977). Errors in motor responding, "rapid" corrections , and false anticipations. *Journal of Motor Behavior*, *9*, 101-111.

Smith, W.M. & Bowen, K.F. (1980). The effects of delayed and displaced visual feedback on motor control. *Journal of Motor Behavior*, *8*, 43-58.

Vince, M.A. (1948). Corrective movements in a pursuit task. *Quarterly Journal of Experimental Psychology*, *1*, 85-103.

Wallace, S.A. & Newell, K.M. (1983). Visual control of discrete aiming movements. *Quarterly Journal of Experimental Psychology*, *35A*, 311-321.

Woodworth, R.S. (1899). The accuracy of voluntary movement. *Psychological Review*, *3*, (2, Whole No. 13).

Zelaznik, H.N., Hawkins, B., & Kisselburgh, L. (1983). Rapid visual feedback processing in single-aiming movements. *Journal of Motor Behavior*, *15*, 217-236.

Approaches to the Study of Motor Control and Learning
J.J. Summers (Editor)

Chapter 11

THE CONTROL OF CATCHING

G.J.P. Savelsbergh
Free University, Amsterdam
University of York

H.T.A. Whiting
University of York

J.R. Pijpers
Free University, Amsterdam

For successful catching access to temporal and spatial information sources is a sine qua non. In this Chapter the means by which temporal and spatial information become available to catchers is discussed and elaborated using concepts and empirical work from both an information-processing and an ecological psychological perspective. Attention is drawn to a number of issues for which satisfactory explanations are still found wanting.

An interesting exercise for students of the history of science is to explore the way in which experimental questions and paradigms reflecting particular theoretical frameworks, prevalent at any one time, change over the years. This is equally true for the relatively young field of Human Movement Science as for the more established sciences. A paradigm example from the former field is provided by the research topic of 'catching behaviour'. Even over the last twenty years or so there is evidence of marked shifts in explanatory frameworks and central questions being asked. Although this Chapter is not orientated towards the history of science per se, it will be necessary to comment, from time to time, on changes in orientation that have motivated a generation of research workers.

The reason why catching behaviour has intrigued certain sections of the scientific community is not difficult to ascertain. Successful one-handed catching, for example, demands conformity to highly constrained spatio-temporal requirements, namely, placing the hand, at the right moment, at the required spatial location and closing the fingers around the ball at the appropriate moment in time. A failure to meet these requirements gives rise to two kinds of error - temporal and spatial (Alderson, Sully, & Sully, 1974). Thus, it is seemly to ask what kind of nervous system would enable the catcher to adequately comply with the very narrow spatial and temporal tolerance bands that success in such behaviour so obviously demands? Although this Chapter is not intended to provide neuropsychological explanations, the search for information sources that guide catching behaviour has obvious implications for those so motivated.

Earlier experiments on catching behaviour - reflecting the theoretical frameworks then current - were conducted within an *information-processing* framework (Fitts & Posner, 1967; Keele, 1968), the objective being to determine, experimentally, the importance of selected *input* variables on task performance (Alderson et al., 1974; Sharp & Whiting, 1974, 1975; Whiting, 1968, 1970; Whiting & Sharp, 1974). Such questions reflected concern about '*the amount*' of information necessary on which to make decisions rather than on the '*nature*' of that information per se. It is difficult to pinpoint the specific aspects of information processing theories that motivated particular workers, although it is reasonably clear that the idea that the human operator processes information in discrete samples - that input information being integrated over a period of time and processed as a single 'sample' or 'chunk' - played a leading role. Such a conception gave rise to the *perceptual moment hypothesis* (Moray, 1970; Whiting, Gill, & Stephenson, 1970) although there was little agreement amongst experimenters about the duration of such a moment. In terms of catching behaviour, the variable most fully addressed, within such a framework, was *viewing time* - its necessary duration and most appropriate moment of occurrence (Whiting, 1968, 1970; Whiting et al., 1970; Whiting & Sharp, 1974).

THE EFFECT OF THE DURATION OF THE VIEWING TIME

While it is a truism that information about the trajectory of a ball in flight is necessary for successful catching behaviour it is also clear that it is not necessary to view the entire trajectory - at least from the point of view of making a successful catch (Whiting, 1968). Information occurring at one stage of the trajectory can be used, in a predictive way, to anticipate the future time and position of the ball. In this respect, it also seems clear that information occurring late in the trajectory of the ball - given the inherent latencies of the perceptual-motor system - cannot contribute towards the catching action. Generally, information about a ball in flight is obtained via the visual system (exceptions being, of course, catching by blind people where auditory information might be used to the same end). What is less clear is how much visual information is necessary and at what stage in the flight path of the ball such information has to be acquired. There are, thus, two considerations - the duration of the viewing period and the section of the trajectory of the ball to which such viewing needs to be directed. To some extent, as will be apparent in what follows, these two considerations are confounded.

The basic paradigm used to explore these two aspects has involved ball projection machines of various kinds and electronic circuitry that allows vision of the ball in flight for controlled periods of time. This has been done in two ways, namely, by illuminating the ball itself or by switching on and off the room lights at predetermined intervals. Either method has its own constraints which makes direct comparisons of results obtained using the two paradigms difficult.

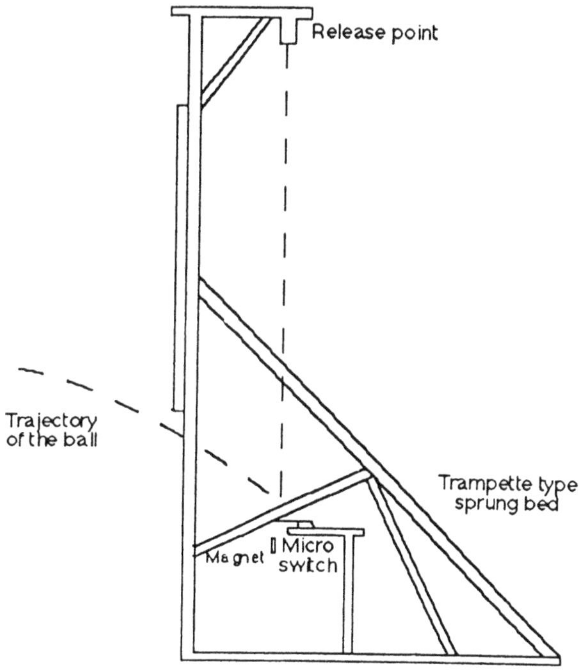

Figure 1. Side elevation of apparatus

Typical of such approaches was the experiment of Whiting et al. (1970) which, in the spirit of the perceptual-moment hypothesis, explored whether or not there were critical time intervals for taking in information about ball flight. A solid perspex ball was caused to enter on to a parabolic flight path by means of the gantry apparatus illustrated in Figure 1.

An electronic device enabled the ball to be illuminated for predetermined temporal intervals - beginning from its time of contact with the trampette - (100, 150, 200, 250, 300, F/L (full light) = 400 ms) of its flight path. The dependent variable for this experiment was restricted to the *number of catches* made - thus limiting inferences about the *quality* of the information provided by the restricted conditions imposed. While it was clear - from the standards of performance shown - that subjects must have obtained both spatial and temporal information from viewing the trajectory of the ball, the relative contribution of these two kinds of information, under the various restricted conditions, was less clear. The results of this experiment are given graphically in Figure 2.

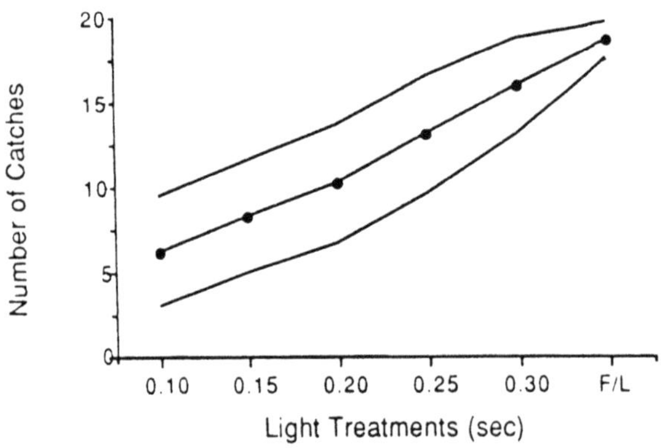

Figure 2. Performance curve - combined means and standard deviation of all subjects (Reprinted with permission from Whiting, H.T.A., Gill, E.B., & Stephenson, J.M. (1970). Critical time intervals for taking in flight information in a ball-catching task. Ergonomics, 13, 265-272).

As can be seen, performance improved - almost linearly - with increasing duration of viewing time thereby questioning the adequacy of information assimilated during a single restricted 'perceptual moment'. Such a statement has, however, to be qualified in the light of the finding of marked individual differences in performance. Some subjects produced results under the 100 and

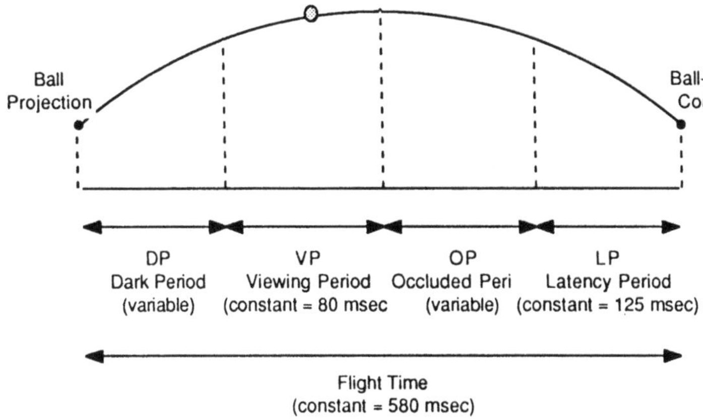

Figure 3. Schematic representation of the experimental paradigm.

150 ms conditions that were remarkably good. Nine had catches of nine or more (out of 20) under the 100 ms condition and 18 subjects achieved this level under the 150 ms condition. Some eighteen years on, Lamb and Burwitz (1988) attempted to replicate this experiment using a similar paradigm. They produced similar findings to those of Whiting et al. (1970) although they reported (in contrast) no further improvement in performance when the viewing time was increased to 300 or 400 ms. There are two comments which need to be made in this respect. In the first place, the status of their catchers was unclear (in the Whiting et al., study all were 'good' catchers on a within-task criterion). Later in the Chapter the importance of this consideration will be explored at some length. In the second place, there were methodological differences between the two studies. While Whiting et al. varied the information available by illuminating the ball (only) in an otherwise dark room for varying periods of time, Lamb and Burwitz by turning the room lights on or off provided background information (in the lighted condition) for their subjects.

In subsequent studies, Whiting and Sharp (1974) returned to the question of the optimal section of the trajectory of the ball at which to provide information. They were able to show that viewing the ball too early or too late in its trajectory - i.e., causing the occluded period (OP) to become too long (> 364 ms) or too short (< 205 ms) - resulted in decreased catching performance. By so doing they drew attention to the importance of the period for which the ball is not seen as well as the period for which it is seen. The former, for example,

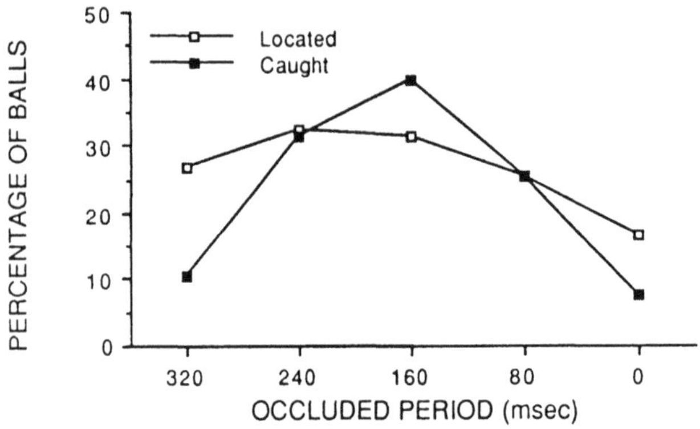

Figure 4. Percentages of all deliveries caught and located as a function of the occluded period (Reprinted with permission from Whiting, H.T.A., & Sharp, R.H. (1974). Visual occlusion factors in a discrete ball catching task. Journal of Motor Behavior, 6, 11-16).

might provide the occasion to process information picked up during the latter.

The point being made can be illustrated by means of the experimental paradigm used (Figure 3) in which DP represents the variable period for which the room was in darkness from the moment of ball projection to the moment at which the room was first illuminated; VP represents the time interval for which the room, and hence the ball, was illuminated; OP and LP represent the remainder of time for which the ball was occluded in flight.

The distinction between OP and LP is conceptual, necessitated by the fact that the period of occlusion following on VP cannot have an effect right up to the moment of ball-hand contact. There is, in fact, an interval preceding this moment - equivalent to a CNS latency plus movement-time - during which, in classical information-processing terms, any change in the stimulus conditions can have no effect on the response of subjects. This interval was taken to be constant and shown to be in the region of 125 ms. Hence the effective occluded period - the variable of interest - is the interval between light offset and the beginning of LP.

In their 1974 experiment, Whiting and Sharp kept VP constant at 80 ms and varied the occluded period between O and 360 ms. They were able to demonstrate that success in ball-catching is significantly affected by the temporal extent of the occluded period following on a constant viewing time (80 ms) of the trajectory of a ball (Figure 4). Thus, confirming the contention of the importance of the occluded period and reinstating the possibility that a 'perceptual-moment' of 80 ms - at an appropriate point of time in the trajectory of the ball, could provide sufficient information on which to make a catching action. The decline in performance between OP = 160 ms and OP = 320 ms, for the dependent variable number of balls caught, suggests that subjects experience increasing difficulty when they have to predict ball flight over successively longer intervals of time. Such an interpretation found support in the, then, topical idea of the decay of information in immediate memory. If, however, the OP effect was due solely to prediction limitations, performance would have been expected to increase as OP changed from 160 to 0 ms. As the trend was, in fact, the reverse, an alternative answer was sought. When sight of the ball is only available *late* in its trajectory, subjects do not have sufficient time to process the necessary flight information. At the same time, they may not have time (invoking classical concepts of reaction time etc.) to translate their perception of the ball's flight into an appropriate response pattern. Both explanations rely on information-processing concepts. While such suggestions seemed appropriate, it was decided to explore the issue further by manipulating both OP and VP (Sharp & Whiting, 1974). There it was demonstrated that both variables and their interaction were significant sources of catching variation (Figure 5).

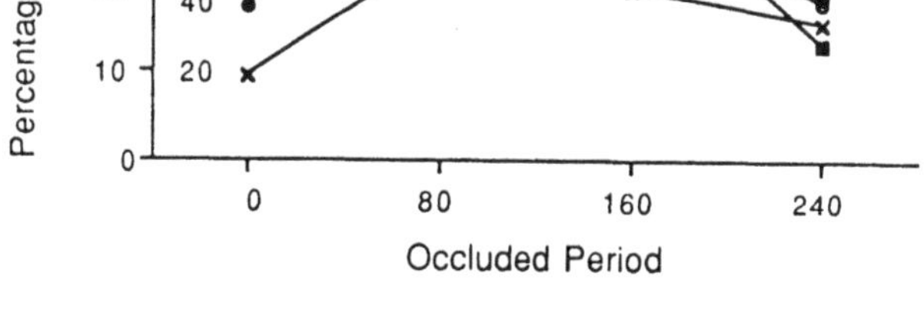

Figure 5. Percentage number off balls caught as a function of viewing and occluded period (Reprinted with permission from Sharp, R.H., & Whiting, H.T.A. (1974). Exposure and occluded duration effects in a ball-catching skill. Journal of Motor Behavior, 3, 139-147).

Generally, the effect of VP diminished as OP was extended. When OP was zero, increases in VP were followed by significant improvement in catching success until VP was 120 ms. Presumably, increasing VP within this range, provided subjects with more time in which both to extract visual information and to select an appropriate response. Unfortunately, it was not possible to differentiate between these processes but it was noticeable that an increase in VP of as little as 20 ms facilitated the entire process.

Although the results of this experiment marked a significant step forward in coming to understand the use of information in catching behaviour it clearly still left much unexplained. Examination of the results of the experiment confirm that even under the most favourable condition used (VP = 160 ms; OP = 80 ms) subjects were still only catching 45% of the balls whereas under normal lighting conditions they were able to catch virtually 100% (the criterion for being selected as a subject).

The need to explain this anomaly posed problems for the design of the subsequent experiment. In principle, an infinite number of combinations of VP, OP, and DP could be used requiring a very large number of subjects. Eventually, based on their experience of a number of experiments and considerations of the position in the trajectory at which information was made available, Sharp and Whiting (1975) opted for a more limited number of combinations of these three variables. They demonstrated that catching success was a discontinuous function of total-time (VP + OP) up to about 120 ms, where a plateau in performance becomes apparent and from 240 up to 320 ms where a second plateau is reached.

The former is in line with the results of the previous experiment and the latter demonstrates how, by extending the total time available for handling information, performance can be raised from +/- 50% of balls caught to +/- 90%. Furthermore - within particular ranges of *total time* - the ratio of VP to OP did not seem to matter much providing VP was not less than about 60 ms.

These experiments not only demonstrated the importance of taking into consideration the total time available (a combination of OP and VP) in providing explanations for catching behaviour, but also the importance of the position in the trajectory of the ball at which such information is made available.

TWENTY YEARS LATER: AN ECOLOGICAL PSYCHOLOGICAL APPROACH

Much of the more recent work on catching makes resort to ecological psychological explanations with the implication that all the information a catcher needs to intercept a ball successfully, is directly available in the optic array (Fitch & Turvey, 1977; Lee, 1976, 1980; Lee & Young, 1986; Savelsbergh, 1990; Savelsbergh & Whiting, 1990; Todd, 1981; Turvey & Carello, 1988; Turvey, 1990). Gibson (1966, 1979) - the founding father of ecological psychology - took as his starting point for a theory of visual perception not a 'retinal image', which is passively sensed and, through inference and recourse to memory, built into a meaningful representation of the world, but the ambient optic array which animals actively sample - picking up the information needed to guide their actions. Clearly, Gibson's position provides a challenge for those experimentalists who had been content to base the interpretation of their findings on more traditional, computational explanations inherent, for example, in information processing approaches. This challenge was accepted in a number of fields particularly, in the present context, in the area of catching behaviour.

PREDICTIVE TEMPORAL INFORMATION

Hints that the ambient optic array - particularly that giving rise to retinal expansion patterns - might provide important information about approaching objects was to be seen in the work of Schiff who showed that expanding shadow projections evoked avoidance behaviour in animals (Schiff, Caviness, & Gibson, 1962; Schiff, 1965). Later, Bower, Broughton, and Moore (1970) reported defensive behaviour in 10 day old infants elicited by approaching objects giving rise to optical expansion (see also Ball & Tronick, 1971, Yonas et al., 1977).

Lee (1976, 1980), developing on his earlier work, demonstrated that the pattern of optical expansion brought about by the relative approach between the actor and the environmental structure of interest - for example, a ball that must be caught - contained predictive temporal information. He was able to demonstrate - mathematically - that the inverse of the relative rate of dilation of the closed optical contour generated by an approaching object (e.g., a ball) in the optic array provides a first order temporal relation between actor and environment, namely the remaining time-to-contact if the speed of relative approach were to remain constant. Since that time, a variety of experimental work has provided evidence that actors can use two dimensional time-to-contact information to regulate their actions (Bootsma & van Wieringen, 1990; Laurent, Dinh Phung, & Ripoll, 1989; Lee, Lishman, & Thomson, 1982; Lee & Reddish, 1981; Savelsbergh, 1990; Savelsbergh, Whiting, & Bootsma, 1991; Sidaway, McNitt-Gray, & Davis, 1989).

That the explanatory usefulness of the parameter 'inverse of the relative rate of dilation' (denoted *tau* by Lee, 1976, 1980) is not confined to situations in which an object approaches with a constant velocity was demonstrated by Lee, Young, Reddish, Lough, and Clayton (1983). They were able to show that explanations based on the premise that subjects gear their actions (punching a dropping ball) to tau and not to the real time-to-contact - in the case of a

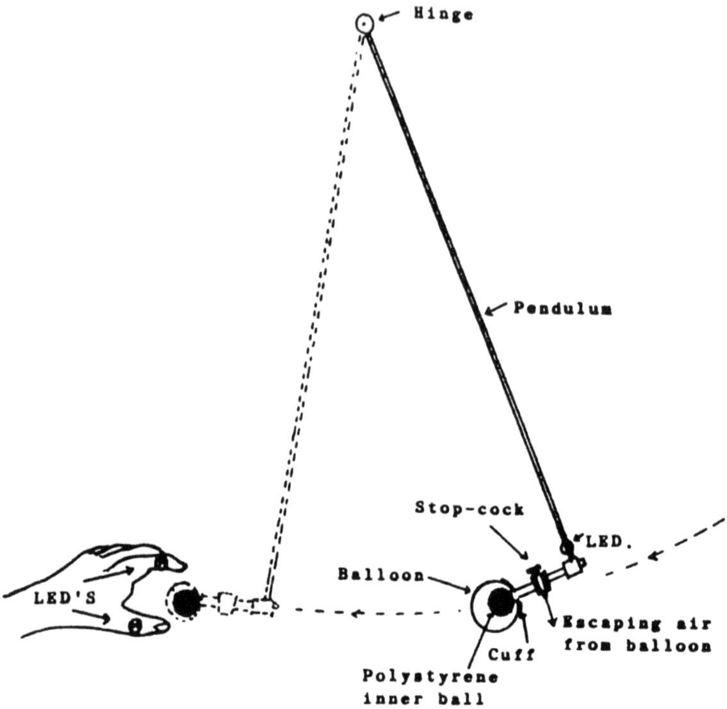

Figure 6. The deflating ball with the enclosed small ball fixed to the pendulum.

discrepancy between the two - brought about by a non-constant relative approach, were consistent with their results.

Elegant as some of these explanations based on the use of tau were shown to be, they did not entirely exclude the possibility of explanations based upon computational procedures. In fact, Abernethy and Burgess-Limerick (this volume), in an extensive review of the relevant literature, were moved to state that unequivocal support for either the distance/velocity (computational) method or the tau (direct perception) method for extracting time-to-contact information has not been forthcoming. They formed the opinion that the two alternative sources of time-to-contact information were complementary rather than competing. While there is a certain merit in the latter statement (the truth of which awaits further experimentation), recent experimental work of Savelsbergh and Whiting (Savelsbergh, 1990; Savelsbergh, Whiting, & Bootsma, 1991; Savelsbergh, Whiting, Pijpers, & Van Santvoord, in preparation) attempted to remove the confounding effects of the availability of information that might be acquired either by computational or by direct perceptual means.

In this experiment subjects were required to catch - one-handed - a ball travelling on a spatially predictable path. Spatial constancy was maintained by attaching the ball to a pendulum (Figure 6). A luminous ball was used in an, otherwise, totally dark room.

Three ball sizes were used - randomised over trials. Two of these were 5.5 cm and 7.5 cm in diameter respectively. A third ball could be made to change its diameter during flight from 7.5 cm to 5.5 cm (see the original article for further information about how the ball was made to deflate). By using this third deflating ball, the provision of non-veridical information - in the sense that the time-to-contact specified by the optical expansion of the approaching ball is not that which would be specified if the ball did not deflate. The ball flight was recorded by means of a video camera with the lens situated at eye level. An analysis of the two-dimensional expansion pattern of the ball on the monitor screen was carried out using a Video Position Analyser which allowed the diameter of the ball to be measured, frame by frame, during its approach. In Figure 7 the relative expansion pattern of the deflating ball and of a constant ball is graphed.

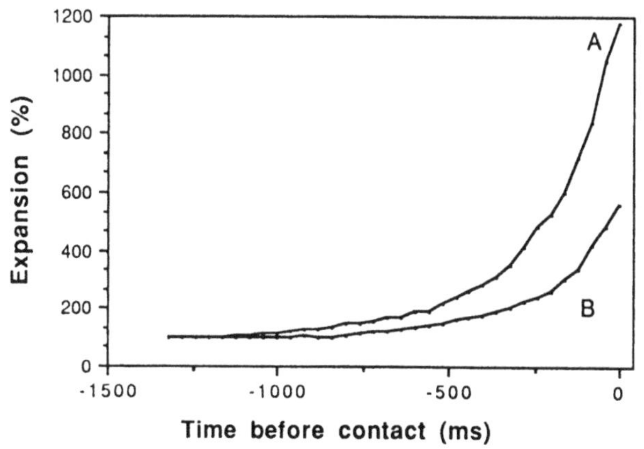

Figure 7. The relative expansion pattern (on a video screen) of the ball of constant size (A) and the deflating ball (B) (Reprinted with permission from Savelsbergh, G.J.P., Whiting, H.T.A., & Bootsma, R.J. (1991). 'Grasping' TAU! Journal of Experimental Psychology: Human Perception and Performance, 17, 315-322).

The analysis confirms that the deflating ball would give rise to a different optical expansion pattern than a ball of which the physical size remained constant.

The results showed that the time of appearance of the maximal closing velocity of the hand was significantly later for the deflating ball than for the

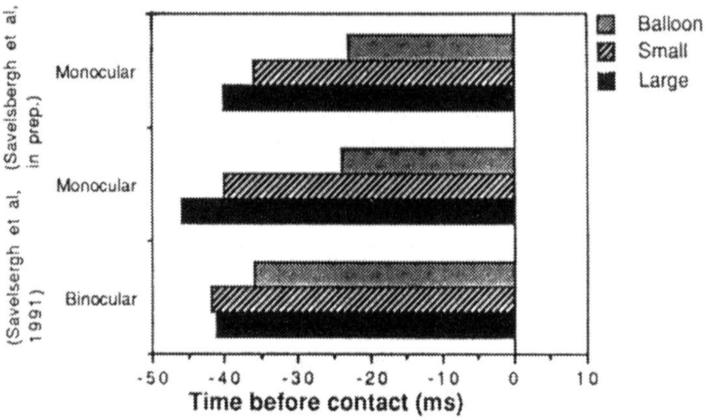

Figure 8. The closing velocities of the fingers for the small (S), large (L) and deflating ball (B) under binocular and monocular (Savelsbergh et al., 1991) and monocular conditions (Savelsbergh et al., in preparartion).

balls of constant size (Savelsbergh, 1990; Savelsbergh et al., 1991: Experiment 1 - binocular vision and Experiment 2 - monocular; Savelsbergh et al., in preparation: monocular vision). The fact that subjects geared their actions to characteristics of the deflating ball and not to its time of arrival based on computation involving position and velocity attests to the use of retinal expansion information in the control of catching actions (see Figure 8).

A second dependent variable sensitive to changes brought about by the deflating ball was the hand aperture - defined as the distance between the thumb and finger. The finding of adjustments to the aperture of the hand in response to the different ball sizes especially the adjustment of the hand to the deflating ball, despite the fact that subjects were not aware of the fact that the ball was deflating during its approach - point not only to a finely attuned perception-action coupling, but strongly indicate that such coupling is based on information specified directly by the relative optical expansion pattern (see Figure 9).

These findings go some way towards providing the kind of confirmation that Abernethy and Burgess-Limerick were seeking but do not deny the possibility that under particular circumstances computational approaches or other information sources might be used.

Elegant as these experiments might be seen to be in providing less equivocal evidence for the use of tau in catching behaviour, it has to be appreciated that catching behaviour also requires the accurate pick up of spatial information (a

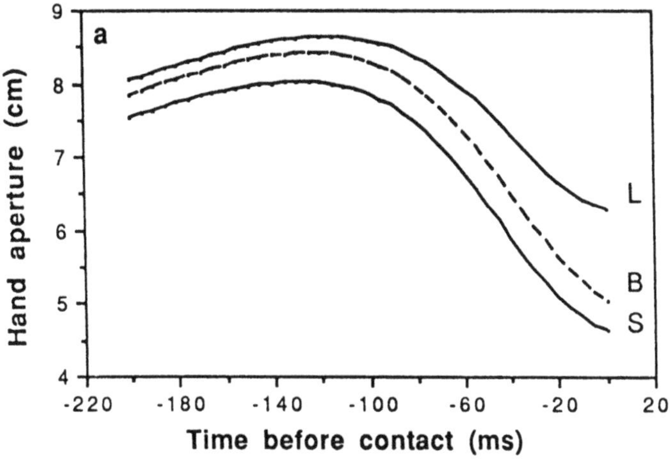

Figure 9. Adjustments to the mean aperture of the hand for large (L), small (S) and deflating ball (B) in the last 200 ms (Reprinted with permission from Savelsbergh, G.J.P., Whiting, H.T.A., & Bootsma, R.J. (1991). 'Grasping' TAU! Journal of Experimental Psychology: Human Perception and Performance, 17, 315-322).

necessity that was obviated in the experiment described by the use of the pendulum). What are the potential sources of information for ensuring that the ball and hand get together at the right place?

SPATIAL INFORMATION SOURCES

Potential (visual) spatial information sources available to the catcher are the hand, the ball, and the context provided by the surrounding environment.

Spatial Information About the Catching Hand.

Why should spatial information about the catching hand be necessary? The rationale generally advanced (see for example Smyth & Marriott, 1982) is that articular proprioception, particularly in the case of novice catchers, is not sufficient to provide accurate information about hand/limb position. Vision of the catching hand may, therefore, be necessary in order to calibrate the proprioceptive system when making one-handed catches. Traditionally (see, for example, Holding, 1965), it was accepted in the literature on motor skill acquisition that while visual control of the effectors may be important in the early stages of learning such monitoring is delegated to the proprioceptive system with extended practice.

In order to empirically explore this issue in the context of catching behaviour a number of different methodological approaches have been used. The Davids and Stratford (1989), Diggles, Grabiner, and Garhammer (1987), Fischman and Schneider (1985), and Smyth and Marriott (1982) studies, for example, excluded vision of the hand by means of a matt black perspex screen - utilising as a control condition a transparent screen (this latter control condition was not used by Diggles et al., 1987, and Fischman and Schneider, 1985). In other experimental work the catcher was required to catch a luminous ball in an otherwise totally dark room, wearing a luminous glove in the 'hand vision' condition and no glove or black glove in the 'no vision of the hand' conditon (von Hofsten, 1987; Rosengren, Pick, & von Hofsten, 1988). Savelsbergh and Whiting in attempting to resolve some of the conflicting findings in the studies cited, used both methodologies (Savelsbergh & Whiting, 1988; Whiting, 1986; Whiting, Savelsbergh, & Faber, 1988).

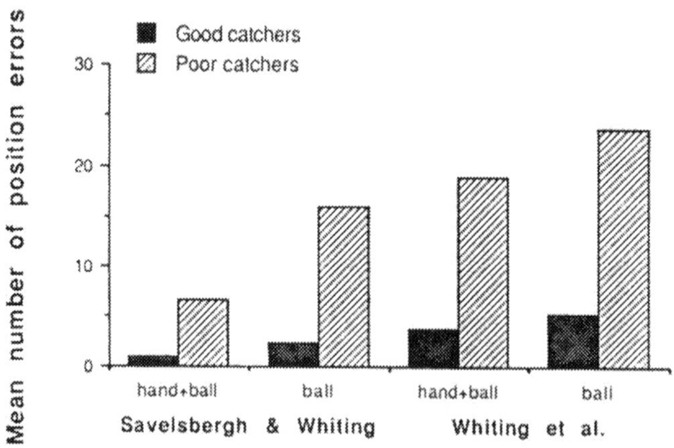

Figure 10. The mean number of position errors for the 'good' and 'poor' catchers under the conditions hand and ball visible, or only the ball visible, in the Savelsbergh & Whiting (1988) and Whiting, Savelsbergh, & Faber (1988) studies.

A number of experiments demonstrated that when vision of the catching hand is prevented, *unskilled* catchers make more spatial errors than do *skilled* catchers (Fischman & Schneider, 1985; Savelsbergh & Whiting, 1988; Whiting,

1986; Whiting et al., 1988; see Figure 10). The fact that 'good' catchers may not need to visually monitor their catching hand for optimal performance, brings into focus the previously cited phenomenon of a transfer (with experience) from visual to kinesthetic monitoring. However, in this respect, the findings of different studies are equivocal. Diggles et al. (1987), for example, concluded that vision of the hand was necessary for all categories of catcher while others found that it was unnecessary for any category of catcher (Davids & Stratford, 1989; Rosengren et al., 1988), or that the absence of such information led to more temporal rather than spatial errors being made (Davids & Stratford, 1989; Fischman & Schneider, 1985). To what can these discrepant findings - using similar paradigms - be attributed? One possibility has been highlighted by Savelsbergh and Whiting (1988; Whiting & Savelsbergh, 1987), namely, the failure to adequately categorise 'good' and 'poor' catchers. Diggles et al. (1987) and Fischman and Schneider (1985), for example, were content to categorise their subjects on the basis of external criteria - success in ball games per se - while Savelsbergh and Whiting (1988) - based on the idea of skill specificity - point to the need to use a within-task criterion (one-handed catching in the laboratory situation). Invoking the latter criterion leads to the conclusion that while relatively 'poor' catchers need to visually monitor their catching hand for optimal performance this is not necessary for 'good' catchers. Thus, lending credence to the idea of a transfer from visual to kinesthetic monitoring (of the catching hand) with extended practice (Whiting & Savelsbergh, in press).

Spatial Information About the Flight of the Ball

A series of experiments by Todd (1981) demonstrated that subjects can accurately predict whether an approaching object, simulated on a computer screen, following a parabolic flight path, will land in front or behind them, even when only part of the ascending flight path is visually available. Todd demonstrated that such information is specified by the ratio (denoted by Turvey & Carello, 1988 the Todd Number) of two time-to-contact components, viz. time-to-contact with the vertical (longitudinal) plane through the point of observation and time-to-contact with the horizontal (sagittal) plane through the point of observation. When the Todd Number (Carello & Turvey, 1989; Turvey & Carello, 1988) is varied, the following predictions can be made:

Tc vertical/Tc horizontal = 1,
the ball will land at the point of observation.
Tc vertical/Tc horizontal > 1,
the ball will land behind the point of observation.

Tc vertical/Tc horizontal < 1,
the ball will land in front of the point of observation (see Figure 11).

Two other sources of predictive spatial information have been suggested, although they have not, experimentally, been addressed as fully. In the first place, Lee (1980; Lee & Young, 1986) noted that an approaching object, that will arrive exactly at the point of observation, generates a stationary focus of expansion in the optic array. A displacing centre of expansion, on the other hand, specifies, quantitatively, the direction of ball flight relative to the observer.

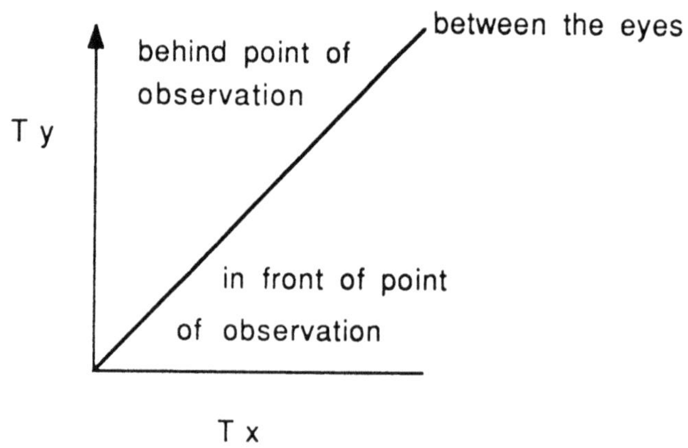

Figure 11. The ratio of two time-to-contact variables indicates where a ball will land relative to the point of observation (adapted from Carello & Turvey, 1989).

It is worth noting that both the aforementioned spatial information sources are available to the catcher whether performing monocularly or binocularly. It should theoretically, therefore, be possible to make accurate spatial judgments about ball flight under monocular conditions. What evidence is there to support such a contention? Experiments conducted by McLeod and his co-workers (McLeod, McLaughin, & Nimmo-Smith, 1986) showed that when subjects were required to hit squash balls which followed a spatially (relatively) unpredictable flight path, more hitting errors (misses) were made under monocular than under binocular vision conditions. When spatial unpredictability was removed (the ball following a constant pathway), and only temporal predictions were required for a successful hit of the ball, no significant differences were found between monocular and binocular conditions. In summary, the McLeod et al. (1986)

study provides evidence for 'indirect' rather than 'direct' pick-up of spatial information. The question might still be asked as to whether there are 'direct' perception explanations of catching performance which can account for spatial accuracy. Savelsbergh and Whiting (in preparation) replicated the McLeod et al. (1986) study for catching, in order to determine under which condition - monocular or binocular - the most catching errors are made. A further intention was to explore the number and nature (temporal or spatial) of the errors made under these vision conditions. Subjects with right hand catching preference took part in the experiment. A ball-projection machine delivered yellow tennis balls with an initial velocity of 8.83 m/s and a ball flight time of approximately 735 ms. Subjects received the six conditions in random order as follows:

Binocular vision
BiLh Catches were required with the left hand.
BiRh Catches were required with the right hand.

Monocular vision
MLeLh Vision of the left eye only, catches were required with the left hand.
MLeRh Vision of the left eye only, catches were required with the right hand.
MReLh Vision of the right eye only, catches were required with the left hand.
MReRh Vision of the right eye only, catches were required with the right hand.

They were allowed thirty training trials under each condition and a rest period of 3 min between conditions. The dependent variables were: number of balls caught out of 30; position errors - a failure to make contact with the ball in the region of the head of the metacarpals; grasp errors - ball makes contact with metacarpal region but grasp is too early or too late. Position and grasp errors were based on video analyses.

The results for the three dependent variables - number of balls caught, number of spatial errors, and number of temporal errors under each condition are reported in Table 1.

The analyses showed that fewer catches and more position errors were made under monocular conditions, while no significant differences were found for temporal errors. The latter finding is consistent with interpretations based on the use of tau, that is, there should be little difference between temporal judgments based on the optical expansion pattern of the ball using monocular or binocular viewing (McLeod et al., 1986). The finding of more spatial errors under the monocular conditions confirms the finding of McLeod et al., (1986). If subjects, in fact, made use of the ratio Tau-horizontal/Tau-vertical - as previously outlined - it would have been possible for them to make accurate spatial judgments under monocular conditions. Since this was not the case what other interpretations are possible? In the first place, it has to be recognised that in spite of theoretical predictions that might be made with respect to the effects of monocular as against binocular vision, the subjects in the study of Todd (1981) used (only) binocular vision in making their judgments. Further, only the early stages of the ball flight trajectory were shown and the judgments required of the subjects (front, behind etc.) might be construed to be more global than those necessary to accurately catch a ball travelling on a relatively unpredictable trajectory. Finely tuned, spatial predictions in the catching task require, in addition to accurate judgments along the longitudinal axis

Table 1. The Mean and Standard Deviations (in parentheses) for the number of catches (out of 30), position errors and grasp errors for the right and left hand under all three vision conditions (binocular (Bi), monocular: right eye open (MRe) and left eye open (MLe)).

	Right hand			Left hand		
	Bi	MRe	MLe	Bi	MRe	MLe
Number of catches	26.3 (3.6)	22.3 (5.2)	21.2 (5.2)	25.2 (4.5)	18.1 (7.5)	20.0 (6.3)
Position errors	1.0 (0.9)	4.1 (2.7)	4.7 (2.4)	1.5 (1.5)	6.2 (5.0)	4.2 (3.8)
Grasp errors	2.7 (3.1)	3.6 (3.7)	4.1 (4.0)	3.3 (3.3)	5.7 (5.1)	5.8 (4.0)

(under/below), accuracy along the transversal axis (left/right) - a situation in which binocular viewing is particularly helpful. When vision with two eyes is available, an image of the ball is projected onto both retinae. Beverley and Regan (1973) argued that the relative velocity of the two images provides a precise cue to the *direction* of motion in depth, and suggested that the brain might be organised to take advantage of this geometrical fact (see Figure 12).

A ball moving sideways produces retinal images that move at the same speeds in the same direction. A ball that will hit the head produces retinal images moving in opposite directions. The ratio of the retinal image velocities is very sensitive when the trajectory passes near to the head. *Distance information* is provided by the fact that the separation between these two images increases when the ball approaches and decreases as the ball goes away (Beverley & Regan, 1973; Regan, 1986). In monocular viewing this information source is not available.

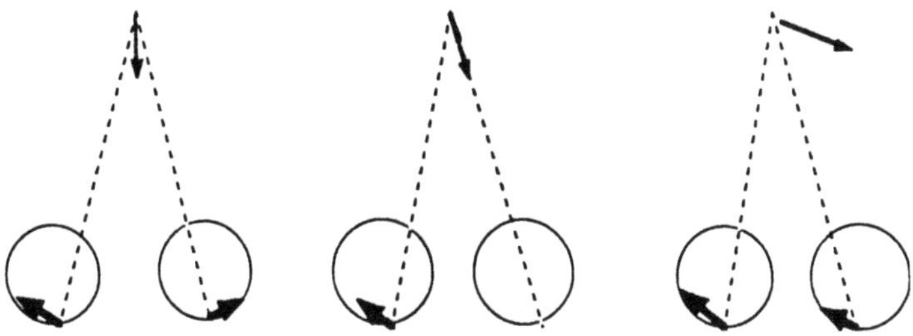

Figure 12. The left and right eyes are depicted looking at a small object whose direction of motion is arrowed. The ratio Vl/Vr between the velocities of the left (Vl) and right (Vr) retinal images unambiguously gives the direction in depth (Adapted from Regan, 1986).

Spatial Information Provided by the Environment

The effect of environmental structure on spatial predictions in catching has been shown in a number of studies (e.g., Rosengren et al., 1988; Savelsbergh & Whiting, 1988, Whiting et al., 1988). In all these studies, catching behaviour was required in a totally dark room with only a ball (luminous) visible. These experiments demonstrated that degrading the environment by reducing the information available leads to an increase in catching errors (Figure 13).

Savelsbergh and Whiting (1988), for example, showed that more spatial and temporal errors were made by both 'poor' and 'good' catchers under the degraded environmental conditions than under the full light condition. What potential information sources does environmental structure provide for the facilitation of spatial judgments?

Fitch and Turvey (1977) argued that powerful information about the path of a ball is provided by the different rates of gain (accretion) and loss (deletion) of optical texture outside the contour of the approaching ball (see Figure 14).

If the background texture is seen to delete equally in all directions, it will hit the catcher 'right between the eyes'. If, the expanding optical contour of the

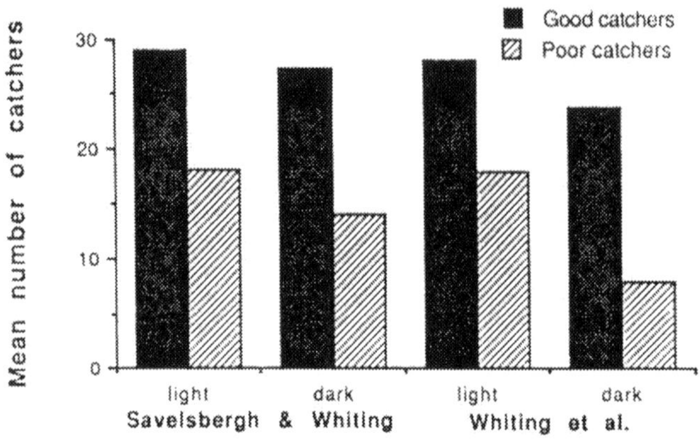

Figure 13. The mean number of catches for the 'good' and 'poor' catchers under the environment light and environment dark condition in the Savelsbergh & Whiting (1988) and Whiting, Savelsbergh, & Faber (1988) study.

ball results in a differing amount of deletion of background texture, the direction of ball flight, relative to the observer is, therein, quantitatively, also specified. Thus, while Todd's and Lee's analyses indicate that predictive spatial information is available from within the expanding optical contour of an approaching ball, Fitch and Turvey (1977) argue that the provision of a textured background enriches the information content of the optic array.

An effect of a background on *spatial* judgments was found in the Rosengren et al. (1988) study (no distinction, however, was made between 'good' and 'poor' catchers). These experiments demonstrated that the presence or absence of a luminescent visual frame in a totally dark room affected catching performance. This frame improved body stability and, therefore, catching success (the effect of the environment on body stabilisation has already been shown in experiments of Lee & Lishman, 1975). In the context of the experiments discussed so far, Savelsbergh (1990) designed an experiment to investigate the effect of different environmental structures on catching - especially on the positioning of the hand.

Fifteen subjects participated in this experiment which was carried out in a specially constructed room 5.9 m long x 1.5 m broad and 2.0 m high. The inside of the room was covered with black, matt surface, heavy weight paper. Mounted in the ceiling of the room was a UV-lamp with a power of 400 watts (Philips UV 400 D). By means of a diaphragm (2 cm broad x 60 cm long) in the ceiling it was possible to illuminate the flight path of a ball (painted with paint sensitive to UV light).

The ball-projection machine projected squash balls at a speed of 10.5 m/s and a ball flight time of approximately 535 ms. The spatial uncertainty of the ball trajectory was, in the vertical plane, from 10 cm to 45 cm and in the horizontal plane 20 cm.

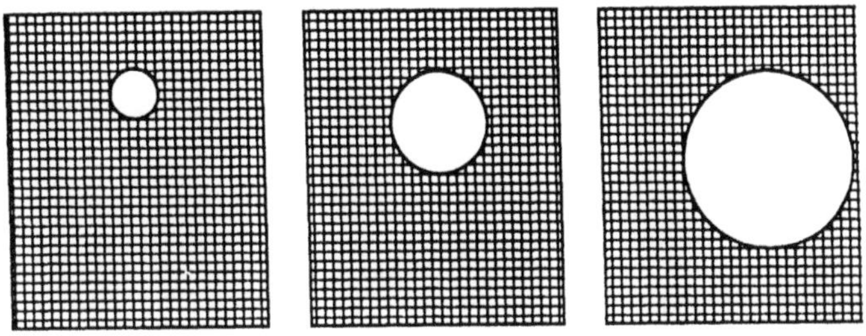

Figure 14. The accretion and decretion of a textured background.

Three light-reflecting (UV) frames were used (Figure 15):

1. **VFS** (Visual Frame Small): The framework consisted of a rectangular luminescent wooden frame of 25 cm x 31 cm and 9 cm thick that was suspended around the ball opening.
2. **VF** (Visual Framework): The framework was constructed from a plastic-coated metal network 1.20 cm broad and 1.85 m long painted with luminescent paint. The mesh was 5 cm x 5 cm. The frame was supported in front of the ball projection machine, an opening of 10 x 20 cm being made to allow free passage of the balls.
3. **VFR**: A framework similar to that used by Rosengren et al. (1988) consisting of 6 luminous strips 5 cm high x 4.5 cm broad. Two of these strips, from the viewpoint of the subject, were on the left hand side and the other four on the right hand side. The strips were attached to a pole (two to one pole and four to another) and were interspersed with black stripes. The distance between the stripes on the left hand pole was 7 cm - the lowest of these being 1.05 m from the ground. For the right hand side pole the lowest strip was 0.57 m from the ground. Between the first and second strip was a distance of 7 cm, between the second and third 67 cm and between the third and fourth, again 7 cm. The poles were 60 cm from one another. The distances between poles and subject were, both, 5.35 m.

Subjects wore transparent protective goggles throughout the experiment and received the following five conditions in random order:

1. Condition **N**: full light - hand, ball, and environment were visible.
2. Condition **VF**: the large frame and the ball were visible.
3. Condition **VFR**: the luminescent frame of Rosengren et al. (1988) and ball were visible.
4. Condition **VFS**: the small frame and the ball were visible.
5. Condition **UVB**: only luminescent ball present in an otherwise totally dark room.

The motivation for these particular frameworks was that they provided a highly structured (N), to a less structured (VF, VFR, VFS) to a hardly structured (dark) environment (UVB). Each condition involved 30 catching trials.

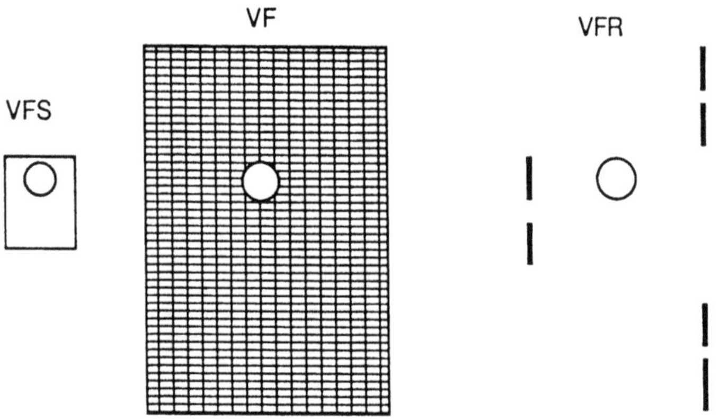

Figure 15. The frameworks used (see text for explanation).

Following a description of the experiment, subjects received 10 training trials - 5 in the light and 5 in the dark (only ball visible). Between conditions was a rest period of five minutes. The dependent variables were the number of balls caught, the number of complete misses (no touch of the ball), and total number of points (catch = 2 points; touch but no catch 1 point, and a complete miss 0 points).

The results of this experiment are reproduced in Table 2. The results showed a significantly better performance in the full light (N) in comparison to all other conditions. Comparing, for all three independent variables, the first five to the last five trials no improvement in catching was found for the full light (N) and **VF** frame. For the other two frames (**VFR** and **VFS**) and the **UVB** an improvement in catching was found. The findings are quite surprising for two reasons: first the **VF** frame does not make any enhancing contribution to ball catching performance even though it provides a highly structured background.

Table 2. Means and Standard Deviations (in parentheses) for the three dependent variables (catches, misses, total number of points) for the first (1-5) and last (26-30) five trials for the five conditions.

	Environmental structure				
	N	VF	VFR	VFS	UVB
Catches					
1-5	2.67 (1.5)	0.33 (0.6)	0.53 (0.6)	0.20 (0.7)	0.47 (0.6)
26-30	2.80 (1.5)	0.87 (1.2)	1.40 (1.1)	1.47 (1.1)	1.33 (1.2)
Misses					
1-5	0.67 (0.7)	2.67 (1.8)	2.53 (1.3)	2.40 (1.5)	2.20 (1.5)
26-30	0.27 (0.4)	2.00 (1.3)	1.53 (1.7)	0.87 (1.0)	0.67 (0.9)
Points					
1-5	7.00 (1.7)	3.07 (2.8)	3.00 (1.6)	3.28 (1.7)	3.27 (1.9)
26-30	7.53 (1.7)	4.00 (2.4)	4.87 (2.4)	5.60 (1.9)	5.67 (1.6)

This lends credence to the idea that the design of the **VF** frame was not conducive to the enhancement of environmental effects. Any potentially facilitating effects of this kind of illuminated framework are probably offset by the negative effects of the particular figure-ground contrasts used. Secondly, it should be appreciated that catching results with the **VFS** and **VFR** were *no better* than those obtained when only the ball was visible (**UVB**). If we have a closer look at the results then it becomes clear that the **VFS** and **UVB** conditions produce similar effects on ball catching performance. Unfortunately, from this experiment it is still not clear why the catching performance in the light is better than in the dark. Further research should focus on the design of background information in experiments of this kind.

CONCLUSIONS AND NEW QUESTIONS

The Effect of the Duration of the Viewing Time

Information about the trajectory of the ball is essential to successful catching, although early experiments of Whiting and his co-workers showed that it is not necessary to view the entire ball trajectory in order to make accurate predictions about the future space-time parameters. When vision of the ball was provided too early or too late in the flight path of the ball catching performance was shown to deteriorate. The enhanced performance effects shown when the viewing period varied from 205-364 ms could provide evidence for the importance of taking into account the section of the trajectory of the ball during which information is, visually, made available. This question has not been adequately pursued (see, however, evidence provided about the importance of information available in the apex of the trajectory of balls in juggling in the studies of Austin (1976) and Beek (1989)).

With respect to the duration of viewing time, Bruce and Green (1985) report an optimal tau margin between 250-300 ms. However, this statement may need to be qualified in terms of the task in question. For example, very early in the flight path of the ball the optical expansion pattern is limited, while late in the flight path the catcher does not have enough time to gear his or her action to any information he or she may be able to pick up. In this respect Lee (1980) has suggested that the 300 ms time-to-contact interval is critical because the necessary movements of catchers tend to be of a fairly constant duration so that it is only necessary to initiate these movements at a specific time-to-contact.

Effects of Viewing the Catching Hand

A number of experiments reviewed produced contradictory findings with respect to the necessity of viewing the catching hand. Some demonstrated that when vision of the catching hand is prevented, *unskilled* catchers make more errors in positioning their hand in the flight path of the ball than do *skilled* catchers (Fischman & Schneider, 1985; Savelsbergh & Whiting, 1988; Whiting et al., 1988). Others (e.g., Diggles et al., 1987) concluded that vision of the hand was necessary for all categories of catcher, or that it was unnecessary for any category of catcher (Davids & Stratford, 1989; Rosengren et al., 1988), or that the absence of such information led to more temporal errors (rather than spatial) being made (Davids & Stratford, 1989; Fischman & Schneider, 1985). Possible explanations of the discrepancies in these findings are the failure to adequately separate 'good' catchers from 'poor' catchers and differences in methodology used (see e.g., Whiting, 1986; Whiting & Savelsbergh, 1987; Whiting et al., 1988). This topic should be pursued further in order to explore long standing questions about the transfer from visual to kinesthetic monitoring as skill develops and questions about the specificity of skill learning (Whiting & Savelsbergh, under review).

Environmental Effects

Studies carried out by Rosengren et al. (1988) and Savelsbergh and Whiting (1988; Whiting et al., 1988) demonstrated the enhancing effect of a structured environment on both *temporal* and *spatial* precision when compared to catching in the dark with only a luminous ball visible. How can these improvements and decrements in temporal and spatial predicitions be explained - particularly, given the departure point of ecological psychologists that all the necessary temporal and spatial information sources are provided by a luminous ball in flight in an otherwise completely dark room. Why then should subjects make more timing errors under the latter condition and why does a structured environment enhance both spatial and temporal judgments?

A study by Cavallo and Laurent (1988) provides a possible explanation of the results obtained for the 'poor' catchers. They suggest that two kinds of time-to-contact information are simultaneously available - *directly* specified by the relative rate of optical expansion and *indirectly* by computation based on information about position and velocity. Unskilled subjects, they suggest, in contrast to skilled, base their judgments on information obtained by the latter means. Thus, the increase in temporal errors for the 'poor' catchers, when moving from the light to the dark, could be a result of the unavailability of distance cues and the consequent negative effects on the computing of time-to-contact from perceived distance and velocity. However, if this explanation is accepted, why is there also an effect on the good catchers?

A number of studies have examined time-to-contact judgments in the absence or presence of background grids (e.g., McLeod & Ross, 1983; Schiff & Detweiler, 1979). Generally, no enhancing effects of less or more structured environments have been found. It should be noted, however, that these studies were not addressed to catching and, furthermore, provided no vision of the path of the approaching object over the last 2 s - a time interval that may provide important information in the control of both catching and striking actions (Bootsma & van Wieringen, 1990; Savelsbergh et al., 1991; Savelsbergh et al., in preparation).

How can we explain the spatial improvement? An effect of the environment on *spatial* judgments was found in the Rosengren et al. (1988) study where it was demonstrated that the presence of a luminescent visual frame in a totally dark room enhanced catching performance. The results of an experiment reported by Savelsbergh (1990, p. 322 this Chapter) showed that despite the presence of a luminous framework in the dark, subjects did not reach the same catching level as in full light. In fact the catching results were the same as when only the luminous ball was visible in a totally dark room. It remains unclear why more catches are made in the full light.

In summary, from experimental studies (e.g., Lee et al., 1983; Savelsbergh et al., 1991; Todd, 1981) and from theoretical considerations (Fitch & Turvey, 1977) it appears that all the ***necessary*** information on which the timing and positioning of the hand and the timing of the grasp in a catching action is made is, in principle, available when *monocular vision of the ball* is provided. Under this circumstance tau (predictive temporal information) and the ratio of 'Tau-vertical/Tau-horizontal' (predictive spatial information) can be derived. However, the fact that more catches were made when a highly textured environment (full light) or when binocular vision was provided, is suggestive that subjects make use of a multiple source strategy in catching. With respect to the monocular/binocular division, one strategy could be the use of information provide by occular disparity and the ratio of retinal image velocities (Beverely & Regan, 1973). However, with respect to the light/dark division a satisfactory explanation is still awaited.

REFERENCES

Abernethy, B. & Burgess-Limerick, Q. (this volume). *Visual information for the timing of skilled movements: a review.*

Alderson, G.J.K., Sully, D.L., & Sully, H.G. (1974). An operational analysis of a one-handed catching task using high speed photography. *Journal of Motor Behavior, 6,* 217-226.

Austin, H.A. (1976). *A computational theory of physical skill*. Unpublished Ph.d thesis, Department of Electrical Engineering and Computer Science, M.I.T., Boston.

Ball, W., & Tronick, E. (1971). Infants responses to impending collision: optical and real. *Science, 171*, 812-820.

Beek, P.J. (1989). *Juggling dynamics*. Amsterdam: Free University Press.

Beverley, K.L., & Regan, D. (1973). Evidence for the existence of neural mechanisms selectively sensitive to the direction of movement in space. *Journal of Physiology, 235*, 17-29.

Bootsma, R.J., & van Wieringen, P.W.C. (1990). Timing an attacking forehand drive in table tennis. *Journal of Experimental Psychology: Human Perception and Performance, 16*, 21-29.

Bower, T.G.R., Broughton, J.M., & Moore, M.K. (1970). Infants responses to approaching objects: An indicator of response to distal variables. *Perception & Psychophysics, 9*, 193-196.

Bruce, V., & Green, P. (1985). *Visual perception: Physiology, psychology and ecology*. Hillsdale, NJ: Lawrence Erlbaum Associates.

Carello, C., & Turvey, M.T. (1989). Ecological physics and baseball's illusions. *PAW review: A technical report of the perceiving-acting workshop in ecological psychology*. University of Connecticut, Storrs.

Cavallo, V., & Laurent, M. (1988). Visual information and skill level in time-to-collision estimation. *Perception, 17*, 623-632.

Davids, K., & Stratford, R. (1989). Peripheral vision and simple catching: The screen paradigm revisted. *Journal of Sports Sciences, 7*, 139-152.

Diggles, V.A., Grabiner, M.D., & Garhammer, J. (1987). Skill level and efficacy of effector visual feedback in ball catching. *Perceptual and Motor Skills, 64*, 987-993.

Fischman, M.G., & Schneider, T. (1985). Skill level, vision, and proprioception in simple one-handed catching. *Journal of Motor Behavior, 17*, 219-229.

Fitch, H.L., & Turvey, M.T. (1977). On the control of activity: Some remarks from an ecological point of view. In D.M. Landers & R.W. Christina (Eds.), *Psychology of motor behavior and sport* (pp. 3-35). Champaign IL: Human Kinetics.

Fitts, P.M., & Posner, M.I. (1967). *Human performance*. Belmont, CA: Brooks-Cole.

Gibson, J.J. (1966). *The senses considered as perceptual systems*. Boston: Houghton Mifflin.

Gibson, J.J. (1979). *The ecological approach to visual perception*. Hillsdale, NJ: Lawrence Erlbaum Associates.

Holding, D.H. (1965). *Principles of training*. London: Pergamon.

Keele, S.W. (1968). Movement control in skilled performance. *Psychological Bulletin, 70*, 387-403.

Lamb, K.L., & Burwitz, L. (1988). Visual restriction in ball catching: A re-examination of earlier findings. *Journal of Human Movement Studies, 14*, 93-99.

Laurent, M., Dinh Phung, R., & Ripoll, H. (1989). What visual information is used by riders in jumping. *Human Movement Science, 8*, 481-501.

Lee, D.N. (1976). A theory of visual control of braking based on information about time-to-collision. *Perception, 5*, 437-459.

Lee, D.N. (1980). Visuo-motor co-ordination in space-time. In G.E. Stelmach & J. Requin (Eds.), *Tutorials in motor behavior* (pp. 281-295). Amsterdam: North-Holland.

Lee, D.N., & Lishman, J.R. (1975). Visual proprioceptive control of stance. *Journal of Human Movement Studies, 1*, 87-95.

Lee, D.N., Lishman, J.R., & Thomson, J.A. (1982). Regulation of gait in long jumping. *Journal of Experimental Psychology: Human Perception and Performance, 8*, 448-459.

Lee, D.N., & Reddish, P.E. (1981). Plummeting gannets: A paradigm for ecological optics. *Nature, 293*, 293-294.

Lee, D.N., & Young, D.S. (1986). Gearing action to the environment. *Experimental Brain Research Series 15*. Berlin: Springer-Verlag.

Lee, D.N., Young, D.S., Reddish, P.E., Lough, S., & Clayton, T.M.H. (1983). Visual timing in hitting an accelerating ball. *Quarterly Journal of Experimental Psychology, 35A*, 333-346.

McLeod, P., McLaughlin, C., & Nimmo-Smith, I. (1986). Information encapsulation and automaticity: Evidence from the visual control of finely timed actions. In M.I. Posner and O.S. Marin (Eds.), *Attention and Performance 11* (pp. 391-406). Hillsdale, NJ: Lawrence Erlbaum Associates.

McLeod, R.W., & Ross, H.E. (1983). Optic-flow and cognitive factors in time-to-collision estimates. *Perception, 12*, 417-423.

Moray, N. (1970). *Attention: Selective processes in vision and hearing*. London: Hutchinson.

Regan, D.M. (1986). The eye in ball games: Hitting and catching. *Proceedings of conference on vision and sport* (pp. 1-33). Haarlem: De Vriesenborch.

Rosengren, K.S., Pick, H.L., & Hofsten, von C. (1988). Role of Visual Information in Ball Catching. *Journal of Motor Behavior, 20*, 150-164.

Savelsbergh, G.J.P. (1990). *Catching Behaviour*. Meppel: Krips Repro.

Savelsbergh, G.J.P., & Whiting, H.T.A. (1990). Omgevingsinformatie en de controle van eenhandig vangen: Een Ecologische Psychologische benadering (Environmental information and the control of one-handed catching: An ecological approach). In P. Wylleman and Y. Vanden Auwele (Eds.), *Proceedings van de studiedagen van de Vlaamse Vereniging voor Sportpsychologie* (pp. 101-123). Leuven: ILO-K.U.L. Belgie.

Savelsbergh, G.J.P., & Whiting, H.T.A. (1988). The effect of skill level, external frame of reference and environmental changes on one handed catching. *Ergonomics, 31*, 1655-1663.

Savelsbergh, G.J.P., & Whiting, H.T.A. (in press) Catching: A motor learning and developmental perspective. In H.Heuer & S. Keele (Eds.), *Motor Skills*. Goettingen: Verlag fur Psychologie.

Savelsbergh, G.J.P., & Whiting, H.T.A. (1991) *The acquisition of catching under monocular and binocular conditions.* Manuscript submitted for publication.

Savelsbergh, G.J.P., Whiting, H.T.A., & Bootsma, R.J. (1991). 'Grasping' TAU! *Journal of Experimental Psychology: Human Perception and Performance, 17.*

Savelsbergh, G.J.P., Whiting, H.T.A., Pijpers, J.R., & Van Santvoord, A.M.M. (1991). The visual guidance of catching (manuscript in preparation).

Schiff, W. (1965). Perception of impending collision: A study of visually directed avoidance behaviour. *Psychological Monograph, 79*, (whole no. 604).

Schiff, W., Caviness, J.A., & Gibson, J.J. (1962). Persistent fear responses in Rhesus monkeys to the optical stimulus of 'looming'. *Science, 136*, 982-983.

Schiff, W., & Detweiler, M.L. (1979). Information used in judging impending collision. *Perception, 8*, 647-658.

Sharp, R.H., & Whiting, H.T.A. (1974). Exposure and occluded duration effects in a ball-catching skill. *Journal of Motor Behavior, 3*, 139-147.

Sharp, R.H., & Whiting, H.T.A. (1975). Information-processing and eye-movement behavior in ball catching skill. *Journal of Human Movement Studies, 1*, 124-131.

Sidaway, B., McNitt-Gray, J., & Davis, G. (1989). Visual timing of muscle preactivation in preparation for landing. *Ecological Psychology, 1*, 253-264.

Smyth, M.M., & Marriott, A.M. (1982). Vision and proprioception in simple catching. *Journal of Motor Behavior, 14*, 143-152.

Todd, J.T. (1981). Visual information about moving objects. *Journal of Experimental Psychology: Human Perception and Performance, 7*, 795-810.

Turvey, M.T. (1990). The challenge of a physical account of actions: A personal view. In H.T.A. Whiting, O.G. Meijer, & P.C.W. van Wieringen (Eds.), *The Natural-Physical Approach to Human Movement* (pp. 57-93). Amsterdam: Free University Press.

Turvey, M.T., & Carello, C. (1988). Exploring a law-based ecological approach to skilled action. In A. M. Colley & J.R. Beech (Eds.), *Cognition and action in skilled behavior* (pp. 191-203). Amsterdam: North-Holland.

von Hofsten, C., (1987). Catching. In H.Heuer & A.P. Sanders (Eds.), *Perspectives on perception and action* (pp. 31-40). Hillsdale, NJ: Lawrence Erlbaum Associates.

Whiting, H.T.A. (1968). Training in a continuous ball throwing and catching task. *Ergonomics, 11*, 375-382.

Whiting, H.T.A. (1970). An operational analysis of a continuous ball throwing and catching task. *Ergonomics, 13*, 445-454.

Whiting, H.T.A. (1986). Isn't there a catch in it somewhere? *Journal of Motor Behavior, 18*, 486-491.

Whiting, H.T.A., Gill, E.B., & Stephenson, J.M. (1970). Critical time intervals for taking in flight information in a ball-catching task. *Ergonomics, 13*, 265-272.

Whiting, H.T.A., & Savelsbergh, G.J.P. (in press). There must be a catch in it somewhere! In G.E. Stelmach & J. Requin (Eds.), *Tutorials in motor learning and performance*. Dordrecht: North Holland.

Whiting H.T.A., & Savelsbergh, G.J.P. (1987). Catch as catch can. *Perceptual and Motor Skills, 65*, 863-866.

Whiting, H.T.A., & Savelsbergh, G.J.P. (1991). An exception that provides the rule! In G.E. Stelmach & J. Requin (Eds.), *Tutorials in neurosciences*. Dordrecht: North Holland (manuscript under review).

Whiting, H.T.A., Savelsbergh, G.J.P., & Faber, C.M. (1988). Catch questions and incomplete answers. In A.M. Colley & J.R. Beech (Eds.), *Cognition and action in skilled behavior* (pp 257-271). Amsterdam: North-Holland.

Whiting, H.T.A., & Sharp, R.H. (1974). Visual occlusion factors in a discrete ball catching task. *Journal of Motor Behavior, 6*, 11-16.

Approaches to the Study of Motor Control and Learning
J.J. Summers (Editor)

Chapter 12

VISUAL INFORMATION FOR THE TIMING OF SKILLED MOVEMENTS: A REVIEW

Bruce Abernethy and Robin Burgess-Limerick
University of Queensland.

The control of many human actions depends on the accurate pick-up of visual information about the time-to-contact (t_c) of approaching objects and surfaces. T_c may potentially be determined by computation of the instantaneous ratio between observer-object (or observer-surface) distance and approach velocity. Alternatively t_c may be picked up directly from the expansion characteristics of closed contours within the optic flow field if the performer is sensitive to a single parameter tau (the inverse of the relative rate of expansion; after Lee, 1976). In this paper we examine the origins of these alternative proposals regarding the pick-up of t_c information, tracing links to traditional and ecological theories of visual perception, in general and the perception of change, in particular. We review empirical evidence derived from tests of the contrasting explanations of t_c and discuss the currently equivocal research evidence in terms of levels of analysis differences between the competing explanations and in terms of the influences of situational context and observer expertise and gender. The capacity of human subjects to optimise their use of available sources of perceptual information for judging impending contact is highlighted as is the necessity to regard the alternative sources of t_c information as complementary rather than competing.

Much of our day-to-day living is dependent upon the visual judgment of coincidence - judgments made so as to intentionally either *avoid* or *engineer* collisions with other objects or surfaces in the environment. Visual information is used to avoid collisions when estimating safe overtaking or braking distances in vehicles, crossing a road as a pedestrian, evading the tackle of an opponent in any of the football codes or dodging overhead branches whilst bush walking. Similar information may be used to deliberately produce coincidence (or collisions) such as when running over uneven terrain, intercepting an errant child, falling an opponent in wrestling, or striking or catching a fast moving ball. In an evolutionary sense the development of such skills (frequently referred to as *coincidence-timing* skills; Stadulis, 1972) may have its origins in the need to avoid predation from other animals while at the same time capturing sufficient food through predation to support growth and reproduction. Natural selection may have thus stimulated the development of dedicated perceptual mechanisms, capable of picking up the information needed to control collision-avoiding and collision-inducing movements (von Hofsten, 1987), and the development of 'smart' perceptual systems (after Runeson, 1977), tightly coupling together the perception and action systems (Turvey & Carello, 1986).

Coincidence-timing skills, at least as they occur in natural settings, have been largely ignored historically as a focal point for the study of either perception or action. From the 1960s onwards the information processing model has dominated experimental psychology and its emphasis upon sequential, independent stage models of human performance (e.g., Stelmach, 1982; Sternberg, 1969) has dictated a research strategy of reductionism, based largely on the recording of reaction times. The principal intent within the information processing model has been to discover the nature of processing *within* given putative processing stages rather than the nature of the links *between* processes. Studies of perception have generally involved tasks in which the responses required are simplistic and atypical of the motor requirements of 'normal' actions (e.g., verbal reports, categorical judgments or key press responses). Conversely studies of movement control have been typically restricted to laboratory paradigms in which the perceptual requirements are deliberately simplified to the point of also being non-representative of 'real world' skills. [The simplified perceptual requirements of Fitts' (1954) popular reciprocal tapping task for examining movement control is a typical example].

Fortunately with the recent burgeoning of interest in ecological psychology, arising from the influential works of J.J. Gibson (1966, 1979), there has been a growing interest in the study of natural skills and a deliberate focus upon coincidence timing as a window to understanding the normal functional coupling and interaction between perception and action. The ecological significance of coincidence-timing skills has resulted in the recent examination of perception-action coupling in a fascinatingly diverse range of human and animal activities. Despite this recent research attention however, still relatively little is known about how visually-guided coincidence-timing skills are controlled and, in turn, how such skills might best be taught or corrected in the face of persistent failure. For example, how should young athletes be taught batting skills, stroke victims re-taught temporal components of gait or learner drivers taught safe overtaking behaviour?

In this particular chapter we focus upon the apparent sensitivity of humans and other animals to visual information specifying the time-to-contact (t_c), using Lee's (1976) term, between either an observer/actor approaching a stationary surface or a moving object approaching a stationary observer. Alternatively referred to as time-to-collision, time-to-go (after Purdy, 1958) or time-to-arrival (Schiff & Oldak, 1990), t_c has been presented as a key optical variable for the initiation of a range of interceptive and avoidance movements and as an essential perceptual variable dictating the selection of appropriate categories of action. We firstly review the evidence to determine if t_c is indeed an important visual variable for the control of coincidence-timing actions. In so doing, we highlight the mediating influence of expertise and gender variables in the performance of coincidence-timing skills. Next we examine different mechanisms which have been proposed for the preferential pick-up of t_c information from the optic flow field (and from the subsequent retinal image). The origins of these proposed mechanisms are traced from contrasting theoretical perspectives on visual perception, in general, and contrasting theoretical views on the perception of change, in particular. In the third section the evidence derived from empirical tests of these different putative mechanisms for t_c extraction is reviewed and in the final section an attempt is made to synthesise this evidence with a view toward summarising conditional support for the competing explanations. In this final section we emphasise the equivocal nature of the existing empirical data, the difficulty/impossibility of devising definitive tests of the competing explanations and the presence of both empirical and anecdotal observations which, perhaps predictably, necessitate the further elaboration of the existing models for t_c pick-up.

SENSITIVITY TO TIME-TO-CONTACT INFORMATION

Evidence for the Selective Pick-up and Utilisation of Time-to-Contact Information

There is quite substantial evidence that humans and other animals are sensitive to/attuned to[1] information about time remaining to contact with approaching

---

[1] Each of the major theoretical viewpoints has associated with it its own unique language and terminology. For example 'attuned to' is very much an expression of ecological psychology whereas discussion of 'processes' and 'mechanisms' implies an information processing framework. As our intent, at least in initially reviewing

objects or surfaces. Across changes in the approach velocity of objects or surfaces the initiation of interceptive movements seems to be consistently geared to t_c rather than to other potential visual control variables such as the animal-object distance or the location of the object or surface in the animal's extracorporeal space. The plummeting gannets studied by Lee and Reddish (1981) or the houseflies studied by Wagner (1982) appear to initiate important actions (in the gannet's case, the folding of its wings to dive through the surface of the water; in the housefly's case, the commencement of deceleration and the extension of the landing gear) not when they are an invariant distance from the surface of interest but rather when the projected t_c with the surface reaches a critical value. The gearing of the animal's action to t_c theoretically allows precise coincidence-timing to be achieved across a range of approach velocities without the necessity for the animal to adjust the duration of its wing-folding or leg-extending movements.

Invariant movement times across a range of altered task conditions have also been demonstrated in a variety of skilled human activities - the apparent advantage of such invariance being the reduction of one degree of freedom from the coincidence-timing task (cf. Bernstein, 1967; Fitch, Tuller, & Turvey, 1982; Turvey, Fitch, & Tuller, 1982). Consistent movement times have been demonstrated across variations in observer-object (or observer-surface) approach velocity (and concomitant variations in the overall time constraints of the task) for the downswing of baseball batters (Hubbard & Seng, 1954), table-tennis players (Bootsma & van Wieringen, 1988; Tyldesley & Whiting, 1975), a field hockey player (Franks, Weicker, & Robertson, 1985) and squash players (Wollstein & Abernethy, 1988), for the release phase of subjects throwing darts at a moving target (Spaeth-Arnold, 1976) and for the knee extension/take-off phase of ski jumpers (Lee & Young, 1985).

Tyldesley and Whiting (1975), in positing an operational timing hypothesis, argued that these consistent movement times were achieved through the use of a motor program (see also Bootsma & van Wieringen, 1988) although it is now clear that alternative explanations of the production of consistent, time-based movements are possible (e.g., Kelso, 1981). Dietz and Noth (1978), in a study in which human subjects were required to fall forward, hands first, from a vertical starting position through a range of between 50° and 80° to a padded platform, observed that the onset of electromyographic activity in the triceps brachii (to break the fall) always occurred at a specific t_c value. Moreover the fact that this coupling of movement initiation to t_c disappeared when subjects

---

the empirical research on t_c, is to remain as detached and theoretically impartial as possible, our use of terms such as 'attuned', 'picked-up', 'processes' and 'mechanisms' should be considered in their most general sense and not as indicative of our allegiance to any particular theoretical viewpoint.

were blindfolded highlighted the visual origin of the controlling t_c information. Similar findings have also recently been presented by Sidaway, McNitt-Gray, and Davis (1989).

Before accepting the evidence for invariant movement times across varying task conditions as definitive evidence for sensitivity to, and use of, visually-derived t_c information as the basis for perception-action coupling in interceptive tasks, some limitations in the existing data base need to be recognised. Of particular concern is the statistical method typically used to imply movement time invariance. Movement time invariance is typically concluded on the basis of the failure of changes in task conditions (particularly observer-object approach velocity) to *significantly* alter movement time. Inferential tests are, however, biased in the direction of accepting the null hypothesis. (The null hypothesis in these cases is the hypothesis supporting invariance). Thus conclusions of movement time invariance on the basis of non-significant approach velocity effects may be unjustified (see Corcos, Agarwal, & Gottlieb, 1985 for discussion of a parallel problem in the tests of some motor control theories). Likewise, the frequent combination of individual subject data into group data has the effect of increasing sample variability and further biasing statistical tests in the direction of demonstrating non-significant differences (see Gentner, 1987 for treatment of a similar problem in the relative timing literature).

Recent studies (Bootsma, 1989; Bootsma & van Wieringen, 1990) indicate that, in fact, relatively small inter-trial variations in the movement trajectories of individual subjects may be of important functional significance. Coincidence-timing accuracy at the point of contact or collision has been shown in these studies to be enhanced relative to accuracy at the point of movement initiation, suggesting that continuous 'on line' corrections can be used throughout an action. The continuous coupling of perception and action to allow movements to be refined during their execution (but still importantly in response to t_c inputs) has been proposed by Bootsma (1988) as more important than the overall maintenance of movement duration consistency. Such a notion is consistent with the (apparently paradoxical) greater movement time variability of experts compared to novices in the backswing phase of many hitting skills (Abernethy, 1984; Burgess-Limerick, Abernethy, & Neal, 1990).

The direct modulation of flight time in gait in response to actual t_c with a specific target surface is a second major source of support for the primacy of t_c information. Lee, Lishman, and Thomson (1982), in a widely cited work on three female long jumpers, demonstrated that the flight times of the final few strides of the jumpers as they 'homed in' on the take-off board were directly modulated in response to t_c with the board. Lee et al. hypothesised that this gait regulation was achieved through control of a single gait parameter viz., the vertical impulse applied during the stance phase. Hay (1988) replicated the Lee et al. experiment with 14 elite male and 14 elite female long jumpers and again observed the presence of visually-based adjustments in foot placement late in the athletes' approaches to the board although no postulations were made as to the precise nature of the visual control parameter. Meeuwsen and Magill (1987) observed similar marked increases in the variability of foot placement in the final two strides (compared to earlier strides) for female gymnasts running up to perform a straight-body handspring vault. The control of foot placement again appeared to be modulated in response to t_c, by altering the duration of the flight phase of gait through adjusting vertical impulse. Interestingly, this adjustment appeared possible without the take-off board being directly foveated. Either information provided continuously from the periphery or information obtained continually and stored in some short term visual store (cf. Thomson, 1983) appears adequate to provide the t_c information needed for late gait adjustments. More recently, Laurent, Dinh Phung, and Ripoll (1989) have demonstrated that the gait of jumping horses is also adjusted by their riders so that the take-off position of the horse for the jump occurs at a set t_c value.

An analogous situation to that involved in adjusting gait to achieve a specific footfall position for take-off in any jumping activity occurs when normal running gait must be adjusted (to avoid stepping on loose stones and other obstacles) when running over uneven terrain. Warren, Young, and Lee (1986) showed that, in a treadmill version of this task, runners could adjust their step length to find appropriate footfall targets through simply adjusting vertical impulse and that the visual information needed for the accurate modulation of this gait parameter was the difference in t_c between two upcoming footfall targets (see also Warren, 1988). To examine gait adaptations further Patla, Robinson, Samways, and Armstrong (1989) had subjects voluntarily adjust their step length in response to visual cues presented at various times during the gait cycle. Direct recording of ground reaction forces (as opposed to indirect inference of kinetics from kinematic recordings; as used by Lee et al., 1983 and Warren et al., 1986) indicated that step length modulation in response to t_c was achieved through alteration in *both* vertical and horizontal impulse. Although the precise nature and magnitude of the horizontal impulse adjustment during gait adaptation is the point of some contention (Patla, 1989; Warren & Yaffe, 1989), and may well vary according to whether treadmill or overground locomotion is examined, the importance of t_c as the visual information source for gait adjustment has not been challenged.

Mediating Variables in the Use of Time-to-Contact Information

The speed and accuracy with which t_c information is picked up visually appears to vary as a function of the observer's developmental age, gender, and expertise. In most cases differences in the ability to pick-up and use t_c

information must be implied from differences in performance on coincidence-timing tasks although some studies particularly directed at t_c information have been conducted. The effect of these mediating variables is important as any theoretical account of how t_c information is detected (at either the computational or algorithmic level; Marr, 1982) must be capable of adequately explaining these effects.

Developmental Age. Despite the capability of humans to respond to impending collision from infancy (e.g., Ball & Tronick, 1971; Bower, Broughton, & Moore, 1970) performance on simple coincidence-timing tasks (usually involving apparent rather than real motion) improves linearly with age (e.g., Bard, Fleury, Carriellec, & Bellec, 1981; Dunham, 1977; Haywood, 1980; Thomas, Gallagher, & Purvis, 1981), reaching adult levels on simple tasks by about age 11-13 and somewhat later on more complex tasks (e.g., see Dorfman, 1977). In tasks such as catching, in which the perception of t_c is crucial for successful performance, it was traditionally thought (Kay, 1969; Williams, 1968, 1973) that 5-6 year old children were capable of estimating ball trajectory with some accuracy but unable to either anticipate the future coincidence point of the ball with the hand or plan their own response times. More recent studies by von Hofsten (1980, 1982, 1983) indicate that predictive reaching to a coincidence point is present in infancy although it is nevertheless apparently true that the capability to pick-up t_c information develops as a function of both age and task-specific experience.

Gender. The evidence concerning gender differences in performance on coincidence-timing skills is somewhat equivocal. Although some studies exist which fail to show any differences in coincidence-timing performance between males and females (e.g., Haywood, 1980; Isaacs, 1983; Stadulis, 1971), the majority of studies indicate both more accurate and more consistent coincidence-timing performance by age-matched male subjects (e.g., Bruce, 1966; Dorfman, 1977; Dunham, 1977; Payne, 1986, 1987; Wrisberg & Mead, 1981; Wrisberg, Paul, & Ragsdale, 1979). Some evidence has been presented of these effects disappearing with practice (Dorfman, 1977), arguing for familiarity as the cause of the gender differences, but such practice effects have been observed only infrequently. Wrisberg and Mead (1983) have suggested that gender differences in coincidence timing performance only occur on tasks in which the movement response requires the use of large muscle groups, hence arguing for a motor rather than a perceptual origin for the gender differences. Recent applied studies in which male and female car drivers are required to verbally estimate t_c with other vehicles over a period of display occlusion, however, indicate systematic gender differences in the *perception* and estimation of t_c. Both McLeod and Ross (1983) and Schiff and Oldak (1990) have demonstrated systematically more accurate estimates of t_c by male subjects which hold regardless of driving experience, the magnitude of actual t_c, viewing time, and the trajectory of approach. As the optic flow field available to both male and female subjects is identical the source of this gender difference in coincidence-timing performance must be sought in either perceptual differentiation differences in information pick-up between males and females or in some subsequent processing mechanism responsible for the "enrichment" of t_c information (cf. Gibson, 1969).

Expertise. Superior coincidence-timing skills are undoubtedly an important component of expert performance in many activities, especially fast ball sports, with experts being capable of operating with precision within smaller time windows than novices (Tyldesley & Whiting, 1975). However attempts to demonstrate systematic expert-novice differences in laboratory coincidence-timing tasks have been generally unsuccessful (e.g., Blundell, 1984; Del Rey, Whitehurst, Wughalter, & Barnwell, 1983). This is apparently because of the ecological differences between the perceptual and response requirements of the natural tasks and the simplistic linear motion and push-button responses used in most laboratory coincidence-timing tasks. The coupling of perceptual and motor information in coincidence-timing tasks appears to be very task-specific. For example, despite the presence of pronounced individual differences on natural tasks such as catching (e.g., Fischman & Schneider, 1985) these differences are not necessarily predictable from specific sport skill (Whiting, Alderson, & Sanderson, 1973; Whiting, Savelsbergh, & Faber, 1988). There has been surprisingly little work on expert-novice differences specifically in the perception/estimation of t_c although Cavallo and Laurent (1988) have recently shown that systematic differences in t_c estimation exist between experienced and beginner drivers. Accounting for expertise and learning effects must be an important pre-requisite for any consolidated theory of how t_c is picked up and processed.

POTENTIAL MECHANISMS FOR ACQUIRING TIME-TO-CONTACT INFORMATION

Contrasting Theories of Visual Perception

Two major theoretical positions have dominated research work in visual perception. The traditional computational (or indirect) perception theories and the ecological (or direct perception) theories differ in terms of their conception of the organisation of the visual system and how it functions in order to provide veridical information about the world. The descriptions of these theoretical positions that follow are necessarily brief and simplified ones and are written in a deliberate attempt to emphasise contrast and polarity. More detailed presentation of these contrasting viewpoints may be found by consulting the protagonistic works of Marr (1982) and Gibson (1979) (for the indirect and direct perception viewpoints respectively). The works of Ullman (1980) and Fodor and Pylyshyn (1981), from an indirect viewpoint, and Turvey (1977), Turvey, Shaw, Reed, & Mace (1981) and Michaels and Carello (1981), from a direct viewpoint, are central readings in these theoretical debates on visual perception.

Indirect (or Computational) Theories of Perception. The traditional view of visual perception has origins that go back at least to Descarte's Corporeal Ideas hypothesis (Reed, 1982). In its modern expression in the information processing model of cognitive psychology the indirect theories view perception as involving an elaborate series of computational processes that take a static, informationally-impoverished, retinal image and enhance it into a rich and accurate representation (or model) of the outside world. Retinal anatomy is such that the retinal image (the working origin for indirect theories of perception) cannot represent the outside world in a simple and precise manner (photoreceptors do not map onto optic nerve fibres in a simple one-to-one ratio, for example). The information leaving the retina via the optic nerve is therefore a mosaic of electrical intensities corresponding only approximately to the light intensities reaching the retina. The correspondence is not complete because the horizontal and amacrine cells act to enhance contrast in adjacent receptor fields. According to the traditional view the raw information carried by the optic nerve lacks the direct detail needed to specify objects in the visual field and to specify the kind of responses needed by the observer. Given the schism between the apparent imprecision of the retinal image and the accurate perception of the 'real world' that we all experience phenomenologically, traditional theorists have concluded that perception must be indirect, requiring substantial enhancement and mediation in the visual cortex through a complex set of computational processes. The performance of complex visual tasks, such as object or pattern recognition, has been seen as necessitating the comparison of current sensory information with templates of previously encountered objects and patterns stored in memory (e.g., Sutherland, 1973). This comparative process invokes the need for central *representation* as an essential feature of an all-encompassing theory of visual perception. Because perception, in its broadest sense, involves development of specific, higher-order knowledge about objects (e.g., the appreciation of the "meaning" in various art forms; Fodor & Pylyshyn, 1981), often not directly linked to the need to perform an immediate action or response, the traditional/indirect theory of visual perception is usually considered to reflect a cognitive perspective.

Because of the nature of the assumptions which underlie the indirect theories of perception, a research orientation is dictated which focuses upon the nature of the computational stages and upon the types of representations and storage needed for seeing to be possible. To this end Marr (1982; Marr & Poggio, 1977), one of the leading contemporary theorists in the computational theory of vision, has suggested that there are at least three levels of explanation (and analysis) which a consolidated theory of vision must address. At the most conceptual level (the *computational* level) an integrated theory of vision must be able to specify the task the visual system must complete, including description of the raw informational sources available to support the task. At the next *(algorithmic)* level, Marr has argued that theorists with a belief in indirect perception must attempt to determine *how* the information available in the retinal image can be processed to meet the computational needs of the task. It is at this level that the specific algorithms, processing mechanisms, and representations needed to solve the computational task have to be discovered and tested. At the *implementational* level the concern must be with the discovery of neural (physiological) mechanisms which allow the algorithms to function.

Research operating from within this indirect perception framework has tended to focus primarily at the algorithmic and implementational levels attempting to understand how systems like feature detectors operate in 'normal' vision (through studies of simple stimuli and illusions) and attempting to develop machine analogues to human vision. Recent advances in cognitive science, especially with the conceptual and software development of neural network and connectionist models (e.g., Hinton & Anderson, 1981; McClelland & Rumelhart, 1985), have provided a link between the algorithmic and implementational levels of analysis and a frontier for further development of the computational model. Parallel developments in the field of expert systems also provide a potential basis for accounting for the known improvements in perception that occur with the accumulation of task-specific experience and knowledge.

Direct Perception Theories. The direct perception view of vision is grounded in Gibson's (1961a, 1979) ecological optics and is thus also frequently referred to as the ecological perspective. The basic premise underlying the Gibsonian view is that the retinal image is not the starting point for seeing; rather the information needed to guide the observer's actions [2] is available in the structure of the light present at a point of observation. Direct perception theorists argue that the structure of the optic array (and the optic flow field generated by relative motion between the observer and objects within the environment) lawfully *specifies inter alia* the layout of the surrounding surfaces, the

---

[2] Within the Gibsonian view the function of perception is to guide action and perception may be defined in totality by this function.

observer's motion relative to those surfaces, and the nature of events occurring within the surrounds. This spatio-temporal information within the optic flow field in turn lawfully specifies the action/response required on the observer/actor's behalf (see Turvey & Carello, 1986). The direct perception perspective, therefore, views the perceptual information available at a point of observation not as static and impoverished but rather as dynamic, rich, and complete. Environmentally-generated optic flow fields and actor-generated dynamic force fields are viewed as causally linked in perception-action cycles (Kugler & Turvey,1987; Turvey, Carello, & Kim,1990) such that the laws of physics, which underlie and describe motion of all types, give rise to laws of ecological optics (for the perception of motion) and these in turn give direct rise to laws of control (specifying the observer/actor's response) (Warren, 1988, 1990). From within such a perspective invoking of internal representations is exchanged for a search for the lawful bases of perception-action systems.

In contrast to the views of computational theorists such as Marr (1982), the direct perception approach, therefore, only recognises effectively two levels of vision - an ecological level (roughly equivalent to Marr's computational level) and a physiological (implementational) level, with the research focus being actively at the first level.[3] The algorithmic level, the level at which any representational processes would exist, is eliminated from the direct perception approach. Opponents of the direct perception view (e.g., Ullman, 1980) have argued that failure to consider such an intermediate level of processing may prevent conceptual and physiological mechanisms being adequately linked, resulting in oversimplification of theory and loss of integral features for a consolidated theory of vision. Such criticisms are largely based on the putative role of representation in perception (e.g., see Bruce & Green, 1990, pp. 387-389 for an extended discussion of this with respect to the levels of analysis issue).

Research from within the direct perception perspective focuses upon the search for invariants within the optic flow field (and the flow fields of other modalities) capable of specifying the essential information to guide action - spatio-temporal invariants to specify direction, speed, and force (in actor-scaled units), and to identify objects and events and the affordances they present for action. Such a focus encourages the use of natural experiments, where the maintenance of the functional links between perception and action is of paramount importance (Lee & Thomson, 1982). Direct perception research also frequently uses the methods from comparative biology and mathematical analyses of optic flow field characteristics (e.g., Warren, 1988, 1990). Evolution is frequently presented as the principal basis for the development of

[3] See Runeson (1977) for a formal statement of this from a direct perception perspective.

specific attunement to optic flow features and hence for learning (Michaels & Carello, 1981). This is in keeping with a fundamental philosophical (and analytical) tenet of ecological realism (Lombardo, 1987) and observer-environment synergy rather than dualism.

Difficult Problems for the Competing Theories. Philosophically the most difficult problem for the indirect theories of visual perception is in explaining veridicality when the perceiver and environment are mutually exclusive entities. Mechanically the most difficult problem for the indirect theories appears to be the sheer computational complexity of existing algorithmic solutions to normal vision. This complexity is (apparently) incongruous with the speed and attention-free nature of the personal experience of normal vision. Recent advances in cognitive science suggest that the computational problems may disappear as more suitable general-purpose algorithms are developed and hardware more closely approximating the potential computational power of the human visual system is developed. The concern remains, however, as to the arbitrary nature of any proposed representations and computations. Ensuring that potentially workable machine solutions to vision are *the* solutions used by biological systems will be a persistently vexing and crucial issue.

The difficult problems for the direct/ecological theories of perception appear to relate to accounting for learning effects without recourse to a memory structure and accounting for the perception of more complex, culturally-determined acts for which conscious knowledge acquisition, storage and representation seems necessary (Bruce & Green, 1990; Fodor & Pylyshyn, 1981). Little advance has also yet been made by direct perceptionists on the implementational level question of accounting for how important invariants are actually picked up (Epstein, Hughes, Schneider, & Bach-y-Rita, 1989).

Reminiscent of the 'motor systems'-'action systems' debates in motor control (Beek & Meijer, 1988; van Wieringen, 1988), each of these contrasting views on visual perception are potentially complementary. In particular, accepting the presence of some form of representation may remove many of the difficult problems facing the direct perception view while recognising the extent of the information contained in reflected light may help alleviate some of the difficulties related to computational workload in the traditional theory. Although some hybrid theories of vision have been presented viewing the differences between the existing theories as largely a levels of analysis problem (e.g., see Ullman, 1980; Young, 1988) consensus on a theory of vision which integrates the direct and indirect approaches is unlikely given the deep philosophical differences which exist between the two positions (cf. Abernethy & Sparrow, Chapter 1, this volume).

Contrasting Views on the Perception of Change

Any theory of visual perception must be capable of explaining how humans (and other animals) perceive both change and non-change in their surrounding environment (Shaw & Pittenger, 1978). The study of the perception of change primarily involves the study of the perception of events. An event is definable as "... a minimal change of some specified type ... wrought over an object or object complex within some determinate region of the space-time continuum" (Shaw & Pittenger, 1978, p. 189). Early interest in explaining the perception of events arose primarily out of studies of motion (Mace, 1985) with more recent interest in events per se arising out of Johansson's (1973) demonstration of the essential role of time in the perception of events of biological significance. This element of time distinguishes events from other purely spatial aspects of perception (Warren & Shaw, 1985). It is of central significance in the performance of coincidence-timing skills.

Theories accounting for change vary according to their compatibility with the more general theories of visual perception. Thus both traditional (indirect) and direct accounts of the perception of change are available (Shaw & Pittenger, 1978).

The Traditional, Indirect View of the Perception of Change. The traditional view of the perception of change is the 'image-comparison model' in which changes in spatial structure (or displacement) from one retinal image to another are believed to provide the basis for the *inference* of motion and change. The image comparison model is an example of the general indirect theory of perception. The determination of change involves representational processes (the original/standard image must be somehow stored, represented, and retrieved from some kind of memory system). It is also dependent on the use of higher order cognitive processes, such as inference, to derive meaning from the nature of object and feature displacements from one retinal image to the next. The assumption of static images as the starting point for the perception of change and the reliance upon cognitive constructs, such as memory and inference, has made this traditional account untenable to theorists with a belief in direct perception.

The Direct View of the Perception of Change. The direct or ecological explanation of the perception of change is grounded in the belief that motion is perceived directly and is not inferred from changes in image displacement between retinal images at different times. The direct perception approach searches for invariants within the optic flow field which are able to specify directly those structural properties of an event that remain constant under conditions of change (so-called structural invariants) and those properties or styles of change which are characteristic of the particular event (so-called transformational invariants) (Pittenger & Shaw, 1975; see also Michaels & Carello, 1981 for examples). It is the possible existence and use of such invariants for specifying the t_c of approaching objects or surfaces which is of greatest interest in the context of this chapter.

Contrasting Accounts of the Visual Perception of Time-to-Contact

Distance/Velocity Computation. Information regarding t_c between the observer and approaching objects or surfaces may be potentially generated by computation of the ratio between the observer-object (or observer-surface) distance and the instantaneous relative velocity of the object or surface, i.e.,

$$t_c = \frac{\text{observer-object distance}}{\text{object approach velocity}}$$

(in the case where the observer is stationary and an object is approaching)

or

$$t_c = \frac{\text{observer-surface distance}}{\text{observer approach velocity}}$$

(in the case where a moving observer approaches a stationary surface).

As a range of cues for the estimation of both distance and velocity exist in most natural settings and as psychological studies of both distance estimation (e.g., Teghtsoonian & Teghtsoonian, 1969, 1970) and velocity estimation (e.g., Evans, 1970; Mashour, 1964; Salvatore, 1968) demonstrate that humans are capable of accurately extracting such information, a distance/velocity computation for detecting t_c appears possible. The presence of neurons in the visual cortex for judging motion in depth (Regan, Beverley, & Cynader, 1979) also provides some implementational level support for this particular algorithmic solution to the computation of t_c (cf. Marr, 1982). This particular approach to t_c determination is frequently referred to as the computational or cognitive approach (Cavallo & Laurent, 1988; Lee & Reddish, 1981; McLeod & Ross, 1983) although the latter term should not be misinterpreted to imply that these computational processes are accessible consciously (cf. Pylyshyn's 1984 notion of cognitive impenetrability).

Relative Distance Change Computation. Cavallo and Laurent (1988) have noted that an alternative computational solution to determining t_c may be derived by basing t_c estimates on distance changes (relative to the absolute observer-object distance) occurring over known time periods i.e.,

$$t_c = \frac{\text{observer-object distance at time 1}}{\text{(observer-object distance difference from time 1-time 2)/(time 1-time 2)}}$$

Cavallo and Laurent note that this method potentially simplifies the amount of data needed to be processed by removing the necessity to constantly assess observer-object distance in absolute terms. It does, however, add the necessity for accurate estimation of time change as a precursor for t_c determination. Access to the equivalent of a real time clock in the central nervous system is therefore essential for the effective functioning of such a procedure for t_c estimates.

Direct Perception Based on Optical Dilation. The potential for "looming" or optical dilation to signal information about the t_c of approaching objects or surfaces was first highlighted by Purdy (1958) and later Carel (1961) and Schiff (1965). In keeping with the strictest tenets of Gibson's (1961a, 1966, 1979) ecological optics, Lee (1974, 1976, 1980a, 1980b) has demonstrated mathematically, that, under conditions of constant approach velocity, t_c can be specified directly from a single parameter available within the optic flow field. This parameter, which Lee termed *tau*, is the inverse of the relative rate of increase in separation between the images of any two points on the approaching object or surface. i.e.,

$$t_c = \frac{\theta_1}{(\theta_2-\theta_1)(t_2-t_1)}$$

where θ_1 and θ_2 are angular separations of the two points on the image at times 1 and 2 (from McLeod & Ross, 1983).

Lee's (1974, 1976) original formulation of *tau* was with respect to a projection surface (at the plane of the retina) although equally and more generally the same property is available as a global property of the optic flow field.

Although formulated specifically with respect to object/surface contact or collision, *tau* is equally applicable in the more general case where any kind of approach relationship exists, including near miss trajectories where no collision occurs (Lee & Young, 1985; Schiff & Oldak, 1990), contact between objects located anywhere in any plane parallel to the plane of observation (i.e., parallel to the retinal plane to which *tau* is generally referenced) (Bootsma, 1988), and contact virtually anywhere within reach providing approach velocity is constant and the direction of the approach path and the interception point are precisely known (Tresilian, 1990). *Tau* has also been proposed as a categorical variable, its value specifying directly to the observer what type of action is needed. Examples have been provided for the use of values of *tau* and *tau* derivatives in determining whether to move forward or to move back to catch a fly ball (Todd, 1981; Turvey & Carello, 1988), to brake or not when driving a motor vehicle (Lee, 1976), to lengthen or shorten stride length to a take-off point (Warren & Kelso, 1985), and to adjust gait or flight to ensure a 'soft' or 'hard' collision (Kim, Turvey, & Carello, 1989; Kugler, Turvey, Carello, & Shaw, 1985; Warren, 1988). (See Solomon, Carello, & Turvey, 1984 for a synthesis). The *tau notio*n is attractive to believers in direct perception because it allows visual support for a whole range of coincidence-timing skills to be provided without the need for cognitive mediation and hence without the imposition of a large computational load on the observer.

There are a number of theoretical lines of argument favouring the *tau* method over the distance/velocity alternative. Among the most convincing is the demonstration that the computation of t_c from monocular distance and velocity requires the exploitation of the same velocity field equations which (earlier) specify t_c through *tau* (Todd, 1981; Tresilian, 1990). Excessive computation to reach a solution already available from component equations appears unduly cumbersome and improbable given the normal parsimony and efficiency which characterises biological processes. Moreover the fewer component processes/computational steps needed to gain a solution the lower is the probability of random error contamination (McLeod, McLaughlin, & Nimmo-Smith, 1986). Tresilian (1990) points out, quite rightly, that detail is sorely lacking for the distance/velocity model as to how the raw distance and velocity information might be picked-up or determined or indeed why absolute distance or velocity information might be of any ecological significance. The exploitation of absolute distance and velocity information seems improbable given the demonstrated superiority of relative over absolute judgments of velocity (Kaufman, 1974; Regan, 1986) and the ready availability of relative but not absolute distance information through the use of ecological scales, such as those provided by eye height (Mark, 1987; Sedgwick, 1973). The next section reveals, however, that the empirical evidence for *tau* utilisation in preference to absolute or relative distance/velocity computations is somewhat less convincing than the theoretical arguments.

Before proceeding to empirical examinations of the competing explanations of t_c pick-up, a caution is necessary against attempting to use the pick-up of t_c as a 'test case' for the efficacy of the more general direct and indirect theories of visual perception. *Tau* has been formulated by theorists with the Gibsonian direct perception view of vision in mind. We have represented *tau* (correctly we believe) as an ecological perspective explanation of t_c perception. However, it remains possible for t_c to be computed using *tau* as the algorithmic level solution (e.g., Buxton & Buxton, 1983). Arguments have been presented to consider *tau,* using the jargon of cognitive psychology, as an 'informationally encapsulated' processor (after Fodor, 1983; see McLeod et al., 1986) embedded within a larger information-processing system. More general arguments have been presented to consider direct perception as an important component (but a component nevertheless) of broader, hybrid views of visual perception (Ullman, 1980). Such a possibility prevents the achievement of clear theoretical resolution and consensus regarding the nature of the visual perception of t_c.

EMPIRICAL TESTS OF MECHANISMS FOR ACQUIRING TIME-TO-CONTACT INFORMATION

Testable Predictions from a Distance/Velocity Computational Model

Most empirical tests of the distance/velocity computational model are based on the assumption that any factor which changes the availability of either distance or velocity cues (and hence which changes the accuracy of the judgment of distance and velocity) should, in turn, systematically influence t_c judgments and coincidence-timing performance.

The Availability of Binocular Cues for Distance Should Enhance Coincidence-Timing Performance. In normal binocular viewing by humans the overlap in the visual fields of the left and right eyes provides a stereoscopic basis for depth and distance perception. Binocular disparity is one of the more powerful information sources for the perception of distance to the extent that disruption to binocular viewing generally causes decrements in distance perception accuracy. An additional advantage of binocular vision is that comparison of the relative velocity of the two retinal images also provides valuable and precise information with regard to the direction of motion in depth (Beverley & Regan, 1973; Regan, Beverley & Cynader, 1979). McLeod et al. (1986) reasoned that if t_c information was dependent on the pre-existence of distance information then performance on coincidence-timing tasks should be impaired if subjects are required to perform the task monocularly rather than binocularly. Conversely if t_c is picked up directly from optical 'looming', as proposed in Lee's (1976) *tau*, then this information should be equally accessible to one eye as to two and coincidence-timing performance under monocular and binocular conditions should be equivalent. Such equivalence can only be expected however if the coincidence-timing task does not involve spatial (directional) uncertainty.

McLeod et al. (1986) compared the monocular-binocular performance of subjects on two different coincidence-timing tasks. In the first, squash balls were dropped vertically toward the subjects, who were required to strike them at targets using bats of varying widths. In the second, balls were projected horizontally across the subjects' visual fields and they were required to coincide a button-press response with the arrival of the ball at a given spatial location. The first task consisted primarily of temporal uncertainty. Subject performance, as assessed from the percentage of successful hits, was not significantly different between the monocular and binocular viewing conditions. A binocular advantage was found on the second task containing both spatial and temporal uncertainty. This led McLeod et al. to conclude that information about binocular displacement plays an essential role in the judgment of the direction of object flight but is non-essential for the judgment of t_c. Comparison between the two conditions, however, may be unjustified given the uncoupling of the natural links between perception and action in the second task (Bootsma, 1989; von Hofsten, 1987).

Abernethy and Crassini (1989) attempted to replicate the McLeod et al. (1986) findings with respect to monocular-binocular equivalence using a coincidence-timing task in which absolutely no spatial uncertainty existed.[4] Apparent motion of between 2.24 $m.s^{-1}$ (5 mph) and 8.94 $m.s^{-1}$ (20 mph) was presented to subjects down a 4.30 m runway and subjects were required to make a thumb-press response to coincide with the 'object's' arrival at the end of the runway. The accuracy of this response was measured. Consistent with the findings of McLeod et al., equivalent coincidence-timing accuracy (as assessed from absolute error) and consistency (as assessed from variable error) were obtained over monocular and binocular viewing. Under monocular viewing, however, subjects systematically made more late responses than they did under binocular viewing, suggesting that deprivation of binocular disparity information causes subjects to slightly but systematically over-estimate tc.[5] Although monocular and binocular performance may appear equivalent in terms of overall accuracy these differences in response bias suggest that different ways of obtaining t_c information may be used under the different viewing conditions.

Contrary to the conclusions of monocular-binocular equivalence reported by McLeod et al. (1986) a number of recent studies in naturalistic settings point

---

[4] Mcleod et al's. first experiment included not only temporal uncertainty but also some spatial uncertainty. The presence of a trend (albeit a non-significant one) in the direction of superior binocular performance on this task meant that it was impossible to determine whether this was a consequence simply of score variability, a consequence of binocular superiority for spatial judgments, or a consequence of a possible binocular advantage for temporal judgments.

[5] Comparisons with the McLeod et al. study cannot be made here because their measure of performance did not consider the direction or type of timing erors made.

towards a binocular advantage, and hence toward tentative support for a computational explanation of t_c determination. In recent studies of catching within our laboratory (Abernethy, Neal, Burgess-Limerick, & Moran, 1990) binocular vision has been shown to provide subjects with an advantage not only with respect to the determination of object direction (as determined from the frequency of positioning errors of the hand) but also with respect to the determination of t_c (as determined from the frequency of grasp errors; cf. Smyth & Marriott, 1982). Cavallo and Laurent (1988), conducted a study in which passengers in a car were required to estimate t_c to a stationary object under conditions of visual occlusion. They observed a binocular superiority which persisted across two different levels of driver/observer experience. Bootsma and van Wieringen (1988) suggest that the deprivation of binocular disparity information may not only influence perception of t_c but that this altered perception may, in turn, directly influence motor properties of the coincidence-timing response. In their study a table tennis player produced slower and longer duration bat downswings under monocular viewing conditions than under binocular viewing conditions. The apparent binocular advantage revealed in many of these field tests may relate to improved distance information (from binocular disparity) although it may be, to some extent, a function of the availability of information binocularly for the detection of motion in depth (Regan et al., 1979) and for the determination of image concordance rather than disparity (Jones & Lee, 1981).

Monocular-binocular tests of t_c mechanisms must necessarily be non-determinant for two reasons. Firstly, the presence of a binocular advantage cannot be definitive evidence for the distance/velocity computational model because binocular vision provides useful information other than that related to the perception of distance. Any binocular advantage may, therefore, be potentially due to the utility of binocular concordance or motion in depth information in t_c judgment and not necessarily due to the facilitation of distance judgment. Secondly, in the event of monocular-binocular equivalence, the distance/velocity computational method cannot be discarded because of the presence of a number of monocular sources of distance information (e.g., texture gradient, background occlusion, accommodative effort), which remain operative when binocular vision is prevented. The presence of a large range of non-stereoscopic animals, such as birds, clearly capable of accurate coincidence-timing judgments (e.g., see Lee & Reddish, 1981) highlights this difficulty and the necessarily non-definitive nature of monocular-binocular comparisons. As Regan and his colleagues have demonstrated (Regan, 1986; Regan & Beverley, 1979) the fundamental differences between monocular and binocular vision are not simple, displaying both substantial individual differences and dependence upon the size and velocity of the object being viewed.

The Availability of Background Features to Enhance Distance Perception Should Enhance Coincidence-Timing Performance. Monocular judgments of distance are generally believed to be influenced by the nature of the surrounding terrain and background with distance perception of objects being altered by the presence or absence of featured (contoured) backgrounds (Hell & Freeman, 1977) and the availability of any external frames of reference. If background texture indeed influences distance perception (see Harvey & Michon, 1974 for some contradictory findings), and if t_c is computed using distance perception as a component then the provision of a textured background should affect the accuracy of t_c estimates. Conversely if t_c is derived from *tau* the nature of the background information should not influence t_c estimates.

Schiff and Detwiler (1979) examined this notion by having both square objects and motor vehicles filmed as they moved on an approach course towards the subject with the nature of the background varied. The objects "approached" at different velocities and the subject's task was to predict, during a period of stimulus occlusion, the exact time of arrival of the object. Schiff and Detwiler found that the estimation of t_c was no different for plain backgrounds (providing few sources of distance information) than for gridded backgrounds (providing enhanced information about distance), arguing against the use of distance information in t_c judgments.

In more recent studies on ball catching Savelsbergh and Whiting (1988) confirmed that the presence of an external frame of reference (in this case a vertical string hung in the subject's field of view) had no enhancing influence on catching performance, as assessed by the number of successful catches and the frequency of temporal and spatial errors. Savelsbergh and Whiting did, however, observe that the loss of background information which occurs when catching in the dark (but with the ball and hand illuminated) disrupts coincidence-timing performance. The number of temporal errors in the catching action increased from the environmentally illuminated to the environmentally dark conditions. As the optical looming caused by the approaching ball is identical in both instances *tau* alone seems an inadequate explanation, in this case, of the pick-up of t_c information for catching. Disruptions to the perception of depth caused by stimulus-background contrast differences between the illuminated and dark conditions (cf. Koslow, 1985) provide a potential explanation of the differences observed.

Clearly there is equivocal evidence with respect to the role of background feature information in coincidence-timing both within and between the existing studies. Whether or not the nature of the background affects coincidence-timing performance appears to depend very specifically on the type of background information provided (or deprived) and the nature of the interception task (especially whether the object is viewed continuously to interception or not).

Viewing Positions Which Enhance the Judgment of Distance and Velocity Should Enhance Coincidence-Timing Performance. At relatively long observer-target distances the optical size changes associated with a moving object or surface are small. In such cases changes in distance and/or velocity of the object or surface are more readily detected (at least in terms of visual thresholds) when the observer is positioned side-on to the direction of motion (i.e., when the motion traverses the visual field) than when the observer is positioned front-on to the direction of motion and the image expands radially as the object or surface approaches. With respect to the visual judgments required in driving a motor vehicle, for example, Hills (1980, p. 201) has noted that

> ...the same physical displacement of a vehicle has a much greater visual effect tangentially than longitudinally. For example, consider a small car, a mini, at a distance of 100 m. If it moves 10 m directly towards an observer, its visual diameter increases by 1 min of arc. On the other hand, a lateral movement of 10 m by the car would result in a visual movement of 170 min arc across the background against which it is seen; it would only have to move 6 cm laterally for a movement of 1 min arc.

If the perception of changes in object distance and velocity is enhanced by a side-on (rather than a front-on) viewing position and if t_c is computed using distance and velocity, then the accuracy of t_c judgments should also be enhanced by side-on viewing. Schiff and Oldak (1990) had subjects predict the time of contact between simulated 'cars' and a barrier under conditions where the approach was seen from front-on, from side-on, or from a viewing angle of 45°. Subjects' estimates of t_c (made over either a 3 or 6 s period of stimulus occlusion immediately prior to contact) were most accurate under the side-on viewing conditions and least accurate under the front-on viewing conditions. This is consistent with computation of t_c from distance and velocity information.

Such findings do not appear generalisable, however. Differences in the accuracy of judging changes in velocity from front-on and side-on viewing positions disappear (Shea & Northam, 1982) when tasks are used in which the observer-target distances are relatively small, the total time to perform the task is reduced to milliseconds rather than seconds, and continuous viewing of the approaching stimulus is available. When coincidence-timing responses are required on tasks in which apparent motion is generated with velocities in the range of 2.24-6.71 $m.s^{-1}$ (5-15 mph) and over viewing times of 320-960 ms coincidence-timing accuracy is generally found to be superior from front-on rather than side-on viewing positions (Abernethy, Crassini, & Burgess, 1989; Payne, 1987). This is contrary to the predictions of a distance/velocity model. Such an observation is more consistent with a *tau* model of t_c and will be discussed in further detail in the next section in which the evidence for *tau* is reviewed. It is difficult to know at this point whether the differences between the findings of Schiff & Oldak (1990) and those of Abernethy et al. (1989) and

Payne (1987) are a function of differences in the nature of the coincidence-timing task (prediction from continuous viewing versus prediction during a period of stimulus occlusion) or differences in the magnitude of the t_c used (ms vs s).

In Cases Where the Observer/Actor Approaches a Stationary Object or Surface, Disruption to Sources of Information for the Perception of Self Velocity Should Detract From Coincidence-Timing Performance. When an observer/actor approaches a stationary object or surface (as in the case of Lee et al.'s (1982) long jumpers or Warren et al's (1986) runners) the computational model for t_c would predict that any loss of information for judging ego-velocity should result in a decrement in coincidence-timing performance. The peripheral visual field (or ambient vision as it is known within the two modes of processing notion, e.g., Leibowitz & Post, 1982) is generally believed to provide the majority of information for determining one's rate of locomotion through the environment (e.g., Brandt, Dichgans, & Koenig, 1973; Dichgans & Brandt, 1978; Paillard, 1980). If this velocity information is used to determine t_c then reduction of the peripheral visual range, using restrictive goggles for example, should disrupt coincidence-timing accuracy.

In support of the computational model, Groeger and Brown (1988) found that restricting the visual field from 40° to 10° resulted in an increase in error on a t_c estimation task. Likewise, Cavallo and Laurent (1988), in a study in which passengers in a car had to predict t_c with a stationary obstacle, found that restricting the visual field to only the 10° of vision around the line of sight produced a decrement in the estimation of t_c for beginner drivers but did not affect the performance of experienced drivers. This suggests that beginner drivers may be dependent on extracting velocity from the optic flow field for use as a component in t_c estimation (as predicted from the traditional computational model). The experienced drivers, however, do not appear to independently pick-up velocity information although their apparent sensitivity to distance information (as indicated by significant binocular-monocular performance differences) perhaps suggests that these drivers may be using the alternative computational method based on *distance change* information.

Like many of the predictions which have been examined, however, the evidence regarding the importance of ego-velocity information for t_c estimates is equivocal. Laurent, Paul, and Cavallo (1988) found that visual field restriction did not impair the ability of runners to adjust their gait patterns in order to produce accurate footfall placements. Decorrelation of peripheral vision (achieved by presenting an optic flow rate beyond that which is generated through self motion alone) did, however, produce gait control changes. Laurent et al. suggested that speed information is actively used in adjusting stride length although such information is not essential; alternative means for accurately picking up t_c information being available in the absence of reliable information about ego-velocity. Laurent et al. (1989) found that restricting the visual field of horse riders to 15° did not significantly affect the rider's regulation of the horse's stride as it approached a jump. Situation specificity and the mediating effect of expertise appear to prevent unequivocal support or rejection of the computational derivation of t_c.

Individual Differences in Distance and Velocity Judgment Should Be Predictive of Skill in Estimating Time-to-Contact. If t_c is computed from distance/velocity ratios then individual differences in the perception of distance and velocity should relate strongly to performance on tasks requiring the use of t_c information. In a recent study in our laboratory Brown (1988) correlated individual scores on a laboratory (Bassin) coincidence-timing task with performance on a standard depth perception task (using the Howard-Dolman apparatus) and on a measure of the difference limen for velocity (cf. Shea & Northam, 1982). Correlations between performance on the coincidence-timing task and both depth perception and velocity discrimination were of extremely low order with the depth perception and velocity perception skills accounting, on average, for less than 10% of the variance on the coincidence-timing task. Such observations are clearly contradictory to a model of t_c estimation in which the accurate perception of distance and velocity information is essential.

Increasing the Time to View Approaching Motion Should Enhance the Accuracy of Time-to-Contact Computation (Assuming Computational Time is a Concern). McLeod and Ross (1983) have suggested that if t_c is computed then restricting the time available to view approaching objects or surfaces (below a threshold level) might be expected to impair the accuracy with which t_c can be estimated. Their rationale for such a prediction was that the computational process must take a finite period to perform and if the viewing time is less than the time needed for computation, estimates of t_c will be necessarily inaccurate. McLeod and Ross found that, in a task in which subjects had to estimate t_c from a film of an approaching moving vehicle, viewing time had no influence on the accuracy of estimating t_c. In their study, however, the shortest viewing time was 2 s - an eternity at least in the world of machine computations where the typical time course for computations is more in the order of microseconds than seconds! When one considers the speed of computational processes running on machines with infinitesimal computational power compared to the human brain the difficulty (impossibility) of attempting to test computational models for t_c estimates using computational time as a limiting variable becomes apparent.

Testable Predictions from a Tau, Direct Perception Model

The Coincidence-Timing Responses Should Be Elicited By Optical Expansion in Absence of Distance/Velocity Changes. If a *tau*-based method for picking up t_c is viable observers must first and foremost be sensitive to information provided by optical expansion or 'looming'. Studies of human infants (Ball & Tronick, 1971; Bower, Broughton, & Moore, 1970; Dunkeld & Bower, 1980; Nanez, 1987; Yonas, 1981; Yonas et al., 1977) along with studies of the young of chickens (Fishman & Tallarico, 1961; Schiff, 1965; Tronick, 1967), turtles (Hayes & Saiff, 1967), monkeys (Schiff, Caviness, & Gibson, 1962), and crabs and frogs (Schiff, 1965) have all systematically revealed the presence of avoidance responses to optical expansion within two-dimensional displays. These responses which occur without any real change in observer-object distance or relative velocity are present essentially from birth and consequently appear to be 'hard-wired' into the visual system. These avoidance responses are only evoked by stimulus 'looming' (they are absent during stimulus contracture) but are present regardless of object shape, magnification rate, and the animal's degree of learning of the association between collision and pain responses (Schiff, 1965). Cortical cells have been located in some animal species which are maximally stimulated by 'looming' optical displays (e.g., Rauschecker, von Grünau, & Poulin, 1987).

Collectively these infant studies reveal that not only are humans and animals sensitive to 'looming' but such optical information is also apparently of immense biological significance, specifying, at the very least, impending collision and danger. Schiff (1965; Experiment 2) noted that, for chickens and crabs at least, rapid rates of expansion were associated with rapid avoidance responses and that the initiation of avoidance behaviours appeared tightly coupled to the time remaining before collision. This observation suggests, in concert with Lee's (1976) later formulation of *tau*, that the information provided by optical expansion specifies not only whether or not collision will occur but also t_c. The presence of alarm responses to 'looming' in animals that have never experienced collision argues firmly for sensitivity to retinal expansion cues being innate; a notion consistent with both the neural evidence (e.g., Rauschecker et al., 1987) and the behavioural evidence (e.g., von Hofsten, 1980, 1982, 1983, 1987) concerning the well developed coincidence-timing skills of human infants. The presence of sensitivity to 'looming' cues in infants and across a range of animal species suggests that this sensitivity is independent of the degree of cortical (and cognitive) development - a finding compatible with a direct perception model of t_c pick-up but incompatible with a computational model dependent on cognitive mediation. Human observers remain sensitive to optical expansion throughout the lifespan. Adult subjects are able to make accurate judgments about the respective t_c of pairs of 'objects' of different size, velocity, and starting distance even when the 'objects' under examination are simply squares on a two-dimensional computer screen (Todd, 1981). This sensitivity holds not only in central vision but also for presentations of optical expansion to the peripheral retina (Stoffgren & Riccio, 1990).

Coincidence-Timing Responses Should Be Geared Directly to Optical Expansion even When Optical Expansion Provides Non-Veridical Information. If *tau* indeed provides the t_c information upon which the timing of skilled actions is based then it should be possible to cause systematic alterations to the time of initiation of interceptive actions by varying directly the optical expansion information. Moreover, in situations where the optical information is non-veridical (and the distance/velocity information is veridical) systematic coincidence-timing errors should be introduceable (Beek, 1986).

In a clever test of this prediction of the *tau* model Savelsbergh, Whiting, and Bootsma (1991) created a somewhat unique situation where the *tau* and distance/velocity methods provided disparate estimates of t_c. Subjects were required to catch, in an otherwise dark room, three different types of luminous ball. Two of the balls were of fixed size (5.5 & 7.5 cm diameter) and the third was a deflating ball which reduced in size from 7.5 to 5.5 cm as it approached the subject. The ball which deflated while approaching provided the essential condition where optical expansion gave a non-veridical estimate of t_c, underestimating actual t_c. In keeping with the utilisation of *tau* rather than a continuous distance/velocity ratio the time of grasp initiation was significantly later for the deflating ball than for the balls of constant size. The same preferential reliance on *tau* rather than veridical distance/velocity information held for monocular and binocular viewing conditions, although the effect was more pronounced under the former condition. For the dark environment, low velocity conditions used in this experiment subjects demonstrated a clear reliance on *tau* rather than distance/velocity methods.

Coincidence-Timing Responses Should Be Most Accurate Under Conditions of Constant Approach Velocity. The estimate of actual t_c provided by *tau* (the inverse of the relative rate of retinal expansion) can only be exact when the rate of approach between the observer/actor and the approaching object or surface is constant. As constant approach velocities are rare in nature *tau*-based estimates of t_c will necessarily contain some degree of imprecision. In particular, when an object is accelerating toward an observer (or vice versa) *tau* will over-estimate actual t_c whereas under conditions of deceleration *tau* will under-estimate actual t_c. The extent of this over- or under-estimation of actual t_c will depend on the duration of the activity. The error is least when actual t_c is relatively small and velocity at contact is high (Lee & Young, 1985). In studies on the wing-closing behaviour of plummeting gannets (Lee & Reddish, 1981) and on human subjects jumping to punch a dropped soccer ball (Lee,

Young, Reddish, Lough, & Clayton, 1983) the initiations of actions have been shown to be delayed until t_c reaches a critical value (or *tau* margin; Lee & Reddish, 1981) at which the inaccuracy in the *tau* estimate is minimal.

Under conditions where the approach velocity between the observer and the object or surface is constant, *tau* should provide an equally accurate estimate of t_c regardless of the absolute magnitude of $t_{c.}$ (Providing, of course, that the extent of retinal expansion is beyond threshold levels). Schiff and Detwiler (1979), however, have shown that when subjects are required to estimate the t_c of approaching objects (either squares or real cars shown on film) during a period of stimulus occlusion, actual t_c is systematically under-estimated. The extent of this under-estimation becomes progressively greater as actual t_c increases. Such observations are consistent with earlier ones made by Carel (1961) and have been since replicated in studies of t_c estimation by car drivers by McLeod and Ross (1983), Cavallo and Laurent (1988), and Schiff and Oldak (1990). McLeod and Ross (1983) and Schiff and Oldak (1990) have demonstrated that the extent of this under-estimation of actual t_c is greater in female than male subjects and Cavallo and Laurent (1988) have shown that the under-estimation is greater in beginners than experienced drivers.

It is worth noting that this systematic under-estimation of actual t_c has only thus far been demonstrated in "vanishing" studies (i.e., studies where continuous vision of the approaching object or surface is not provided) and in studies where the nature of the task dictates collision avoidance as a more desirable error than collision engineering. The under-estimation of t_c in such studies may, therefore, be interpretable in terms of the use of an inbuilt "margin-of-safety" (Gibson, 1961b; Hills, 1980), with beginner drivers and female subjects being more inclined to err on the conservative side than experienced drivers and male subjects. In any case the consistent nature of the under-estimation of t_c made in such tasks suggests that if *tau* is providing the basis for subjects' estimates of actual t_c (as the absence of distance enhancement effects in such studies might suggest; Schiff & Detwiler, 1979) *tau* must contain a proportional constant error of some type.

Coincidence-Timing Responses Should Be Most Accurate When Coincidence Has To Be Judged to the Frontal Eye Plane. Lee's (1976, 1980a) formulation of *tau* provides a direct estimate of actual t_c only under those conditions where the approaching object or surface is on a direct collision course with the observer or on a near miss path (von Hofsten & Lee, 1983). T_c is referenced specifically to the plane of observation (i.e., the frontal eye plane of the observer). In the case of directly approaching motion where coincidence needs to be made in front of the eye plane (e.g., in the case of catching a ball in front of the body with outstretched arms) t_c to the point of interception is not specified directly by *tau* and presumably information other than that provided by optical expansion is needed (cf. von Hofsten, 1987). Information about the time needed for the object to traverse the distance from the interception point to the frontal eye plane is necessary in such cases, as is the scaling of t_c information to the limb dimensions of the actor.

As *tau* only provides accurate t_c information to the frontal eye plane, if *tau* is the sole source of t_c information, coincidence timing accuracy should be directly related to the proximity of the plane of interception to the frontal eye plane. In a simple coincidence-timing experiment in our laboratory subjects viewed directly approaching apparent motion from a front-on position with the approach velocity varied from 2.24 to 6.71 $m.s.^{-1}$ (5-15 mph). The subject's task was to make a manual response to coincide with the arrival of the 'object' at a point 15 cm, 65 cm, or 115 cm forward of the plane of observation. Contrary to the expectations from a *tau*-based model of t_c estimation the proximity of the plane of coincidence to the frontal eye plane had no significant influence on the accuracy, consistency, or bias within the coincidence-timing responses.

Coincidence-Timing Responses Should Be Most Accurate When Judgments Have To Be Made of Approaching Rather Than Transverse Motion. The *tau* model predicts t_c should be more accurately picked up when the object or surface approaches the observer directly (giving rise to genuine optical expansion) than when the observer is viewing motion side-on and the image moves across the visual field rather than expanding. Studies involving continuous viewing of an approaching object have found that front-on viewing is superior to side-on viewing for coincidence-timing accuracy (Abernethy, Crassini, & Burgess, 1989; Payne, 1987). Such differences exist even though differences in sensitivity to velocity information are not apparent on the same type of task (cf. Shea & Northam, 1982) - a finding also consistent with the tau model. However, the differences in accuracy between front-on and side-on viewing positions are, while nevertheless significant, surprisingly small and arguably trivial (absolute error differences in the Payne and Abernethy et al. studies were in the order of only 5-10 ms). One reason that these differences may be as small as they are is that *tau* or *tau*-like information may in fact be available in both instances. Whereas the front-on viewing position provides t_c information through optical expansion in the classical *tau* sense (Lee, 1976), Bootsma (1988) has demonstrated that when two objects approach each other on a collision course on a plane parallel to the frontal eye-plane (as occurs in these side-on viewing manipulations) t_c may be specified by a *tau*-like optical parameter viz., the inverse of the relative rate of constriction of the optical gap separating, in this case, the moving object and the stationary target. Performance differences from front-on and side-on may, therefore, be simply due to subjects' greater experience with judging directly approaching motion; there being more front-on judgments of biological significance needed in 'real world' activities. Comparisons of timing accuracy between front-on and side-on viewing positions thus provide an inconclusive means of discriminating the *tau* and distance/velocity explanations of the pick-up of t_c information.

AN ATTEMPT AT SYNTHESIS AND SUMMARY

Unequivocal support for either the distance/velocity (computational) method or the *tau* (direct perception) method for extracting t_c information is not forthcoming from the literature. In part this equivocality may reflect the difficulty (perhaps impossibility) of empirical separation of the two approaches and the possibility that a levels of analysis argument can always be invoked to make key findings interpretable from either viewpoint (cf. Young, 1988). The overriding lack of uniformity and generalisability in the empirical findings and the apparently powerful effects of task specificity also suggest that, in part, the equivocal findings are a consequence of the range of different paradigms used to examine the efficacy of the respective t_c models. For example, whether or not the observer is provided with continuous vision of the approaching object or surface, or whether rather subjects are forced to estimate t_c over a period of stimulus occlusion appears to have a powerful influence on the conclusions which are reached. Bias in the direction of underestimation of actual t_c, for instance, is more apparent in studies using the 'vanishing' paradigm than studies allowing continuous viewing of the approaching motion. Likewise the duration of approaching motion which is available for detecting t_c appears to be important with the *tau* method more favoured in situations where t_c is short (Cavallo & Laurent, 1988) or avoidance is required (Schiff, 1965), while cognitive strategies seem more probable when estimates of t_c over periods of greater than a few seconds are required (Schiff, 1986, p. 258).

An important consideration in assessing the 'weight' which should be placed on any one piece of empirical research evidence must relate to the ecological validity of the experiment, i.e., the extent to which the experiment maintains normal rather than altered viewing conditions and the extent to which the coincidence-timing task involves the perception and the production of interceptive actions which are natural rather than simulated. Ecological validity is especially important in examining 'real-world' coincidence-timing skills because the use of artificial coincidence-timing tasks can substantially underestimate the coincidence-timing capabilities of subjects (e.g., see Ebbeson, Parker, and Konĕcni, 1971; von Hofsten, 1987; and especially Runeson, 1977). Mean timing errors on contrived laboratory coincidence-timing tasks are commonly in the order of 20-50 ms (e.g., Abernethy & Crassini, 1989; Blundell, 1984; Haywood, 1980; Payne, 1987) whereas performance on apparently more complex but natural hitting and catching actions occur within time windows in the order of 4-10 ms (Alderson, Sully, & Sully, 1974;

Bootsma & van Wieringen, 1990; McLeod et al., 1986; Tyldesley & Whiting, 1975).

Ecologically valid 'natural' experiments have been prompted more by a direct perception view of vision than by the traditional computational view. However, it needs to be noted that the interpretability of naturally occurring phenomena by direct perception notions is not necessarily disproof of the computational alternatives. Simulated laboratory coincidence-timing tasks may, in fact, interfere more with naturally available sources of distance and velocity information than they do with optical expansion information (Cavallo & Laurent, 1988). This may bias the interpretation of t_c extraction in the direction of supporting the ecological (*tau*) explanation rather than the traditional (distance/velocity) explanation. In either case implications to coincidence-timing in the 'real world' from studies using apparent motion need to be made cautiously given the specificity of subject responses to apparent motion (Allen & Kolers, 1981) and the specificity of perception-action couplings (Bootsma, 1989). In all types of coincidence-timing experiments close scrutiny also needs to be maintained over the movement (response) kinematics to ensure that any alterations to normal viewing conditions do not alter the characteristics of the ensuing action (cf. Bootsma & van Wierengen, 1988).

The only 'safe' conclusion available from the research evidence to date is that t_c estimation from distance/velocity computation and from *tau* does not fit a simple 'either-or' solution. The direct and computational methods appear to function rather in a complementary fashion (cf. Cavallo & Laurent, 1988; Laurent et al., 1988, 1989). Subjects use whatever information is available in the particular task setting. Humans appear to generally use distance and velocity information when such information is available (e.g., under conditions of binocular viewing or side-on observation) but are nevertheless capable of maintaining reasonable t_c estimates on the basis of *tau* when distance and velocity cues are reduced (e.g., under conditions of monocular viewing or viewing of two-dimensional displays). Situational context seems crucial. It appears, as Cutting (1986, p. 247) suggested , that:

> ...perceptual systems do their best in different ways under different circumstances ... perceptual systems may use different sorts of information at different times, even when performing the same apparent task and when all sources equally specify the object or event perceived.

Although *tau* is the generally favoured explanation of t_c pick-up in the literature[6], and the most direct empirical comparison of the two methods

---

[6] Much of the evidence frequently cited as supportive of *tau* (e.g., the Lee et al., 1982 study of long jumping; Wagners's 1982 study on the landing of house flies) is equally interpretable from a distance/velocity model. Studies frequently cited as evidence for *tau* are rather evidence for human sensitivity to t_c information rather

(Savelsbergh et al., 1991) supports preferential usage of *tau* over the distance/velocity method, it also appears true that *tau* is infrequently used alone. Reliable distance and speed information is also apparently generally used when available (Cavallo & Laurent, 1988; Laurent et al., 1988). Situations can be created where there is no optical expansion (i.e., where *tau* is ambiguous) yet accurate coincidence-timing performance is still possible. Von Hofsten (1987), for example, points out that it is possible to catch an object which circles the head at a constant radial distance from the eyes even though no 'looming' is provided by the object. In a similar vein it is apparent that in fast ball sports, for example, there is information available prior to the occurrence of ball flight (and hence prior to optical expansion information) which is useful in informing a skilled performer not only where but when the ball will arrive (Abernethy & Russell, 1987a). Such information available from the preparatory actions (postural configurations) of the opposing player is picked up better by experts than by novices (Abernethy, 1990; Abernethy & Russell, 1987b) and can be shown to be specified in the kinematics of the opponent's actions (Abernethy & Packer, 1989).

As is the case with other aspects of motor control and learning (see Abernethy & Sparrow, this volume) a central and as yet unresolved question with respect to coincidence-timing skills relates to accounting for the effects upon performance of observer characteristics such as gender and expertise. In particular the issue of *how* the well-documented improvements in t_c pick-up with practice proceed remains a vexing one. This issue appears as a potentially crucial one for testing not only the efficacy of the competing t_c models, but also, more generally, the efficiency of competing explanations of perceptual learning (cf. Gibson, 1969).

ACKNOWLEDGMENTS

Appreciation is expressed to Peter Beek for helpful comments on an earlier draft of this paper. Preparation of this manuscript was supported in part from funds available from Australian Research Council Grant No. A78832056 awarded to the first author and to Dr. R.J. Neal.

---

than any particular mechanism through which t_c may be extracted.

REFERENCES

Abernethy, B. (1984). Skill in cricket batting: Laboratory and applied evidence. In M.L. Howell, & B.D. Wilson (Eds.), *Proceedings of the VIIth Commonwealth and International Conference on Sport, Physical Education, Recreation and Dance, Vol. 7, Kinesiological Sciences*, Brisbane, September, 1982 (pp. 35-50). Brisbane: University of Queensland.

Abernethy, B. (1990). Expertise, visual search and information pick-up in squash. *Perception, 19*, 63-77.

Abernethy, B. & Crassini, B. (1989). Perception-action coupling in a simple coincidence-timing task. In D. Vickers, & P.L. Smith (Eds.), *Human information processing: Measures, mechanisms and models* (pp. 143-154). Amsterdam: Elsevier.

Abernethy, B., Crassini, B., & Burgess, R. (1989). Is there a dedicated processor for time-to-contact information? (Abstract). *International Journal of Neuroscience, 46*, 29.

Abernethy, B., Neal, R.J., Burgess-Limerick, R., & Moran, M. (1990, January). *The visual timing of skilled movements*. Paper presented at the Commonwealth and International Conference on Physical Education, Sport, Health, Dance, Recreation and Leisure, Auckland.

Abernethy, B., & Packer, S. (1989). Perceiving joint kinematics and segment interactions as a basis for skilled anticipation in squash. In C.K. Giam, K.K. Chook, & K.C. Teh (Eds.), *Proceedings of the 7th World Congress in Sport Psychology*, Singapore, (pp. 56-58). Singapore: International Society of Sport Psychology.

Abernethy, B., & Russell, D.G. (1987a). Expert-novice differences in an applied selective attention task. *Journal of Sport Psychology, 9*, 326-345.

Abernethy, B., & Russell, D.G. (1987b). The relationship between expertise and visual search strategy in a racquet sport. *Human Movement Science, 6*, 283-319.

Alderson, G.H.K., Sully, D.J., & Sully, H.G. (1974). An operational analysis of one-handed ball catching using high speed photography. *Journal of Motor Behavior, 6*, 217-226.

Allen, P.G., & Kolers, P. A. (1981). Sensory specificity of apparent motion. *Journal of Experimental Psychology: Human Perception and Performance, 7*, 1318-1326.

Ball, W. & Tronick, E. (1971). Infant responses to impending collision. *Science, 171*, 818-820.

Bard, C., Fleury, M., Carriére, L., & Bellec, J. (1981). Components of the coincidence-anticipation behavior of children aged from 6 to 11 years. *Perceptual and Motor Skills, 52*, 547-556.

Beek, P.J. (1986). Perception-action coupling in the young infant. In M.G. Wade & H.T.A. Whiting (Eds.), *Motor development in children: Aspects of co-ordination and control* (pp. 187-196). Dordrecht: Martinus Nijhoff.

Beek, P.J., & Meijer, O.G. (1988). On the nature of 'the' motor-action controversy. In O.G. Meijer, K. Roth (Eds.), *Complex movement behaviour: 'The' motor-action controversy* (pp. 157-185). Amsterdam: North-Holland.

Bernstein, N. (1967). *The coordination and regulation of movements*. Oxford: Pergamon Press.

Beverley, K.I., & Regan, D. (1973). Evidence for the existence of neuronal mechanisms selectively sensitive to the direction of movement in space. *Journal of Physiology*, *235*, 17-29.

Blundell, N.L. (1984). Critical visual-perceptual attributes of championship level tennis players. In M.L. Howell, & B.D. Wilson (Eds.), *Proceedings of the VIIth Commonwealth and International Conference on Sport, Physical Education, Recreation and Science. Vol. 7. Kinesiological Sciences* (pp. 51-59). Brisbane: University of Queensland.

Bootsma, R.J. (1988). *The timing of rapid interceptive actions*. Doctoral dissertation, Free University, Amsterdam: Free University Press.

Bootsma, R.J. (1989). Accuracy of perceptual processes subserving different perception-action systems. *Quarterly Journal of Experimental Psychology*, *41A*, 489-500.

Bootsma, R.J., & van Wieringen, P.C.W. (1988). Visual control of an attacking forehand drive in table tennis. In O.G. Meijer, & K. Roth (Eds.), *Complex movement behaviour: The 'motor-action' controversy* (pp. 189-199). Amsterdam: North-Holland.

Bootsma, R.J., & van Wieringen, P.C.W. (1990). Timing an attacking forehand drive in table tennis. *Journal of Experimental Psychology: Human Perception and Performance*, *16*, 21-29.

Bower, T.G.R., Broughton, J.M., & Moore, M.K. (1970). Infant responses to approaching objects: An indicator of response to distal variables. *Perception & Psychophysics*, *9*, 193-196.

Brandt, T., Dichgans, J., & Koenig, E. (1973). Differential effects of central versus peripheral vision on egocentric and exocentric motion perception. *Experimental Brain Research*, *16*, 476-491.

Brown, P.H. (1988). *Visual coincidence timing: An examination of two conflicting models through individual subject differences*. Unpublished Honours thesis, University of Queensland.

Bruce, R.D. (1966). *The effects of variations in ball trajectory upon catching performance of elementary school children*. Unpublished doctoral dissertation, University of Wisconsin, Madison.

Bruce, V., & Green, P. (1990). *Visual perception: Physiology, psychology and ecology* (2nd. ed.). London: Lawrence Erlbaum Associates.

Buekers, M., Pauwels, J., & Meugens, P. (1988). Temporal and spatial anticipation in twelve-year-old boys and girls. In A.M. Colley & J.R. Beech (Eds.), *Cognition and action in skilled behaviour* (pp. 283-292). Amsterdam: North-Holland.

Burgess-Limerick, R., Abernethy, B., & Neal, R.J. (1990). *Expertise and functional variability in the performance of a field hockey drive*. Manuscript submitted for publication.

Buxton, B.F., & Buxton, H. (1983). Monocular depth perception from optical flow by space-time signal processing. *Proceedings of the Royal Society of London: Series B, 217*, 27-47.

Carel, W.L. (1961). Visual factors in the contact analog. Publication R61ELC60, General Electric Company Advanced Electronics Center, Ithaca, NY.

Cavallo, V., & Laurent, M. (1988). Visual information and skill level in time-to-collision estimation. *Perception, 17*, 623-632.

Corcos, D.M., Agarwal, G.C., & Gottlieb, G.L. (1985). A note on accepting the null hypothesis: Problems with respect to the mass-spring and pulse-step models of motor control. *Journal of Motor Behavior, 17*, 481-487.

Cutting, J.E. (1986). *Perception with an eye for motion*. Cambridge, MA: MIT Press.

Del Rey, P., Whitehurst, M., Wughalter, E., & Barnwell, J. (1983). Contextual interference and experience in acquisition and transfer. *Perceptual and Motor Skills, 57*, 241-242.

Dichgans, J., & Brandt, T. (1978). Visual-vestibular interaction: Effects on self-motion and postural control. In R. Held, H.W. Leibowitz, & H.L. Teuber (Eds.), *Handbook of sensory physiology. Vol. III*. Heidelberg: Springer.

Dietz, V., & Noth, J. (1978). Pre-innervation and stretch responses of triceps brachii in man falling with and without visual control. *Brain Research, 142*, 576-579.

Dorfman, P.W. (1977). Timing and anticipation: A developmental perspective. *Journal of Motor Behavior, 9*, 67-79.

Dunham, P. (1977). Age, sex, speed and practice in coincidence-anticipation performance of children. *Perceptual and Motor Skills, 45*, 187-193.

Dunkeld, J., & Bower, T.G.R. (1980). Infant responses to impending collision. *Perception, 9*, 549-554.

Ebbesen, E.G., Parker, S., & Konĕcni, V.J. (1977). Laboratory and field analyses of decisions involving risk. *Journal of Experimental Psychology: Human Perception and Performance, 3*, 576-589.

Epstein, W., Hughes, B., Schneider, S., & Bach-y-Rita, P. (1989). Perceptual learning of spatio-temporal events: Evidence from an unfamiliar modality. *Journal of Experimental Psychology: Human Perception and Performance, 15*, 28-44.

Evans, L. (1970). Automobile speed estimation using movie film simulation. *Ergonomics*, *13*, 231-237.

Fischman, M.G., & Schneider, T. (1985). Skill level, vision, and proprioception in simple one-handed catching. *Journal of Motor Behavior*, *17*, 219-229.

Fishman, R., & Tallarico, R.B. (1961). Studies of visual perception: II. Avoidance reaction as an indicator response in chicks. *Perceptual and Motor Skills*, *12*, 251-257.

Fitch, H.L., Tuller, B., & Turvey, M.T. (1982). The Bernstein perspective: III. Tuning of coordinative structures with special reference to perception. In J.A.S. Kelso (Ed.), *Human motor behavior: An introduction* (pp. 271-281). Hillsdale, NJ: Lawrence Erlbaum Associates.

Fitts, P.M. (1954). The information capacity of the human motor system in controlling the amplitude of movement. *Journal of Experimental Psychology*, *47*, 381-391.

Fodor, J.A. (1983). *The modularity of mind: An essay on faculty psychology*. Cambridge, MA: MIT Press.

Fodor, J.A. & Pylyshyn, Z.W. (1981). How direct is visual perception? Some reflections on Gibson's "Ecological Approach". *Cognition*, *9*, 139-196.

Franks, I.M., Weicker, D., & Robertson, D.G.E. (1985). Kinematics, movement phasing and timing of a skilled action in response to varying conditions of uncertainty. *Human Movement Science*, *4*, 91-105.

Gentner, D.R. (1987). Timing of skilled motor performance: Tests of the proportional duration model. *Psychological Review*, *94*, 255-276.

Gibson, E.J. (1969). *Principles of perceptual learning and development*. New York: Appleton-Century-Crofts.

Gibson, J.J. (1961a). Ecological optics. *Vision Research*, *1*, 253-262.

Gibson, J.J. (1961b). The contribution of experimental psychology to the formulation of the problem of safety -- A brief for basic research. *Behavioral approaches to accident research* (pp. 77-89). New York: Association for the Aid of Crippled Children.

Gibson J.J. (1966). *The senses considered as perceptual systems*. Boston: Houghton-Mifflin.

Gibson, J.J. (1979). *The ecological approach to visual perception*. Boston: Houghton-Mifflin.

Groeger, J.A., & Brown, I.D. (1988). Motion perception is not direct with indirect viewing systems. In A.G. Gale et al. (Eds.), *Vision in vehicles II* (pp. 27-34). Amsterdam: North-Holland.

Harvey, L.O., Jr., & Michon, J.A. (1974). Detectability of relative motion as a function of exposure duration, angular separation, and background. *Journal of Experimental Psychology*, *103*, 317-325.

Hay, J.G. (1988). Approach strategies in the long jump. *International Journal of Sport Biomechanics*, *4*, 114-129.

Hayes, W.N., & Saiff, E.I. (1967). Visual alarm reactions in turtles. *Animal Behavior*, *15*, 102-108.

Haywood, K.M. (1980). Coincidence-anticipation across the life span. *Experimental Aging Research*, 6, 451-462.

Hell, W., & Freeman, R.B., Jr. (1977). Detectability of motion as a factor in depth perception by monocular movement parallax. *Perception & Psychophysics*, 22, 526-530.

Hills, B.L. (1980). Vision, visibility and perception in driving. *Perception*, *9*, 183-216.

Hinton, G.E., & Anderson, J.A. (Eds.) (1981). *Parallel models of associative memory*. Hillsdale, NJ: Lawrence Erlbaum Assoicates.

Hubbard, A.W., & Seng, C.N. (1954). Visual movements of batters. *Research Quarterly*, *25*, 42-57.

Isaacs, L. (1983). Coincidence-anticipation timing in simple catching. *Journal of Human Movement Studies*, *9*, 195-201.

Johansson, G. (1973). Visual perception of biological motion and a model for its analysis. *Perception & Psychophysics*, *14*, 201-211.

Jones, R.K., & Lee, D.N. (1981). Why two eyes are better than one: The two views of binocular vision? *Journal of Experimental Psychology: Human Perception and Performance*, 7, 30-40.

Kaufman, L. (1974). *Sight and mind: An introduction to visual perception*. New York: Oxford University Press.

Kay, H. (1969). The development of motor skills from birth to adolescence. In E.A. Bilodeau (Ed.), *Principles of skill acquisition* (pp. 33-57). New York: Academic Press.

Kelso, J.A.S. (1981). Contrasting perspectives on order and regulation in movement. In J. Long, & A. Baddeley (Eds.), *Attention and performance IX* (pp. 437-458). Hillsdale, NJ: Lawrence Erlbaum Associates.

Kim, N-G., Turvey, M.T., & Carello, C. (1989). Optical information for the prospective control of contacts with surrounding surfaces. *Perceiving-Acting Workshop Review*, *4*, 6-9 (Technical Report of the Center for the Ecological Study of Perception and Action, University of Connecticut, Storrs, CT).

Kugler, P.N., & Turvey, M.T.(1987). *Information, natural law and the self-assembly of rhythmic movements*. Hillsdale, NJ: Lawrence Erlbaum Associates.

Kugler, P.N., Turvey, M.T., Carello, C., & Shaw, R.E. (1985). The physics of controlled collisions: a reverie about locomotion. In W.H. Warren, Jr., & R.E. Shaw (Eds.), *Persistence and change* (pp. 195-229). Hillsdale, NJ: Lawrence Erlbaum Associates.

Laurent, M., Dinh Phung, R., & Ripoll, H. (1989). What visual information is used by riders in jumping? *Human Movement Science*, *8*, 481-501.

Laurent, M., Paul, P., & Cavallo, V. (1988). How is gait visually regulated when the head goes faster than the legs? *Journal of Motor Behavior, 20,* 301-316.

Lee, D.N. (1974). Visual information during locomotion. In R.B. MacLeod, & H.L. Pick, Jr. (Eds.), *Perception: Essays in honor of James J. Gibson* (pp. 250-267). Ithaca & London: Cornell University Press.

Lee, D.N. (1976). A theory of visual control of braking based on information about time-to-collision. *Perception, 5,* 437-459.

Lee, D.N. (1980a). Visuo-motor coordination in space-time. In G.E. Stelmach, & J. Requin (Eds.), *Tutorials in motor behavior* (pp. 281-295). Amsterdam: North-Holland.

Lee, D.N. (1980b). The optic flow field: The foundation of vision. *Philosophical Transactions of the Royal Society of London, 290,* 169-179.

Lee, D.N., Lishman, J.R., & Thomson, J.A. (1982). Regulation of gait in long jumping. *Journal of Experimental Psychology: Human Perception and Performance, 8,* 448-459.

Lee, D.N., & Reddish, P.E. (1981). Plummeting gannets: A paradigm of ecological optics. *Nature, 293,* 293-294.

Lee, D.N., & Thomson, J.A. (1982). Vision in action: The control of locomotion. In D.J. Ingle, M.A. Goodale, & R.J.W. Mansfield (Eds.), *Analysis of visual behavior* (pp. 411-433). Cambridge, MA: MIT Press.

Lee, D.N., & Young, D.S. (1985). Visual timing of interceptive action. In D. Ingle, M. Jeannerod, & D.N. Lee (Eds.), *Brain mechanisms and spatial vision* (pp. 1-30). Dordrecht: Martinus Nijhoff.

Lee, D.N., Young, D.S., Reddish, P.E., Lough, S., & Clayton, T.M.H. (1983). Visual timing in hitting an accelerating ball. *Quarterly Journal of Experimental Psychology, 35A,* 333-346.

Leibowitz, H.W., & Post, R.B. (1982). The two modes of processing concept and some implications. In J.Beck (Ed.), *Organization and representation in perception* (pp. 343-363). Hillsdale, NJ: Lawrence Erlbaum Associates.

Lombardo, T.J. (1987). *The reciprocity of perceiver and environment: The evolution of James J. Gibson's ecological psychology.* Hillsdale, NJ: Lawrence Erlbaum Associates.

Mace, W.M. (1985). Johansson's approach to visual event perception - Gibson's perspective. In W.H. Warren, Jr., & R.E.Shaw (Eds.), *Persistence and change* (pp. 55-65). Hillsdale, NJ: Lawrence Erlbaum Associates.

Mark, L.S. (1987). Eyeheight scaled information about affordances: A study of sitting and stair climbing. *Journal of Experimental Psychology: Human Perception and Performance, 13,* 361-370.

Marr, D. (1982). *Vision: A computational investigation into the human representation and processing of visual information.* San Francisco: W.H. Freeman & Co.

Marr, D., & Poggio, T. (1977). From understanding computation to understanding neural circuitry. *Neuroscience Research Program Bulletin, 15*, 470-488.

Mashour, M. (1964). *Psychophysical relations in the perception of velocity*. Stockholm: Almqvist & Wiksell.

McClelland, J.L., & Rumelhart, D.E. (1985). Distributed memory and the representation of general and specific information. *Journal of Experimental Psychology: General, 114*, 159-188.

McLeod, P., McLaughlin, C., & Nimmo-Smith, I. (1986). Information encapsulation and automaticity: Evidence from the visual control of finely timed actions. In M.I. Posner, & O. Marin (Eds.), *Attention and performance XI* (pp. 391-406). Hillsdale, NJ: Lawrence Erlbaum Associates.

McLeod, R.W., & Ross, H.E. (1983). Optic-flow and cognitive factors in time-to-collision estimates. *Perception, 12*, 417-423.

Meeuwsen, H., & Magill, R.A. (1987). The role of vision in gait control during gymnastics vaulting. In T.B. Hoshizaki, J.H. Salmela, & B. Petiot (Eds.), *Diagnostics, treatment and analysis of gymnastic talent* (pp. 137-155). Montreal: Sport Psyche Editions.

Michaels, C.F., & Carello, C. (1981). *Direct perception*. Englewood Cliffs, NJ: Prentice-Hall.

Nanez, J.E. (1987). *Perception of impending collision in 3- to 6-week old infants*. Doctoral dissertation, University of Minnesota.

Paillard, J. (1980). The multi-channeling of visual cues and the organization of a visually guided response. In G.E. Stelmach, & J. Requin (Eds.), *Tutorials in motor behavior* (pp. 259-279). Amsterdam: North-Holland.

Patla, A.E. (1989). In search of laws for the visual control of locomotion: Some observations. *Journal of Experimental Psychology: Human Perception and Performance, 15*, 624-628.

Patla, A.E., Robinson, C., Samways, M., & Armstrong, C.J. (1989). Visual control of step length during overground locomotor: Task-specific modulation of the locomotor synergy. *Journal of Experimental Psychology: Human Perception and Performance, 15*, 603-617.

Payne, V.G. (1986). The effect of stimulus runway length on coincidence-anticipation timing performance. *Journal of Human Movement Studies, 12*, 289-295.

Payne, V.G. (1987). Effects of angle of stimulus approach on coincidence-anticipation timing performance. *Journal of Human Movement Studies, 13*, 383-390.

Pittenger, J.B., & Shaw, R.E. (1975). Aging faces as viscal-elastic events: Implications for a theory of non-rigid shape perception. *Journal of Experimental Psychology: Human Perception and Performance, 1*, 374-382.

Purdy, W.C. (1958). *The hypothesis of psychophysical correspondence in space perception*. Unpublished doctoral dissertation, Cornell University.

Pylyshyn, Z.W. (1984). *Computation and cognition: Toward a foundation for cognitive science*. Cambridge, MA: MIT Press.

Rauschecker, J.P., von Grünau, M.W., & Poulin, C. (1987). Centrifugal organization of direction preferences in the cat's lateral suprasylvian visual cortex and its relation to flow field processing. *Journal of Neuroscience*, *7*, 943-958.

Reed, E. (1982). Descartes' corporeal hypothesis and the origin of scientific psychology. *Review of Metaphysics*, *35*, 731-752.

Regan, D. (1986). The eye in ballgames: hitting and catching. In *Proceedings of conference on vision and sport* (pp. 7-32). Haarlem: De Vriesenborch.

Regan, D., & Beverley, K. (1979). Binocular and monocular stimuli for motion-in-depth, changing-disparity and changing-size inputs feed the same motion-in-depth stage. *Vision Research*, *19*, 1331-1342.

Regan, D., Beverley, K., & Cynader, M. (1979). The visual perception of motion in depth. *Scientific American*, *241*, 122-133.

Rosengren, K.S., Pick, H.L., & von Hofsten, C. (1988). Role of visual information in ball catching. *Journal of Motor Behavior*, *20*, 150-164.

Runeson, S. (1977). On the possibility of "smart" perceptual mechanisms. *Scandinavian Journal of Psychology*, *18*, 172-179.

Salvatore, S. (1968). The estimation of vehicular velocity as a function of visual stimulation. *Human Factors*, *10*, 27-32.

Savelsbergh, G.J.P., & Whiting, H.T.A. (1988). The effect of skill level, external frame of reference and environmental changes on one-handed catching. *Ergonomics*, *31*, 1655-1663.

Savelsbergh, G.J.P., Whiting, H.T.A., & Bootsma, R.J. (1991). 'Grasping' tau. *Journal of Experimental of Psychology: Human Perception and Performance*, *17*, 315-322.

Schiff, W. (1965). Perception of impending collision: A study of visually directed avoidant behavior. *Psychological Monographs: General and Applied*, *79*, Whole No. 604.

Schiff, W. (1986). *Perception: An applied approach*. Acton, MA: Copley.

Schiff, W., Caviness, J.A., & Gibson, J.J. (1962). Persistent fear responses in rhesus monkeys to the optical stimulus of 'looming'. *Science*, *136*, 982-983.

Schiff, W., & Detwiler, M.L. (1979). Information used in judging impending collision. *Perception*, *8*, 647-658.

Schiff, W., & Oldak, R. (1990). Accuracy of judging time-to-arrival: Effects of modality, trajectory, and gender. *Journal of Experimental Psychology: Human Perception and Performance*, *16*, 303-319.

Sedgwick, H. (1973). The visible horizon: A potential source of visual information for the perception of size and distance. *Dissertations Abstract International*, *34*, 1301B-1302B. (University Microfilms No. 73-22530).

Shaw, R.E., & Pittenger, J. (1978). Perceiving change. In H.L. Pick & E. Saltzman (Eds.), *Modes of perceiving and processing information* (pp. 187-204). Hillsdale, NJ: Lawrence Erlbaum Associates.

Shea, C.H., & Northam, C. (1982). Discrimination of visual linear velocities. *Research Quarterly for Exercise and Sport*, *53*, 222-225.

Sidaway, B., McNitt-Gray, J., & Davis, G. (1989). Visual timing of muscle preactivation in preparation for landing. *Ecological Psychology*, *1*, 253-264.

Smyth, M.M., & Marriott, A.M. (1982). Vision and proprioception in simple catching. *Journal of Motor Behavior*, *14*, 143-152.

Solomon, J., Carello, C., & Turvey, M.T. (1984). Flow fields: The optical support for skilled activities. In W.F. Straub & J.M. Williams (Eds.), *Cognitive sport psychology* (pp. 129-139). Lansing, NY: Sport Science Assocs.

Spaeth-Arnold, R.K. (1976). Skill acquisition under variable temporal constraints: Cinematographic analysis of movement organization. *Journal of Human Movement Studies*, 2, 98-113.

Stadulis, R.E. (1971). *Coincidence anticipation behavior of children*. Unpublished doctoral dissertation, Columbia University.

Stadulis, R.E. (1972). Motor skill analysis: Coincidence-anticipation. *Quest*, *XVII*, 70-73.

Stelmach, G.E. (1982). Information-processing framework for understanding motor behavior. In J.A.S. Kelso (Ed.), *Human motor behavior: An introduction* (pp. 63-91). Hillsdale, NJ: Lawrence Erlbaum Associates.

Sternberg, S. (1969). The discovery of processing stages: Extensions of Donders' method. In W.G. Koster (Ed.), *Attention and Performance II. Acta Psychologica*, *30*, 276-315.

Stoffgren, T.A., & Riccio, G.E. (1990). Responses to optical looming in the retinal center and periphery. *Ecological Psychology*, 2, 251-274.

Sutherland, N.S. (1973). Object recognition. In E.C. Carterette, & M.P. Friedman (Eds.), *Handbook of perception, Volume III: Biology of perceptual systems*. (pp. 157-185). London: Academic Press.

Teghtsoonian, M., & Teghtsoonian, R. (1969). Scaling apparent distance in natural indoor settings. *Psychonomic Science*, *16*, 281-283.

Teghtsoonian, M., & Teghtsoonian, R. (1970). Scaling apparent distance in natural outdoor settings. *Psychonomic Science*, *21*, 215-216.

Thomas, J.R., Gallagher, J.D., & Purvis, G.J. (1981). Reaction time and anticipation time: Effects of development. *Research Quarterly for Exercise and Sport*, *52*, 359-367.

Thomson, J.A. (1983). Is continuous visual monitoring necessary in visually guided locomotion? *Journal of Experimental Psychology: Human Perception and Performance*, 9, 427-443.

Todd, J.T. (1981). Visual information about moving objects. *Journal of Experimental Psychology: Human Perception and Performance*, 7, 795-810.

Tresilian, J.R. (1990). Perceptual information for the timimg of interceptive action. *Perception*, *19*, 223-239.

Tronick, E. (1967). Approach responses of domestic chicks to an optical display. *Journal of Comparative and Physiological Psychology*, *64*, 529-531.

Turvey, M.T. (1977). Contrasting orientations to the theory of visual information processing. *Psychological Review*, *84*, 67-88.

Turvey, M.T., & Carello, C. (1986). The ecological approach to perceiving-acting: A pictorial essay. *Acta Psychologica*, *63*, 133-155.

Turvey, M.T., & Carello, C. (1988). Exploring a law-based ecological approach to skilled action. In A.M. Colley, & J.R. Beech (Eds.), *Cognition and action in skilled behaviour* (pp. 191-203). Amsterdam: North-Holland.

Turvey, M.T., Carello, C., & Kim, N-G. (1990). Links between active perception and the control action. In H. Haken, & M. Stadler (Eds.), *Synergetics of cognition* (pp. 269-295). Berlin: Springer-Verlag.

Turvey, M.T., Fitch, H.L., & Tuller, B. (1982). The Bernstein perspective: I. The problems of degrees of freedom and context conditioned variability. In J.A.S. Kelso (Ed.), *Human motor behavior: An introduction* (pp. 239-252). Hillsdale, NJ: Lawrence Erlbaum Associates.

Turvey, M.T., Shaw, R.E., Reed, E.S., & Mace, W.M. (1981). Ecological laws of perceiving and acting: In reply to Fodor and Pylyshyn (1981). *Cognition*, *9*, 237-304.

Tyldesley, D.A. , & Whiting, H.T.A. (1975). Operational timing. *Journal of Human Movement Studies*, *1*, 172-177.

Ullman, S. (1980). Against direct perception. *Behavioral and Brain Sciences*, *3*, 373-415.

van Wieringen, P.C.W. (1988). Discussion: Self-organization or representation? Let's have both! In A.M. Colley, & J.R. Beech (Eds.), *Cognition and action in skilled behaviour* (pp. 247-253). Amsterdam: North-Holland.

von Hofsten, C. (1980). Predictive reaching for moving objects by human infants. *Journal of Experimental Child Psychology*, *30*, 369-382.

von Hofsten, C. (1982). Eye-hand coordination in newborns. *Developmental Psychology*, *18*, 450-461.

von Hofsten, C. (1983). Catching skills in infancy. *Journal of Experimental Psychology: Human Perception and Performance*, *9*, 75-85.

von Hofsten, C. (1987). Catching. In H. Heuer, & A.F. Sanders (Eds.), *Perspectives on perception and action* (pp. 33-46). Hillsdale, NJ: Lawrence Erlbaum Associates.

Wagner, H. (1982). Flow-field variables trigger landing in flies. *Nature*, *297*, 147-148.

Warren, W.H., Jr. (1988). Action modes and laws of control for the visual guidance of action. In O.G. Meijer, & K. Roth (Eds.), *Complex movement behaviour: 'The' motor-action controversy* (pp. 339-380). Amsterdam: North-Holland.

Warren, W.H., Jr. (1990). Perception-action coupling. In H. Bloch & B.I. Bertenthal (Eds.), *Sensory-motor organizations and development in infancy and early childhood* (pp. 23-37). Netherlands: Kluwer.

Warren, W.H., Jr., & Kelso, J.A.S. (1985). Work group on perception and action. In W.H. Warren, Jr., & R.E.Shaw (Eds.), *Persistence and change* (pp. 269-281). Hillsdale, NJ: Lawrence Erlbaum Associates.

Warren, W.H., Jr., & Shaw, R.E. (1985). Events and encounters as units of analysis for ecological psychology. In W.H. Warren, Jr., & R.E. Shaw (Eds.), *Persistence and change* (pp. 1-27). Hillsdale, NJ: Lawrence Erlbaum Associates.

Warren, W.H., Jr., & Yaffe, D.M. (1989). Dynamics of step length adjustment during running: A comment on Patla, Robinson, Samways, and Armstrong (1989). *Journal of Experimental Psychology: Human Perception and Performance, 15*, 618-623.

Warren, W.H., Jr., Young, D.S., & Lee, D.N. (1986). Visual control of step length during running over irregular terrain. *Journal of Experimental Psychology: Human Perception and Performance, 12*, 259-266.

Whiting, H.T.A., Alderson, G.J.K., & Sanderson, F.M. (1973). Critical time intervals for viewing and individual differences in performance on a ball-catching task. *International Journal of Sport Psychology, 4*, 155-166.

Whiting, H.T.A., Savelsbergh, G.J.P., & Faber, C.M. (1988). "Catch" questions and incomplete answers. In A.M. Colley, & J.R. Beech (Eds.), *Cognition and action in skilled behaviour* (pp. 257-271). Amsterdam: North-Holland.

Williams, H.G. (1968). *The effects of systematic variation of speed and direction of object flight and skill and age classifications upon visuo-perceptual judgments of moving objects in three-dimensional space.* Unpublished doctoral dissertation, University of Wisconsin.

Williams, H.G. (1973). Perceptual-motor development in children. In C.B. Corbin (Ed.), *A textbook of motor development* (pp. 111-148). Dubuque, IA: William C. Brown.

Wollstein, J.R., & Abernethy, B. (1988). Timing structure in squash strokes: Further evidence for the operational timing hypothesis. *Journal of Human Movement Studies, 15*, 61-79.

Wrisberg, C.A., & Mead, B.J. (1981). Anticipation of coincidence in children: A test of schema theory. *Perceptual and Motor Skills, 52*, 599-606.

Wrisberg, C.A., & Mead, B.J. (1983). Developing coincident-timing skill in children: A comparison of training methods. *Research Quarterly for Exercise and Sport, 54*, 67-74.

Wrisberg, C.A., Paul, J.H., & Ragsdale, M.R. (1979). Subject gender, knowledge of results, and receptor anticipation. *Research Quarterly, 50*, 699-708.

Yonas, A. (1981). Infants' responses to optical information for collision. In R.N. Aslin, J.R. Alberts, & M.R. Peterson (Eds.), *Development of perception:*

Psycho-biological perspectives. Volume 2: The visual system (pp. 313-334). New York: Academic Press.

Yonas, A., Bechtold, A.G., Gordon, F.R., McRoberts, G., Novcia, A., & Sternfels, S. (1977). Development of sensitivity to information for impending collision. *Perception & Psychophysics*, *21*, 97-104.

Young, D.S. (1988). Describing the information for action. In O.G. Meijer, & K. Roth (Eds.), *Complex movement behaviour. 'The' motor-action controversy* (pp. 419-437). Amsterdam: North-Holland.

PART IV

MOVEMENT DISORDERS

Approaches to the Study of Motor Control and Learning
J.J. Summers (Editor)

Chapter 13

NEUROMOTOR CONTROL AND DOWN SYNDROME

J. Greg Anson
University of Otago

The cause of Down syndrome is as yet unknown; its neuropathology is well described and the physical characteristics are distinct. Although the effect of DS on motor control appears to parallel that observed in other similarly mentally retarded individuals, there are notable unique exceptions, particularly with respect to speed of responding. The results of our experiments indicate the involvement of both peripheral and central mechanisms in the slower reaction time observed in DS individuals. A distal-proximal pattern of movement initiation, however, suggests a complex relationship between central and peripheral mechanisms in DS individuals. We can only speculate on the reason for this difference at this time and hope that future research, with the cooperation of our DS participants, will elucidate the mechanism(s) underlying the apparent reversal in the sequence of muscle activation.

> One of the fundamental goals of kinesiology is to elucidate the neurological control strategies underlying movement *(Ramos, Stark, & Hannaford, 1989, p. 231).*

With an endorsement by the 101st Congress of the United States, the decade of the 90's will be known as the "decade of the brain" (IBRO News, 1989); a significant event given the last such endorsement for scientific research was the International Geophysical Year in 1958. This focus coupled to the rapidly evolving interest in the application of chaos theory to the study of the behaviour of biological systems heralds a most exciting era for motor control research, perhaps the most promising since the publication (translation) of *The*

Coordination and Regulation of Movement (Bernstein, 1967). Without doubt the effects of this evolution of knowledge will flow on and over to the general area of motor behaviour including movement disorders. This chapter will take the perspective that knowledge of motor control in other than normal conditions is enhanced when the abnormalities are contrasted against the characteristics of motor control described as normal. Specifically, the focus is on Down syndrome and the effect of this genetic disorder on motor control, particularly its influence on the Down syndrome individual's capacity to initiate and perform rapid movements. The chapter contains four sections: 1) An overview of aetiological and pathological literature on Down syndrome; 2) a review of experimental work in Down syndrome related to neuromotor control; 3) discussion of the specific effects of Down syndrome on neuromotor reaction time; and 4) possible directions for future research.

DOWN SYNDROME: AN OVERVIEW

This section describes the aetiological, pathological, and general behavioural characteristics of Down syndrome (DS) including brief reference to the study of DS through specific animal models. Although the prevalence of Down syndrome has increased, and the incidence is unlikely to decrease in the near future (Wishart, 1988), relatively little is known about the underlying mechanisms of motor control despite frequent descriptions of DS motor behaviour (Henderson, 1985). Best estimates of incidence vary between 1:600 (Wishart, 1988) and 1:1000 (Pisarchick, 1987) live births. Extrapolation to the local scene in New Zealand predicts approximately 50 Down syndrome babies born per year. With improved postnatal care the prevalence is likely to increase rather than decrease. Survival beyond the age of 10 years has increased from 36.8% (1944-1945) to 86.0% (1966-1975) (Fryers, 1986) and mean life expectancy is currently 55-60 years (Epstein, 1987; Fryers, 1986; Patterson, 1987). But what is Down syndrome? Down syndrome is: "...the set of physical, mental, and functional abnormalities that result from trisomy 21, the presence in the genome of three rather than the normal two chromosomes 21." (Epstein, 1987, p. 336).

According to Patterson (1987) the clinical characteristics were first described in 1866 by English physician, Dr J.H. Langdon Down (1828-1896), although the condition had reportedly been observed since the 9th Century. The distinctive physical characteristics apparently led Langdon Down to use the term mongolism in his original description of the syndrome, a term which remained in common use until quite recently.

Aetiology

The cause of DS is not known but numerous candidate agents have been suggested including radiation, gene mutation, viruses, auto immune mechanisms, aged gametes, drugs, and other chemicals (Patterson, 1987; Pisarchick, 1987; Wishart, 1988). The most "reliable" predictor remains maternal age with the likelihood of women over 35 years of age giving birth to DS babies (Spreen, Tupper, Risser, Tuokko, & Edgell, 1984) being much greater. It is worth noting, however, that 60% of DS babies are born to women who have no known "predisposing genetic or environmental factors" (Wishart, 1988, p. 9).

Down syndrome is a genetic disorder represented by chromosomal dysgenesis. Less than 4% of DS results from inheritance, about 1% is due to mosaicism and 95% occurs because of non-dysjunction (failure of meiosis) of the chromosome during gamete formation. Interestingly, chromosome 21 is the smallest of the 23 chromosomes (containing about 1.5% of genetic material) and the portion of the long arm of chromosome 21 believed to be involved in DS represents only about 10-20% of the total. For such a minuscule biological quantity the effects on the individuals growth, development, and motor control are analogous to the effects of drift-netting on the fish population of the South Pacific Ocean. At the neurocellular level, knowledge about DS is being gained from the study of murine trisomy 16 - the mouse analogue of human trisomy 21. Observations include differences in cellular proliferation, and decreased numbers of cortical neurons (Blue, Molliver, & Gearhart, 1984; Oster-Granite, 1986).

Among the most evident physical characteristics of human DS are inner epicanthic folds, flatness of the bridge of the nose, midfacial hypoplasia, reduced stature, and tongue protrusion (particularly in the very young) (Epstein, 1987). In addition to central nervous system deficits (structural and functional) Down syndrome individuals are vulnerable to other abnormalities including congenital heart disease (nearly 40%), intestinal tract obstruction, increased susceptibility to infection, increased (compared to normal) likelihood of developing childhood leukemia, and increased susceptibility to stroke and respiratory infection (Epstein, 1987; Fryers 1986). Beyond 40 years of age dementia similar to that of Alzheimer disease is likely to develop and in combination with the existing mental retardation, produces an increased loss of mental function (Dalton & Crapper-McLachlan, 1986; Kemper, 1988; McGeer, McGeer, Suzuki, & Norman, 1984; Patterson, 1987; Zemlan, Thienhaus, & Bosmann, 1986).

Neuropathology

A thorough review of the neuropathological aspects of Down syndrome is beyond the scope of this chapter and is available elsewhere (see for example, Epstein, 1987; Fryers, 1986; Kemper, 1988; Patterson, 1987). In brief, brain weight which may be normal at birth, diminishes by up to 24% during early development with the cerebellum (especially middle lobes) and brainstem being particularly affected (Epstein, 1987; Kemper, 1988). Brain size is also reported to be diminished as are the number of synaptic spines, dendritic intersections, neurons, and convolutions in the cerebral surface. Poor myelination of descending tracts and brain-stem neurons, and decreased neural connections in motor cortex, basal ganglia, cerebellum, and brain-stem are cited by Shumway-Cooke and Woollacott (1985) as characteristic of DS.

Although the relationship between structural abnormality and functional impairment in DS is unclear (Spreen et al., 1984), the implications of cerebellar and brainstem pathology for motor control are potentially significant given their perceived role in the timing and coordination of motor performance (Ghez & Fahn, 1985).

Epstein describes three "salient clinical abnormalities of the nervous system" associated with Down syndrome. They are hypotonia, mental retardation, and progressive loss of mental function resulting from dementia in those who live into the fifth decade. So-called hypotonia is recognisable after birth ("floppy baby" syndrome) and particularly during the early years of development. Mental retardation is generally moderate but can vary from mild to severe and appears to be influenced by environmental events such as home-based upbringing vs institutionalised care (Champion, 1987; Wisniewski, Miezejeski, & Hill, 1988).

DOWN SYNDROME: NEUROMOTOR CONTROL

A substantial literature exists which collectively describes many characteristics of motor behaviour of individuals with Down syndrome (see Henderson, 1985 for an excellent review). However, with the exception of postural and equilibrium control (Haley, 1987; Parker & Bronks, 1980; Parker, Bronks, & Snyder, 1986; Shumway-Cook & Woollacott, 1985; Woollacott & Shumway-Cook, 1986) there has been relatively little effort directed toward investigating the mechanisms underlying motor control in DS, although the need for this approach has been implied if not categorically stated: "What is possibly required is an explanation which takes account of the delays inherent at the neuromotor level" (Henderson, 1985, p. 211).

Perhaps the lack of productive research in this area is less surprising given the difficulty of resolving the debate about which variables affecting motor control are commanded by the nervous system (Stein, 1982). Recently, Gottlieb and colleagues (Gottlieb, Corcos, & Agarwal, 1989) emphasised the difficulties surrounding an adequate description of "what is controlled" in their depiction of the inherent variability of human movement which depends upon the initial state of a variety of elements including: limbs, muscles, nervous system, and decision processes which specify parameters. In a provocative statement Gottlieb et al., offer the suggestion that the controlled variable is the "neural input to the alpha motor neuron pool" (p. 193). In contrast to the scarcity of research on mechanisms of motor control in DS there has been a considerable contribution to the description of DS motor behaviour. This section will describe briefly the characteristics of sensory acuity and hypotonia in DS then summarise research which has focused on: 1) Posture, locomotion, and equilibrium; 2) practice; 3) information processing; and 4) manual task performance.

Sensory Acuity. Making sense of the literature on motor control in DS is a challenge as few clear patterns exist beyond general observations. The influence of modality specific sensory acuity effects, paints a picture of equivocality. Kinaesthetic sense has been reported as more useful (Anwar, 1983; Davis & Kelso, 1982), less useful (Johnson & Olley, 1971), and not different (Komiya, 1973) from vision for DS in manual tasks. Visual processing as assessed by evoked potential analysis is reported to be slower in DS (Yellin, Lodwig, & Jerison, 1979). Poor control and/or integration of proprioceptive input was cited as a reason for failure of DS participants to modulate grip force (Cole, Abbs, & Turner, 1988). Greater susceptibility to auditory than to visual distraction in a recall task (Marcell & Armstrong, 1982) and delayed processing of auditory information (Lincoln, Courchesne, Kilman, & Galambos, 1985) have also been described. While the presence of generally decreased sensory acuity in DS compared to mentally retarded non-DS individuals (Clausen, 1968) has some support, the suggestion that neuromotor function in DS is notably poorer because of sensory deficit (Cole et al., 1988; Courchesne, 1988) is not clearly substantiated.

Hypotonia. One of the most frequently cited characteristics of DS, particularly in infancy is "floppy baby" syndrome attributable to the presence of diminished muscle tone (Wisniewski, Miezejeski, & Hill, 1988). It is easily recognisable from birth through the early years (Epstein, 1987) and has served as a causal explanation for slowness in reaction time (Anwar & Hermelin, 1979), developmental deficit in the use of equilibrium reactions (Haley, 1987), increased oscillatory movement in a limb positioning task (Davis & Kelso, 1982), and diminished strength in young (aged 4 - 15 years) DS participants (Morris, Vaughan, & Vaccaro, 1982). However, the influence of hypotonia on motor behaviour in and beyond early childhood has recently been questioned

(Shumway-Cook & Woollacott, 1985). By definition a muscle exhibiting no tone (hypotonic) would be expected to demonstrate no electrical activity, yet Shumway-Cook and Woollacott reported normal stretch reflex activity in young DS children in response to translational and rotation perturbations of standing posture. Furthermore, maintenance by DS subjects of joint stiffness during a joint-angle torque-positioning task was taken as evidence against the presence and influence of hypotonia (Davis & Kelso, 1982). In a later experiment (Davis & Sinning, 1987), a lack of difference between DS and mentally retarded (non-DS) subjects on elbow flexor stiffness assessment was interpreted as further evidence against hypotonia in DS. However, an actual assessment of muscle tone of the participants was not reported in either experiment. In sum, the role of hypotonia in accounting for movement disorders in DS individuals can no longer be considered a default explanation when alternatives fail.

Posture, Locomotion, and Equilibrium

The development of posture, locomotion, and equilibrium in DS is almost always delayed but frequently it is eventually achieved. As stated by Henderson "...they walk, run, climb, and ride bicycles; most learn to dress, go to the toilet and eat tidily" (Henderson, 1985, p. 193) and yet a characteristic of DS motor behaviour is clumsiness of unknown nature and extent (Frith & Frith, 1974). Recent research has begun to shed light on the underlying mechanisms of posture, locomotion, and equilibrium in DS. The development of walking is characterised by poor heel-toe mechanisms, exaggerated abduction of the lower limb, delayed temporal components, and an increased variability of walking patterns. These developmental delays are possibly due to arrested or retarded neural development (Parker & Bronks, 1980; Parker, Bronks, & Snyder, 1986). The neuromuscular mechanisms underlying maintenance of standing posture in DS have also been investigated. In contrast to control subjects and "normal" developmental patterns, DS demonstrate longer, long-loop reflexes, absence of synergistic muscle activity, and lack of adaptation to perturbation. Perhaps surprisingly, young DS children showed normal latency stretch reflex activity which would not be predicted if hypotonic influences were present (Shumway-Cook & Woollacott, 1985; Woollacott & Shumway-Cook, 1986). Near normal reflex latencies in DS were also described by Latash, Corcos, and Gottlieb (1989) for responses to perturbations during a rapid elbow flexion task.

Performance by DS subjects on tasks involving static balance showed them to be not different from mentally age-matched and chronologically age-matched subjects and superior to them on a test of dynamic balance (Le Blanc, French, & Schultz, 1977). It has been reported that DS individuals have an enhanced appreciation of music and sense of rhythm yet this anecdotal observation does not appear to have withstood empirical validation. Although some capacity to improve on gross motor tasks involving music and rhythm was reported (Stratford & Ching, 1989) DS individuals were not different from mentally retarded non-DS persons. With respect to the achievement of developmental milestones and the role of early intervention programs, the accomplishment of DS children remains delayed with least progress occurring in gross motor skills and expressive language (Champion, 1987). Are DS individuals really slower to respond and perform developmental motor tasks or is this effect ameliorated with extensive practice?

Does Practice Improve Motor Performance in Down Syndrome?

Insufficient practice can be invoked to explain almost any deficit in motor control in DS individuals or others diagnosed as mentally or motorically retarded. This view and its delimitations was expressed succinctly by Newell (1989) who proposed that the practice explanation; "...can be an irritating hypothesis to researchers because proponents of this practice view can always argue, that more practice is needed" (p. 44). It is an ubiquitous explanation which leaves as many questions unanswered as it purports to address. How much practice is sufficient to assess the real effect of an independent variable? Should a "final" description consider a relatively unvarying performance as reflecting the motor capability of the individual regardless of the magnitude of error or time delay? Kerr and Blais (1988) suggested that a minimum of 100 responses (trials) and preferably not less than 400 were required to assess effects in reaction time and/or movement time tasks. From the perspective of practice DS motor control research presents a mixed bag. Practice was reported to have no effect on tracking and tapping tasks (Frith & Frith, 1974; Henderson, Morris, & Frith, 1981); not facilitate improvement in reaction time (Kerr & Blais, 1985), and not to facilitate modulation of grip force in a lifting task (Cole et al., 1988). Paradoxically practice has been shown to improve performance on reaction time (after 2400 responses) without effecting changes in movement time (Kerr & Blais, 1987) *and* to improve performance on movement time without altering reaction time (Kerr & Blais, 1988). Similar observations in studies of the mentally retarded (non-DS) were reported by Wade and colleagues in experiments utilising large numbers of trials and several days of practice (Hoover, Wade, & Newell, 1981; Wade, Hoover, & Newell, 1984; Wade, Newell, & Wallace, 1978). Interestingly, Hoover et al., reported the performance of mentally retarded persons to be amenable to task-component specific practice. That is, if task instruction was focused on the reaction time component it improved and, likewise, if focused on the movement speed segment, movement time improved, although the task itself was "simple" (reacting from a switch and reaching to a target).

Maybe the real issue is the extent to which insufficient practice disguises the true residual deficit from effects due to environmental or experiential influences (Worringham, 1989). It is clear within the limitations of the literature reviewed that DS individuals, although capable of showing improvement, are slower developmentally and exhibit poorer motor performance even when considerable amounts of practice are involved (Kerr & Blais, 1987). Perhaps one reason for the equivocal results of practice effects is related to the difficulty of determining whether some parts of the neuromuscular system are more amenable to practice effects than others. Observable motor performance, for example, may be a consequence of information processing failure - a central nervous system deficit - and less dependent on faulty musculoskeletal parameters.

Information Processing Deficits Affect Motor Performance

In portraying DS motor performance one of the most all encompassing characteristics is slowness (Henderson, 1985), and the object of much of the research has been directed toward determining the cause of slowness. It is not just a matter of mental retardation as DS performance is frequently described as slower than that revealed by the non-DS mentally retarded (Berkson, 1960c, Blais & Kerr, 1986; Clausen, 1968; Frith & Frith, 1974; Spreen, et al., 1984). So where is the block? Hypotonia cannot be assumed to explain all the delay, and problems of sensory acuity cannot absorb the universal observation of slowness. Within the general scheme of an information processing model then, the block could be associated with one or more of the following stages: stimulus recognition, response selection, motor programming, or response execution. Alternatively the stages may be intact but, in the presence of reduced attentional capacity, not function satisfactorily. At the cellular level a reduction in the number of noradrenergic and cholinergic cells in the locus coeruleus and/or substantia innominata was not sufficient to explain the observed mental deficiency (McGeer, et al., 1984), although in the animal model (murine trisomy 16) fewer information processing modules and fewer cells per module were reported (Blue et al., 1984). At the brain-functional level, evoked response potential analysis reveals a different profile for DS individuals compared to controls and similarly mentally retarded subjects. Processing of auditory information was reported to be slower, accompanied by altered distribution of scalp recorded potentials (Lincoln et al., 1985) and occurrence of increased amplitude signals (Karrer, 1989; Yellin, Lodwig, & Jerison, 1980). Increased amplitude and latency of visual evoked potentials has also been reported (Yellin et al., 1979). Results like these led Courchesne (1988) to infer that the mechanisms involved in temporal integration and information storage were abnormal, and to postulate that increased amplitude signals could be due to decreased inhibitory control leading to decreased selectivity and specificity of responsiveness. It is as though DS individuals are unable to engage the necessary filtering process to screen out non-significant stimuli.

At the behavioural level, information processing difficulties have been attributed to an attentional deficit (Blais & Kerr, 1986; Dunst, 1988), memory deficit (Anwar & Hermelin, 1979; Cole, et al., 1988; Marcell & Armstrong, 1982), and perceptual dysfunction (Clausen, 1968; Spreen et al., 1984; Stratford, 1980). Lack of, or extremely delayed development of motor programs with a greater dependency on feedback has been proposed to explain information processing deficits as measured in reaction or response time tasks (Frith & Frith, 1974; Henderson, Morris, & Ray, 1981). The question of deficit-uniqueness and DS is not resolved within the information processing literature, with claims that the similarities between DS and other mentally retarded individuals are greater than the differences (Johnson & Olley, 1971). Nettlebeck and Brewer (1976) comment on information processing difficulties in general for mental retardation, and suggest that the increased time and variability is due to delays in information accumulation and translation of the stimulus to selection of the response.

In summary, we are left with a somewhat confused picture as to the uniqueness of information processing-motor performance deficits in DS. While many deficits have been claimed as significant characteristics of DS, the only one of substance appears to be that of slowness, which is greater in DS than in control groups of subjects matched for mental age, functional age, developmental age, and chronological age. This slowness is characteristic of some information processing tasks, but is it also prevalent in the motor component of fine (as compared to gross) motor tasks? This question will be addressed in the next section within the context of simple manual tasks.

Down Syndrome and Performance on Manual Tasks

The results of the experiments described in this section come exclusively from tasks involving tracking, lifting, tapping, sorting, or copying (drawing or model construction). Performance is measured in terms of accuracy (errors) and/or time.

Compared to appropriately matched control subjects, DS individuals were slower on pursuit and continuous tracking tasks (Blais & Kerr, 1986; Frith & Frith, 1974; Henderson, 1985; Kerr & Blais, 1985) but made fewer errors. According to Henderson, Morris, & Firth (1981), DS subjects seemed to treat continuous tracking as a discontinuous aiming task. This interpretation has additional appeal in light of the idea that DS persons are unable to utilise motor programs and, therefore, function in an increasingly feedback dependent mode (Frith & Frith, 1974). In a finger tapping task DS subjects were slower than normal controls and not different from similarly mentally retarded subjects (Elliott, 1985); but demonstrated more variable performance (Elliott, Weeks, & Jones, 1986; Henderson, 1985). In a similar experiment involving two-plate tapping, DS subjects were reported to be able to increase speed but only at the expense of accuracy. While, on a grasp and lift task (Cole et al., 1988) and a reach-lift-transport manoeuvre (Nativ & Abbs, 1989) DS participants displayed slower (x2 to x3) performance, and an inability to modulate the force of their grip despite different frictional coefficients. Force exerted always exceeded that required for the task.

Performance of DS individuals on tasks requiring shape recognition using the hands was poorer when stereognostic feedback rather than visual feedback was permitted (O'Connor & Hermelin, 1961). In a drawing test requiring copying, DS subjects did better with kinaesthetic feedback than with vision, compared to non-DS mentally retarded controls (Anwar, 1983). However, Komiya (1973) employed a similar task and found no difference between the performance of DS subjects and that of controls. DS subjects had difficulty replicating a 5-block display from a model and on a retest situation demonstrated no improvement in performance (Stratford, 1980). In the same experiment Stratford conducted a test of recognition in which three models were constructed by the experimenter, one of which was identical to the stimulus model. DS participants had little difficulty recognising the correct shape. From this Stratford concluded that the difficulty for DS subjects lay in the manipulative component of the task and not at the perceptual level.

With the exception of the continuing persistent theme of slowness coupled to increased variability, the motor performance characteristics of DS individuals on manual tasks present no clearer picture than that described for other aspects of the motor domain.

DOWN SYNDROME AND REACTION TIME

The time required to complete a discrete response is frequently used as an index of the performers capability to produce a speeded response. Reaction time is the interval from the onset of an imperative stimulus to the initiation of a movement, whereas response time includes, in addition to reaction time, the duration of the movement. Reaction time is described as simple (simple reaction time) when the subject knows precisely what response to make before the stimulus occurs but does not know the exact time of stimulus onset. Choice reaction time is the delay measured when a subject is required to respond to one of two or more stimuli, thus response selection cannot be determined until the stimulus is presented. Choice reaction time contains added delay due to decision and possibly programming processes. Simple reaction time (SRT), which is assumed to reflect the fastest capacity of the neuromuscular system to initiate a movement, can be fractionated into central and peripheral components using electromyography (EMG). This technique gives an accurate measure of the duration from stimulus recognition to the onset of change in activity in the muscle of interest.

Given that the theme of slowness is a consistently reported characteristic of DS, it should not be surprising to find that lengthened reaction time is the rule rather than the exception. What is puzzling is the persistent finding that DS reaction times are slower than those exhibited by similarly mentally retarded (non-DS) individuals. In fact, Berkson (1960c) reported DS reaction times to be considerably longer than those of severely subnormal and subnormal subjects.

The principal research theme in our laboratory focuses on the investigation of neuromotor mechanisms underlying simple reaction time. Recently, we (Anson, 1989a,b; Anson & Davis, 1988; Anson & Gorely, 1990; Gorely & Anson, 1990) began a series of experiments to investigate the underlying mechanisms of SRT in DS. A brief review of the DS-reaction time literature is in order before discussing some of the results from our own studies. The literature exemplifies the findings discussed earlier. DS individuals seem to have excessively slow and more variable reaction times even in SRT studies wherein decision making is minimal. The following discussion refers primarily to experiments in which SRT was the principal dependent measure.

Only one paper (MacKay & Bankhead, 1983) has reported no difference in SRT among groups of subjects including DS, mentally retarded (non-DS), and epileptics. The SRT values, however, were very long (greater than 1500 ms) in all cases. A substantial number of studies have reported longer SRT for DS subjects than for similarly mentally retarded non-DS control subjects (Berkson, 1960c; Blais & Kerr, 1986; Davis, Ward, & Sparrow, 1988; Johnson & Olley, 1971; Kerr & Blais, 1987, 1988; Lincoln et al., 1985; Miezejeski, 1974). Increases in SRT for DS subjects varied from 25% to greater than 300%. The effect of practice has been referred to previously. With respect to SRT the data are equivocal. Extensive practice has produced reductions in SRT with no apparent change in the accompanying movement time (Kerr & Blais, 1987) and paradoxically reductions in movement time with no effect on SRT (Kerr & Blais, 1988). A clue to the cause of this paradoxical observation is found in the results of studies described earlier, with non-DS mentally retarded individuals (Hoover et al., 1981; Wade et al., 1978; 1984). In spite of component-specific intervention, much practice, and the ability to make use of advance information, SRT was reported to be slower than that achieved by control subjects (Wade et al., 1978). These findings point to a failure in the neuromuscular mechanism involved in processing the information.

One way to address the problem of failure in the neuromuscular mechanism is to examine the central and peripheral elements of SRT separately using the fractionation technique (Weis, 1965). Although Yellin and colleagues (Yellin et al., 1979, 1980) assessed visual and auditory evoked potentials in DS individuals, they did not use this technique in a SRT setting, nor did they utilise EMG to separate the peripheral component of muscle activation time. To date we are aware of just one report which has applied the fractionation technique to measuring SRT in DS. In an unpublished paper Davis and colleagues (1988) reported fractionated SRT to visual, auditory, and visual + auditory stimuli. They used an elbow extension task with subjects receiving 10 trials under each stimulus condition. Their results indicated that DS subjects were slower than non-DS retarded and normal control subjects and this slowness occurred in both the central (premotor time) and peripheral (motor time) elements of SRT. However, given the paucity of trials in each condition, it is not surprising that high variability was reported.

In an attempt to gain some understanding of the mechanisms underlying DS we have utilised an SRT paradigm which permits predictions of the memory drum theory of neuromotor reaction time (Henry & Rogers, 1960; Sternberg, Monsell, Knoll, & Wright, 1978) to be tested. This approach allows empirical investigation of the inference that DS individuals are slower because they cannot develop and/or utilise motor programs (Frith & Frith, 1974; Henderson, 1985; Kerr & Blais, 1985, 1987). Succinctly, memory drum theory predicts that SRT will increase as a function of the greater neuromotor programming requirements imposed by increasingly complex movements. It is argued that longer SRT reflects the additional readout time and/or storage capacity required by the programming process. This process is defined specifically as "...the translation of the stored program into organised motor nerve commands to the muscle..." (Henry, 1981, p. 301) or more generally as "...the acquisition, storage, selection, and read-out of complex temporal-spatial sequences of motor command signals" (Loeb, 1987, p. 692). Without the advantage of motor programming, SRT would be predicted to increase and a greater dependency on peripheral feedback would occur.

Fractionation of SRT permits the effects of movement complexity to be quantified as central (affecting the premotor time - PMT), peripheral (affecting the motor time - MOT), or both. Thus in DS, if the delay principally involves a deficit in motor programming, the PMT fraction would be predicted to reflect most of the increase. If the delay is due to hypotonia, strength decrement, or other peripheral variable such as inertia of the limb (Anson, 1982, 1989), then the MOT fraction would be greater. Because the SRT paradigm permits maximum use of advance preparation (preprogramming), under conditions in which the movement required is simple, that is, unidirectional with minimal accuracy constraints (e.g., pointing one finger at a large target), fractionated SRT should reflect the shortest neuromuscular delay and minimal post-stimulus information processing constraints.

In an exploratory experiment (Anson, 1989b; Anson & Davis, 1988) we measured SRT in DS and control subjects to a "simple" and a "complex" aiming task. The simple task required subjects to respond to an imperative auditory stimulus by pointing as quickly as possible at a large (25 cm^2) brightly coloured target. In the complex task, two targets of the same size but different colours were used and subjects were asked to point to each in turn as quickly as possible. To add incentive and assist in maintaining attention a candy bar was attached to the centre of each target. Myoelectric activity was recorded via disposable AgAgCl surface electrodes from the right anterior deltoid and biceps brachii muscles. Photo-transistor light emitting diode switches recorded SRT at the elbow and index finger. Data were captured on FM-tape for later analysis. Problems with some EMG data prevented a complete off-line analysis of fractionated SRT but three important observations were noted: 1) SRT for DS participants was generally more than twice as long as that for control subjects; 2) delays were proportionately similar in premotor and motor time for the anterior deltoid muscle for all groups; and 3) DS subjects demonstrated a distal-to-proximal sequencing of movement initiation (i.e., SRT measured at the index finger was shorter than SRT measured at the elbow). The latter was an unexpected and, as far as we know, not previously reported result. Normally the initiation sequence for rapid movement is proximal to distal (Grimm, 1983; Jeannerod, 1988) or synergistic such that the whole limb moves as a unit (Anson, 1982). Data from control groups revealed no effect of complexity on SRT. In the DS group there was a slight tendency for SRT to be shorter in the "complex" response setting.

In a follow-up experiment (Anson & O'Connor, 1989) we looked at the patterns of sequencing of muscle activation in three DS subjects. Tasks from the first experiment were modified to include measurement of movement time (striking the target) and a condition in which two targets were hit in succession to provide three levels of complexity (1 = pointing at a target; 2 = striking one target; 3 = striking two targets in succession). The results were similar to those obtained in Experiment 1. DS subjects were slower, more variable, and demonstrated a distal-to-proximal pattern of movement initiation. Furthermore, the trend was reproduced in the PMT data; onset of change in activity of extensor indicis muscle preceded that for biceps and anterior deltoid muscles. Not only were the EMG onset latencies indicative of a distal-to-proximal initiation sequence, but the EMG envelopes describing the profile of muscle activation during and beyond the MOT interval appeared different from those of non-DS subjects. Preliminary analysis of the EMG data revealed a ramp-like onset to change in muscle activity in DS subjects compared to a step-like change observed in control non-DS subjects.

Why do Down syndrome individuals demonstrate a distal-to-proximal initiation pattern? We interpreted our fractionated SRT results as follows: If DS individuals are unable to form and/or utilise motor programs (Anwar, 1983; Frith & Frith, 1974; Kerr & Blais, 1985, 1987) to produce fast reaction times, then perhaps they are more likely to be dependent on feedback at all stages of responding. We proposed that distal-proximal sequencing might be a reflection of such feedback dependency. Initial movement of the distal segment would provide visual confirmation that the movement was under way, so-to-speak, and then shoulder flexion (anterior deltoid) could be implemented to propel the limb toward the target. This strategy could be analogous to an aim, then fire approach involving serial organisation, as opposed to the synchronous, synergistic organisation typical of control subjects. If this explanation is correct then occlusion of visual feedback would be expected to disrupt DS information processing even more, resulting in longer and more variable reaction times.

The hypothesis that removal of visual feedback would cause greater disruption of DS information processing and result in longer SRT was investigated in a third experiment. In the non-vision condition visual feedback was removed by having participants wear comfortably fitting opaque goggles. In addition to the manipulation of visual feedback, the protocol was modified to include double the number of trials per condition to assess the effect of extended practice. Two control groups were tested, one matched with DS subjects for chronological age (CA), and one matched with DS for mental age (MA) based on the assessment of mental age in DS using the Peabody Picture Vocabulary Test. There were four subjects in each group, the sample size being determined by the number and availability of the DS participants. Each subject received a total of 192 SRT trials, 96 with visual feedback, 96 without visual feedback. Within each level of visual feedback there were 32 trials (4 blocks of 8 trials each) at each level of complexity. In summary, the design was a Groups (3) x Complexity (3) x Practice (2) x Vision (2) with repeated measures on all within subjects factors. The results presented in this paper represent analysis of data from the 2nd (Early Practice) and 4th (Late Practice) blocks for each level of complexity and vision respectively.

Participants were seated in a dental chair which provided full body support and minimised the need for significant postural stabilisation during response initiation. A verbal warning (READY!) preceded the onset of an imperative auditory stimulus by 1-2 seconds. Participants were frequently reminded and encouraged to respond as rapidly as possible. Trials on which subjects initiated a response before stimulus onset were considered errors and repeated at the end of the block. As detailed analysis of EMG profiles is currently in progress, only the fractionated SRT results will be described. In general, there were no significant effects for complexity, vision, or practice. For DS subjects, mean SRT and PMT tended to be faster (shorter duration) in the "most complex" condition (striking two targets in succession) and in the absence of visual feedback. In contrast, the CA and MA control groups demonstrated a very slight tendency toward increased SRT and MOT with increasing complexity, and performance was not affected by a change in visual feedback. It is likely that the limited sample size and considerable variability evident in the DS data contributed to the lack of statistically significant effects. In subsequent analyses

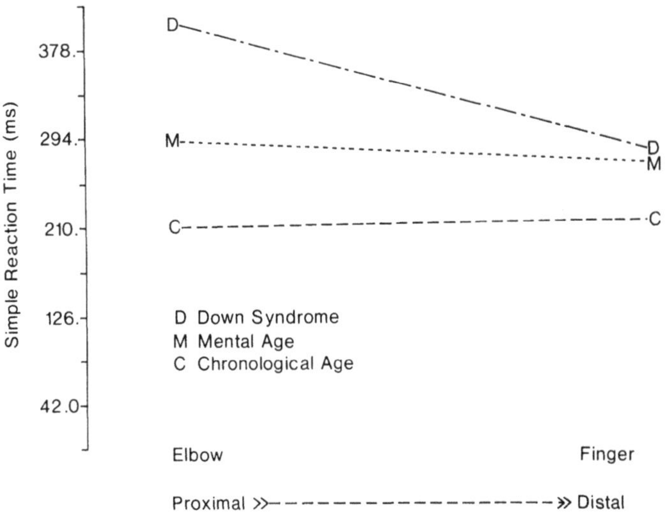

Figure 1. Mean simple reaction time in milliseconds of CA, MA, and DS groups recorded at the elbow (proximal) and finger (distal) reaction time switches.

the data were collapsed across the complexity, practice, and visual feedback factors and the effect of group x reaction time switch location (elbow vs finger) on SRT; group x muscle (anterior deltoid vs biceps vs extensor indicis) on PMT; and group x muscle on MOT were examined.

Figure 1 shows the mean SRT for the elbow and finger switches for the three groups. There was a significant interaction between group and switch location, $F(2, 9) = 54.95$, $p < .05$. Mean SRT differed between elbow switch and finger switch location for the DS group, but not for the CA and MA groups. Distal-proximal sequencing of response initiation was clearly evident for the DS group, whereas synchronous initiation was characteristic of the CA and MA groups.

The pattern of change in PMT for each group across the anterior deltoid, biceps, and extensor indicis muscles is shown in Figure 2. The main effect of group was significant, $F(2, 9) = 4.32$, $p < .05$, and post hoc analyses indicated that the DS and MA groups were significantly slower than the CA group, but not different from one another. The main effect for muscles was not significant but a distal-proximal pattern was evident in the DS data (see Figure 2); mean PMT for extensor indicis being shorter than that of anterior deltoid. Note that the average PMT for the DS group more closely resembled that of the MA

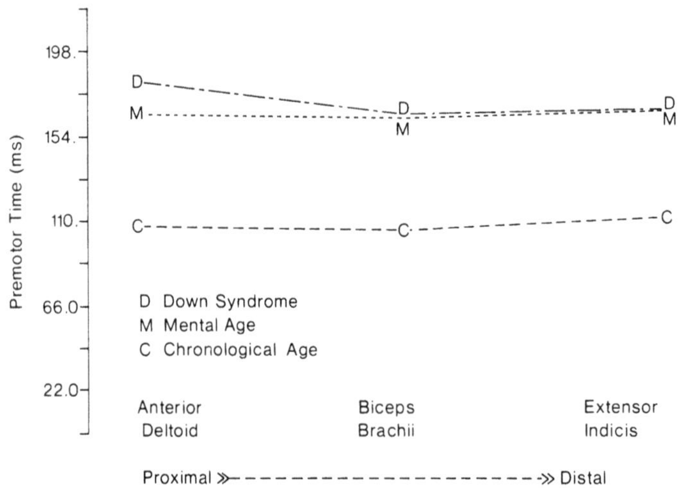

Figure 2. Mean premotor time in milliseconds of CA, MA, and DS groups for anterior deltoid (proximal), biceps, and extensor indicis (distal) muscles.

group than the CA group. This suggests that delayed information processing may be the source of the slow SRT observed in DS subjects.

Figure 3 presents the mean MOT for each group across the three muscles, in proximal to distal order. The Group x Muscle interaction was significant, $F(4, 18) = 37.73$, $p < .05$, but ordinal (Keppel, 1982), thus the main effects were analysed. Both the between groups difference and the main effect for muscles were significant, $F(2, 9) = 10.29$, $p < .05$, and $F(2, 18) = 39.69$, $p < .05$, respectively. Post hoc simple effects analyses revealed that the DS group was significantly slower than the CA and MA groups and this difference was confined to the comparison between groups for the anterior deltoid muscle. Although the trend of DS being slower than control groups continued across muscles it was not significant between groups at biceps or extensor indicis. Interestingly, the pattern of change for reaction time in the MA control group indicated that in young children (5 to 8 years) slower times were due more to central processing delays than to delays in the time course of muscle activation. The proportion of SRT made up of PMT is greater for the MA group than the CA group (Figure 2), while MA group MOT is similar to that of the CA group (Figure 3). The distal-proximal sequencing observed in DS subjects for both SRT and PMT measures was clearly evident in the MOT results. As shown in Figure 3, MOT for the anterior deltoid muscle was markedly slower than for the biceps and extensor indicis muscles. In contrast, there was virtually no change across muscles for the CA and MA groups.

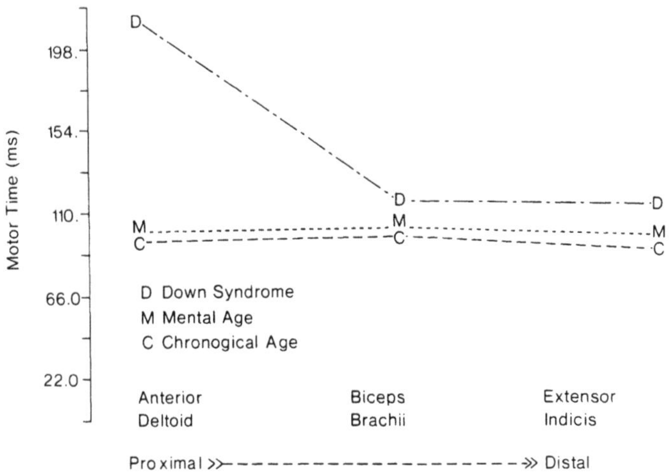

Figure 3. Mean motor time in milliseconds of CA, MA, and DS groups for anterior deltoid (proximal), biceps, and extensor indicis (distal) muscles.

What do the results tell us about neuromotor control in Down syndrome? Before attempting to answer this question let us consider the results of the two control groups. Collectively, their movement initiation was faster than the DS group with the MA group consistently slower than the CA group in SRT, PMT, and MOT. This latter observation demonstrates the influence of neuromotor development and maturation on SRT. Specifically, speed of information processing develops more slowly than the ability of muscles to become active quickly. Premotor time for MA subjects makes up about 10% more of the SRT interval than is the case for CA subjects. The independent variables of practice, complexity, and visual feedback produced no significant effect on performance. The tasks were very easy to execute rapidly. Although similar results were obtained for DS subjects, there was a trend toward faster SRT in the absence of vision and when complexity increased. It is possible that the challenge of the more complex task (hitting two 25 cm^2 styrofoam targets in quick succession) facilitated motivation and readiness to respond. The decreased SRT in the absence of vision also raises the possibility that multimodal sensory input could detrimentally affect information processing capacity in DS individuals (an inverse explanation to that of sensory deprivation). What may have been regarded as redundant by non-DS subjects could have contributed to sensory overload in the case of DS subjects. Thus removal of vision may have reduced the sensory load and facilitated attention leading to the slightly shorter SRT in this condition. Of course, as there was no significant effect of visual feedback, this hypothesis must be regarded as speculative, but arguably not without merit.

Clearly the most striking result obtained in all our experiments has been the distal-proximal ordering of the initiation sequence in DS subjects. According to Grimm (1983) "...the hierarchical design of the CNS has, at all levels and in all circumstances, a fundamental priority: Before voluntary movement of any kind, stabilisation of posture comes first" (p. 3). In control group subjects this strategy was seen in the presence of either proximal-distal ordering, or a synchronous initiation of movement presumably based on postural stability provided by the support of the dental chair. Why was it not present in DS? Three tentative explanations are offered: 1) The apparent mis-ordering is a consequence of DS pathology; 2) DS individuals invoke the distal-proximal sequencing as a deliberate strategy; and/or 3) the observation of mis-ordering is a function of the design and data acquisition specific to the experimental procedure.

A Consequence of Pathology? The neuropathology of DS includes diminished weight of the cerebellum (Epstein, 1987; Kemper, 1988). Given the involvement of the cerebellum in timing and coordination, it does not seem unreasonable to expect cerebellar deficits to impact on motor control (Brooks, 1986; Ghez & Fahn, 1985). For example, if the cerebellum functions in the efference copy or corollary discharge mode to check the operation of a motor program, then cerebellar dysfunction could disrupt the comparator process resulting in an overall slowing of information processing. Also poor myelination of the descending tracts, another pathological characteristic of DS, may contribute to loss of integrity of motor neuron conduction. We are not aware, however, of any studies of nerve conduction velocity in DS individuals which would be needed to test this hypothesis.

A Deliberate Strategy? To account for the distal-proximal sequencing observed in DS individuals in terms of a deliberate strategy requires acceptance of the idea that DS individuals are able to program responses, at least in part, in advance of stimulus onset. We have no reason to believe from our data that this is not the case. If DS subjects were unable to preprogram responses we would have expected marked increases SRT with increased response complexity, and when visual feedback was removed. A ready-aim-fire strategy, for example, could be implemented by raising the finger to line up the target (extension of the index finger and flexion of the elbow) before advancing the arm toward the target. If this strategy was adopted it would be expected to influence PMT for anterior deltoid as much, if not more, than MOT. Figures 2 and 3, however, show that this was not the case. The MOT for the anterior deltoid muscle in DS subjects was proportionately much more lagged than was PMT. Perhaps the "intensity" of the neural message or the format of motor unit recruitment is faulty in DS individuals and although the onset of change in EMG in the anterior deltoid muscle occurs, it does not do so with sufficient speed to generate the torque required for rapid shoulder flexion. The plausibility of this explanation awaits, in part, completion of the EMG profile analysis.

A Product of Experimental Procedure? A third explanation suggests that the distal-proximal sequencing occurs as a consequence of either excessive cocontraction following stimulus onset or the presence of antagonist muscle activity (e.g., posterior deltoid and triceps) which prevents and/or slows the activation of the agonist muscles. At this time we have no data to support this interpretation but the following analogy is offered as a feasible example. Consider if you will, the 100 metre sprinter who is ready for the starters gun. In preparation the sprinter exerts a good deal of force against the blocks to assist in rapid propulsion at the onset of the gun's firing (stimulus onset). In our experiment this is equivalent to pushing the responding elbow against the support and the forearm against the arm rest to gain purchase prior to stimulus onset. This strategy, however, is unlikely to be beneficial to reaction time as the preparatory force (and muscle activity) would need to be inhibited to initiate movement in the required direction; this action would take time at the likely cost of increasing SRT.

Further research is clearly needed to determine the source of the distal-proximal sequencing observed among individuals with DS.

POSSIBLE DIRECTIONS FOR FUTURE RESEARCH

An obvious direction for future research is to determine the effect of antagonist muscle activity on the initiation of rapid movement. This research should utilise both electromyographic and kinematic analysis to measure the temporal components and characteristics of muscle activation. For example, we are currently examining the EMG profiles for each muscle within individual subjects. Differences between subjects (and groups) in the shape of the EMG envelope for the MOT interval and the time to peak EMG should provide data from which some conclusions can be drawn about the influence of hypotonia and/or muscle contraction on the underlying mechanism of neuromotor reaction time in DS. A second question involves the delays in DS due to decision making and its effect on the central and peripheral components of information processing. Initially this issue could be addressed using simple movements but in a choice reaction time (CRT) paradigm employing EMG and the fractionation technique. Further research should examine the interaction between decision making and specific response requirements including accuracy, displacement, and direction. The interaction of displacement and accuracy in a Fitts' Law situation would permit quantification of the response in terms of Index of Difficulty and this parameter in combination with the measurement of fractionated reaction time would provide a comprehensive view of decision making and performance characteristics. Perhaps one of the most promising directions for future research would be to employ the instrumentation and EMG measurement procedure to assess SRT for activities more closely allied to "activities of daily living."

ACKNOWLEDGMENTS

Preparation of this chapter was supported in part by a New Zealand University Grant's Committee, Grant No. 88/086 and University of Otago Research Grants: No. 808 & No. 814. The experimental work with Down syndrome individuals could not have been completed without the dedicated help of Trish Gorely whose assistance is gratefully acknowledged. Thanks also to Teresa Keast for assistance with data analysis. We gratefully acknowledge the help and support provided by our Down syndrome and control group participants.

REFERENCES

Anson, J.G. (1982). Memory drum theory: Alternative tests and explanations for the complexity effects on simple reaction time. *Journal of Motor Behavior*, *14*, 228-246.

Anson, J.G. (1989a). Effects of moment of inertia on simple reaction time. *Journal of Motor Behavior*, *21*, 60-71.

Anson, J.G. (1989b). Down syndrome: Neuromotor programming and fractionated reaction time. In M.L. Latash (Ed.), *Proceedings of a Conference Sponsored by the Down's Syndrome Research Fund* (pp. 6-13). Chicago, IL: Rush-Presbyterian St. Luke's Medical Center.

Anson, J.G., & Davis, S.A. (1988). Neuromotor programming and Down syndrome. *International Journal of Neuroscience*, *40*, 82.

Anson, J.G., & Gorely, P.J. (1990). Down syndrome: Movement control and performance variability. *Commonwealth and International Conference on Physical Education, Sport, Health, Dance, Recreation and Leisure*, Abstract.

Anson, J.G., & O'Connor, H.M. (1989). Down syndrome: Initiation of discrete rapid movements. *International Journal of Neuroscience*, *46*, 36.

Anwar, F. (1983). The role of sensory modality for the reproduction of shape by the severely retarded. *British Journal of Developmental Psychology*, *1*, 317-327.

Anwar, F., Hermelin, B. (1979). Kinesthetic movement after-effects in children with Down's syndrome. *Journal of Mental Deficiency Research*, *23*, 287-297.

Berkson, G. (1960a). An analysis of reaction time in normal and mentally deficient young men. I. Duration threshold experiment. *Journal of Mental Deficiency Research*, *4*, 51-58.

Berkson, G. (1960b). An analysis of reaction time in normal and mentally deficient young men. II. Variation of complexity in reaction time tasks. *Journal of Mental Deficiency Research*, *4*, 59-67.

Berkson, G. (1960c). An analysis of reaction times in normal and mentally retarded young men. III. Variation of stimulus and of response complexity. *Journal of Mental Deficiency Research*, *4*, 69-77.

Bernstein, N. (1967). *The coordination and regulation of movements.* Oxford, UK: Pergamon Press.

Blais, C. & Kerr, R. (1986). Probability information in a complex motor task with respect to Down syndrome. *Journal of Human Movement Studies*, *12*, 183-194.

Blue, M.E., Molliver, J.D., & Gearhart, J.D. (1984). Abnormalities of cortical development in murine trisomy 16, an animal model for Down's syndrome. *Society Neuroscience Abstracts*, *10*, *Part* 2, 953.

Brooks, V.B. (1986). *The neural basis of motor control.* New York: Oxford University Press.

Champion, P. (1987). An investigation of the sensorimotor development of Down's syndrome infants involved in an ecologically based early intervention programme: A longitudinal study. *The British Journal of Subnormality*, *33*, 88-99.

Clausen, J. (1968). Behavioral characteristics of Down syndrome subjects. *American Journal of Mental Deficiency*, *73*, 118-126.

Cole, K.J., Abbs, J.H., & Turner, G.S. (1988). Deficits in the production of grip forces in Down syndrome. *Developmental Medicine and Child Neurology*, *30*, 752-758.

Courchesne, E. (1988). Physioanatomical considerations in Down syndrome. In L. Nadel (Ed.), *The Psychobiology of Down syndrome* (pp. 291-313). Cambridge, MA: M I T Press.

Dalton, A.J., & Crapper-McLachlan, D.R. (1986). Clinical expression of Alzheimer's disease in Down's syndrome. *Psychiatric Perspectives on Mental Retardation*, *9*, 659-670.

Davis, W.E., & Kelso, J.A.S. (1982). Analysis of "invariant characteristics" in the motor control of Down's syndrome and normal subjects. *Journal of Motor Behavior*, *14*, 194-212.

Davis, W.E., & Sinning, W.E. (1987). Muscle stiffness in Down syndrome and other mentally handicapped subjects: A research note. *Journal of Motor Behavior*, *19*, 130-144.

Davis, W.E., Ward, T., & Sparrow, W.A. (1988). *Fractionated reaction times and movement times of Down syndrome and other adults with mental retardation*. Manuscript submitted for publication.

Dunst, C.J. (1988). Stage transitioning in the sensorimotor development of Down's syndrome infants. *Journal of Mental Deficiency Research, 32*, 405-410.

Dupont, A., Vaeth, M., & Videbech, P. (1986). Mortality and life expectancy of Down's syndrome in Denmark. *Journal of Mental Deficiency Research, 30*, 111-120.

Elliott, D. (1985). Manual asymmetries in the performance of sequential movement by adolescents and adults with Down syndrome. *American Journal of Mental Deficiency, 90*, 90-97.

Elliott, D., Weeks, D.J., & Jones, R. (1986). Lateral asymmetries in finger-tapping by adolescents and young adults with Down syndrome. *American Journal of Mental Deficiency, 90*, 472-475.

Epstein, C.J. (1987). Down syndrome. In G. Adelman (Ed.), *Encyclopedia of Neuroscience* (pp. 336-337). Boston, MA: Birkhauser.

Frith, U., & Frith, C.D. (1974). Specific motor disabilities in Down's syndrome. *Journal of Child Psychology and Psychiatry, 15*, 293-301.

Fryers, T. (1986). Survival in Down's syndrome. *Journal of Mental Deficiency Research, 30*, 101-110.

Ghez, C., & Fahn, S. (1985). The cerebellum. In E.R. Kandel & J.H. Schwartz (Eds.), *Principles of neuroscience* (2nd ed.), (pp. 502-521). New York: Elsevier.

Gorely, P.J., & Anson, J.G. (1990). Down syndrome: Fractionated simple reaction time and motor control. *Commonwealth and International Conference on Physical Education, Sport, Health, Dance, Recreation and Leisure*, Abstract.

Gottlieb, G.L., Corcos, D.M., & Agarwal, G.C. (1989). Strategies for the control of voluntary movements with one mechanical degree of freedom. *Behavioral and Brain Sciences, 12*, 189-250.

Greenwald, C.A., & Leonard, L.B. (1979). Communicative and sensorimotor development of Down's syndrome children. *American Journal of Mental Deficiency, 84*, 296-303.

Grimm, R.J. (1983). Program disorders of movement. In J.E. Desmedt (Ed.), *Motor control mechanisms in health and disease* (pp. 1-11). New York: Raven Press.

Gunasingham, V., & Akuffo, E.O. (1988). The significance of atlanto-axial instability in Down's syndrome. *Journal of Mental Deficiency Research, 32*, 501-505.

Haley, S.M. (1987). Sequence of development of postural reactions by infants with Down syndrome. *Developmental Medicine and Child Neurology, 29*, 674-679.

Henderson, S.E. (1985). Motor skill development. In D. Lane & B. Stratford (Eds.), *Current approaches to Down syndrome* (pp. 187-218). London: Holt, Rhinehart & Winston.

Henderson, S.E., Morris, J., Ray, J. (1981). Performance of Down syndrome and other retarded children on the Cratty Gross-Motor Test. *American Journal of Mental Deficiency*, *85*, 416-424.

Henderson, S.E., Morris, J., & Frith, U. (1981). The motor deficit in Down's syndrome children: A problem of timing? *Journal of Child Psychology & Psychiatry*, 22, 233-245.

Henry, F.M. (1981). The evolution of the memory drum theory of neuromotor reaction. In G.A. Brooks (Ed.), *Perspectives on the academic discipline of physical education* (pp. 301-322). Champaign, IL: Human Kinetics.

Henry, F.M., & Rogers, D.E. (1960). Increased response latency for complicated movements and a "memory drum" theory of neuromotor reaction. *Research Quarterly*, *31*, 448-458.

Hoover, J.H., Wade, M.G., & Newell, K.M. (1981). Training moderately and severely mentally retarded adults to improve reaction and movement times. *American Journal of Mental Deficiency*, *85*, 389-395.

Jeannerod, M. (1988). *The neural and behavioural organization of goal-directed movements*. Oxford: Oxford University Press.

Johnson, J.T., & Olley, J.G. (1971). Behavioral comparisons of mongoloid and nonmongoloid retarded persons: A review. *American Journal of Mental Deficiency*, *75*, 546-559.

Karrer, R. (1989). Movement-related brain potentials: Implications for motor control in the mentally retarded and Down syndrome. In M.L. Latash (Ed.), *Proceedings of the Motor Control in Down syndrome Conference* (pp. 19-21). Chicago, IL: Rush-Presbyterian St Luke's Medical Center.

Kemper, T.L. (1988). Neuropathology of Down syndrome. In L. Nadel (Ed.), *The psychobiology of Down syndrome* (pp. 269-289). Cambridge, MA: MIT Press.

Keppel, G. (1982). *Design and analysis: A researcher's handbook* (2nd ed.). Englewood Cliffs, NJ: Prentice-Hall.

Kerr, R. & Blais, C. (1985). Motor skill acquisition by individuals with Down syndrome. *American Journal of Mental Deficiency*, *90*, 313-318.

Kerr, R. & Blais, C. (1987). Down syndrome and extended practice of a complex motor task. *American Journal of Mental Deficiency*. *91*, 591-597.

Kerr, R. & Blais, C. (1988). Directional probability information and Down syndrome: A training study. *American Journal on Mental Retardation*, 92, 531-538.

Komiya, M. (1973). Comparative studies of Down's syndrome and physiologically mentally retarded children on figure-copying ability. *Japanese Journal of Special Education*, *11*, 31-38.

Latash, M.L., Corcos, D.M., & Gottlieb, G.L. (1989). Kinematic and electromyographic characteristics of single-joint elbow movements in Down syndrome subjects. In M.L. Latash (Ed.), *Proceedings of the Motor Control in Down syndrome Conference* (pp 22-29). Chicago, IL: Rush-Presbyterian St Luke's Medical Center.

Le Blanc, D., French, R., & Schultz, B. (1977). Static and dynamic balance skills of trainable children with Down's syndrome. *Perceptual and Motor Skills*, *45*, 641-642.

Lincoln, A.J., Courchesne, E., Kilman, B.A., & Galambos, R. (1985). Neuropsychological correlates of information-processing by children with Down syndrome. *American Journal of Mental Deficiency*, *89*, 403-414.

Loeb, G.E. (1987). Motor control. In G. Adelman (Ed.), *Encyclopedia of Neuroscience* (pp. 690-692). Boston, MA: Birkhauser.

MacKay, D.N., & Bankhead, I. (1983). Reaction times of Down's syndrome and other mentally retarded individuals. *Perceptual and Motor Skills*, *56*, 266.

Maisto, A.A., & Sipe, S. (1980). Effects of stimulus probability on encoding by mentally retarded and non-retarded persons. *American Journal of Mental Deficiency*, *84*, 577-581.

Marcell, M.M., & Armstrong, V. (1982). Auditory and visual sequential memory of Down syndrome and nonretarded children. *American Journal of Mental Deficiency*, *87*, 86-95.

McGeer, P.L., McGeer, E.G., Suzuki, J., & Norman, M. (1984). Cholinergic and noradrenergic systems in aging, Alzheimer's disease and Down's syndrome. *Society Neuroscience Abstracts*, *10*, *Part* 2., 995.

Miezejeski, C.M. (1974). Effect of white noise on the reaction time of mentally retarded subjects. *Journal of Mental Deficiency*, *79*, 39-43.

Morris, A.F., Vaughan, S.E., & Vaccaro, P. (1982). Measurement of neuromuscular tone and strength in Down's syndrome children. *Journal of Mental Deficiency Research*, *26*, 41-46.

Nativ, J., & Abbs, J.H. (1989). Goal-directed arm movements in Down syndrome. In M.L. Latash (Ed.), *Proceedings of the Motor Control in Down syndrome Conference* (pp. 36-42). Chicago, IL: Rush-Presbyterian St Luke's Medical Center.

Nettlebeck, T., & Brewer, N. (1976). Effects of stimulus-response variables on the choice reaction time of mildly retarded adults. *American Journal of Mental Deficiency*, *81*, 85-92.

Newell, K.M. (1989). Down's syndrome and motor control: Comments and notes. In M.L. Latash (Ed.), *Proceedings of the Motor Control in Down syndrome Conference* (pp. 43-46). Chicago, IL: Rush-Presbyterian St Luke's Medical Center.

Nieminen, K., & Rapoport, S.I. (1986). Electrical membrane properties of cultured fetal dorsal root ganglia neurons from normal human and Down's syndrome. *Society Neuroscience Abstracts*, *12*, *Part* 2., 1360.

O'Connor, N., & Hermelin, B. (1961). Visual and stereognostic shape recognition in normal children and mongol and non-mongol imbeciles. *Journal of Mental Deficiency Research*, *5*, 63-66.

Oster-Granite, M.L. (1986). Dr Down and his syndrome. *Society Neuroscience Abstracts*, *12*, *Part 1*., 170.

Parker, A.W., & Bronks, R. (1980). Gait of children with Down syndrome. *Archives of Physical Medicine and Rehabilitation*, *61*, 345-350.

Parker, A.W., Bronks, R., & Snyder, C.W. (1986). Walking patterns in Down's syndrome. *Journal of Mental Deficiency Research*, *30*, 317-330.

Patterson, D. (1987). The causes of Down syndrome. *Scientific American*, *257*, 2, 42-48.

Pisarchick, S.E. (1987). Down's syndrome. In C.R. Reynolds & L. Mann (Eds.), *Encyclopedia of special education* (Vol 1), (pp. 541-543). New York: Wiley.

Ramos, C., Stark, L., & Hannaford, B. (1989). Time optimality, proprioception, and the triphasic EMG pattern. *Behavioral and Brain Sciences*, *12*, 231-232.

Seyfort, B., & Spreen, O. (1979). Two-plated tapping performance by Down's syndrome and non-Down's syndrome retardates. *Journal of Child Psychology and Psychiatry*, *20*, 351-355.

Shumway-Cook, A., & Woollacott, M.H. (1985). Dynamics of postural control in the child with Down syndrome. *Physical Therapy*, *65*, 1315-1322.

Spreen, O., Tupper, D., Risser, A., Tuokko, H., & Edgell, D. (1984). *Human developmental neuropsychology*. New York: Oxford University Press.

Stein, R.B. (1982). What muscle variable(s) does the nervous system control in limb movements? *Behavioral and Brain Sciences*, *5*, 535-540.

Sternberg, S., Monsell, S., Knoll, R.L., & Wright, C.E. (1978). The latency and duration of rapid movement sequences: Comparisons of speech and typewriting. In G.E. Stelmach (Ed.), *Information processing in motor control and learning* (pp. 117-152). New York: Academic Press.

Stratford, B. (1979). Discrimination of size, form and order in Mongol and other mentally handicapped children. *Journal of Mental Deficiency Research*, *23*, 45-53.

Stratford, B. (1980). Perception and perceptual-motor processes in children with Down's syndrome. *The Journal of Psychology*, *104*, 139-145.

Stratford, B., & Ching, E.Y.Y. (1989). Responses to music and movement in the development of children with Down syndrome. *Journal of Mental Deficiency Research*, *33*, 13-24.

Wade, M.G., Hoover, J.H., & Newell, K.M. (1984). Training reaction and movement times of moderately and severely mentally retarded persons in aiming movements. *American Journal of Mental Deficiency*, *89*, 174-179.

Wade, M.G., Newell, K.M., & Wallace, S.A. (1978). Decision time and movement time as a function of response complexity in retarded persons. *American Journal of Mental Deficiency*, *83*, 135-144.

Weathers, C. (1983). Effects of nutritional supplementation on IQ and certain other variables associated with Down syndrome. *American Journal of Mental Deficiency*, *88*, 214-217.

Weiss, A.D. (1965). The locus of reaction time change with set, motivation and age. *Journal of Gerontology*, *20*, 60-64.

Wishart, J.G. (1988). Early learning in infants and young children with Down syndrome. In L. Nadel (Ed.), *The psychobiology of Down syndrome* (pp. 7-50). Cambridge, MA: MIT Press.

Wisniewski, K.E., Miezejeski, C.M., & Hill, A.L. (1988). Neurological and psychological status of individuals with Down syndrome. In L. Nadel (Ed.), *The psychobiology of Down syndrome* (pp. 315-343). Cambridge, MA: MIT Press.

Woollacott, M.H., & Shumway-Cook, A. (1986). The development of postural and voluntary motor control systems in Down's syndrome children. In M.G. Wade (Ed.), *Motor skill acquisition and the mentally handicapped: Issues in research and training* (pp. 45-71). Amsterdam: North-Holland.

Worringham, C.J. (1989). Inferring motor deficits in Down syndrome: The role of practice. In M.L. Latash (Ed.), *Proceedings of the Motor Control in Down syndrome Conference* (pp. 47-49). Chicago, IL: Rush-Presbyterian St Luke's Medical Center.

Yellin, A.M., Lodwig, A.K., & Jerison, H.J. (1979). Effects of rate of repetitive stimulus presentation on the visual evoked brain potentials of young adults with Down's syndrome. *Biological Psychiatry*, *14*, 913-924.

Yellin, A.M., Lodwig, A.K., & Jerison, H.J. (1980). Auditory evoked brain potentials as a function of interstimulus interval in adults with Down's syndrome. *Audiology*, *19*, 255-262.

Zemlan, F.P., Thienhaus, O.J., & Bosmann, H.B. (1986). Increased chromosome 21q22.1 marker in Alzheimer's disease and Down's syndrome. *Society Neuroscience Abstracts*, *12*, *Part* 2., 1314.

Approaches to the Study of Motor Control and Learning
J.J. Summers (Editor)

Chapter 14

THE MOVEMENT APPROACH: A WINDOW TO UNDERSTANDING THE CLUMSY CHILD

Dawne Larkin & Deborah Hoare
University of Western Australia

Poorly coordinated children who have difficulty learning and performing motor skills manifest many different profiles. Given the complexity of the multiple subsystems that interact in the organisation of tasks, it is not surprising that there is uncertainty as to the nature of the movement dysfunctions. The information processing approach has investigated perceptual and cognitive processes contributing to the problems with movement organisation. The neurobehavioural approach has been used to explore aberrant movement and subtypes of dysfunction in various subsystems that contribute to the organisation of motor behaviour. No matter what the source of the problem, it is apparent in the emergent movement. The final focus here is on the movement processes that are impaired in the clumsy child. Problems are apparent in coordination and control. However individual differences in movement profiles have indicated that subtypes may be recognised at the movement level of analysis.

There has been limited analyses of the inefficient movement processes that contribute to the awkward actions of children with movement dysfunctions. Studies of the underlying myoelectric activity that support action and modulate the reactions of the moving system have received sparse attention. Even fewer studies have actually explored changes in the movement patterns of these motor learning disabled children during skill acquisition. The distributed control approach to the organisation of movement indicates that control could be degraded by dysfunction in any contributing subsystem. Neurophysiological studies provide support that lesioning or cooling of different areas of brain can degrade movement initiation, direction, amplitude, velocity, acceleration, force, sequencing, and timing. Investigation of the kinematic, kinetic, and myoelectric patterns underlying the task outcomes can help to identify the different problems that contribute to awkward movement and promote a deeper understanding that can concomitantly improve remediation protocols.

In this chapter we explore approaches to understanding children who have difficulty learning or performing motor skills. Following this introduction there is a brief review of the information processing and the neurobehavioural perspectives on clumsy movement. The final section includes a review of work focusing on the movement processes which contribute to the inefficient outcomes. Our understanding of the movement dysfunctions manifest by this population has emerged from these perspectives and present a somewhat haphazard but complementary body of knowledge. In consequence the categorisation attempted here is somewhat arbitrary.

Children who have difficulty learning and performing skills that most children achieve with relative ease are labelled in many ways. Terms such as clumsiness, dyspraxia, motor impairment and movement dysfunction are used synonymously throughout this paper to refer to this group. However, attempts have been made to define dyspraxia as a subcategory within a general category of mild movement disorder (Ayres, 1979; Denckla, 1984; Gubbay, 1975). The problems encountered with a more succinct definition of dyspraxia were clearly discussed by Denckla (1984).

We do not know what causes the awkward movement of children who do not have an identifiable neural dysfunction. Many theorists and clinicians have suggested multiple causality (Gubbay, 1975; Morris & Whiting, 1971). Subclinical conditions have been considered as causes of the discoordinate movement (Illingworth, 1963; Ingram, 1963) including minimal cerebral dysfunction (Ayres, 1979; Wigglesworth, 1963). Subtypes are hypothesised at the process level, particularly the sensori-integrative (Ayres, 1979), the perceptuo-motor level (Dare & Gordon, 1970; Hulme, Biggerstaff, Moran, & McKinlay, 1982; Laszlo & Bairstow, 1985a), and at the task level (Hoare & Larkin, 1989). Although the motor tasks used to identify subtypes have been loaded differentially in terms of underlying processes, they have all relied on outcome measures such as error, time taken, or distance achieved.

It has also been considered that the movement difficulties simply reflect performance at the lower end of the normal distribution of movers (Ingram, 1963). Developmental delay has been suggested as an explanation of the poor control and coordination. Kalverboer (1975) and van Dellen (1986) have addressed this issue by attempting to differentiate dysmaturity and dysfunction.

Clinical observations suggest that there are a group of inefficient movers who by comparison to their peers, respond rapidly to a movement program. These children may be movement deprived (Morris & Whiting, 1971) but identification at present is post hoc rather than a priori. Implicit in the notion of developmental delay or deprivation is the consideration that the clumsy child may in fact 'catch up'. However identification, remediation, and support during the 'delay' period are important to prevent the development of inappropriate patterns in the fundamental skills generally acquired during this time.

By contrast it is apparent that many movement problems are marked by qualitatively different rather than delayed myoelectric (Williams, Fisher, & Tritschler, 1983) and movement patterns (Hoare, 1987; Larkin, Hoare, Phillips, & Smith, 1987). It is important that we define more precisely how these movement problems vary and if there are consistent subtypes at any level of observation, be it task, underlying movement, or perceptuo-motor process.

It is likely that we may never identify all the factors that contribute to this apparently heterogeneous condition. However, more systematic inquiry of the movement processes (Davis, 1984) in combination with the morphological and fitness components that contribute to unsuccessful movement outcome is necessary. Without this research, we cannot identify whether the different patterns of movement deficit manifest by poorly coordinated children reflect specific motor disabilities (Lockwood, Larkin, & Wann, 1987) or the interaction between subtypes, strategies, and experience.

THE INFORMATION PROCESSING APPROACH AND MOVEMENT DYSFUNCTION

The information processing approach to motor control has provided a vehicle for exploring the processes perturbed in developmental clumsiness (Hulme & Lord, 1986; Hulstijn & Mulder, 1986; Laszlo & Bairstow, 1985a; van Dellen & Geuze, 1988). This model has limitations as it is a somewhat linear representation of human motor performance. It has, however, been an appropriate framework to use given our current understanding of clumsiness.

Using the information processing model, attempts have been made to relate deficiencies in receptor modalities to motor problems in children. Motor output normally requires some processing of perceptual information. If this is impaired in any manner then motor skills may reflect this. Decisions based upon inadequate perceptual input and error detection imply that correction during performance may also suffer. Perceptual research has primarily addressed vision and kinaesthesis as they are the dominant sensory contributors to motor performance.

Visual Perception and Movement Dysfunction

A series of studies by Hulme and colleagues has consistently related visual perceptual deficits to motor problems in clumsy children (Hulme et al., 1982;

Hulme, Smart, & Moran, 1982; Lord & Hulme, 1987a; Lord & Hulme, 1988). Using a line length matching task, clumsy children were found to be less accurate than normal children in both visual, kinaesthetic, and cross modal matching (Hulme et al., 1982). The deficit in visual perception correlated with performance on a small battery of motor tests, whereas kinaesthetic and cross modal sensitivity did not. Further research using a variety of measures has shown that difficulties occurred in visuo-spatial perception of area, slope, spatial position, and linear length that were not due to visual acuity problems (Lord & Hulme 1987a).

When perceptual input conditions were systematically varied to determine the effect on drawing performance, the clumsy children were inferior to that of a control group (Lord & Hulme, 1988). When the children were required to draw the same object without sight the results were similar. If poor visual perception was contributing to the motor problem one would expect that in the absence of vision the performance difference between the two groups would be smaller. The results suggest, therefore, that impaired visual monitoring during drawing was not a contributing factor to the inferior performance of clumsy children. Overall, there is a certain amount of ambiguity in this series of studies. The extent to which visual perceptual problems contributed to movement dysfunction was not clearly established. Much of the evidence was based on correlations.

Kinaesthesis and Movement Dysfunction

Hume and colleagues were unable to show that kinaesthetic perception was correlated with motor skill in clumsy children. In contrast, Laszlo and coworkers have reported consistent relationships between kinaesthesis and motor behaviour. Poor kinaesthetic sensitivity has been shown to correlate with difficulties in writing and drawing in children (Bairstow & Laszlo, 1981). Laszlo and Bairstow (1983) also found that kinaesthetic training improved the drawing performance of children identified by low kinaesthetic ability. During the development of a kinaesthetic sensitivity test (Laszlo & Bairstow, 1985b) it was noted that, for their age, the performance of clumsy children was inferior. In a subsequent study (Laszlo, Bairstow, Bartrip, & Rolfe, 1988) a group of 40 clumsy children, when trained kinaesthetically over several hours, improved their posttest motor performance.

The relationship between kinaesthesis and motor development has been somewhat inconclusive. Lord and Hulme (1987b) have shown that clumsy children could not be distinguished from a group of age matched controls using kinaesthetic testing. Furthermore, there was no consistent relationship between kinaesthesis and motor development in these children. Elliott, Connolly, and Doyle (1988) found that the relationship between kinaesthesis and motor performance was a function of maturation and that the two were not associated independent of age. Sugden and Wann (1987) could not establish a clear relationship between kinaesthesis and motor performance in children with learning and movement difficulties.

It is apparent from the work of Laszlo and colleagues that dyskinaesthesis could be contributing to the motor problems of clumsy children. However, theoreticians who focus on facilitation of underlying sensory processes often hypothesise that a global and non specific activation will lead to an improvement in general motor performance. A transfer of process information is assumed across tasks. Kinaesthesis, however, varies according to movement (Loeb, 1984) and task requirements. Clarifying these demands may elucidate the relationships with motor performance.

We still have much to learn about the role of vision and kinaesthesis in the movement problems of clumsy children. Contrasting results only serve to reemphasise the need to consider the heterogeneity of the population. These inconsistencies may reflect the varying characteristics of the samples used.

Movement Dysfunction and Response Selection, Programming and Execution

The preceding discussion focused on the sensory input stage of the information processing paradigm. Cognitive, central, and motor response processes have been addressed by others. The emphasis has been on breakdown in response selection, programming, and/or response execution.

Van Dellen (1986) varied precuing in a choice reaction time task in order to differentiate response selection from response programming. Clumsy children were found to be slower and less accurate than age matched control children. The increase in reaction time was greater when direction was not cued and the response direction was incompatible with the stimulus direction. The clumsy children also demonstrated an increased reaction time when neither extent or direction were cued. Movement time was longer in the incompatible condition but it did not differentiate the clumsy from the control group. It appeared that clumsy children had more difficulty in the translation of the stimulus code to the response code than normal children, particularly as the amount of information increased.

Hulstijn and Mulder (1986) also reported that children with minor motor difficulties had increased reaction times when drawing simple lines and more complex patterns. The children found difficulty in performing the task quickly and relied heavily on visual feedback. This is in contrast to the findings of Lord and Hulme (1988) who suggested that poor visual monitoring did not contribute to inefficient performance in their sample of clumsy children. Although movement time did not discriminate the group with minor motor difficulties from normal controls, error scores did and may have reflected an inability to utilise stored motor programs or a problem with response execution.

Schellekens, Scholten, and Kalverboer (1983) looked at response time and movement organisation in hand movements of children with minor neurological dysfunction. The slower responses of these children, when compared to control subjects, were attributed to difficulties in the planning and control of hand movements. The initial movement was shorter (in the open loop phase), suggesting that preprogramming was less efficient in these children. In addition, the overall movement time was longer and they required more corrections towards the end of the movement. Similar results have been reported by Forsstrom and von Hofsten (1982) in a study of children with motor impairments. An interesting observation was that when reaching for moving targets motor impaired children took their inability to time their actions into account by aiming the movements ahead of the target in order to intercept it effectively.

Looking at the movement production can provide valuable insights when there are no apparent movement time differences. For example, Kalverboer and Brouwer (1983) reported similar total times on a visuo-motor task (fitting shapes into matching apertures) for boys grouped according to neurological status. Although the poorer groups had faster motor activity, it was accompanied by "more additional movements, misplacements, and major deviations at insertion" (Kalverboer & Brouwer, 1983, p. 83).

The information processing model has been used extensively as a basis to further our understanding of developmental movement dysfunctions. It has proved to be a useful model to work from as the components can be differentially loaded to determine their contribution to movement. Nevertheless, the above research has demonstrated some inconsistent findings. The parallel exploration of the movement processes has the potential to elucidate some of the incongruity.

There is one overriding difficulty with research in this area: the profiles of the groups vary. Some inconclusive findings may be resolved by defining samples more stringently. Identification of subtypes of clumsiness could control for the varying characteristics within and between samples used, and provide some explanation for the discrepant results.

NEUROBEHAVIOURAL APPROACHES AND MOVEMENT DYSFUNCTION

Neurobehavioural approaches to the study of clumsy movement have tended to use developmental apraxia and agnosia (Gubbay, 1975) or dyspraxia (Cermak, 1985) as the terminology of choice. The movement information reported has predominantly been qualitative description of aberrant motion using neurological terms (Denckla, 1984; Gubbay, 1975). By contrast to the simpler movements often used in information processing research, tasks evaluated and researched have been based on experience with brain damage, representative of hypothesised neurofunctions (Ayres, 1979; Denckla, 1974; Paine, Werry, & Quay, 1968), or age appropriate motor behaviour (Denckla, 1984).

Motor Impairments

Neurological descriptions of the awkward movement of children have provided a basis for movement subtypes based on subclinical recognition. For example, Ingram (1964) refers to varying categories of mild cerebral palsy as being recognisably or abnormally clumsy with the mildly diplegic having clumsy gait. Undoubtedly some of these children are not identified by neurological examination and simply labelled as clumsy. In experimental work using motor impaired groups, subtypes of movement dysfunction are included. For example, Forsstrom and von Hofsten (1982) described the movement style of some group members as athetotic, some ataxic, and others as exhibiting combinations of these styles.

Other problems seen that typify motor control difficulties include extraneous movement. Often with gross motor movement it appears to occur more as a reaction to segmental and intersegmental forces rather than as athetotic or choreic movement. Synkinaesis and overflow movements are also apparent at ages when they are considered inappropriate (Denckla, 1984).

In addition to these problems of mobility, the inability to maintain positions or postures has been described in the clumsy child. Morris and Whiting (1971) related this to the neurological dysfunction termed motor impersistence which has been more closely associated with right hemisphere deficits in adults (Fisher, 1956). Difficulties regularly reported with standing balance have been attributed to sensory integrative dysfunction (Ayres, 1979) as well as more complex disharmony between sensory and motor interactions (De Quiros & Schrager, 1978).

Subtypes of Dyspraxia

From a neurobehavioural perspective, emphasis has also been placed on the contribution of sensory processes to clumsy movement. Ayres (1979) described developmental dyspraxia as a motor planning deficit resulting from sensory integrative dysfunction and manifested as poor coordination. The degradation of vestibular, proprioceptive, and tactile integration contributing to clumsiness. By contrast, Denckla (1984) discusses a variety of definitions of developmental dyspraxia.

Adult apraxia has been considered to be a breakdown in learned actions, while developmental dyspraxia has been regarded as a problem with learning actions. Adult apraxia results from brain damage, whereas developmental apraxia does not show evidence of this type of trauma (Knuckey, Apsimon, & Gubbay, 1983). Nevertheless, the adult models have provided directions for a theoretical framework with different types of dyspraxia.

Constructional apraxia (Benton, 1967/1985) described in adult patients, for example, has a behavioural parallel in some dyspraxic children. Difficulties with construction of two and three-dimensional structures and the copying and drawing of shapes have been reported (Brenner, Gillman, & Farrell, 1968), sometimes accompanied by finger agnosia (De Ajuriaguerra & Stambak, 1969).

The more obscure types of apraxia that impair axial movements and gait have warranted little attention despite the apparent difficulties experienced by clumsy children when performing locomotor tasks (Larkin & Raynor, 1989). Apraxia of gait has been described in terms of limb apraxia of the legs and feet where bilateral leg movements may be more impaired (Meyer & Barron, 1960). Movement difficulties of the face and trunk may accompany those of the limbs (Poeck, 1985; Poeck, Lehmkuhl, & Willmes, 1982). Similar problems are observed in the movement of clumsy children. However, the lack of specific movement description has hampered comparison, and the extrapolation from the adult to the developing child is difficult.

De Ajuriaguerra and Stucki (1969) indicated that two types of dyspraxic children have difficulties with body image, those with severe motor problems and those with affective problems. Ayres (1979) proposed a strong link between dyspraxia and the disordered 'body percept' by focusing on sensory integrative dysfunction. A problem with tactile processing, or proprioceptive dysfunction may result in a failure to update the changing position of body and limbs during movement. Vestibular dysfunction was also hypothesised to contribute to the disrupted body percept. These sensory disturbances were seen as contributing to the motor planning disorder. Ayres described a number of movement related problems which reflected vestibular deficit. Symptoms considered to accompany vestibular underactivity included ambimanuality, left-right confusion, difficulty with gross and fine motor skills, and impaired balance. Over-reaction to vestibular stimulation was also hypothesised to interfere with the performance of movement by making a child posturally or gravitationally insecure (Ayres, 1979). The over-reaction resulted in constant fear of moving above the ground or on stairs and slopes, and a dislike of rapid or spinning movement. Ayres suggested that the fear was a much greater threat than the actual likelihood of falling, in contrast to the underactive vestibular disorder where the child constantly falls but has very little reaction to it.

Difficulty producing movements requiring interaction with extrapersonal space has also been attributed to underlying neural disorder. Ayres (1979) suggested that the sensory integration disorder could lead to movement problems when dysfunction at the cortical level interfered with the development of spatial maps which were necessary for dealing with activities in personal and extrapersonal space.

Although subtypes of dyspraxia are implied in the foregoing neurobehavioural descriptions, the subtyping of developmental dyspraxia was explicitly researched by Ayres, Mailloux, and Wendler (1987) and Conrad, Cermak, and Drake (1983). The tasks selected to elucidate subtypes were drawn from different adult models. However, both studies used children with learning rather than motor learning disabilities. The failure to identify subtypes could be related to the assumption that the learning disability (sensory integrative disorder) would be accompanied by a motor planning disorder. Additional problems arise from operationalising the definitions of dyspraxia (Denckla, 1984).

The neurobehavioural literature suggests subtypes of movement dysfunction even within the broad context of dyspraxia. If we hypothesise that movement dysfunctions are a reflection of 'minimal cerebral dysfunction' (Ayres, 1979; Wigglesworth, 1963), it would be necessary to hypothesise subtypes to accommodate damage to different functional subsystems with deficits in the movement processes reflected in movement production as well as different types of tasks. The movement profiles shown by children with motor planning or execution problems should be different from those with sensory disorders, if these theoretical models are viable. Hoare, who is currently carrying out an investigation of subtypes with children grouped according to whether their movement is "normal" or "clumsy", should be able to classify subgroups in terms of their performance on tasks differentially loaded according to modality and movement type. Preliminary findings indicate that this is the case (Hoare & Larkin 1989).

DISTRIBUTED CONTROL OF MOVEMENT

An underlying theme that influences our research comes from studies of motor control that support distributed organisation of movement (Arbib, 1972; Mountcastle & Edelman, 1978). The neurofunctional subsystems of the brain seem to be committed to the organisation of relatively specific aspects of movements or tasks (Roland, 1984). It is obvious that such a complex and dynamic system could both obscure or sustain multiple movement dysfunctions of a relatively mild nature, with somewhat complex implications for motor learning, assessment, and remediation.

Despite the very limited understanding of brain function and its relationship to behaviour, these understandings have always influenced approaches to assessment and remediation. Theoretical ideas of the distributed organisation of movement and the supporting research are suggestive of subtypes of movement dysfunction and provide direction for exploring movement deficiencies. Nevertheless damage to a subsystem which may be crucial to the performance of a task, redundant or irrelevant for a different task, and cause interference with other motor tasks, means that under different task demands performance could be impaired, unperturbed, or improved (Arbib, 1972). A complicating problem may be that variable strategies available to solve the action could obscure a deficit.

Along with the notion of distributed control of movement by the brain, notions of reciprocity and redundancy (Davis, 1976) may have relevance for the educator or therapist. The notion of reciprocity suggests that there are reciprocal neural networks that are active in more than one role. Failure to automate movement or damage to such a network would limit available strategies and possibly lead to inconsistencies in task production under different circumstances. By contrast, the concept of redundancy has been put forward (Davis, 1976) to accommodate duality of function which may allow recovery of movement through alternate subsystems.

The presence of multiple representation of muscles and limbs in different combinations may make possible limited redundancy in the system. However, somatotopy can also support damage and consequent breakdown in specific limbs without decrement in other areas. The clumsy child with specific lower limb problems may fall into a category that requires topological considerations.

Hypothesising Movement Dysfunctions

A relevant example of distributed control is demonstrated by separate cortical subsystems for reciprocal and coactive control of movement. Humphrey and Reed (1983) reported that some cortical neurons were activated in relation to reciprocal activity of flexor or extensor activity while different neurons (subsystems) were related to cocontractive activity. Furthermore, the type of motor unit activity varied with the frequency demands of the movement and the reciprocal activity of flexor and extensor muscles.

What can this information contribute for those who are trying to understand subtle problems in the production of movement? If such a predictive mode is generated to maintain static balance, the cocontractive mode of the flexors and extensors around the joints should prime the fast twitch motor units so that they respond to disturbances by rapidly initiating a compensatory reaction on a relatively stiff joint. This would limit sway and assist in maintenance of balance. Williams, McClenaghan, and Ward (1985) suggested that by comparison to normally developing children, slowly developing children used more reciprocal than cocontractive control in the maintenance of standing. They did not appear to be using a predictive mode. This may account for the very slow responses of many clumsy children to disturbances, with a resultant inability to hold static balance.

We could hypothesise a subtype of movement dysfunction where cocontraction is a problem. If cocontraction is used in the early phase of skill development to limit the degrees of freedom (Bernstein, 1967) and reduce external perturbations, including those which are a function of the physical forces created by the movement itself, the learning of new skills would be difficult. A different problem with movements and motor learning would be predicted if a subsystem involved in reciprocal activity was impaired.

There are a number of functional subsystems where non-optimal activity may contribute to different movement problems. The proprioceptors provide an example by way of their complex contribution to the organisation of movement. Muscle spindle afferents respond specifically to position, velocity, and changes in length of muscles. Their responses also vary according to the type of contraction. Eccentric responses are differentiated from concentric responses (Loeb, 1984). Despite the fact that their signals come from the muscle, the information appears to be interpreted in terms of joint adjustments and positions (Matthews, 1982, for review).

The varying responses of subjects to proprioceptive illusions induced by vibration of muscles emphasises the interdependence between motor and sensory subsystems. Undoubtedly the absence of efferent discharge in Lackner's (1988) vibration experiments contributed to bizarre interpretations of joint positions and changes in size and position of body parts. Just how the efferent and afferent information is integrated in the learning and performance of neuromotor tasks is a complex and unresolved issue (Partridge, 1979). However, the occurrence of proprioceptive illusions when efferent information is unavailable indicates that subtypes involved of movement dysfunction could arise from malfunction of the subsystems in the identification of active body parts. A problem with active body positioning could involve motor-sensory disturbances and require different identification and remedial procedures that a closely related subtype such as dyskinaesthesis, where the sensory subsystem is implicated.

When attempting to categorise movement dysfunctions, relationships to the external environment should be considered as well as movement requirements. For example, different functional subsystems were indicated when blood flow in the parietal lobe changed according to whether movements were carried out in intrapersonal or extrapersonal space (Roland, 1984). The premotor area was strongly activated by non-routine tasks relying on sensory input. Prefrontal cortex activity varied according to whether the information used to generate movement involved language, perceptions, or internal volition (Roland, 1984). These functionally defined subsystems support the notion of motor dysfunction subtypes and could help explain the different profiles of clumsiness (Hoare & Larkin, 1989). However, devising tests to identify the separate contributions of functional subsystems to the organisation of movements and tasks is obviously complex.

Despite the subtlety of the movement dysfunctions, we use the information from brain-behaviour studies to guide our observations. Exploration of movement guided by ideas of functional subsystems may elucidate subtypes of movement dysfunctions in children. Motor control relies on the integration of multiple subsystems. Interplay and balance between subsystems contribute to the smooth production of movement. Imbalance between subsystems may affect the fine tuning of the movement. The neurobehavioural studies also support a need to look at elements of the movement such as timing, movement direction, speed, amplitude, and force. Movement analysis in conjunction with a breakdown of the task elements may provide information about underlying processes that are probably less global than those we currently use.

A MOVEMENT EMPHASIS ON MOVEMENT DYSFUNCTION

The focus on the movement of clumsy children has been indirectly influenced by the complexity of the acting system. Attempting to deal with the interaction between the neuromotor subsystems, the energetics, and the environmental constraints is awesome. By exploring the production of fundamental locomotor skills we have been able to eliminate some perceptual demands and focus on segmental, intersegmental, and interlimb performance. Our ongoing intent is to carefully describe the movement processes of the children experiencing difficulties with motor control.

We hope to identify whether the breakdown appears in: the sequencing of the activity as measured by the ordering of limb segments; the timing of the activity as indicated by the time flow of initiations of segments, and the timing of peak velocities; the amplitude of the movement; the speed of the movement; or the force parameters. Movement subtypes may be identified and further our understanding of factors contributing to the degraded acquisition and performance of skills. Exploring kinematics has provided more information about movement production, and increased our understanding of the underlying motor control deficits.

In this section we focus on the movement processes, for no matter what the cause of the breakdown, it emerges in the movement. First, we will review our own studies of locomotion which compare poorly coordinated children with normally and well coordinated children. Secondly, drawing upon the studies of other researchers, we will provide a broader view of the information that has emerged from focusing on movement processes.

Our studies of locomotion have provided empirical support for the notion that clumsy children have problems with the control of force, amplitude, and tempo of movement (Walton, Ellis, & Court, 1962). However, coordination may be impaired as well as control. The studies involved three tasks, running (Larkin & Raynor, 1989; Raynor, 1989), jumping (Hoare, 1987; Larkin, Hoare, Phillips, & Smith, 1987), and hopping (Larkin et al., 1987; Phillips, 1987). The tasks were selected because they are fundamental skills (Wickstrom, 1983) that have meaning for the child (culturally relevant) and provide the basis for more complex game skills. Additionally, despite exposure and practice, they are not well performed by the majority of clumsy children. We also had a concern that the clumsy child may maintain inefficient locomotor habits unless intensive teaching and feedback were provided. Their patterns are perceived as awkward and expose the children to peer ridicule.

To date our cinematographic studies have been confined to children ranging in age from 5 to 8 years. The choice of these age groups was influenced by the children that we work with and the importance of this age band for the development of fundamental skills. The children described in all of the following studies were functioning in ordinary schools, although some had specific learning disabilities apart from their motor learning disability. With one exception the McCarron Neuromuscular Development battery (McCarron, 1982) was used to identify the movement proficiency of the populations.

All filming of locomotor trials was done with a Locam high speed camera set at 100 frames per second. The x-y coordinates obtained from lower limb joint centres provided the raw data which was filtered at 4 or 6 Hz before segmental and endpoint kinematics were obtained, including displacement and velocity. Our quantitative focus was confined to the right lower limb in the running and jumping studies, the preferred hopping leg in the initial study of the hop, and both limbs in the second hopping study. Because the poorly coordinated groups demonstrated instability of the trunk, head, and arms which resulted in rotational movements, qualitative analysis was considered the appropriate method to describe these body segments.

Running

The study of running involved poorly coordinated and well coordinated 7-year-old girls and boys (Larkin & Raynor, 1989; Raynor, 1989). This age was selected because there is fair agreement in the limited literature that the movement pattern should be mature by this age (Fortney, 1980; Wickstrom, 1983), although Bernstein (1967) suggested that mature gait was reached around 12 years. Ages at which mature patterns are achieved in movement skills are quite variable (Bloomfield, Elliott, & Davies, 1979). For this reason it is appropriate to select well coordinated children to provide the model of what an optimal system can do. The well coordinated 7-year-old runners presented a relatively mature movement pattern and aesthetically pleasing performance, providing an excellent model to compare to the discoordinate patterns.

During a 50 metre run, when the poorly coordinated children ran as fast as they could, their performance was characterised by a decreased stride length and an increased stride time when compared to their well coordinated peers. We have no data from comparative studies with this population, however adults with gait apraxia have demonstrated some similar adjustments when walking. Reduced velocity of walking was accounted for by decreased stride length and increased stride time (Knutsson & Lying-Tunell, 1985).

For poor runners, the percentage of cycle time spent in support was greater, whereas the percentage of time in the swing phase was less. The amplitude of their movements undoubtedly contributed to the decreased swing time and stride length. During the swing phase of the run, the clumsy runners had limited flexion and extension of the hip and knee and a smaller range of movement. Knutsson and Lying-Tunell (1985) reported that adults with gait apraxia also had a reduced ratio of swing to stance phase which could be partially accounted for by the continuous activation of antigravity muscles throughout the gait cycle. The adult gait apraxia was further characterised by poor push-off and reduced angular displacements.

Peak segmental velocities were lower in the poorly coordinated groups for the thigh and the leg during the support phase. The findings were similar during the swing phase where the velocity difference was also apparent in the foot. Although the lower peak velocities could result from a coping strategy, it is more likely that inefficiency of the underlying muscular activity is contributory. The electromyographic study of Williams and colleagues (Williams, Fisher, & Tritschler, 1983) support such an hypothesis.

The coordination difficulties experienced by the children were highlighted by the relatively later initiation of ankle extension during the support phase. This slower initiation was interpreted as a reflection of inefficient dynamic balance. It could also represent a general problem with extensor movements in the propulsive phase of locomotor movements. Difficulties were also experienced in the propulsive phase of the jump where dynamic balance loading would be somewhat less, and in the continuous stationary hop where it would be increased. Overactive anti-gravity muscles need to be eliminated as a possible explanation.

In the running study, we were also interested in whether clumsy females would produce a similar or different movement profile to male peers. In the movement analysis, however, no differences were apparent (Raynor, 1989). Using a visuo-motor task, Kalverboer and Brouwer (1983) report minor differences between sexes attributable to slower performance of the girls from the group with the lowest neurological optimality scores. However, these slower times were recorded when the children were not under time stress.

Jumping

The findings from two studies of the standing broad jump with poorly coordinated children are reviewed here. Study 1 compared two normally performing groups with two groups of poorly coordinated children (Larkin et al., 1987). At each coordination level the groups were aged 5 to 6 and 7 to 8 years. There were four boys in each group. The poorly coordinated groups in this study were identified using the Stott, Moyes, and Henderson (1972) battery. Study 2 compared a group of 5 and 7-year-old well coordinated boys with poorly coordinated groups of the same age (Hoare, 1987). There were ten boys in each group. Despite the difference in control criteria (normal and well coordinated) the two studies provided comparable information.

The outcome measure of distance jumped clearly differentiated the poorly coordinated children from normally and well coordinated peers. The poorly coordinated groups were relatively inconsistent with a greater difference between their best and worst performance.

The initial preparation for the jump is referred to as the unweighting phase. It extends from the start of movement until the knees reach maximal flexion. Differences in hip and knee flexion did not clearly differentiate between the groups of children (Hoare, 1987; Larkin et al., 1987). Nevertheless, in both studies the poorly coordinated children did not prepare as well as the normally coordinated children. Their limited knee flexion (significantly less for the poorly coordinated 7-8 year olds in Study 1) during the preparatory phase of the jump restricted the range of movement through which force could be developed by sequential segmental extensions in the propulsive phase of the jump. In the second study this was very obvious. By comparison with their well coordinated peers, the poorly coordinated boys had a limited movement range at the hip, knee, and ankle during propulsion (Hoare, 1987).

The reduced movement range was accompanied by less extension of the knee and hip at take off for the poorly coordinated when compared to their well coordinated peers. However in both studies, the mean extension at the ankle of the older poorly coordinated boys was less than that of any other group. This difference was not apparent with the younger poorly coordinated group. The pattern was suggestive of a performance deterioration in the older poorly coordinated jumpers. Having to move a heavier and taller body with a poorly tuned neuromotor system may have repercussions on performance that could reflect coping strategies rather than a further degradation in the neuromotor system. The effect of weight has been demonstrated in a study of spastic paretic patients. These subjects showed an improvement in joint angular displacements, stride length, and timing of EMG patterns while walking with support that reduced body weight by 40% (Visintin & Barbeau, 1989).

The sequence of initiation of segmental extensions provided some insight into coordination. Of the well coordinated boys, 80% initiated extension at the hip, followed by the ankle, and then the knee. This was similar to the mature pattern reported by DiRocco, Clark, and Phillips (1987) where initial heel extension preceded knee extension. This pattern allows the jumper to extend the body further forward at takeoff and contributes to a more optimal performance. The remaining 20% had sequential or simultaneous extension of hip, knee, and ankle. Only 40% of the poorly coordinated group used the hip, ankle, then knee initiation sequence so prevalent among the well coordinated group. Sequential initiation at the hip followed by the knee then the ankle was used by 30% of this group, while 15% used simultaneous extension. Two of the remaining 7-year-old poorly coordinated children initiated an early extension at the hip and a late, but simultaneous, extension at the knee and ankle, while a lone 7-year-old child had early extension of the hip and knee followed by late extension at the ankle.

Coordination during propulsion was poor, and the qualitative analysis showed that the inefficient strategies responsible varied across individuals. These differences in initiation and order of sequential extensions are suggestive of subtypes of movement problems. The difficulties with sequencing and timing may reflect a specific problem in the organisation of movement.

Landing patterns of these children were inefficient, while the well coordinated children provided a model of control available at this developmental age. The clinician and educator are well aware of the heavy landings of the clumsy child, however movement processes that contribute to this problem have received limited attention. Landing patterns are of particular concern as they are basic to all locomotor tasks. The inability to smoothly absorb the forces exerted throughout the body when landing results in jarring and may contribute to joint deterioration and soft tissue injury. The limited flexion of the limbs during landing certainly constrains the dissipation of momentum.

Just prior to landing the clumsy children demonstrated limited ventroflexion of the head by contrast to the well coordinated group who appeared to throw their heads forward which facilitated the forward movement of their centre of gravity. The data showed that the poorly coordinated children had less flexion at the hip and knee at the point of impact, indicative of a failure to prepare for landing. Limited dissipation of momentum resulted from the strategy predominant among the poorly coordinated group. They took a similar time to move through a shorter movement range than their well coordinated peers. Their more conservative movements could reflect an attempt to simplify the action by limiting the degrees of freedom, or it may reflect an inability to accommodate or utilise the external force field (Bernstein, 1967).

Qualitative analysis of the arm actions revealed that 75% of the clumsy children were asymmetrical at landing. Only 10% of the well coordinated group demonstrated this lack of control. In this instance it was clear that the poorly coordinated were unable to constrain excessive degrees of freedom.

Landing is considered to be preprogrammed rather than reflexive (Melvill Jones & Watt, 1971a, b). Difficulties experienced in achieving a smoothly executed landing may represent problems with planning, a difficulty in the fine tuning of the neuromotor system, or a perturbation during jumping. When landing, the necessary predictive organisation was inadequate in the discoordinate groups.

The landing patterns clearly differentiated between the two levels of coordination. The poorly coordinated children were considered to have a different quality of movement pattern rather than demonstrating a developmentally delayed pattern. Generally the jumping patterns of the poorly coordinated 7-year-olds could not be described as similar to children with a less mature pattern.

Hopping

Hopping was studied in two experiments. The initial study (Larkin et al., 1987) involved a normal population, the second study (Larkin, Phillips, Hoare, & Smith, 1988; Phillips, 1987) involved the same 5 and 7-year-old boys who performed in the jumping study. Hopping was of interest not only for its pragmatic value for the child (the hop is seen as a task used to arrest perturbations, as well as a movement of play), but also for its unusual asymmetric development which has been considered useful as a predictor of later clumsiness (Denckla, 1984). Initially children will have a preferred leg for hopping. Denckla (1974) reported that left to right hopping performance differences decreased from age 5 to age 7. By age 7, 90% of the children sampled were capable of hopping with minimal performance differences between legs. The hopping task provided a natural activity to explore whether asymmetry of performance would be prolonged in the child with neuromotor delay or a subclinical asymmetric motor dysfunction. The children hopped on the spot on a Kistler force platform. Although the children were asked to perform six high hops in a row, this was not possible for all children on the preferred and non-preferred foot.

For both legs, the poorly coordinated boys spent relatively more time in the support and propulsive phase of the hop than in the flight phase. The decreased flight time of the clumsy boys can be attributed to lower vertical velocities and the decreased extension of the hip at take off on the preferred and non-preferred side. On the non-preferred side the limited extension of the knee and ankle also contributed to the shorter flight time (Phillips, 1987).

Force plate data revealed that the poorly coordinated group had a lower impulse on the preferred and the non-preferred leg, but the lower peak ground reaction force normalised by body weight was clearly apparent only for the non-preferred leg (Larkin et al., 1988). The force data from the poorly coordinated child reflected a lack of strength and coordination. At this stage of our enquires we are unable to disassociate the contribution of each of these factors, however the limited extension of the hip, knee, and ankle apparent on the non-preferred leg undoubtedly contributed to the lower peak force. Attempts to measure strength in the poorly coordinated are probably confounded by the coordination problem when traditional multi-segmented movements such as the broad jump are used.

The poorer performance outcomes of the poorly coordinated children were accompanied by a reduced range of segmental movement, particularly in the propulsive phase of the jump and hop and the swing phase of the run. Lower peak segmental velocities were apparent in the run during the support phase and the run and the jump during the flight phase. The poorly coordinated groups spent relatively longer time in the support phase of the hop and the run with relatively less time in the swing phase of the run and the flight phase of the hop.

Qualitative analysis also made a contribution to our understanding of the problems experienced by these inefficient movers. Different patterns of segmental initiations were apparent with a few of the poorly coordinated children that were suggestive of ordering problems and timing problems. The quantitative data showing a different pattern of initiation of extension in the support phase while running (Raynor, 1989) provided more general support for the latter problem.

Other Studies

Other researchers who have focused on movement processes have reported differences between motor impaired children and normal controls. Williams et al. (1983) explored underlying muscular activity during static balance tasks. Whereas the control group showed a reduction in average EMG amplitude with increasing age from 4 to 8 years, this decrease was not apparent in the slowly developing group. Between the impaired and control groups within each age band, the patterns of activity were quite different. In a further study, Williams et al. (1985) reported decreased cocontraction in the EMG patterns of the awkward children. The child with sufficient information about environmental perturbations can predict postural instability and produce early postural adjustments through anticipated and preplanned motor responses (Keshner, 1983). It seems that the clumsy child with postural deficits is unable to maintain postural stability as a function of internal perturbations rather than any external interference. Delays in postural feedback have been reported (Haas, Diener, Rapp, & Dichgans, 1989). Long loop responses to postural disturbances were later in children with motor and mental delays than children who were functioning normally at school.

The difficulty that clumsy children have learning motor skills has often been reported, however few studies have actually explored the changes that occur with learning. Marchiori, Wall, and Bedingfield (1987) followed the progress of two physically awkward boys for 6 weeks who were practising 200 hockey shots each week. Filming procedures were used to monitor their progress every two weeks. In an initial comparison with two control boys, the velocity of the puck did not clearly distinguish between the awkward and control boys. However, the awkward children showed discontinuous movement as observed from the angular velocity of the moving stick. The inconsistency remained even after 1200 practice trials.

Although inconsistency in outcome measures has been noted in clumsy children, kinematic analysis has provided a more detailed description of the movement problem. The increased movement elements reported in the hand trajectory of motor impaired children (Geuze & Kalverboer, 1987; Shellekens et al., 1983) appear to represent a similar problem to the discontinuous movement in the velocity trace of the moving stick (Marchiori et al., 1987). The velocity trace appears similar to that reported by Brooks (1986) for non-programmed movements during the early stages of learning.

The lack of consistency in the performance of movements (Geuze & Kalverboer, 1987; Larkin et al., 1987; Marchiori et al., 1987) would be confusing and the motor-sensory match from the movement task would be inadequate to promote learning for the clumsy child. Even in the normally performing child, the acquisition of skill is limited if feedback is not complemented by good teaching (Alexander, 1941/1986) or coaching.

Dysfunction in the execution phase of the movement would affect the development of predictive strategies. The inability to reliably generate the desired outcome, manifest by inconsistency in the movement could interfere with the development of motor control feedforward strategies. Efference copy and corollary discharge may contribute to difficulties in tuning movement. However, where there is a general breakdown in the neuromotor system, we would predict that the deficit would be apparent in all movements and tasks predominantly requiring this function. It would be independent of topology.

We have also attempted to identify other movement related factors that may contribute to difficulties learning and performing motor skills. For example, if the lowered motor fitness of the clumsy child (Larkin & Hoare, 1990b) results from the movement problem, the effect can contribute to further movement degradation. The hypotonicity seen in a number of children with movement dysfunctions, may be a function of the initial problem or a secondary problem emerging from withdrawal hypoactivity. It may be related to the low strength demonstrated by these children when compared to norms for their age group (Larkin & Hoare, 1990b).

Similarly, the lack of flexibility seen in a portion of these children may be a primary or secondary problem. A bimodal distribution found in our clinical sample (Larkin & Hoare, 1990b) where the children were hypoflexible and hyper extensible suggests both possibilities.

In our studies we have also measured other anthropometric characteristics of the poorly and well coordinated samples. The poorly coordinated groups have consistently been more endomorphic than their well coordinated peers (Larkin, Hoare, & Kerr, 1989; Raynor, 1989).

These problems with fitness and size would be more apparent in gross motor skills. Size changes may be of importance in understanding the interrelationship between cause and effect. If, for example, we assume a developmental lag in the nervous system as a cause of movement dysfunction, we cannot ignore that the interaction between increased physical size and an immature neuromuscular system may lead to complications in the organisation of movement. Something as unusual as a failure of the neuromuscular system to respond to the demands of increased growth and size, hypothesised to occur in the normally growing child (Sargeant, 1989), could contribute to the low estimates of anaerobic power seen in clumsy children (Raynor, 1989). With the exception of force measures we have not been able to clearly establish a link between size and performance of the poorly coordinated groups.

THE TASK APPROACH

The concepts of task specificity (Henry, 1968) and 'task specific devices' (Bingham, 1988) appear to have some relevance for children who have a general problem learning motor tasks. With explicit teaching and motivation, these children are able to achieve an acceptable level of task performance, i.e., they may learn to land efficiently in specific contexts but the ability to land well does not generalise across tasks or contexts. Skill achievement is somewhat isolated.

Teaching tasks is one approach that can be taken with the clumsy child. Theoretically this approach assumes specificity of motor skill performance, with the task as an emergent of the multiple subsystems that are required to perform. There is a certain amount of indeterminacy hypothesised within the neuromotor system which will contribute to the use of different strategies to achieve similar performance outcomes. For simplicity, we can assume that a number of sensory modalities can contribute differentially to the organisation of a specific task, and the predominance of a modality varies according to the bias of the individual or the teaching approach taken. For example, the task of walking on a balance beam could be approached by the teacher focusing the child on a visual cue or alternatively on tactile and kinaesthetic cues. One approach may be more appropriate than the other if there is a degradation in a particular sensori-motor modality.

Unfortunately with the clumsy child, at the task level, we see the inappropriate transfer of information between tasks. An example is the combination of a star and broad jump when the two are taught within the same lesson but not necessarily consecutively. The separation of the legs during elevation and landing may be superimposed on the broad jump. This is typical of perseveration and interference seen in some forms of adult apraxia.

If difficulty with transfer is a problem experienced by some dyspraxic/clumsy children, then facilitating sensorimotor processes in one task or context, may have a negative influence on tasks that might be assumed to have predominantly the same sensorimotor requirements. For example, the gravity receptors activated on the trampoline are just the same as those activated when jumping down from a box or balance beam. The movement organisation required to deal with the landing surfaces, however, are quite different. Even in the normally coordinated child, the motor set established while landing on the trampoline interferes with the ability to land safely on the ground when jumping from the trampoline. Unless there is a change in motor set, the interference from the previous task can contribute to the perseveration of the movement pattern established by the repetitive action established on the trampoline, with rather negative consequences as the mover fails to absorb the ground reaction forces of the inflexible surface.

SUMMARY

Movement dysfunction is the primary indicator for identifying the clumsy child. Despite this obvious focus toward movement breakdown, research has been predominantly directed toward perceptuo- and sensori-motor processes. We have currently been exploring the problems experienced by this population from a number of perspectives including movement processes, sensori-motor and perceptuo-motor processes, as well as task performances. These approaches contribute in different ways to further our understanding of the motor control problems experienced by these children. In isolation these perspectives can provide a biased view.

A number of questions that arise from the subtypes hypothesised earlier, focus on the emergent movement, for it is the movement that clearly identifies these children. From a movement organisation perspective, what subtypes of movement dysfunction might we be able to predict? Are there identifiable variations in the movement profiles of these children, that will help us to identify the underlying dysfunctions? For example, is there a group that are unable to time segmental interactions to produce an orderly and efficient summation of the lower limbs? Are there subgroups that are able to coordinate lower limbs but have difficulty when it comes to the upper and lower limb linkage? Certainly the clinician regularly experiences this type of discoordination. At the movement level, what is it that distinguishes the slowly moving subgroup from those who are able to move quickly but not well? Using theoretical perspectives on the organisation of movement, we may eventually predict and identify different types of disordered processes which will help us to understand the movement dysfunctions.

REFERENCES

Alexander, F.M. (1941/1986). *The universal constant in living*. Centerline Press.

Arbib, M.A. (1972). *The metaphorical brain.* New York: Wiley-Interscience.

Ayres, J.A. (1979). *Sensory integration and the child.* Los Angeles: Western Psychological Services.

Ayres, J.A., Mailloux, Z.K., & Wendler, C.L.W. (1987). Developmental dyspraxia: Is it a unitary function? *Occupational Therapy Journal of Research, 7*, 93-110.

Bairstow, P.J., & Laszlo, J.I. (1981). Kinaesthetic sensitivity to passive movements and it's relationship to motor development and motor control. *Developmental Medicine and Child Neurology, 23*, 606-616.

Benton, A.L. (1985). Constructional apraxia and the minor hemisphere. In L. Costa & O. Spreen. (Eds.), *Studies in neuropsychology* (pp. 119-130). New York: Oxford University Press. (Reprinted from *Confinia Neurologica*, 1967, *29*, 1-16).

Bernstein, N. (1967). *The coordination and regulation of movements*. Oxford: Pergamon.

Bingham, G.P. (1988). Task specific devices and the perceptual bottleneck. *Haskins Laboratories Status Report on Speech Research, SR93/9*, 221-246.

Bloomfield, J., Elliott, B.C., & Davies, C.M. (1979). Development of the soccer kick: A cinematographic analysis. *Journal of Human Movement Studies, 5*, 152-159.

Brenner, M.W., Gillman, S., & Farrell, M.F. (1968). Clinical study of eight children with visual dysfunction and education problems. *Journal of Neurological Sciences, 6*, 45-61.

Brooks, V.B. (1986). *The neural basis of motor control*. New York: Oxford University Press.

Cermak, S. (1985). Developmental dyspraxia. In E.A. Roy (Ed.), *Neuropsychological studies of apraxia and related disorders* (pp. 225-248). Amsterdam: North-Holland.

Conrad, K.E., Cermak, S.A., & Drake, C. (1983). Differentiation of praxis among children. *American Journal of Occupational Therapy, 37*, 466-473.

Dare, M.T., & Gordon, N. (1970). Clumsy children: A disorder of perception and motor organisation. *Developmental Medicine and Child Neurology, 12*, 178-185.

Davis, W.E. (1984). Motor ability assessment of populations with handicapping conditions: Challenging basic assumptions. *Adapted Physical Activity Quarterly*, *1*, 125-140.

Davis, W.J. (1976). Organizational concepts in the central motor networks of invertebrates. In R.M. Herman, S. Grillner, & P.S.G. Stein (Eds.), *Neural control of locomotion* (pp. 265-293). New York: Plenum Press.

De Ajuriaguerra, J., & Stambak, M. (1969). Developmental dyspraxia and psychomotor disorders. In P.J. Vinken & G. Bruyn (Eds.), *Handbook of Clinical Neurology*, (Vol. 4. pp. 443-464). Amsterdam: North-Holland.

De Ajuriaguerra, J., & Stucki, J-D. (1969). Developmental disorders of the body schema. In P.J. Vinken & G. Bruyn (Eds.), *Handbook of Clinical Neurology*, (Vol. 4. pp. 392-406). Amsterdam: North-Holland.

Dellen, T. van (1986). *Response processing and movement organisation in clumsy children: An experimental approach*. Proefschrift, Rijksuniversiteit te Gronigen.

Dellen, T. van, & Geuze, R.H. (1988). Motor response processing in clumsy children. *Journal of Child Psychology and Psychiatry*, *29*, 480-500.

Denckla, M.B. (1974). Development of motor co-ordination in normal children. *Developmental Medicine and Child Neurology*, *16*, 729-741.

Denckla, M.B. (1984). Developmental dyspraxia: The clumsy child. In M.D. Levine & P. Satz (Eds.), *Middle childhood: Development and dysfunction*. (pp. 245-260). Baltimore: University Park Press.

De Quiros, J.B., & Schrager, O.L. (1978). *Neuropsychological fundamentals in learning disabilities*. San Rafael, CA: Academic Therapy.

DiRocco, P.J., Clark, J.E., & Phillips, S.J. (1987). Jumping coordination patterns of mildly mentally retarded children. *Adapted Physical Activity Quarterly*, *4*, 178-191.

Elliott, J.M., Connolly, K.J., & Doyle, A.J.R. (1988). Development of kinaesthetic sensitivity and motor performance in children. *Developmental Medicine and Child Neurology*, *30*, 80-92.

Fisher, M. (1956). Left hemiplegia and motor impersistence. *Journal of Nervous and Mental Diseases*, *123*, 201-218

Forsstrom, A., & von Hofsten, C. (1982). Visually directed reaching of children with motor impairments. *Developmental Medicine and Child Neurology*, *24*, 653-661.

Fortney, V.L. (1980). *The kinematics and kinetics of the running pattern of two, four-, and six-year-old children* [Microform]. Ann Arbor MI: University Microfilm International.

Geuze, R.H. & Kalverboer, A.F. (1987). Inconsistency and adaptation in timing of clumsy children. *Journal of Human Movement Studies*, *13*, 421-432.

Gubbay, S.S. (1975). *The clumsy child: A study of developmental apraxic and agnosic ataxia*. London: W.B. Saunders.

Haas, G., Diener, H.C., Rapp, H., & Dichgans, J. (1989). Development of feedback and feedforward control of upright stance. *Developmental Medicine and Child Neurology*, *31*, 481-488.

Henry, F.M. (1968). Specificity v generality in learning motor skill. In R.C. Brown & G.S. Kenyon (Eds.), *Classical studies on physical activity*. (pp. 328-331). Englewood Cliffs, NJ: Prentice Hall.

Hoare, D. (1987). *Jumping patterns of poorly co-ordinated children*. Unpublished honours thesis, University of Western Australia. Nedlands, W.A.

Hoare, D., & Larkin, D. (1988, August). *Movement differences between poorly coordinated boys and their well coordinated peers*. Paper presented at the XXIV International Congress of Psychology, Sydney, N.S.W.

Hoare, D., & Larkin, D. (1989). Subtypes of dyspraxia in children. [Abstract]. In S.A. Dunlop & M.G. Grounds (Eds.), *Transactions of the Tenth Annual Neuroscience Colloquium of Western Australia*. Fremantle, W.A.

Hulme, C., Biggerstaff, A., Moran, G., & McKinlay, I. (1982). Visual, kinaesthetic and cross-modal judgements of length by normal and clumsy children. *Developmental Medicine and Child Neurology*, *24*, 461-471.

Hulme, C., & Lord, R. (1986). Clumsy children: A review of recent research. *Child: Care, Health and Development*, *122*, 256-269.

Hulme, C., Smart, A., & Moran, G. (1982). Visual perceptual deficits in clumsy children. *Neuropsychologia*, *20*, 475-81.

Hulstijn, W., & Mulder, T. (1986). Motor dysfunctions in children. Towards a process-oriented diagnosis. In H.T.A. Whiting & M.G. Wade (Eds.), *Themes in motor development* (pp. 109-126). Dordrecht: Martinus Nijhoff.

Humphrey, D.R., & Reed, D.J. (1983). Separate cortical systems for control of joint movement and joint stiffness: Reciprocal activation and coactivation of antagonist muscles. In J.E. Desmedt (Ed.), *Motor control mechanisms in health and disease* (pp. 347-372). New York: Raven Press.

Illingworth, R.S. (1963). The clumsy child. *Little Club Clinics in Developmental Medicine*, *10*, 26-27.

Ingram, T.T.S. (1963). Chronic brain syndromes in childhood other than cerebral palsy, epilepsy and mental defect. *Little Club Clinics in Developmental Medicine*, *10*, 10-17.

Ingram, T.T.S. (1964). *Paediatric aspects of cerebral palsy*. Edinburgh: Livingstone Ltd.

Kalverboer, A.F. (1975). *A neurobehavioural study in pre-school children*. London: William Heinemann Medical Books.

Kalverboer, A.F., & Brouwer, W.H. (1983). Visuo-motor behaviour in pre-school children in relation to sex and neurological status: An experimental study on the effect of 'time-pressure'. *Journal of Child Psychology & Psychiatry*, *24*, 65-88.

Keshner, E.A. (1983). *Organization of equilibrium reactions in children under varying conditions of spatial and temporal uncertainty*. Unpublished doctoral dissertation, Columbia University, New York.

Knuckey, N.W., Apsimon, T.T., & Gubbay, S.S. (1983). Computerized axial tomography in clumsy children with developmental apraxia and agnosia. *Brain and Development*, *5*, 14-19.

Knutsson, E., & Lying-Tunell, U. (1985). Gait apraxia in normal-pressure hydrocephalus: Patterns of movement and muscle activation. *Neurology*, *35*, 155-160.

Lackner, J.R. (1988). Some proprioceptive influences on the perceptual representation of body shape and orientation. *Brain*, *111*, 281-297.

Larkin, D., & Hoare, D. (1990a, January). Movement dysfunctions in clumsy children. [Abstract]. *Commonwealth and International Conference on Physical Education, Sport, Health, Dance, Recreation & Leisure, Auckland, N.Z.*

Larkin, D., & Hoare, D. (1990b). *Understanding and teaching children with movement dysfunctions*. Manuscript submitted for publication.

Larkin, D., Hoare, D., & Kerr, G. (1989, June). *Structure/function interactions: A concern in the movement impaired child.* Poster presentation at the 7th International Symposium on Adapted Physical Activity, Berlin (Abstract No.: 159).

Larkin, D., Hoare, D., Phillips, S., & Smith, K. (1987). Children with impaired co-ordination: Kinematic profiles of jumping and hopping movements. In D.E. Jones & T. Cuddihy (Eds.), *Progress through refinement and innovation*. (pp. 67-72). Brisbane: CAE Press.

Larkin, D., Phillips, S., Hoare, D., & Smith, K. (1988, August). *Performance asymmetry in poorly coordinated children.* Paper presented at the XXIV International Congress of Psychology, Sydney, N.S.W.

Larkin, D., & Raynor, A. (1989). Locomotor limitations exhibited by the clumsy child. [Abstract]. In S. A. Dunlop & M. G. Grounds (Eds.), *Transactions of the Tenth Annual Neuroscience Colloquium of Western Australia* (p. 39). Fremantle, W. A.

Laszlo, J.I., & Bairstow, P.J. (1983). Kinaesthesis: It's measurement, training and relationship to motor control. *Quarterly Journal of Experimental Psychology*, *35a*, 411-421.

Laszlo, J.I., & Bairstow, P.J. (1985a). *Perceptual-motor behaviour: Developmental assessment and therapy*. London: Holt, Rinehart & Winston.

Laszlo, J.I., & Bairstow, P.J. (1985b). *Test of kinaesthetic sensitivity*. London: Holt, Rinehart & Winston.

Laszlo, J.I., Bairstow, P.J., Bartrip, J., & Rolfe, U. (1988). Clumsiness or Perceptuo-motor dysfunction. In A.M. Colley & J.R. Beech (Eds.), *Cognition and action in skilled behaviour* (pp. 293-309). Amsterdam: North-Holland.

Lockwood, R.J., Larkin, D., & Wann, J.P. (1987). Specific motor disabilities. In R.J. Lockwood (Ed.), *Physical education and disability* (pp. 80-86). Parkside, South Australia: ACHPER.

Loeb, G.E. (1984). The control and responses of mammalian muscle spindles during normally executed motor tasks. In R.L. Terjung (Ed.), *Exercise and Sport Sciences Reviews* (Vol. 12, pp. 157-204). Lexington, MA: Collamore Press.

Lord, R., & Hulme, C. (1987a). Perceptual judgements of normal and clumsy children. *Developmental Medicine and Child Neurology*, *29*, 250-257.

Lord, R., & Hulme, C. (1987b). Kinaesthetic sensitivity of normal and clumsy children. *Developmental Medicine and Child Neurology*, *29*, 720-725.

Lord, R., & Hulme, C. (1988). Visual perception and drawing ability in clumsy and normal children. *British Journal of Developmental Psychology*, *6*, 1-9.

Marchiori, G.E., Wall, A.E., & Bedingfield, E.W. (1987). Kinematic analysis of skill acquisition in physically awkward boys. *Adapted Physical Activity Quarterly*, *4*, 305-315.

Matthews, P.B.C. (1982). Where does Sherrington's "muscular sense" originate? Muscles, joints, corollary discharges? *Annual Review of Neurosciences*, *5*, 189-218.

McCarron, L.T. (1982). *McCarron assessment of neuromuscular development* (rev. ed.). Dallas: Common Market Press.

Melvill Jones, G., & Watt, D.G.D (1971a). Observations on the control of stepping and hopping movements in man. *Journal of Physiology*, *219*, 709-727.

Melvill Jones, G., & Watt, D.G.D (1971b). Muscular control of landing from unexpected falls in man. *Journal of Physiology*, *219*, 729-737.

Meyer, J.S., & Barron, D.W. (1960). Apraxia of gait: A clinico-physiological study. *Brain*, *83*, 261-284.

Morris, P.R., & Whiting, H.T.A. (1971). *Motor impairment and compensatory education*. London: G. Bell & Sons.

Mountcastle, V., & Edelman, G.M. (1978). *The mindful brain*. Cambridge, MA: MIT Press.

Paine, R.S., Werry, J.S., & Quay, H.C. (1968). A study of 'minimal cerebral dysfunction'. *Developmental Medicine and Child Neurology*, *10*, 505-520.

Partridge, L.D. (1979). Muscle properties: A problem for the motor controller physiologist. In R.E. Talbot & D.R. Humphrey (Eds.), *Posture and movement*. (pp. 189-229). New York: Raven Press.

Phillips, S.E. (1987). *Exploring lateral differences in poorly and well coordinated populations on the hopping task*. Unpublished honours thesis, University of Western Australia. Nedlands, W.A.

Poeck, K. (1985). Clues to the nature of disruptions to limb praxis. In E. A. Roy (Ed.), *Neuropsychological studies of apraxia and related disorders*. (pp. 99-109). Amsterdam: North-Holland.

Poeck, K., Lehmkuhl, G., & Willmes, K. (1982). Axial movements in ideomotor apraxia. *Journal of Neurology and Psychiatry*, *45*, 1125-1129.

Raynor, A.J. (1989). *A comparison of the coordination and gender differences in the running pattern of seven year old children.* Unpublished honours thesis, University of Western Australia, Nedlands, W.A.

Roland, P.E. (1984). Organisation of motor control by the normal human brain. *Human Neurobiology*, 2, 205-216.

Sargeant, A. (1989). Short-term muscle power in children and adolescents. *Advances in Paediatric Sport Sciences*, *3*, 41-65.

Schellekens, J.M.H., Scholten, C.A., & Kalverboer, A.F. (1983). Visually guided hand movements in children with minor neurological dysfunction: Response time and movement organisation. *Journal of Child Psychology and Psychiatry*, *24*, 89-102.

Stott, D., Moyes, F., & Henderson, S. (1972). *Test of motor impairment.* Ontario: Brook Education Publishing.

Sugden, D., & Wann, C. (1987). The assessment of motor impairment in children with moderate learning difficulties. *British Journal of Educational Psychology*, *57*, 225-236.

Visintin, M., & Barbeau, H. (1989). The effects of body weight support on the locomotor pattern of spastic paretic patients. *Canadian Journal of Neurological Sciences*, *16*, 315-325.

Walton, J.N., Ellis, E., & Court, S.D.M. (1962). Clumsy children: Developmental apraxia and agnosia. *Brain*, *85*, 603-612.

Wickstrom, R.L. (1983). *Fundamental motor patterns* (3rd ed.). Philadelphia: Lea & Febiger.

Wigglesworth, R. (1963). The importance of recognising minimal cerebral dysfunction in paediatric practice. *Little Club Clinics in Developmental Medicine*, *10*, 34-38.

Williams, H.G., Fisher, J.M., & Tritschler, K.A. (1983). Descriptive analysis of static postural control in 4, 6, and 8 year old normal and motorically awkward children. *American Journal of Physical Medicine*, *62*, 12-26.

Williams, H.G., McClenaghan, P.E.D., & Ward, D.S. (1985). Duration of muscle activity during standing in normally and slowly developing children. *American Journal of Physical Medicine*, *64*, 171-189.

Approaches to the Study of Motor Control and Learning
J.J. Summers (Editor)

Chapter 15

MOTOR CONTROL CONSIDERATIONS FOR ASSESSMENT AND REHABILITATION OF MOVEMENT DISORDERS

Judith L. Charlton
Victoria College, Burwood

Recent advances in the study of motor control have, as yet, had little impact on the field of neuromotor rehabilitation. This chapter reviews motor control issues relevant to assessment and rehabilitation of movement disorders. A theoretical framework for the processes responsible for skilled actions is elaborated with particular emphasis on organisation, control and coordination of actions involving the upper limb. The chapter draws together empirical studies describing spatiotemporal characteristics of both pathological and non-pathological actions involving prehension and object manipulation. Evidence is presented for atypical limb trajectories in one apraxic subject. Implications for the use of kinematic measures for clinical assessment, monitoring recovery and establishing strategies for restoration of normal movement patterns are discussed.

Much has been written about neuromotor disorders with respect to localisation of lesions and characterisation of movement difficulties. However, with the exception of Roy (1982, 1983) and Paillard (1982), the study of movement dysfunction has, in the past, been addressed with scant regard to motor control theory. Moreover, motor control research has had negligible impact on clinical assessment and rehabilitation practices. Notwithstanding the importance of neuropsychological and neurophysiological studies in understanding motor dysfunction, the study of processes determining the control and coordination of non-pathological actions has much to contribute to both assessment and therapeutic strategies.

This chapter will focus upon hemiplegia and apraxia, two disorders of voluntary motor control resulting from neurological damage, such as a cerebrovascular accident (CVA), closed head injury or a brain tumour. Discussion will be primarily directed towards disruptions to upper limb function in reaching and grasping and other complex gestural and manipulative actions.

Hemiplegia is a unilateral movement disorder, characterised by uncoordinated, stereotypic movement with abnormal muscle strength and tone and varying degrees of associated loss of sensation. The symptoms arise from damage originating in the contralateral areas of the brain including the sensorimotor cortex, involving Brodmann areas 4 and 6, as well as the internal capsule.

Brunnstrom (1970) has described the sequelae of motor recovery in hemiplegia in terms of a six stage process. The onset of hemiplegia is characterised by flaccidity and a total loss of voluntary action. In Stage 2, spasticity develops with the typical resting posture in the upper extremity of "shoulder girdle retraction, shoulder adduction, elbow flexion and forearm pronation" (O'Sullivan, Cullen, & Schmitz, 1981, p. 146). Voluntary control of so called *movement synergies* is achieved to varying levels in Stage 3. Among rehabilitation professionals, much emphasis has been placed on assessment of synergies, defined by Duncan and Badke (1987a) as "functionally related patterns of muscle contractions" (p. 137). Upper limb control first appears in a stereotypic flexor pattern, identified by elbow flexion, forearm supination, external rotation and abduction of the shoulder, and retraction and elevation of the shoulder girdle. Next, the extensor synergies are reinstated, with stereotyped movements involving elbow extension, forearm pronation, internal rotation and adduction of the shoulder, and protraction of the shoulder girdle. In Stage 4, spasticity declines and greater flexibility of movement patterns may develop using combinations of movements other than those dictated by the flexor and extensor synergies. Brunnstrom describes Stage 5 as the acquisition of more difficult movement combinations; although it is recognised that not all patients will achieve this stage. Finally, in Stage 6, individual joint movements and full restoration of normal coordination are observed.

In contrast to hemiplegia, the difficulties encountered in apraxia cannot be accounted for by abnormalities in muscle strength or tone. Heilman (1979) characterises apraxia as a disorder of "learned skilled movements, not caused by weakness, akinesia, deafferentation, abnormality of muscle tone or posture, abnormal movements such as tremors or chorea, intellectual deterioration, poor comprehension or uncooperativeness" (p. 159). Difficulties arise in particular, in complex tasks or series of actions (Kimura, 1982; Roy, 1981). The disorder is thought to be reflected in actions requiring fine motor control using distal musculature more than actions requiring only proximal limb segments and gross motor control (Haaland, Porch, & Delaney, 1980). Furthermore, apraxia is primarily manifested when pantomiming actions in a clinical setting. The same actions are performed more successfully in their natural context, in the presence of appropriate objects and environmental cues.

Numerous classifications and explanations of apraxia have been offered in an attempt to align what is known about the localisation of brain areas damaged and the resulting movement errors exhibited (see De Renzi, 1985; Faglioni & Basso, 1985; Roy, 1982 for more thorough reviews). Apraxia has most frequently been associated with left hemisphere lesions. Liepman was perhaps the first to suggest a prominent role of the left hemisphere in controlling movements (1905, cited in Faglioni & Basso, 1985). More specifically, Faglioni and colleagues (1985) have identified potential loci of various forms of apraxia as parietal (angular and supramarginal gyri and parieto-occipital areas) and frontal association areas, premotor cortex, as well as intra- and inter-hemispheric pathways connecting these centres.

Our understanding of the recovery processes in apraxia and hemiplegia has been retarded by the subjective nature of clinical assessment and the loose terminology used to evaluate recovery of function. In the following section, a brief review of the various traditional approaches as well as more recent developments in movement assessment is presented.

Evaluation of movement disorders can be categorised into three distinct approaches, differing essentially in terms of the type of information provided. The first approach involves the evaluation of fundamental capacities of the motor system such as muscular strength, muscle tone, and joint range of motion, and reflex activity. The second approach examines the movement outcome and considers aspects such as speed, accuracy, and the level of independence with which the desired action has been achieved. Thirdly, movement disorders can be measured in terms of temporal and spatial characteristics of the movement pattern itself.

ASSESSMENT OF FUNDAMENTAL CAPACITIES

Tests of fundamental capacities of the neuromuscular system have a vital role to play in identifying specific deficits as well as planning therapeutic strategies. These measures are particularly useful in the early stages of recovery of hemiplegia when functional actions are not possible. For example, resistance to passive movement of a limb by a clinician provides information about muscle tone. Joint range of motion (ROM) is commonly used as a measure of maximal joint mobility in stroke patients with limb paralysis. Tests of muscular strength provide information regarding the residual capacity of a muscle to produce tension.

Among the most widely accepted approaches to motor assessment for both clinical and research purposes are those developed by Brunnstrom (1970) and

Bobath (1978). Both authors emphasise that muscle strength and range of motion of the hemiplegic limb vary according to factors such as the particular limb posture or movement adopted. For example, a patient may have full range of wrist extension when the fingers and elbow are flexed but a limited range of wrist extension when the fingers and elbow are extended. Thus, it is important to examine strength and ROM within designated postures or movement contexts. To illustrate this, Brunnstrom's (1970) assessment includes measures of active joint range of the shoulder girdle, shoulder, elbow, and forearm when reaching up to scratch behind the ear and then again, when reaching in a forward and downward direction.

A major criticism of both Brunnstrom's (1970) and Bobath's (1978) tests is that they fail to provide clinicians with objective, quantifiable data (Duncan & Badke, 1987b; Fugl-Meyer, Jaasko, Leymen, Olsson, & Steglind, 1975). For example, Brunnstrom (1970) states that:

> ...active joint ranges may be recorded as 0, 1/4, 1/2, 3/4 or full range. At joints where such estimates are difficult, the ranges may be recorded as zero, incomplete, or complete. For elbow flexion it is convenient to record the joint angle as obtuse, 90 degrees, or acute (p. 144).

More recently, Fugl-Meyer addressed the need to establish quantitative, standardised tests of motor function in patients with hemiplegia. One aspect of the Fugl-Meyer's method of evaluation involves a comparison of passive range of motion in the hemiplegic and non-affected limbs. In this test, passive elbow flexion is given a standard numerical rating of 0 for "only a few degrees of range-of-motion; 1: (for) decreased passive range-of-motion; 2: (for) normal passive range-of-motion" (Fugl-Meyer et al., 1975, p. 19).

The most useful information regarding muscular strength following neurological damage, comes from neurophysiological studies at the level of the motor unit. In a recent review of this research, Duncan and Badke (1987a) attribute the reduction in force output in hemiplegia to one or more of the following factors: "(1) the number of motor units recruited, (2) the type of motor units recruited, and (3) the motor unit discharge frequency" (p. 142). Although a more detailed discussion of this research is not within the scope of this chapter, clinicians should be aware of the potential of integrating knowledge of patterns of muscle activation with other kinds of measures, particularly those describing movement patterns of limbs.

Outcome Measures

Another method of evaluation is to measure how closely the patient's action achieves a predetermined goal. Schmidt (1988a, p. 51) refers to this as measurement of movement outcome.

Speed and spatial accuracy are commonly used outcome measures. Pointing tasks similar to the Fitts tapping task (Fitts, 1954), such as the finger-nose test (Fugl-Meyer et al., 1975), provide the clinician with a relatively crude measure of accuracy in achieving a desired end location.

More precise error measures such as Constant Error (CE) are useful in determining inherent biases in the motor control system in actions involving temporal or spatial accuracy, while Variable Error (VE) describes the patient's consistency in achieving the desired goal. Although widely used in motor control research, these error measures are not commonly used in a clinical setting.

In addition to the examination of fundamental capacities of the motor system and a general neuropsychological examination to rule out muscular weakness and intellectual disorders, apraxia is determined using more global measures of performance outcome. Typically, the apraxia examination assesses performance of learned actions or gestures under three conditions: pantomiming an action according to the clinician's verbal command; imitation of a gesture demonstrated by the clinician; and using real objects appropriate for the task. Various quantitative scoring systems have been employed to rate the severity of apraxia (Dabul, 1979; De Renzi, Motti, & Nichelli, 1980). Roy has drawn attention to the shortcomings of these kinds of outcome measures and suggests that "a clear understanding of the disorder will only develop through careful observation of the nature of the patients' performances" (Roy et al., 1985, p. 403). Roy and colleagues (1985) present a case for more detailed qualitative information about performance and have developed a Limb Praxis Error System to assess the types of errors in apraxic performance. This system attempts to do more than simply characterise the outcome of the action. It provides a means of characterising the pattern of movement and, as such, will be further discussed in the third category of measurements.

In the assessment of hemiplegia, Brunnstrom (1978), Bobath (1978), and Fugl-Meyer and colleagues (Fugl-Meyer et al., 1975) are concerned with performance of movements that form the flexor and extensor synergies, as well as movements combining synergies and movements out of synergy. For example, Fugl-Meyer examines voluntary and independent shoulder joint movement; the desired outcome being shoulder flexion from 90-180 degrees, with the elbow extended and the forearm in the mid-position. A three-point scoring system is used to denote "faultless" motion, or the appearance of elbow flexion or shoulder abduction, either during the motion, or prior to the shoulder movement. While such measures provide information regarding patients' ability to perform specified movements or more functional actions such as grasping an object, limited information is gained about the quality of the action performed.

Clinicians concerned with determining rehabilitation goals assess functional ability in tests of Activities of Daily Living (ADL). ADL scales are designed to describe or quantify the level of independence (or the severity of disability) in performance of basic self-care activities such as dressing, grooming, and eating.

Unlike many tests of movement outcome, ADL scales involve assessment of residual movement abilities in a functional context. Perhaps the most widely accepted ADL scale used in assessment of stroke patients is the Barthel Index (Mahoney & Barthel, 1965). Typical items in this test include categorisation of feeding skills according to whether they can be achieved with help (food needs to be cut) or independently.

Although the Barthel Index is claimed to be both reliable and valid (Granger, Albrecht, & Hamilton, 1979; Granger, Dewis, & Peter, 1979; Gresham, Phillips, & Labi, 1980; Law & Letts; 1989) the major shortcoming of this and other scales of ADL is that they permit compensatory actions. For example, a hemiplegic patient may achieve independence in feeding by using the non-affected arm. Thus, a successful performance, in this instance, tells the therapist nothing about the patient's ability to control and coordinate the affected limb. Another major shortcoming of tests of ADL is the relatively crude scales of measurement, rendering the examination useless for evaluation of long term recovery and efficacy of treatments (Lough, Wing, Fraser, & Jenner, 1984).

The ability to compensate for various movement disabilities raises an important consideration for assessment and therapeutic practice. Goldstein (1948) has identified two distinct rehabilitation strategies. The first is described as a process of restoration of pre-morbid function by relearning old movement strategies (restitution). The second involves compensation for loss of skills by learning new strategies (substitution). If the overriding goal of rehabilitation is to regain functional independence regardless of the quality of movement, the most informative measures of the recovery process are those that determine whether or not a desired action has been achieved. That is, outcome measures. On the other hand, if the primary rehabilitation goal is to restore neuromotor function to its pre-morbid quality, measurements must be more concerned with the pattern of the entire action, not simply the outcome.

One might argue that if a patient is able to drink a glass of water without assistance and without spilling the contents of the glass, the desired outcome has been achieved. Clearly an acceptable level of spatial accuracy has been demonstrated in lifting the glass to the mouth without spilling its contents. Furthermore, the patient's thirst has been satisfied, independent of any assistance. However, a more sophisticated analysis of the quality or pattern of the arm action, such as the path of the hand or the changes in shoulder and elbow joint motion, may provide more helpful information for determining strategies for restoration of normal patterns of movement. The measurement of movement patterns is discussed below.

Measures of Movement Pattern

Traditionally, measures of fundamental capacities and movement outcome have been used almost exclusively by clinicians in the evaluation of movement dysfunction. However, over the past decade, there has been a move in motor control research to describe performance in terms of spatiotemporal characteristics of various limb segments, from initiation of the action to final goal achievement.

The Limb Praxis Error System (Roy et al., 1985) provides a useful research and clinical instrument for qualitative evaluation of apraxia. This system comprises 10 categories of errors, including temporal (delayed responses), spatial (e.g., plane of movement), and form errors (e.g., formation of hand posture). Using this system, each gesture or action is described by a list of error types from the beginning to the end of the action.

More detailed descriptions of actions in terms of displacement, velocity, and acceleration of body segments are collectively called kinematic measures (for an overview of kinematic measurement, see Schmidt, 1988a). Soechting and Lacquaniti (1981) suggest that the trajectory profiles, describing spatial and temporal aspects of movement, provide important information concerning organisation and control of skilled movements. More specifically, Marteniuk and colleagues state that "trajectory profiles are important because if they remain invariant over various task demands, this is support for a movement organisation system (i.e., an internal representation) that is both general and abstract" (Mackenzie, Marteniuk, Jeannerod, Athenes, & Dugas, 1987, p. 366). The question of how general and abstract the action plan is will be addressed later in the chapter. The approach adopted by Marteniuk is that by systematically manipulating variables such as action goals, precision demands, and the number of movement sequences, one can begin to identify those factors which limit or constrain the way actions are controlled and organised. Similar constraints will be reflected in similar organisation and control strategies. By the same logic, similarities and differences in normal and pathological movement trajectories can be determined in order to make inferences about disruptions to organisation and control of actions.

While the techniques are currently available to provide more detailed accounts of motor dysfunction and the motor recovery process, it is essential that these assessment procedures are implemented in a manner that respects current knowledge of how actions are controlled and coordinated. In the following discussion, a brief overview of action plans is presented, with an example to illustrate normal motor control of the upper limb. This review, will focus on those environmental and task-related constraints that determine the temporal and spatial characteristics of action.

THE ACTION SYSTEM

Current theories about mechanisms and processes responsible for skilled actions have described a dynamic interface between performer and environment. Several authors have highlighted the role of two subsystems of an action system. The first subsystem is conceptual in nature and comprises knowledge about the action, objects, or tools and how components of the action are sequenced. The second subsystem, a production system, is procedural in nature and comprises production rules for generating action (Anderson, 1982; Roy, 1983).

I have selected the term *action system*, not with the intention of fuelling the controversy surrounding the distinction between Action and Motor Theories (Marteniuk, MacKenzie, & Leavitt, 1988; Schmidt, 1988b), but rather to emphasise that what is being planned by the system is not a collection of movements per se, but actions with a specific goal, to be achieved within a specific context.

Influenced by Bernstein's (1967) notion of a coalitional style of control, Roy (1983) suggests that the action programs, for which the production subsystem is responsible, are not specific to any one muscle. The act of prehension, for example, involves the regulation of many planes of motion (degrees of freedom) at the shoulder, elbow, wrist, carpal, metacarpal, and interphalangeal joints. An economic solution, it is suggested, is to have an action system that organises the various limb segments involved in movement of a limb in such a way that they are constrained to work as a unit. Alternatively, muscles acting at various joints may be organised into groups, constrained to act as a functional unit, thus reducing the number of individual variables to be controlled and coordinated (Kelso, 1982; Turvey, 1977). Indeed, there is some support for the notion that goal-oriented plans may be carried out by consistent patterns of activation of functional muscle synergies (Cordo & Nashner, 1982; Grillner, 1975; Lee, 1980).

There has been a great deal of debate surrounding the nature of the representation of action. Indeed some authors have argued against the notion of central storage of knowledge for actions (Michaels & Carello, 1981). The view presented here, is that a knowledge base for actions is built up from past experiences and is stored as some form of internal representation that is specific to a given action or class of actions.

Thus, while the idea of muscle specific commands continues to lose favour, empirical support is accumulating for an action-specific view of organisation and control. In this context, *action* or *task* is defined as "the interaction of the performer with the environment under given movement goals" (Marteniuk et al., 1987, p. 377). Consistent with the idea of functional units of action or muscle synergies, Schmidt (1982) suggests that action plans may include general rules for the sequencing, phasing and relative forces generated by muscles operating in a given action. These general rules may be thought of as invariant features of the plan. The performer may select parameters such as the overall duration, overall force, and the limb used, to execute a given action under a specific set of cues.

Several major sources of information have been proposed that might be important in constraining the way an action is performed. These include intentions or goals, on-line body position information, environmental context (including perceived object properties), physical or anatomical properties of the performer, and internalised information about past action experiences such as sensory consequences of actions and knowledge of functional use of objects (Abbs, Gracco, & Cole, 1984; Marteniuk et al., 1987; Roy, 1983).

The pathway of information flow in the action system is not simply a unidirectional route from stimulus to central processor and back to the effector units. Rather, processing is proposed to be distributed throughout the nervous system in a multi-level flexible hierarchy (Allport, 1980). Higher levels, it is suggested here, direct the course of action at an abstract level, with motivation or intent playing an important role in initiating the idea or goal for an action. Lower levels are thought to fill in the detailed adjustments according to the constraints of the specific environmental context. Within this multi-level control mechanism there exists the potential for control to shift from one level to another, depending on the particular set of external or internal constraints (Roy, 1983).

Consistent with this action system explanation is Arbib's (1985) description of a coordinated control program. Arbib highlights the role of environmental properties such as object size, shape, texture, orientation, and location that are incorporated into an internal model, a perceptual schema, which provides identification of parameters relevant for the control system. The control system, which Arbib terms a motor schema, is thought to use the relevant parameters in conjunction with on-line visual and proprioceptive feedback in order to achieve its goals. The extent to which actions are determined by pre-programmed commands or by feedback sampled during the movement is subject to some debate and undoubtably depends on specific task demands. Evidence for the interaction of both strategies in aiming and prehension actions is discussed in the next section.

In order to explain control of complex actions involving many limb segments, Arbib (1985) suggests that combinations of motor schemas are interwoven to achieve a coordinated control program. Arbib's model of a coordinated control program has been used to explain empirical findings of interdependence of a limb transport component, defined as the trajectory of a wrist marker, and a hand manipulation component, or aperture formed between markers on the thumb and index finger, during a reach and grasp action (Jeannerod, 1984). The model is elaborated further in the following section in the context of a complex goal-directed manipulative skill.

To this point in the discussion, the terms *control* and *coordination* have yet to be defined. Indeed, in motor control literature, the two terms have been used somewhat indiscriminantly. This poses a particular problem for rehabilitation professionals who seek to accurately assess and monitor improvement in control and coordination. In this respect, recent attempts to operationally define and distinguish between the terms are particularly welcomed (Kugler, Kelso, & Turvey, 1982; Newell, 1985).

In the action system described above, control refers to the regulation or parameterisation of the functional units involved in the action. Coordination refers to the particular relationship that links individual components of an action. Thus, a well-coordinated action can presumably be described in terms of some spatial and/or temporal relationship among the various joints or limb segments involved. The more "skilful" the action, the more closely its plan approximates some set of optimal values of controlled parameters and some optimal relationship among limb segment movements. It follows, that in order to understand disruptions to skilled actions both control and coordination characteristics should be examined.

Prehension and Object Manipulation - Organisation, Control and Coordination

Let us now consider how an action system, such as that outlined above, might be used to explain the processes involved in prehension and object manipulation. This issue will be addressed with reference to empirical evidence from research on control and coordination of non-pathological actions.

Voluntary actions such as stirring a cup of coffee with a spoon must at some stage in the organisation be 'conceived' (Allport, 1980; Paillard, 1982). This abstract notion of an idea for an act is intentional or motivational in nature; an elusive concept, yet its existence must be acknowledged in order to understand how the more tangible aspects of the action unfold. If the primary goal is to satisfy thirst, the appropriate action may be to use the spoon to first stir the coffee and then to direct the cup to the mouth. Thus stirring the coffee may be thought of as a sub-goal in preparing to drink the coffee. One can then see how the intent and its composite sub-goals, might play an important role, not only in initiating the idea for the action, but in constraining the way in which the action unfolds.

Consider for example, two different goals: (1) stirring and drinking coffee, and (2) scooping food from a bowl and eating. Clearly, in achieving each of these goals, two very different limb trajectories will be produced. Less intuitively, however, the intents implicit in the stirring and scooping actions may also constrain the performance of the initial reaching movement, whereby the wrist is transported towards the spoon. Evidence for this idea comes from the work of Marteniuk and colleagues (1987). These authors found differences in wrist transport trajectories when subjects were required to reach, grasp, and either throw an object into a large container or carefully fit it into a slot. Subjects took longer to perform the initial reach and grasp and spent a greater proportion of time in deceleration when the goal for the entire action required 'fitting'.

Similarly, Fisk and Goodale (1989) manipulated another kind of action goal in order to determine the effects on programming and execution of actions. In this study, subjects performed pointing actions under three different instructional conditions which were interpreted as three different action goals: pointing as quickly as possible, as accurately as possible, or both quickly and accurately. When subjects performed with a speed objective, a significantly smaller proportion of the total movement time was spent in deceleration as compared with both the accuracy and speed/accuracy goals. Thus, goals which incorporate prioritising speed and accuracy affect the characteristics of the limb trajectory, predominantly in the deceleration phase where it is presumed that adjustments or corrections are made under feedback control.

Next let us consider how perception of environmental cues might interact with the action goal. Conceivably, the head, eyes, and trunk will orient towards the objects of interest. This will allow for the object properties to be identified, such as the shape of the spoon handle or the extent to which the coffee cup is filled. In order to identify relevant properties, the performer must draw upon knowledge of spoons and their function. The information the performer has about his or her own body and its location with respect to the spoon, and information about the spoon and its uses, together will constrain the type of grasp that is implemented. Indeed, several researchers have demonstrated that kinematic properties of grasp (e.g., the maximum aperture attained) are sensitive to object size (Jeannerod, 1984; Marteniuk, MacKenzie, & Leavitt, 1988). Furthermore, the size of objects has also been found to influence wrist trajectories in prehension and pointing in such a way that when precision demands were increased (i.e., decreasing the size of objects), a proportionately longer deceleration phase of the wrist transport component was observed (MacKenzie et al., 1987; Marteniuk et al., 1987).

The control or regulation of the reaching, grasping and stirring action is determined by the specific context and demands of the task. If there is an urgent need to quickly satisfy thirst, the action will be performed faster. Similarly, the movement may be speeded up and performed more forcefully if the coffee mug was sturdy and large, but a more delicate action may be generated when a fine china cup is used.

An important issue not considered to this point in the action example is coordination of body segments. In the context of our stirring action, the performer must not only orient the head and trunk in the direction of the spoon and cup, but must coordinate the position of the trunk with movement of the various segments of the upper limb as they reach towards the spoon. Although researchers study a single transport component, in fact this component is comprised of action at both the shoulder and elbow joints. In the above example of the very thirsty performer, while the urgency implicit in the goal may demand that the speed of the reaching action be increased, the phase relations of the component limb segments may remain invariant.

Some of the most important studies that have contributed to our understanding of limb segment coordination have been conducted by Soechting, Lacquaniti, and Terzuolo (1986); Lacquaniti, Soechting, and Terzuolo, (1986); Soechting and Lacquaniti, (1981). For example, Lacquaniti, Soechting, and Terzuolo (1986) demonstrated a tight coupling of shoulder and elbow movements for pointing and drinking actions as expressed by linear relationships between the elbow and shoulder angles. Sparrow, Donovan, van Emmerik, and Barry, (1987) have presented some useful ways of characterising changes in relative joint motion using cross-correlation techniques (see also Chapter 5, this volume). For example, similarities and differences in angle-angle plots can be measured in terms of shape, size, and orientation. While such measures are helpful in quantifying the degree of similarity of intra-limb coordination during prehension, the functional significance of these features of coordination must be interpreted according to the specific task demands.

In the act of reaching to grasp a spoon, not only is there a need to control and coordinate proximal limb segments, but as these movements unfold, the hand must be opened, preshaped and subsequently closed around the spoon thus achieving the goal. It can be seen, therefore, that the action requires certain movements to be performed in sequence and others in parallel.

Indeed, Jeannerod (1981), in a systematic investigation of reaching and grasping actions, identified two distinct yet interacting functional components of the action system. Jeannerod highlighted a temporal coordination between the first component, the transport component, which directs the limb toward the target, and the second component, the manipulation component, wherein the grasping action is effected. Consistent with Soechting and Lacquaniti's (1981) findings, Jeannerod identified within the transport component, an initial fast, ballistic period. This is presumed to be a pre-programmed impulse carrying the limb toward the target. This is followed by a slower period presumably where visual information is used to make the fine adjustments needed to home-in on the target.

Temporal coordination of the transport and manipulation components must be such that the hand is opened prior to reaching the object's location. More precisely, Jeannerod (1981, 1984) has observed that maximum grasp aperture occurs at the onset of the slow, homing-in phase of the transport component. Although it is recognised that efficient prehension is characterised by parallel performance of wrist transport and preparation of the fingers for grasp, other researchers have not reported the precise temporal coordination noted by Jeannerod.

In addition to the temporal organisation of reaching and grasping documented by Jeannerod (1981, 1984), Wing, Turton, and Fraser (1986) have found evidence for spatial organisation links between transport and manipulation components. These authors demonstrated that if the wrist is not accurately directed towards the object, the grasp aperture will be adjusted to compensate for impending spatial error.

In summary, the action system presented here is thought to comprise a number of functional components (such as transport and manipulation components) whose control systems interact and influence one another in a flexible fashion. Execution of the action is thought to be influenced by the action goal, and both stored information about the properties of the performer's body, objects, and their functions, as well as feedback processes providing sensory information about the position of limb segments. The research into normal motor control and coordination presented here is not exhaustive. The intention is to provide some insight into the characteristics of movement patterns during reaching, grasping, and object manipulation. It is proposed that rehabilitation professionals might use this knowledge to guide their observations, methods of assessment and ultimately their understanding of movement disorders.

Disruptions to the Action System

Although the location of cerebral lesions may be vastly different, control and coordination of the upper limbs are clearly disrupted in both hemiplegia and apraxia. Although there is much variability in hemiplegic movement patterns, the characteristic features of fine finger control and motion at the shoulder and elbow joints are typically described as "stereotypic, uncoordinated, inflexible, and non-functional" (Duncan & Badke, 1987a, p. 135). In apraxia, spatial and temporal errors in action sequences involving complex coordination and fine hand posturing have been identified (Friesen, 1986; Haaland et al., 1980; Roy, 1981). These kinds of errors have also been commonly reported in clinical observations. For example, hammering may be demonstrated as a rhythmical pounding action in an inappropriate plane, or waving good-bye may be performed with the hand in a fist posture. Given that apraxics are usually able to recognise that a depicted action is spatially incorrect, Roy (1983) indicates that this is suggestive of a disruption of the production subsystem. Furthermore, apraxia is characterised by errors in miming tool or object use. Performance often improves when appropriate context (actual tool) is provided. This has been attributed to a conceptual subsystem problem; that is, an inability to evoke the pertinent knowledge of tool shape, size, or function (Roy, 1983).

Despite the availability of appropriate technologies and the surge of interest in understanding the spatial and temporal characteristics of reaching and grasping in non-disabled children and adults, few studies have explored the movement patterns of hemiplegia and apraxia. The following review will present some recent attempts to use measures of movement patterns to understand disruptions to motor control and coordination.

In one of the first studies of its kind, Lough, Wing, Fraser, and Jenner (1984) described a longitudinal study of recovery of function in the hemiplegic upper limb following cerebrovascular accident. Holding the handle of an arm support device, subjects performed a reaching action, aligning the handle to a target. Movements were performed as fast as possible. With the forearm resting on a mobile arm support, subjects were able to reach forward freely, without the need to hold the upperarm in an elevated position against gravitational forces. Trajectories of the affected limb were compared with those of the unaffected limb. Preliminary results for a single subject with left side involvement were reported.

Bare in mind that detailed clinical descriptions of the movement recovery process in hemiplegia indicate that flexor synergies appear before extensor synergies and actions requiring more flexible combinations of joint motion appear much later in the course of recovery, if at all (Brunnstrom, 1970). Lough and colleagues (1984) point out that the midline extension required for their reaching task demanded this kind of flexible combination of adduction of the shoulder (part of the flexor synergy) and extension of the elbow (part of the extensor synergy). Although this sequence of recovery is well documented, the spatial and temporal patterns of these actions are little understood. Thus, the reaching action studied here was of particular therapeutic interest.

Trajectories of the handle (part of the arm support, gripped by subject) and key kinematic measures were recorded at 2, 6, and 10 weeks post-CVA. For the purpose of this discussion, the reader should consider the handle trajectories to be comparable with the wrist trajectories reflecting the transport of the wrist to a target. At two weeks post-CVA, displacement profiles indicated marked deviations of more than 10 cm from a straight line path between the starting point and the target. Indeed, for the individual trajectory presented, the wrist followed a zig-zag path, with 5 major direction changes before reaching the target. The movement was slow (3.1 s) with a peak velocity of .8 m/s. At 6 weeks post-CVA, the path of the wrist was more direct, with much smaller deviations of less than 4 cm from a straight line to the target. Total movement time decreased dramatically (to less than 500 ms) and peak speed reached 1.6 m/s. Ten weeks post-CVA, the hemiplegic limb reportedly reached higher peak speeds but a great deal of time was spent making small corrections at the end of the movement to accurately reach the target.

Curiously, although it is recognised that the results were preliminary, Lough and colleagues did not present resultant velocity or acceleration profiles. Such data may have provided greater insight into disruptions to control strategies alluded to here. Consider, for example, a recovery process represented by fundamentally similar shapes of wrist trajectories with relative time spent in acceleration and deceleration remaining invariant but with peak speed increasing as a function of recovery. This may suggest that the same base wrist trajectory (same program) was implemented, but, later in recovery, the basic trajectory was scaled or parameterised by increasing the muscular forces, thereby increasing the peak speed.

On the basis of the displacement-time data, however, it is more likely that the fundamental shape of the trajectory did in fact change over the recovery process, suggesting that fundamental differences in strategies were adopted. More specifically, as recovery progressed, the path of the wrist in the early phase of the movement may be interpreted as adoption of a control strategy which initiates a relatively accurate impulse projecting the hand in a much more direct manner towards the target, with minor feedback-based corrections required only in the final part of the movement. Again, such interpretations may be made more convincingly with the help of acceleration profiles.

Although Lough and colleagues expressed concern for understanding the recovery of coordination in a multi-joint action they did not report data that would allow them to make inferences about the relationship between shoulder and elbow joint motion. Clearly, there is a need for more research in this area to provide directions for rehabilitation professionals in their assessment of control and coordination of the hemiplegic upper limb.

In a similar study, Lough (1987), examined the nature of wrist trajectories of four hemiplegic patients in a pointing task. The action essentially involved either flexion or extension at the elbow joint. Subjects rested their wrist in a cradle and moved between designated targets by sliding the cradle along a track. Of primary interest, was the use of vision to monitor the action. Thus, subjects performed the action both with and without vision of the arm.

Lough reported the general finding that the actions of the stroke patients were slow and halting, as indicated by the multiple peaks of the velocity profiles. In contrast, actions of the patients' unaffected limb and those of the non-brain damaged control subject were represented by movement trajectories with a singular velocity peak. When differences between performance of flexion and extension of the affected limb were compared across the two visual conditions, some most interesting results emerged. Accuracy was consistently high in the flexion action when vision was withdrawn. In contrast, when vision was withdrawn in the extension action, the outcome of the action, the pattern of the action, and the pattern of muscular contraction were noticeably affected.

More specifically, Lough reports that when vision was withdrawn, extension actions were slow and jerky and patients consistently undershot the target. Furthermore, analysis of the EMG data for the extension actions revealed the expected activity of the agonist, triceps, throughout the movement, but undesirable activity in the antagonist group (biceps). Visual monitoring of the limb reduced the level of biceps cocontraction and movements were more accurate, faster, and smoother. In light of the EMG data for the no vision condition, Lough questions whether the interpretation of feedback-based corrections can explain the jerky trajectories of the extension actions performed by the affected limb. Alternatively, it is suggested here that when vision is not available, the hemiplegic patients adopt a pre-programmed control strategy that appears to specify an ineffective pattern of agonist-antagonist contraction. Regrettably, a comparison of velocity profiles for the two visual conditions was not presented. This may reveal helpful information for determining the mode of control adopted. For example, it would be of interest to determine whether sub-movements were made throughout the entire duration of the extension action, or whether they were primarily evident at the end of the action. On the basis of what is known about normal aiming movements, we might expect sub-movements to be evident primarily at the end of the movement when vision was available. This would suggest a relatively accurate pre-programming of the initial impulse carrying the limb towards the target, with visual feedback-based corrections to home-in on the target.

Thus, while Lough's study makes an important contribution in demonstrating the potential of visual information to improve performance of hemiplegic limbs, there is more that could be determined from a detailed comparison of the fundamental shape of the limb trajectories under the two visual conditions.

Some of the most significant contributions to understanding disruptions to upper limb function have come from the work of Jeannerod (1986a, 1986b). Of particular interest is a case study in which Jeannerod (1986a) examined prehension in a child with hemiplegia. Although it is not clear whether the results can be generalised to adult hemiplegia, the methodology and interpretation of results demonstrate a useful approach for assessment of movement disorders. Results indicated that the general shape of the patient's transport component, did not differ noticeably from normal. Although Jeannerod does not address this issue, the trajectory of the affected limb appears to be scaled differently with much greater peak speed to that of the unaffected side. These kinds of differences might be associated with difficulty in regulating the overall forces produced by muscles acting at the shoulder joint, the elbow joint, or both. Alternatively, an inappropriate balance of forces produced by agonist and antagonist muscles in the proximal arm segments might explain these differences in performance speed. An electromyographic analysis together with an examination of the relationship between motion at the elbow and shoulder joints would be useful in addressing these hypotheses.

In addition, Jeannerod (1986a) reports that the kinematic profiles of the manipulation component (aperture between the index finger and thumb, plotted over time) revealed aspects of the grasp that differed considerably from those of normal subjects. More specifically, Jeannerod found that the index finger extended in an exaggerated fashion during the preshaping of the grasp and there was a notable inability to form a grip or closure of the index finger and thumb around the object.

Several authors have reported on the timing of recovery of motion in the various segments of the upper limb (Fugl-Meyer et al., 1975; Bard & Hirschberg, 1965; Twitchell, 1951). There is some support for a recovery pattern that proceeds from proximal to distal, while others suggest that restoration of hand function is independent of recovery of proximal joint motion. The assessment of hemiplegic limb trajectories in both pointing and prehension actions provide a useful model for studying the nature of the recovery process for the control and coordination of proximal and distal limb segments.

On the basis of converging evidence for difficulties in complex coordination and fine hand manipulation in apraxia, Charlton (1988) conducted a systematic examination of the characteristics of movement patterns during performance of reaching and prehension. Complexity of intersegmental limb coordination was manipulated by increasing the number of limb segments and the degree to which fine hand posture and orientation were required. Two apraxics and three non-brain-damaged control subjects, matched by age and gender, participated in the study.

Coordination complexity was manipulated in four experimental conditions. Condition 1, "reach", required subjects to reach forward and place a rod, held vertically in the hand, through a vertically oriented slot. In Condition 2, "reach-orient", subjects reached forward, placing the rod through a slot oriented at 45 degrees to the left of vertical. This condition thus required orientation of the distal limb segment in addition to the reaching action. In Condition 3, "reach-orient-grasp", subjects reached forward and grasped a rod, oriented at 45 degrees. Condition 4, "reach-orient-grasp-stir", was similar to Condition 3, but subjects were required to stir an imaginary cup of coffee once they grasped the rod. The transport component (reach) was examined in all four conditions and the manipulation component (grasp) was examined in Conditions 3 and 4. Neither the lifting of the rod, designating the end of Condition 3, nor the lifting and stirring action of Condition 4 were analysed.

For the purpose of presenting an approach to recording differences in limb trajectories as a function of neuromotor disorder, only left hand performances of one apraxic and one control subject are reported here. The apraxic subject was a 60 year old male who had suffered a CVA of the left hemisphere approximately three years prior to testing. Both subjects performed with their left, non-dominant arm. This was appropriate because the apraxic subject was unable to perform any functional task with the right (contralesional) limb due to dense hemiplegia and subsequent contractures.

The WATSMART (Waterloo Spatial Motion Analysis and Recording Technique) system provided three dimensional spatial coordinates of arm

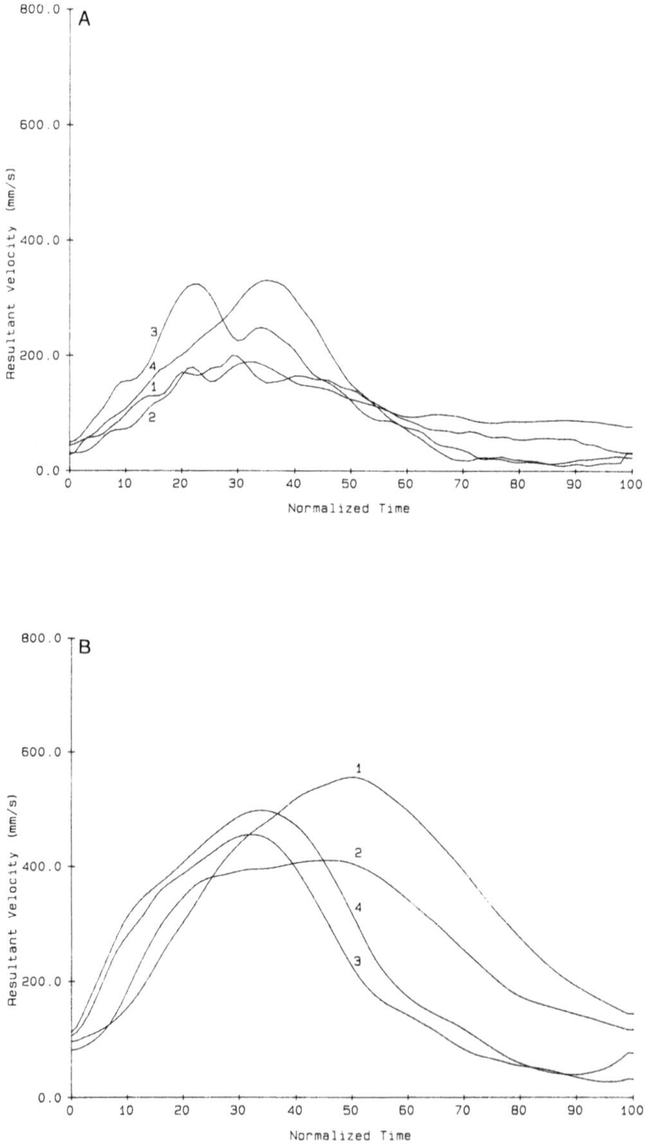

Figure 1. Mean resultant velocity profiles, normalised in time, for apraxic subject (A) and control subject (B) for Condition 1: "reach", Condition 2: "reach-orient", Condition 3: "reach-orient-grasp" and Condition 4: "reach-orient-grasp-stir".

movements. The transport component was described in terms of wrist resultant velocity and acceleration profiles and elbow and shoulder joint phase relations. The manipulation component was described by thumb-index finger aperture profiles. A detailed description of the experimental setup and results for other variables manipulated in this series of experiments are documented elsewhere (Charlton, Roy, Marteniuk, & Mackenzie, in preparation).

Analysis of mean wrist resultant velocity profiles indicated that the apraxic subject was significantly slower, exhibiting smaller peak speeds for all conditions. There was no systematic effect of complexity. However, both subjects were slowest in Condition 3, with the apraxic taking an average of 2.423 seconds and the control taking 1.209 seconds to complete the "reach-orient-grasp" action.

Normalised trajectories presented in Figure 1, show very different shapes for the apraxic and control subject. Note the presence of multiple peaks in Conditions 1 and 2 for the apraxic subject. Thus, comparisons based on percent time spent in acceleration and deceleration are not particularly meaningful since they fail to capture the fundamental differences of irregularities in trajectory shape. Differences in trajectory shape are further highlighted in the acceleration profiles. The acceleration profiles presented in Figure 2 indicate that the apraxic subject made more frequent adjustments of acceleration and deceleration

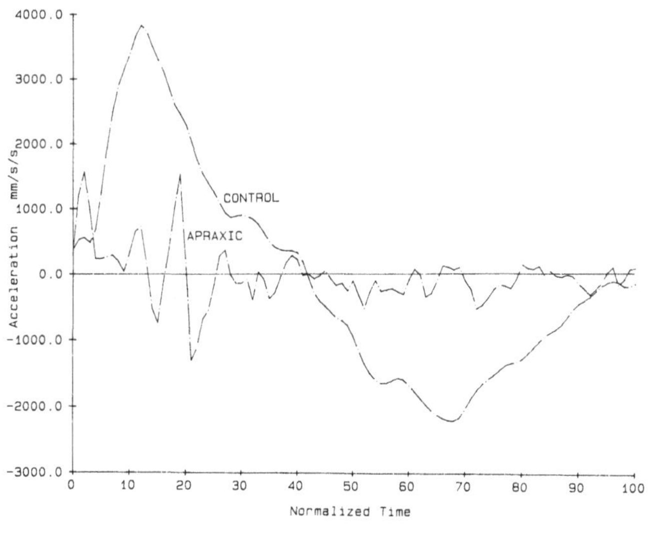

Figure 2. Representative acceleration profiles, normalised in time, for apraxic and control subjects for the "reach" action.

than the control subject, suggesting reliance upon a feedback guidance strategy throughout the action. The angle-angle diagrams in Figure 3 reveal the relative motion at the shoulder and elbow joints. Notably, in the two more complex conditions, the apraxic subject extends at the elbow and flexes at the shoulder joint through a greater range of motion than the control subject. This is a curious finding, given that the movement amplitude was constant across all conditions and was identical for both subjects. The most likely explanation is that the control subject achieved the same actions by leaning forward with the trunk, thereby reducing the range of motion required at the shoulder and elbow joints. These differences in patterns of coordination may reflect an inability of the apraxic subject to coordinate trunk movement with movement of proximal and distal limb segments.

In the conditions requiring both reaching and grasping components, the apraxic subject adopted a notably wider maximum aperture and spent a longer proportion of the total movement time in closure of the fingers around the rod. The apraxic's wide aperture was clearly inappropriate to the size of the rod (15 mm). This might suggest difficulties in using contextual cues of the rod (e.g., shape, size, or location) or in comparing such cues with stored information from past actions in order to execute an appropriate grasp. Alternatively, the wide aperture of the apraxic subject might be explained by a compensatory strategy for spatial errors in guiding the hand to the rod. That is, the wider the aperture, the greater the tolerance for error in directing the hand to the target location. Note also, in the aperture profiles presented in Figure 4, that the apraxic subject completed the grasp relatively early but had particular difficulty in transferring to the next component of the task which involved stirring the imaginary cup of coffee.

For the particular apraxic subject described above, rehabilitation strategies might focus upon improving force production to increase speed of movement. Therapists may also emphasise smooth transitions between successive parts in multi-phase tasks. Finally, cognitive strategies may be helpful for directing attention towards critical contextual features of objects.

In an experiment designed to examine apraxic limb trajectories as a function of the effect of environmental context, Charlton et al. (in preparation) compared reaching and grasping performance using a rod and imaginary cup versus a real spoon and cup of coffee. In reaching for the rod, many important contextual cues were not available. Indeed, there was a need for subjects to draw upon stored knowledge (from the conceptual subsystem) of the properties and functions of spoons and cups to assist in organising an appropriate action. In contrast, appropriate contextual cues were available in the task using the real spoon and cup. Implicit in this task then, was the need for subjects to use available cues about the shape and size of the spoon handle, the location and shape of the cup, and the extent to which the coffee filled the cup.

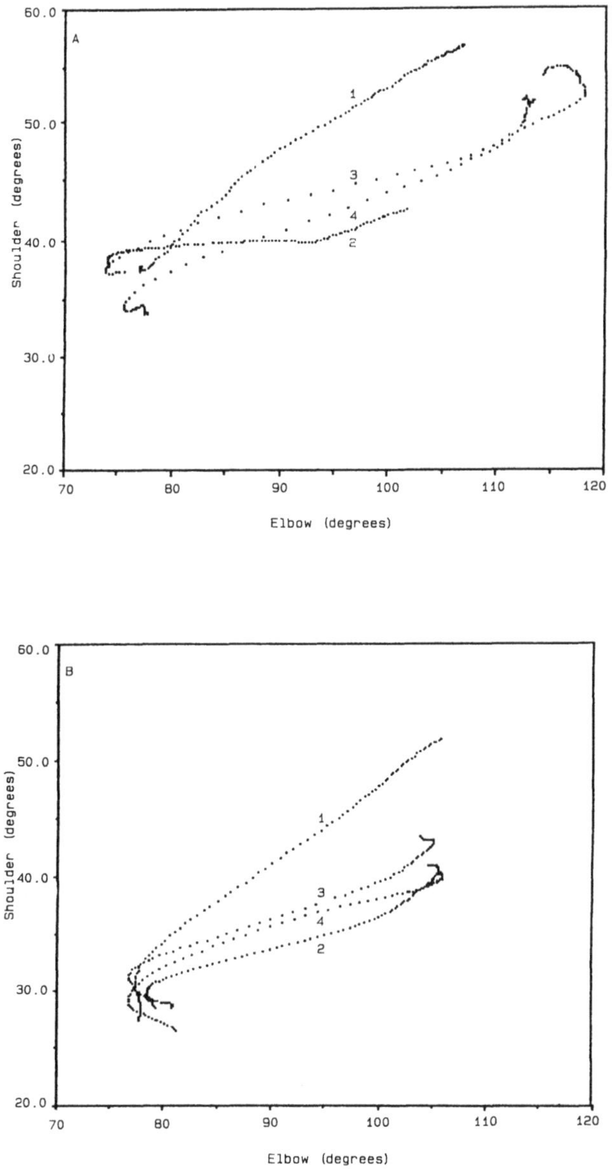

Figure 3. Angle-angle diagrams of representative trials of reaching actions for apraxic subject (A) and control subject (B) for Conditions 1 to 4. Note that "shoulder" refers to forward flexion at the shoulder joint and "elbow" refers to extension at the elbow joint. The start of the action can be identified on the left most end of each profile.

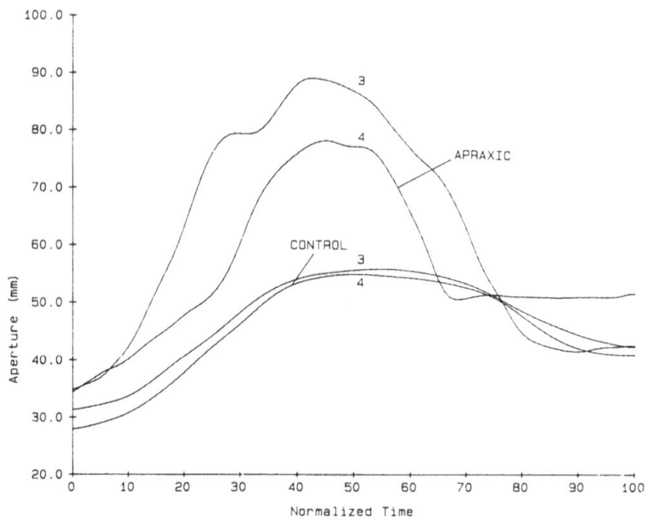

Figure 4. Mean aperture profiles, normalised in time, for apraxic subject and control subject for Condition 3: "reach-orient-grasp" and Condition 4: "reach-orient-grasp-stir".

In general, the kinematic characteristics for the transport and manipulation components of the prehension action supported the well documented clinical observations of improvements in gestural performance when real objects are provided. That is, apraxics' transport and manipulation components were more like those of the non-brain-damaged control subjects when the real object was used.

One of the most interesting findings was the apraxics' smoother wrist trajectories when reaching for the real spoon. A comparison of the exemplary acceleration profiles presented in Figure 2 with those for the same subjects presented in Figure 5 indicates that the apraxic made fewer adjustments, and in particular, fewer zero acceleration crossings, when reaching for the real spoon. The authors suggest that appropriate contextual cues enable apraxics to use a control strategy that is more like that of non-brain-damaged subjects, with an initial impulse carrying the limb towards the spoon in an open-loop fashion and a second phase wherein sensory feedback is used to make corrective adjustments to home-in on the spoon.

This experiment (Charlton et al., in preparation) represents a preliminary examination of movement patterns associated with apraxia. While there are well documented clinical reports for more successful performance of gestures

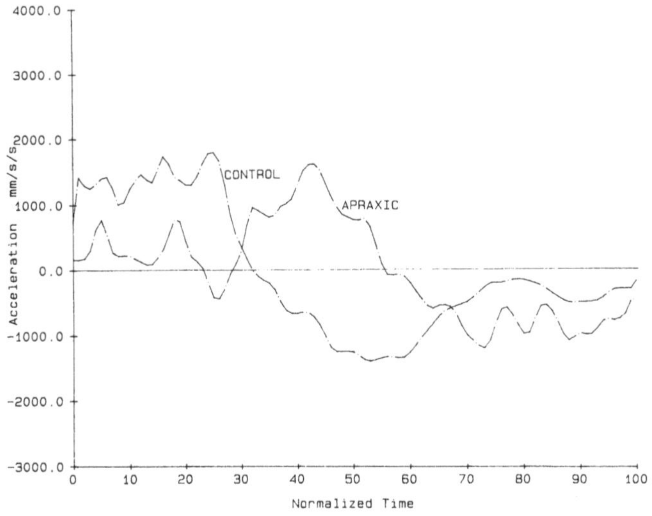

Figure 5. Representative acceleration profiles, normalised in time, for apraxic and control subjects for the task of grasping a real spoon to stir a real cup of coffee.

when real objects are used rather than pantomimed, the kinematic characteristics described here shed more light on the nature of different underlying strategies adopted.

CONCLUSION

Motor control research has much to contribute to clinical assessment and rehabilitation of neuromotor disorders. In particular, there is significant merit in the use of kinematic measurements to characterise differences in spatial and temporal features of movement patterns. This chapter has emphasised the need to evaluate differences between pathological and normal movement trajectories within a theoretical framework of organisation and control of actions. The preliminary studies presented have provided insight into the nature of the disorders of hemiplegia and apraxia, allowing for speculation about disruptions to underlying action control strategies.

REFERENCES

Abbs, J.H., Gracco, V.L., & Cole, K.J. (1984). Control of multimovement coordination sensorimotor mechanisms in speech motor programming. *Journal of Motor Behavior, 16,* 195-231.

Allport, D.A. (1980). Patterns and actions: Cognitive mechanisms are content-specific. In G. Claxton (Ed.), *Cognitive psychology* (pp. 26-64). London: Routledge & Kegan Paul.

Anderson, J.R. (1982). Acquisition of cognitive skill. *Psychological Review, 89,* 369-406.

Arbib, M.A. (1985). Schemas for the temporal organization of behavior. *Human Neurobiology, 4,* 63-72.

Bard, G., & Hirschberg, G.G. (1965). Recovery of voluntary motion in upper extremity following hemiplegia. *Archives of Physical Medicine and Rehabilitation, 46*, 567-572.

Bernstein, N. (1967). *The coordination and regulation of movements.* Oxford: Pergamon Press.

Bobath, B. (1978). *Adult hemiplegia: Evaluation and treatment.* London: William Heinemann Medical Books.

Brunnstrom, S. (1970). *Movement therapy in hemiplegia.* NY: Harper & Row.

Charlton, J.L. (1988). Disruptions to limb praxis: A kinematic analysis. *Dissertation Abstracts International, 48,* 2883, B.

Charlton, J.L., Roy, E.A., Marteniuk, R.G., & MacKenzie, C.L. (in preparation). A kinematic analysis of prehension in apraxia.

Cordo, P.J., & Nashner, L.M. (1982). Properties of postural adjustments associated with rapid arm movements. *Journal of Neurophysiology, 47,* 287-302.

Dabul, B. (1979). *Apraxia battery for adults.* C.O. Publications.

De Renzi, E. (1985). Methods of limb apraxia examination and their bearing on the interpretation of the disorder. In E.A. Roy (Ed.), *Neuropsychological studies in apraxia and related disorders* (pp. 45-64). Amsterdam: North-Holland.

De Renzi, E., Motti, F., & Nichelli, P. (1980). Imitating gestures. A quantitative approach to ideomotor apraxia. *Archives of Neurology, 37,* 6-10.

Duncan, P.W., & Badke, M.B. (1987a). Determinants of abnormal motor control. In P.W. Duncan, & M.B. Badke (Eds.), *Stroke rehabilitation: The recovery of motor control* (pp. 135-159). Chicago: Yearbook Medical Publishers Inc.

Duncan, P.W., & Badke, M.B. (1987b). Measurement of motor performance and functional abilities following stroke. In P.W. Duncan, & M.B. Badke (Eds.), *Stroke rehabilitation: The recovery of motor control* (pp. 199-221). Chicago: Yearbook Medical Publishers Inc.

Faglioni, P., & Basso, A. (1985). Historical perspectives on neuroanatomical correlates of limb apraxia. In E.A. Roy (Ed.), *Neuropsychological studies in apraxia and related disorders* (pp. 3-44). Amsterdam: North-Holland.

Fisk, J.D., & Goodale, M.A. (1989). The effects of instructions to subjects on the programming of visually directed reaching movements. *Journal of Motor Behavior, 21,* 5-19.

Fitts, P.M. (1954). The information capacity of the human motor system in controlling the amplitude of movement. *Journal of Experimental Psychology, 47,* 381-391.

Friesen, H.I. (1986). *Interrater reliability and error patterns of a modified scoring system for limb apraxia.* Unpublished master's thesis, University of Waterloo.

Fugl-Meyer, A., Jaasko, L., Leyman, I., Olsson, S., & Steglind, S. (1975). The post-stroke hemiplegic patient: A method of evaluation of physical performance. *Scandinavian Journal of Rehabilitation Medicine, 7,* 13-31.

Goldstein, K. (1948). *Language and language disorders.* NY: Grune & Stratton.

Granger, C.V., Albrecht, G.L., & Hamilton, B.B. (1979). Outcome of comprehensive medical rehabilitation: Measurement by PULSES profile and Barthel Index. *Archives of Physical Medicine Rehabilitation, 60,* 145-154.

Granger, C.V., Dewis, L.S., & Peter, N.C. (1979). Stroke rehabilitation: Analysis of repeated Barthel Index measures. *Archives of Physical Medicine Rehabilitation, 60,* 14-17.

Gresham, G.E., Phillips, T.F., & Labi, M.L.C. (1980). ADL status in stroke: Relative merits of three standard indexes. *Archives of Physical Medicine Rehabilitation, 61,* 355-358.

Grillner, S. (1975). Locomotion in vertebrates: Central mechanisms and reflex interaction. *Physiological Review, 11,* 189-200.

Haaland, K.Y., Porch, B.E., & Delaney, H.D. (1980). Limb apraxia and motor performance. *Brain and Language, 9,* 315-323.

Heilman, K. (1979). Apraxia. In K.M. Heilman, & E. Valenstein (Eds.), *Clinical neuropsychology* (pp. 159-185). New York: Oxford University Press.

Jeannerod, M. (1981). Intersegmental coordination during reaching at natural visual objects. In J. Long, & A. Baddeley (Eds.), *Attention and performance IX* (pp. 153-168). Hillsdale, N.J: Lawrence Erlbaum Associates.

Jeannerod, M. (1984). The timing of natural prehension movements. *Journal of Motor Behavior, 16,* 235-254.

Jeannerod, M. (1986a). The formation of finger grip during prehension. A cortically mediated visuomotor pattern. *Behavioural Brain Research, 19,* 99-116.

Jeannerod, M. (1986b). Mechanisms of visuomotor coordination: A study in normal and brain-damaged subjects. *Neuropsychologia, 24,* 41-78.

Kelso, J.A.S. (1982). Concepts and issues in human motor behavior: Coming to grips with the jargon. In J.A.S. Kelso (Ed.), *Human motor behavior: An introduction* (pp. 21-58). Hillsdale, NJ: Lawrence Erlbaum Associates.

Kimura, D. (1982). Left hemisphere control of oral and brachial movements and their relation to communication. *Philosophical Transactions of the Royal Society of London, B298,* 135-149.

Kugler, P.N., Kelso, J.A.S., & Turvey, M.T. (1982). On the control and coordination of naturally developing systems. In J.A.S. Kelso, & J.E. Clark (Eds.), *The development of movement coordination and control* (pp. 5-78). New York, London: Wiley.

Lacquaniti, F., Soechting, J.F., & Terzuolo, C. (1986). Path constraints on point-to-point arm movements in three-dimensional space. *Neuroscience, 17,* 313-324.

Law, M., & Letts, L. (1989). A critical review of Scales of Activities of Daily Living. *The American Journal of Occupational Therapy, 43,* 522-528.

Lee, W.A. (1980). Anticipatory control of postural and task muscles during rapid arm flexion. *Journal of Motor Behavior, 12,* 185-196.

Lough, S. (1987). Visual control of arm movement in the stroke patient. *International Journal of Rehabilitation Research, 10,* 113-119.

Lough, S., Wing, A.M., Fraser, C., & Jenner, J.R. (1984). Measurement of recovery of function in the hemiparetic limb following stroke: A preliminary report. *Human Movement Science, 3,* 247-256.

MacKenzie, C.L., Marteniuk, R.G., Dugas, C., Liske, D., & Eickmeier, B. (1987). Three dimensional movement trajectories in Fitts' task: Implications for control. *Quarterly Journal of Experimental Psychology: Human Experimental Psychology, 39A,* 629-647.

Mahoney, F.I., & Barthel, D.W. (1965). Functional evaluation: The Barthel Index. *Md. State Medical Journal, 14,* 61-65.

Marteniuk, R.G., MacKenzie, C.L., Jeannerod, M., Athenes, S., & Dugas, C. (1987). Constraints on human arm movement trajectories. *Canadian Journal of Psychology, 41,* 365-378.

Marteniuk, R.G., MacKenzie, C.L., & Leavitt, J.L. (1988). Representational and physical accounts of motor control and learning: Can they account for the data? In A.M. Colley, & J.R. Beech (Eds.), *Cognition and action in skilled behaviour.* Amsterdam: North-Holland.

Michaels, C.F., & Carello, C. (1981). *Direct perception.* New York: Prentice-Hall.

Newell, K.M. (1985). Coordination, control and skill. In D. Goodman, R.B. Wilberg, & I.M. Franks (Eds.), *Differing perspectives in motor learning, memory and control* (pp. 295-317). Amsterdam: North-Holland.

O'Sullivan, M.S., Cullen, K.E., & Schmitz, T.J. (1981). *Physical rehabilitation: Evaluation and treatment procedures.* Philadelphia: F.A. Davis Company.

Paillard, J. (1982). Apraxia and the neurophysiology of motor control. *Philosophical Transactions of the Royal Society of London. B298,* 111-134.
Roy, E.A. (1981). Action sequencing and lateralized cerebral damage: Evidence for asymmetries in control. In J. Long, & A. Baddeley (Eds.), *Attention and performance IX* (pp. 487-498). Hillsdale, NJ: Lawrence Erlbaum Associates.
Roy, E.A. (1982). Action and performance. In A. Ellis (Ed.), *Normality and pathology in cognitive function* (pp. 265-298). New York: Academic Press.
Roy, E.A. (1983). Neuropsychological perspectives on apraxia and related disorders. In R.A. Magill (Ed.), *Memory and control of action* (pp. 293-320). Amsterdam: North-Holland.
Roy, E.A., Square, P.A., Adams, S., & Friesen, H. (1985). Error movement notation system. *Semiotic Inquiry, 5,* 402-412.
Schmidt, R.A. (1982). The schema concept. In J.A.S. Kelso (Eds.), *Human motor behavior: An introduction* (pp. 219-235). Hillsdale, NJ: Lawrence Erlbaum Associates.
Schmidt, R.A. (1988a). *Motor control and learning: A behavioral emphasis (2nd Ed.).* Champaign, IL: Human Kinetics Publishers.
Schmidt, R.A. (1988b). Motor and action perspectives on motor behavior. In O.G. Meijer, & K. Roth (Eds.), *Complex movement behavior: "The" motor-action controversy* (pp. 3-44). Amsterdam: North-Holland.
Soechting, J.F., & Lacquaniti, F. (1981). Invariant characteristics of a pointing movement in man. *Journal of Neuroscience, 1,* 710-720.
Soechting, J.F., Lacquaniti, F., & Terzuolo, C. (1986). Coordination of arm movements in three-dimensional space. Sensorimotor mapping during drawing movement. *Neuroscience, 17,* 295-311.
Sparrow, W.A., Donovan, E., van Emmerik, R., & Barry, E.B. (1987). Using relating motion plots to measure changes in intra-limb and inter-limb coordination. *Journal of Motor Behavior, 19,* 115-129.
Turvey, M.T. (1977). Preliminaries to a theory of action with reference to vision. In R. Shaw, & J. Bransford (Eds.), *Perceiving, acting and knowing* (pp. 211-265). Hillsdale, N.J: Lawrence Erlbaum Associates.
Twitchell, T.E. (1951). The restoration of motor function following hemiplegia in man. *Brain, 74,* 443-480.
Wing, A.M., Turton, A., & Fraser, C. (1986). Grasp size and accuracy of approach in reaching. *Journal of Motor Behavior, 18,* 245-260.

Approaches to the Study of Motor Control and Learning
J.J. Summers (Editor)

Chapter 16

THE CONTRIBUTION OF MOVEMENT DISORDERS RESEARCH TO THEORIES OF MOTOR CONTROL AND LEARNING

James G. Phillips
Monash University

George E. Stelmach
Arizona State University

The present paper discusses the potential contribution of the study of movement disorders to the understanding of motor control and learning. The study of movement disorders may serve to establish the function of specific brain structures involved in movement control. Such an approach provides information about the actual mechanisms (rather than information from simulated mechanisms) and permits a view of important converging lines of evidence in the study of motor control. In this review, methods of examining neuropathological syndromes are described, as well as associated disruptions of motor functioning. In addition, the emerging isomorphism between neurophysiological and cognitive-psychological accounts of motor control is illustrated in a discussion of the role of the basal ganglia in the control of movement. Specifically, two models of basal ganglia function are outlined, as viewed in the context of Parkinson's and Huntington's diseases. The literature suggests that the basal ganglia have a role in the initiation and maintenance of movement forces. Ultimately, a study of movement disorders, focused upon those issues regarding the control of movement, may be a catalyst for new theories while challenging the present ones.

The present Chapter will outline how a study of movement disorders can contribute to the understanding of motor control. The study of the disorders of movement caused by damage to the central nervous system dramatises the computational role of the brain in motor control. In particular, such investigations, may enable researchers to trace the site of damage to a specific structure in the brain. Eventually, through consistent experimental results, verification of those symptoms expected as indicators of a given deficit may be possible, and knowledge of the functional role of the specific part of the brain associated with that deficit may become apparent. Thus, the study of movement disorders provides an exciting approach to the study of motor control when evidence of the impaired structure can be linked to the process of movement coordination.

APPROACHES TO THE STUDY OF MOTOR CONTROL

A number of paradigms have been employed to investigate the central control of movements. The nature of the motor program has been inferred, for example, from reaction times, and from patterns of response invariance. The assumptions underlying these methods of studying the motor program, however, have been questioned.

Reaction Time. Henry and Rogers (1960) suggested that computational processes occur during the response latency which enable the programmed control of movement. In such a case, the complexity of motor programs could be inferred from the latency before a response is initiated (the reaction time - RT). This basic assumption is problematic, however, and cannot be justified on the basis of reaction time alone. Indeed, the appropriateness of the RT paradigms has been open to debate (e.g., Goodman & Kelso, 1980; Klapp, Wyatt, & Lingo, 1974), and the computational nature of the response latency period has been challenged. For example, Carlton, Carlton, and Newell (1987) have suggested that the response latency may be a function of *force development*, rather than the result of *computational processes*.

Response Invariance. Schmidt (1985) has suggested that the nature of motor programs may be inferred from invariant features of movement, contending that those features which are invariant are those represented within a motor program. However, the nature of these invariances has been questioned by Gentner (1987) and Wann and Nimmo-Smith (1990). The search for invariant features has disregarded, in the main, the biological mechanisms upon which movement is based (Abbs & Connor, 1989); some invariant features may result from *anatomical and biomechanical constraints*, rather than any form of *central representation*.

MOVEMENT DISORDERS

Damage to specific brain structures can cause various impairments in movement coordination. Indeed the classic picture of a basal ganglia disorder is one of progressively deteriorating motor coordination with relatively intact mental functioning, as in Parkinson's disease (Parkinson, 1817). Such a dissociation of functioning suggests that the basal ganglia play a role in the coordination of movement.

Important developments in the understanding of the neurotransmitter systems involved in Parkinson's disease (Stahl, 1986), and advances in brain imaging technology (Martin & Calne, 1986), have stimulated interest in the study of movement disorders. It is hoped that current advances will lead to an ability to better localise and examine the function of brain structures involved in movement coordination, in real time (see Posner, Pea, & Volpe, 1982); to determine the location of structural damage and to identify functional loss, both require expertise in neurophysiology, neurology, and experimental psychology (see Phillips, Muller, & Stelmach, 1989).

The *localisation of brain function* requires minute study. The brain is a distributed control system (Edelman & Mountcastle, 1979; Stelmach & Diggles, 1982), consisting of a large number of serial and parallel connections. The redundancy of such a distributed system means that local lesions only degrade, rather than destroy, system function. Consideration must be given to the neural flow of activity during the movement production. Specifically, to the inputs relayed by structures such as the basal ganglia and cerebellum; to the processing of these inputs; and, ultimately, to the brain structures affected by the process. Indeed, Marsden (1982) has suggested that damage to a given brain structure causes impairment not only in that structure, but also in the other structures it innervates. Thus, there is a loss of those functions associated with the damaged structure (negative symptoms), as well as an excess of activity in other functions of the central nervous system (positive symptoms), due to a loss of inhibitory control. Marsden has suggested that to understand the unimpaired function of a particular brain structure, which has sustained damage, researchers should observe those functional losses occurring as a consequence of that damage.

The *identification of functional impairment*, however, requires considerable methodological expertise. Movement provides the basis for human expression, and diseases such as Parkinson's disease and Huntington's disease affect basal ganglia function, which, in turn, may disrupt speech, writing, posture, and even patients' mood states (Lohr & Wisniewski, 1987; Swerdlow & Koob, 1987). Neuromuscular control is multifaceted. Performance in complex tasks depends on a number of processes, the disturbance of function may result from any of the following: (1) natural age-related decline; (2) deficits in higher cognitive processes (e.g., depression, dementia); (3) side effects of drug therapy (e.g., dyskinaesia, confusion); (4) biomechanical changes (e.g., rigidity, change in body mass); or (5) deficits in the coordination of movements (e.g., programming, feedback guidance).

Ultimately, confounding issues must be addressed to avoid faulty inferences about functional impairment (Brown & Marsden, 1986a; Gordon & Illes, 1987; Phillips, Muller, & Stelmach, 1989).

In the remainder of this Chapter, which considers specific functional deficits caused by Parkinson's and Huntington's disease, a number of issues are discussed that should be taken into account in the attempt to identify those brain structures involved in movement control, specifically, the role of the basal ganglia in the movement coordination.

PARKINSON'S DISEASE AS A MODEL OF BASAL GANGLIA FUNCTION

The basal ganglia mediate between higher and lower brain structures, receiving inputs from cortical areas and the substantia nigra, and innervating thalamic and mid-brain nuclei (DeLong, Georgopoulos, & Crutcher, 1983; Gunilla, Oberg, & Divac, 1985). The damage associated with Parkinson's disease tends to be localised pharmacologically, appearing to affect more than one neurotransmitter system; however, it most specifically interferes with dopaminergic functioning, i.e., a loss of the dopaminergic cells in the substantia nigra that project to the basal ganglia (Forno, 1982; Hornykiewicz, 1982). Therefore, it follows that there is also a disturbance of basal ganglia function. Marsden (1982) has suggested that movement impairment caused by Parkinson's disease provides the best model for inferring motor function of the basal ganglia.

Symptoms of Parkinson's Disease

In general, although patients with Parkinson's disease initially may exhibit unilateral symptoms, they exhibit bilateral symptoms as the disease progresses. In later stages of the disease impairment in postural reflexes and gait is evident (Hoehn & Yahr, 1967; Jankovic, 1987). The cardinal symptoms of Parkinson's disease are:

Akinesia: a difficulty in the initiation of movement (DeAjuriaguerra, 1975);
Bradykinesia: a slowness in executing movement (Hallett & Khoshbin,1980);
Rigidity: resistance to the passive stretch of muscles (McLellan,1981);
Tremor: a tremor at rest around 4 to 5.5 Hz (Gresty & Findley,1981).

Marsden (1982) has suggested that positive symptoms, such as tremor and rigidity, are due to the loss of inhibitory influences within the basal ganglia, but reasons that basal ganglia function may best be understood through examination of the loss of function, that is, the negative symptoms of akinesia and bradykinesia (Marsden, 1982, 1984, 1985). Most of the research effort to date, has been devoted to the study of akinesia and bradykinesia. It is possible to consider these symptoms separately, as they tend to be independent of one another (Zetusky, Jankovic, & Pirozzolo, 1985).

Examination of disturbances in the initiation and execution of movement caused by Parkinson's disease may provide an understanding of basal ganglia function; in particular, an overview of functional losses may be gained from observing patients' handwriting. While handwriting in Parkinson's disease patients tends to be slower and smaller than that in normals, it does not reflect the serious shape disorders of handwritten letters found in patients with certain forms of neuropsychological dysfunction such as dysgraphia (Margolin, 1984). The symptoms associated with Parkinsonian handwriting would not appear to result from deficits in distance judgment, as Stelmach, Phillips, and Chau (1989) found that patients could accurately judge distances (see also Brown & Marsden, 1986b; Della Sala, Lorenzo, Giordano, & Spinnler, 1986). Such observations suggest that patients have motor programs which are intact, but have difficulty in preparing specific parameters of movement (Marsden, 1982).

Further questions may be answered through the use of electromyography. The observed slowness of movement is not the result of a definite cocontraction of agonist and antagonist muscles (Hallett, 1983). Hallett, Shanani, and Young (1977) have observed that Parkinsonian patients have normal triphasic patterns of muscle activation (agonist, antagonist, agonist), but require more cycles of activity to produce movement. There appear to be deficits in the scaling of the size and/or duration of bursts of muscle activity.

The foregoing observations suggest that although patients with Parkinson's disease do not exhibit impaired motor programs overall, they do show difficulty specifying some of the parameters for these programs (Marsden, 1984). The task of researchers has been to document the effect of Parkinson's disease on the selection and preparation of response parameters.

Akinesia: Preparatory Processes

Since Flower's (1976) initial observations of tracking performance in Parkinson's disease patients, there have been a number of papers considering the preparatory processes in these patients (see Phillips, Muller, & Stelmach, 1989). The present discussion will be limited to recent, systematic examinations of preparatory processes using reaction time paradigms (i.e., Rafal, Inhoff, Friedman, & Bernstein, 1987; Sheridan, Flowers, & Hurrell, 1987; Stelmach, Worringham, & Strand, 1986). Response latencies have been used as an index of the difficulty in movement preparation. Researchers reason that if disproportionate difficulty in movement preparation is exhibited in patients with Parkinson's disease it should be evident from longer response latencies (Stelmach, Worringham, & Strand, 1986; Wing & Miller, 1984).

Stelmach et al. (1986) examined Parkinson's patients' ability to prepare the parameters of direction, arm, and extent, using Rosenbaum's (1980) precuing paradigm. Although patients took longer in movement preparation, and were slower in execution, they did not find that any specific parameter was more difficult to prepare than another. In addition, patients seemed to specify movement parameters at about the same rate as did normal subjects.

Similar results were found by Sheridan et al. (1987) in simple and choice tasks that tested patients' ability to prepare movements of different lengths and for different target widths. Although Sheridan et al. found that patients with Parkinson's disease had longer premotor times, a result suggesting that problems were central in origin, they did not discover that one specific parameter was more of a problem for patients than another.

Rafal et al. (1987) observed the ability of patients with Parkinson's disease to prepare repetitive tapping sequences of varying lengths. They found that both response and movement times were longer for patients, and that patients, like normal subjects, required more time to prepare longer movement sequences. On the other hand, patients did not demonstrate disproportionate difficulty in the preparation of a specific movement parameter.

It is perhaps surprising that results from experiments assessing preparatory processes have not linked deficits in the control of a specific movement parameter to Parkinson's disease. Such observations have led researchers to consider: (1) whether Parkinson's disease causes non-specific deficits in attentional processes; and (2) whether patients rely less upon advance preparation of movement, and more upon feedback guidance.

Non-specific Deficits in Attentional Processes. Poorly identified deficits in the preparation of specific movement parameters in Parkinson's disease patients have led some researchers to suggest that patients have non-specific deficits in their ability to prime or alert themselves (Brown & Marsden, 1988; Cools, Van Den Bercken, Horstink, Van Spaendonck, & Berger, 1984; Stern & Mayeux, 1986).

Non-specific attentional deficits have been observed in patients with Parkinson's disease by Cools et al. (1984), Flowers and Robertson (1985), Lees and Smith (1983). Cools et al. (1984) and Flowers and Robertson (1985) found, in particular, that patients showed impairment in developing and changing their cognitive set in conceptual tasks. Patients do not exhibit the signs of "warming-up" during the acquisition of a skill (Frith, Bloxham, & Carpenter, 1986) that normal subjects do. Similarly, Worringham and Stelmach (1990) found that patients required more practice to benefit from advance information, in a simple reaction-time task.

Certain experimental results suggest that Parkinson's disease patients are unable to direct and maintain attention. For example, patients benefit less from warning signals than do normal subjects (Bloxham, Dick, & Moore, 1987; Bloxham, Mindel, & Frith, 1984), and do not use precues to the same extent as normal subjects (Wright, Burns, Geffen, & Geffen, 1990). It is suspected, however, that these nonspecific deficits could be a function of depressed mood and motivation; depression has been reported in patients with Parkinson's disease by (Mayeux, Williams, Stern, & Core, 1984). Indeed, there are similarities between symptoms associated with Parkinson's disease, and those associated with depression (e.g., lack of initiative, tiredness) (Levin, Llabre, & Weiner, 1988). It is possible that certain non-specific attentional deficits are reactive, that is, they are a function of the depression caused by a progressive debilitating disease (Dakof & Mendelsohn, 1986; Gotham, Brown, & Marsden, 1986; Taylor, Saint-Cyr, Lang, & Kenny, 1986).

The relative importance of cognitive deficits, and motor deficits is highlighted during symptom fluctuations that patients experience during the "on-off" phases of "difficult" sinemet therapy (Lees, 1989; Marsden, 1980; Obeso, et al., 1989); changes in motor functioning are far more noticeable than those in cognitive functioning during these symptom fluctuations (Brown, Marsden, Quinn, & Wyke, 1984; Girotti et al., 1986; Starkstein, Esteguy, Berthier, Garcia, & Leiguarda, 1989). Although on-off fluctuations are related to affect/arousal level, they do not dominate the clinical picture of these patients (Knight, Godfrey, & Shelton, 1988), as do the far greater motor changes (Brown et al., 1984).

The initial presenting symptoms of Parkinson's disease are disruptions of motor control. Goldenberg (1990) has considered whether problems of attentional control could explain the difficulty patients have in performing two motor tasks at once. They reasoned that although motor tasks are disrupted when patients are required to share their attention, this does not necessarily mean that patients have attentional deficits, rather they may require greater amounts of attention to control their movements. To establish whether patients with Parkinson's disease have a general attentional deficit, Goldenberg required that patients perform non-motor tasks (verbal, visuo-spatial, memory), singly or concurrently. Both patients with Parkinson's disease and control subjects showed a decline in performance when performing tasks concurrently, but the degree of decline did not differ between groups. A general attentional deficit was not demonstrated. Non-specific attentional deficits do not readily explain or assist in the understanding of the motor control deficits in patients with Parkinson's disease.

Reduced Reliance Upon Advance Preparation in Parkinson's Disease. Identification of specific deficits in preparatory processes caused by Parkinson's disease, has proved to be difficult. However, it is not thought, that a consideration of non-specific attentional deficits will lead to an understanding of the impairment in the initiation and execution of movement. Instead, it may be necessary to consider the detrimental impact of Parkinson's disease on the *functional role* of preparatory processes, whereby the amount of on-line control required during movement is reduced. Both Flowers (1976) and Marsden (1982) have suggested that Parkinson's disease forces patients to rely less upon the advance preparation of movement, and more upon feedback guided control of movement. This view is supported by Evarts, Teravainen, and Calne (1981), who reported that prolonged reaction time in patients with Parkinson's disease is less reliable than prolonged movement time. Thus, assessment of the preparatory processes in patients with Parkinson's disease is complicated, because patients *may not be preparing* movement in the same manner as normal subjects (Marsden, 1984).

This shift in the mode of movement control may be seen in an experiment by Stelmach, Worringham, and Strand (1987). Stelmach et al. considered how normal subjects and patients with Parkinson's disease prepared sequences of repetitive tapping movements. In normal subjects, response times increase with the number of taps required in a given response sequence, indicating that subjects programmed their responses in advance. In contrast, response times of patients with Parkinson's disease did not increase with the number of taps in a response sequence. In addition, patients showed longer movement times, a finding which suggests that patients controlled their movements during execution rather than preparing them in advance. Similar observations were made by Stelmach, Phillips, and Chau (1989). They found that patients, performing a repetitive tapping task, prepared for two taps in advance when there was a straightforward link between stimulus and response, but not when the link between stimulus and response was more complicated. It is probably during more difficult movements that patients shift from the advanced preparation of movement to the control of movement during execution.

Parkinson's disease disrupts movement preparation, and in so doing, illustrates the functional importance of preparatory processes. Patients do not appear to prepare sequences of movements in advance, their movements being slow and jerky, and instead, control movement during execution. Such a shift in the mode of movement control, creates difficulty to making inferences about the adequacy of preparatory processes in these patients. Deficits in patients' control of movement may be inferred rather from execution of movement; patients would be expected to have difficulty controlling parameters of movement associated with the primary deficits caused by Parkinson's disease. Clinically, Parkinson's disease appears to cause problems in those processes involved in the parameterisation of movement, particularly movement length and duration. Bradykinesia in patients with Parkinson's disease, with respect to movement length and duration will be discussed in the next section.

Bradykinesia: Movement Execution

Most characteristics of bradykinesia may be observed in the kinematics of movement in Parkinson's patients. For example, Phillips, Stelmach, and Teasdale (1989) found trends illustrative of the deficits seen in movement of patients with Parkinson's disease. Patients were required to independently modulate spatial and temporal aspects of their handwriting. While they showed control of movement length and duration, they demonstrated difficulty with the precise control of movement forces:

1. They could not move as fast as control subjects (see Baroni, Benvenuti, Fantini, Pantaleo, & Urbani, 1984; Berardelli, Dick, Rothwell, Cay, & Marsden, 1986).
2. They experienced difficulty in modulating movement velocities, tending not to be able to control movement lengths independently of movement durations (see Draper & Johns, 1964; Flowers, 1976).
3. Movements were jerky and irregular (see Hallett & Khoshbin, 1980).
4. The acceleration phase of movements tended to be prolonged (see Wing, 1989).

The clinical picture of shorter and slower movements in patients with Parkinson's disease could occur in a number of ways: (1) through central processing difficulty in accessing programs and *sequencing movements*, thus causing problems maintaining ongoing movement; (2) through central difficulty with the *scaling of muscle activity*; or (3) through *rigidity and tremor*, reducing movement extent, and increasing irregularity of movement.

Movement Sequencing in Patients with Parkinson's Disease. There is evidence that patients with Parkinson's disease are unable to coordinate more than one movement at a time. For example, Benecke, Rothwell, Dick, Day, and Marsden, (1986, 1987) had subjects simultaneously flex an arm and squeeze a manipulandum with the same limb. The patients could not superimpose or sequence movements normally, as was evident from the dramatic increases observed in movement times.

In an experiment by Stelmach, Garcia-Colera, and Martin (1989), it was considered whether the deficits observed in sequential control of movement could be a function of damaged force control. Specifically, Stelmach et al. considered whether patients with Parkinson's disease could perform sequential finger-tapping movements of increasing complexity. In two separate sessions, subjects were required to tap at a fast (200 ms) or slow (600 ms) rate under a number of conditions in which stress and force components were varied within a movement sequence: no stress on a tap; simple RT (advance knowledge of stress position); and choice RT (no advance knowledge of stress position). Both the introduction of a stressed tap and the uncertainty of its position adversely affected RT, intertap interval, and error rates. These results demonstrate that impaired sequential movement could result from force control deficits.

Patients with Parkinson's disease clearly exhibit deficits in the execution of movement sequences. These deficits are confounded, however, when patients are required to vary their *movement forces*. This suggests that simple additive deficits in the production of movement forces maybe causing the observed deficits in complex movement sequences (see Phillips, Muller, & Stelmach, 1989).

Force Control in Patients with Parkinson's Disease. The observed slowness and irregularity of movements in patients with Parkinson's disease could result from deficits in control of basic movement parameters such as length, duration, or force (Phillips, Stelmach, & Teasdale, 1989; Stelmach, Teasdale, Phillips, & Worringham, 1989; Stelmach & Worringham, 1988; Teasdale, Phillips, & Stelmach, 1990). Experimental results from our laboratory suggest that observed slowness and irregularity of movement may be due to impairment in initiation and maintenance of appropriate movement forces.

A series of experiments have examined the force control of patients with Parkinson's disease. Stelmach and Worringham (1988) addressed the control of movement forces in patients with Parkinson's disease in an isometric force production task. Patients were required to produce forces at 25%, 50%, and 75% of the maximum force they could produce. While patients produced some variability in forces, they were as accurate as control subjects. The fact that visual feedback was not available during force production, suggests that patients had an accurate "internal model" of the required forces. Force production was considered in more detail in a subsequent experiment (Stelmach et al., 1989), in which patients were required to produce forces at 15%, 30%, 45%, and 60% of the maximum force they could produce. Again, while patients took longer to reach their peak forces, they produced forces as accurately as control subjects. Patients, however, had more irregular force-time curves, characterised by jerkiness of force production.

Teulings and Stelmach (1991) considered the regularity, relative to the variability, of features in patients' movement trajectories (Signal to Noise Ratio). The Signal-to-Noise Ratio (SNR) provides an index of the efficiency of the control of various aspects of movement trajectories such as duration, size, and peak acceleration of handwriting movements. While patients exhibited normal SNR for features such as movement duration, they showed lower SNR for the peak acceleration of movement, suggesting impaired force control.

Hallett and Khoshbin (1980) proposed a mechanism for the observed irregularities in the movement of patients with Parkinson's disease: bradykinesia results from difficulty in energising agonist muscles, such that patients require a number of cycles of agonist and antagonist muscle activity to complete a movement. Hallett and Khoshbin's energisation hypothesis, therefore, suggests that patients with Parkinson's disease would require *more bursts of muscle activity for faster or longer movements*.

Recent evidence, however, indicates that the energisation hypothesis may not be correct (Berardelli, Dick, Rothwell, Day, & Marsden, 1986; Teasdale, et al., 1990). Berardelli et al. (1986) speculated that the multiple cycles of muscle activity seen in Parkinson's disease have a central, rather than a peripheral, site. They considered patients' muscle activity during movements of the wrist through 15 and 60 degrees. The size of agonist bursts increased in a normal fashion with movement size (although not scaled for task demands), suggesting that the muscles themselves were not saturated.

Force control deficits have been reported to occur during movements of various lengths and durations (Baroni et al., 1984; Berardelli et al., 1986). In particular, it has been reported that patients *cannot* voluntarily control the speed of their movements (Berardelli, Accornero, Argenta, Meco, & Manfredi, 1986; Draper & Johns, 1964). On the other hand, in our experiments, patients showed slow, but comparatively accurate, control of forces during isometric tasks (Stelmach et al., 1989; Stelmach & Worringham, 1988). It was, therefore, necessary to consider patients' control of movement duration in more detail.

Teasdale et al. (1990) asked patients to move at various percentages of a previously determined maximum speed (10% faster, the same speed, 30% slower, and 60% slower). Although patients were slower in movement, and showed irregularity in muscle activity, they exhibited control over movement times and could increase movement speed (within limits) when required. Whereas Hallett and Khoshbin (1980) suggested that patients with Parkinson's disease would require more bursts of muscle activity for faster or longer movements, Teasdale et al. (1990) found that patients showed more bursts of muscle activity for movements of longer duration only. It appears that the observed deficits in Parkinsonian movement are not a function of the energisation of muscles, but rather of scaling of muscle activity.

Rigidity and Tremor as Determinants of Bradykinesia. Studies of force control in patients with Parkinson's disease have repeatedly shown that patients can modulate movement forces, but that their movements are slow, jerky, and irregular. These consistent findings of slowness and jerkiness could be manifestations of the Parkinsonian symptoms of rigidity and tremor.

Parkinsonian *rigidity* may impede maintenance of fast, smooth movement. In patients with Parkinson's disease there is a heightened background muscle activity, creating a stiffness and resistance to movement. Caligiuri (1987) considered whether aberrations of movement in the orofacial system were a function of increased muscle tone. Measurements of movement and labial muscle rigidity were made in patients with Parkinson's disease. Their orofacial movements were of lower amplitude and velocity; however, there was no statistical relationship between labial rigidity and degree-of-movement abnormality. In addition, if there is a relationship between rigidity and speed of movement it would appear to be weak (Evarts et al., 1981) and unlikely to be the sole cause of motor slowing.

While motor slowing is unlikely to be a function of rigidity, observed jerkiness and irregularity of movement may be a function of Parkinsonian *tremor*. Nakamura, Nagasaki, and Narabayashi (1978) observed that sequential movements were entrained by a characteristic rhythm approximately the frequency of Parkinsonian tremor. They had patients perform finger taps in synchrony with a periodic stimulus. Patients exhibited difficulty at certain frequencies: at some critical frequency, between 2.5 and 5 Hz, control of tapping deteriorated, and between roughly 5 and 6 Hz, hastening of movement developed, independent of the stimulus. Such data suggest that tremor may be associated with the jerkiness of movement seen in patients with Parkinson's disease.

On the other hand, tremor is probably not the *sole* determinant of the irregularity observed in the movement of patients with Parkinson's disease. Parkinsonian tremor characteristically occurs at rest (Young, 1985) and is much less noticeable during movement (see Lakie & Mutch, 1989). Furthermore, Phillips, Stelmach, and Teasdale (1991) have provided some evidence indicating that jerkiness of movement in patients with Parkinson's disease is not the result of tremor. They examined the handwriting of patients with Parkinson's disease who showed minimal tremor. While these patients demonstrated characteristic jerkiness of movement, they did not exhibit a higher proportion of handwriting velocity in the ranges associated with tremor (5 to 8 Hz), as revealed by spectral analysis.

Parkinson's disease appears to cause deficits in the smooth production of movement forces (Stelmach et al., 1989; Stelmach & Worringham, 1988; Teasdale et al., 1990), rather than in the control of parameters such as movement length or duration (Philllips, Stelmach, & Teasdale, 1989; Stelmach, Worringham, & Strand, 1986). These deficits would explain patients' difficulty in performing movement sequences.

Functional Disturbances Caused by Parkinson's Disease. In summary, Parkinson's disease: disrupts the preparation of movement, especially evident in more complex movement sequences; causes slow, irregular movements in patients; (both motor control deficits are unlikely to be the result of disturbed higher cognitive or biomechanical processes); and, in some way, disrupts processes involved in the scaling of movement, i.e., patients show deficits in the production of smooth movement forces. Such deficits indicate the involvement of the basal ganglia in the production and maintenance of movement forces. These findings need to be verified and extended by other models of basal ganglia function. The following section discusses Huntington's disease as still another context for the study of basal ganglia function.

HUNTINGTON'S DISEASE AS A MODEL OF BASAL GANGLIA FUNCTION.

Huntington's disease is a hereditary disorder with a 50% chance of transmission from affected parent to offspring (Breakefield & Bressman, 1986; Hayden, 1981). Onset is insidious, generally occurring in the third decade of life; death usually follows within fourteen to seventeen years. The disease is thought to be a glutamate-dependent neurotoxic process, producing substantial reductions in dopaminergic neurons (Borison, Hitri, & Diamond, 1986). While causal mechanisms are as yet unclear, it may be said that multiple neurotransmitter systems are affected; specifically, the disease is associated with enhanced dopaminergic activity and reduced cholinergic activity (Borison et al., 1986; Graybiel, 1989; Young, Albin, & Penney, 1989). Huntington's disease causes a progressive atrophy, first in the basal ganglia, then in cortical structures (Lebrun-Grandie et al., 1989; Martin & Calne, 1986).

Symptoms of Huntington's Disease

In the early stage of Huntington's disease, mood, personality (Hayden, 1981), and visuo-spatial disturbances have been reported (Jossiassen, Curry, & Mancall, 1983). While changes in mood and personality are usually the first signs of the disease, disturbance of movement is the most obvious clinical feature (Hayden, 1981; Lohr & Wisniewski, 1987). Jerkiness and lack of coordination develop, followed by choreiform movement. In addition, there are disturbances of speech, gait, and swallowing (Hayden, 1981). In fact, many patients die as a result of respiratory problems caused by swallowing (Hayden, 1981; Still & Goldschmidt, 1986). Eventually, the disease causes depression and progressive dementia (Lohr & Wisniewski, 1987). The following motor symptoms are associated with Huntington's disease:

Chorea - involuntary movement resulting from random, irregular, rapid contractions in any combination of muscles (Hallett, 1983; Marsden, Obeso, & Rothwell, 1983).

Akinesia and Bradykinesia - difficulty in the initiation and execution of movement (Hefter, Homberg, Lange, & Freund, 1987; Thompson et al., 1988).

Rigidity and Hypotonia - both enhanced and reduced muscle tone are reported depending upon the age of the patient (Hayden, 1981; Lohr & Wisniewski, 1987).

As discussed below, Huntington's disease, in its early stages, provides two potential models for basal ganglia function:

1. A consideration of *choreiform movement* may provide additional insight into the dopaminergic systems within the basal ganglia; and
2. A consideration of the *akinesia and bradykinesia* caused by Huntington's disease may provide insight into the function of structures within the basal ganglia.

Chorea: Functional Excess

While Parkinson's disease is associated with reductions in the activity of dopaminergic neurotransmitter systems, Huntington's disease is in part associated with enhanced activity in dopaminergic neurotransmitter systems (Stahl, 1986). Whereas Parkinson's disease responds to treatment with dopamine agonists, aspects of Huntington's disease respond to treatment with dopamine antagonists (Young et al., 1989). Indeed, excess use of dopamine agonists produces choreiform movements, such as seen in Huntington's disease, and excess use of dopamine antagonists produces Parkinson-like symptoms. This suggests that Huntington's disease may serve as a model for basal ganglia function (Young et al., 1989). An understanding of excess movement, related to the dopaminergic system, as it operates in chorea, should provide a indication of basal ganglia function.

An overview of functional excess caused by chorea may be gained from an examination of handwriting in patients with Huntington's disease. Handwriting is intact in the early stages of the disease, but becomes slow and laborious, and may even increase in size, as the disease progresses. At first, patients show some difficulty with the shape and slant of letters, and eventually, prominent distortions of letter shape (Podoll, Caspary, Lange, & North, 1988). Present are considerable variations in the amount of force used during writing which is disrupted by pauses and choreic jerks (Podoll et al., 1988). These disruptions are unlikely to be the result of language impairment, as Huntington's disease does not appear to cause specific linguistic deficits (Ludlow, Connor, & Bassich, 1987; Podoll et al., 1988; Wallesch & Fehrenbach, 1988). However, in later stages of the disease, patients do show omission, perseveration (repetition), and substitution of letters, all of which may be attributable to the progressive, dementing nature of the disease (Podoll et al., 1988). Early on in the disease, programs for complex movement, such as speaking (Podoll et al., 1988; Wallesch & Fehrenbach, 1988), and writing (Podoll et al., 1988), would appear to be intact, but *general movement is disrupted by a variety of involuntary movement.*

Choreiform movement is difficult to characterise electromyographically, exhibiting reflexive, ballistic, and tonic patterns of muscle activity. Indeed

Hallett (1983) reported that patients may show any pattern of activity in any muscle at any time. Marsden, Obeso, and Rothwell, (1983) considered choreiform movement in patients with Huntington's disease, in whom they observed continuous change in activity from one muscle to another, and, within an individual muscle, from one pattern of activation to another. Muscle activation in chorea ranged from very brief bursts (50 to 200 ms) to prolonged contractions (2 seconds) (Thompson et al., 1989). Muscle activity is not correctly sequenced, as cocontractions occur which interfere with voluntary movement (Thompson et al., 1989). Kinematic analysis also reveals that choreiform movement lacks a clear pattern. Myers and Falek (1979) used an accelerometer to assess resting hand tremor in control subjects and in patients with Huntington's disease. Whereas the normal subjects had a dominant tremor frequency, the patients with Huntington's disease showed intermittent bursts of tremor at no consistent frequency.

Lohr and Wisniewski (1987) have suggested that chorea may be the result of: (1) inappropriate release of reflexes; or (2) inappropriate release of fragments of motor programs. Long latency *reflexes* are associated with voluntary movement. A number of temporally distinct reflex components are elicited when a loaded muscle, or a voluntary movement is perturbed (Lee & Tatton, 1978). Early components of the reflex response have been related to the spinal-stretch reflex, while the components of longer latency have been related to higher structures within the central nervous system (Lee & Tatton, 1978; Marsden, Rothwell, & Day, 1983). Reduced or absent long-latency reflexes have been reported in the hands and wrists of patients with Huntington's disease (Abbruzzese, et al., 1990; Noth, Podoll, & Friedmann, 1985; Thompson et al., 1989). As in this disease there are abnormalities in the reflexes associated with voluntary movement, Lohr and Winiewski (1987) suggested that chorea may be the result of an inappropriate release of reflexes. This hypothesis, however, is not supported by experiments by Abbruzzese et al., (1990), and Huttunen and Homberg (1990). Abbruzzese et al., (1990) examined long-latency reflexes in the wrist. The size of the long-latency stretch reflex was reduced in patients with Huntington's disease. The reduced size of long-latency reflexes tended to be related to hypotonia, but was not related to duration of the disease, or to severity of chorea. Huttunen and Homberg (1990) also failed to find a relationship between long-latency reflexes and chorea in an experiment examining the maintenance of balance during posture perturbations. Although patients with Huntington's disease had delayed onset of stabilising long latency reflexes, these delays did not correlate with severity of chorea.

An alternative hypothesis is that chorea is the result of a haphazard activation of *motor programs* (Lohr & Wisniewski, 1987). As choreiform movement ranges in appearance from "reflex" to "ballistic" to "tonic" (Hallett, 1983), it would seem that the basal ganglia have a role in muscle selection and regulation of both *reflex and voluntary movement* activity. In Huntington's disease heightened dopaminergic activity increases the likelihood that any muscle or movement will be activated.

In summary, chorea is characterised by random patterns of muscle activation, and the functional excess associated with it, suggests that the basal ganglia have a general role in the initiation and maintenance of muscle activity.

Akinesia and Bradykinesia Caused by Huntington's Disease

Whereas Parkinson's disease affects dopaminergic cells in the substantia nigra projecting to the striatum, Huntington's disease causes atrophy of neurons in the caudate nucleus within the basal ganglia (Graybiel, 1989; Lebrun-Grandie et al., 1989). Therefore, Huntington's disease may provide information about the role of the caudate nucleus in the control of movement; specifically, the loss of function (akinesia, bradykinesia) caused by Huntington's disease may indicate the unimpaired function of the caudate nucleus (Brown & Marsden, 1986a; Thompson et al., 1988).

Akinesia has been reported in Huntington's disease (Hefter et al., 1987; Podoll et al., 1988; Thompson et al., 1988). Indeed, choreiform movement is not the earliest symptom of the disease, nor is it the best indicator of functional impairment (Hayden, 1981; Shoulson & Fahn, 1979). The symptom of akinesia has been found to be a better predictor of functioning than severity of chorea (Girotti, Morano, Soliver, Geminiani, & Scigliano, 1988; Hefter et al., 1987).

Reaction time tends to be longer in patients with Huntington's disease (Girotti et al., 1988; Hefter et al., 1987; Lasker, Zee, Hain, Folstein, & Singer, 1987). As with Parkinson's disease, however, findings of prolonged reaction time in patients with Huntington's disease are less reliable than those findings of prolonged movement time (Ludlow et al., 1987; Hefter et al., 1987). This may be because involuntary choreiform movement, affects the initiation of voluntary movement. For example, Lasker et al., (1987) found patients had difficulty in suppressing eye saccades in a simple RT task. On the other hand, as in the case of Parkinson's disease, it would appear that patients with Huntington's disease tend to control movements during execution, rather than preparing them in advance (Bradshaw et al., 1990).

Bradykinesia does not arise from cortical deficits or problems of peripheral conduction (Homberg & Lange, 1990). Stimulation of the motor cortex shows that central motor conduction to upper and lower extremity muscles is normal in patients with Huntington's disease (Homberg & Lange, in press).

Hefter et al. (1987) examined muscle activity during ballistic movement in the fingers of patients with Huntington's disease. The normal agonist-antagonist pattern was maintained in these patients, suggesting that the ability to select proper muscle groups was unimpaired. However, patients required longer to attain peak force. Hefter et al. reported a linear relationship between contraction time and contraction amplitude in their patients, i.e., movement of greater amplitude required longer contraction time. As most patients were not on any medication, the observed bradykinesia was unlikely to be the result of treatment with dopamine antagonists.

Thompson et al. (1989) examined muscle activity, during simple and complex movement, in the wrists of patients with Huntington's disease. Although slower than control subjects, patients could perform simple wrist flexions (15 and 60 degrees). Movement was characterised by slow, prolonged contractions. Central deficits in the activation of movement were indicated, as patients had additional difficulty performing more complex, simultaneous or sequential movement (squeezing hand and flexing elbow). The observed slowness of movement, probably, was not the result of a proprioceptive deficit, as speed of movement was not related to abnormalities in somatosensory-evoked potentials (stimulation of median nerve of wrist), nor to any component of long-latency reflexes elicited in the wrist.

Whereas in Parkinson's disease there exists impairment in the scaling of size of initial agonist bursts (requiring additional cycles of activity), in Huntington's disease there exists impairment in the development of muscle activity, and prolongation of bursts of muscle activity. These latter observations suggest that the caudate nucleus has a role in the activating muscle contractions.

CONCLUSION

In this chapter we have been discussed some of the ways in which movement-disorders research may lead to a better understanding of the brain structures involved in movement control. A study of movement disorders may provide information about how movements are actually represented and controlled, and is an exercise in the application of data from clinical cases to motor control and learning. Movement disorders dramatise issues in the control of movement, and provide a window through which we can examine the role of brain structures in motor control. The basal ganglia would appear to have a role in the initiation and maintenance of movement forces, the neocerebellum, in specifying the endpoints of movement (Phillips, Muller, & Stelmach, 1989), and parts of the cortex, in the specification of spatial orientation (see Poizner et al., 1990).

A consideration of movement disorders may provide converging evidence for theoretical entities proposed by motor control theorists. For example, Parkinson's and Huntington's diseases illustrate the importance of *preparatory processes* to the smooth, fast execution of movement. These movement disorders also allow a discussion of representation; a *generalised representation* of movement is intact, but the scaling is disrupted. In Parkinson's disease, handwriting may be reduced in size, while in Huntington's disease it may be magnified. On the other hand, movement disorders may illustrate the importance of biomechanical factors; Parkinsonian tremor provides a clear example of *entrainment* of movement (Frischer, 1989; Nakamura et al., 1978).

Perhaps the most important role of movement disorders is as that of a powerful tool for the study of neurophysiological and biomechanical bases of motor control (Abbs & Connor, 1989). Application of advanced kinematic techniques may be especially beneficial in investigations of movement disorders. For example, certain frequencies from spectral analysis of movement velocities (e.g., Meulenbroek & Van Galen, 1989) may be related to tremors associated with specific brain structures (Young, 1985), and measures of ballisticity (Meulenbroek & Van Galen, 1989) may be validated in patients with known motor control deficits (Hallett & Khoshbin, 1980). Again, studies of movement disorders, focused upon the current issues in motor control, may engender new paths of research, while challenging already existing theories.

ACKNOWLEDGMENT

Preparation of this Chapter was supported by a grant from the National Institute of Neurological Diseases and Stroke NS 17421.

REFERENCES

Abbruzzese, G., Dall'Agata, D., Morena, M., Spadavecchia, L., Ratto, S., & Favale, E. (1990). Impaired habituation of long-latency stretch reflexes of the wrist muscles in Huntington's disease. *Movement Disorders, 5*, 32-35.

Abbs, J.H., & Connor, N.P. (1989). Motor coordination for functional human behaviors: Perspectives from a speech motor base. In S.A. Wallace (Ed.), *Perspectives on the coordination of movement* (pp. 157-183). Amsterdam: North-Holland.

Baroni, A., Benvenuti, F., Fantini, L., Pantaleo, T., & Urbani, F. (1984). Human ballistic arm abduction movements: Effects of L-dopa treatment in Parkinson's disease. *Neurology, 34*, 868-876.

Benecke, R., Rothwell, J.C., Dick, J.P.R., Day, B.L., & Marsden, C.D. (1986). Performance of simultaneous movements in patients with Parkinson's disease. *Brain, 109*, 739-757.

Benecke, R., Rothwell, J.C., Dick, J.P.R., Day, B.L., & Marsden, C.D. (1987). Simple and complex movements off and on treatment in patients with Parkinson's disease. *Journal of Neurology, Neurosurgery, and Psychiatry, 50*, 296-303.

Berardelli, A. Accornero, N., Argenta, M., Meco, G., & Manfredi, M. (1986). Fast complex arm movements in Parkinson's disease. *Journal of Neurology, Neurosurgery, and Psychiatry*, *49*, 1146-1149.

Berardelli, A., Dick, J.P.R., Rothwell, J.C., Day, B.L., & Marsden, C.D. (1986). Scaling of the size of the first agonist EMG burst during rapid wrist movements in patients with Parkinson's disease. *Journal of Neurology, Neurosurgery, and Psychiatry*, *49*, 1273-1279.

Bloxham, C.A., Dick, D.J., & Moore, M. (1987). Reaction times and attention in Parkinson's disease. *Journal of Neurology, Neurosurgery, and Psychiatry*, 50, 1178-1183.

Bloxham, C.A., Mindel, T.A., & Frith, C.D. (1984). Initiation and execution of predictable and unpredictable movements in Parkinson's disease. *Brain*, *10*, 371-384.

Borison, R.L., Hitri, A. & Diamond, B.I. (1986). Biochemical and pharmacological aspects of movement disorders in Huntington's disease. In N.S. Shah & A.G. Donald (Eds.), *Movement disorders* (pp. 275-292). New York: Plenum Press.

Bradshaw, J.L., Phillips, J., Dennis, C., Mattingley, J.B., Andrewes, D., Chiu, E., Pierson, J. & Bradshaw, J.A. (in press). *Initiation and execution of movement sequences in those suffering from and at risk of developing Huntington's disease. Journal of Clinical and Experimental Neuropsychology.*

Breakefield, X.O., & Bressman, S. (1986). Molecular genetics of movement disorders. In C.D. Marsden & S. Fahn (Eds.), *Movement disorders* 2. (pp. 33-62). London: Butterworths.

Brown, R.G. & Marsden, C.D. (1986a). Neuropsychology and cognitive function in Parkinson's disease: An overview. In C.D. Marsden & S. Fahn (Eds.) *Movement disorders 2* (pp. 99-123). London: Butterworths.

Brown, R.G., & Marsden, C.D. (1986b). Visuospatial function in Parkinson's disease. *Brain*, *109*, 987-1002.

Brown, R.G. & Marsden, C.D. (1988). Internal versus external cues and the control of attention in Parkinson's disease. *Brain*, *111*, 323-345.

Brown, R.G., Marsden, C.D., Quinn, N., & Wyke, M.A. (1984). Alterations in cognitive performance and affect-arousal stage during fluctuations in motor function in Parkinson's disease. *Journal of Neurology, Neurosurgery, and Psychiatry*, *47*, 454-465.

Caligiuri, M.P. (1987). Labial kinematics during speech with patients with Parkinsonian rigidity. *Brain*, *110*, 1033-1044.

Carlton, L.G., Carlton, M.J., & Newell, K.M. (1987). Reaction time and response dynamics. *Quarterly Journal of Experimental Psychology*, *39A*, 337-360.

Cools, A.R., Van Den Bercken, J.H.L., Horstink, M.W.I., Van Spaendonck, K.P.M., & Berger, J.J.C. (1984). Cognitive and motor shifting aptitude disorder in Parkinson's disease. *Journal of Neurology, Neurosurgery, and Psychiatry*, *47*, 443-453.

Dakof, G.E., & Mendelsohn, G.A. (1986). Parkinson's disease: The psychological aspects of a chronic illness. *Psychological Bulletin*, *99*, 375-387.

DeAjuriaguerra, J. (1975). The concept of akinesia. *Psychological Medicine*, *5*, 129-137.

Della Sala, S.D., Lorenzo, G.D., Giordano, A., & Spinnler, H. (1986). Is there a specific visuo-spatial impairment in Parkinsonians? *Journal of Neurology, Neurosurgery, and Psychiatry*, *49*, 1258-1265.

DeLong, M.R., Georgopoulos, A.P., & Crutcher, M.D. (1983). Cortico-basal ganglia relations and coding of motor performance. In J. Massion, J. Paillard, W. Schultz, & M. Wiesendanger (Eds.), *Experimental Brain Research: Supplementum: Vol. 7. Neural coding of motor performance* (pp. 30-400). Berlin: Springer.

Draper, I.T., & Johns, R.S. (1964). The disorders of movement in Parkinsonism and the effect of drug treatment. *Bulletin of the John Hopkins Hospital*, *115*, 465-480.

Edelman, G.M., & Mountcastle, V.B. (1979). *The mindful brain.*Cambridge, MA: The MIT Press.

Evarts, E.V., Teravainen, H., & Calne, D.B. (1981). Reaction time in Parkinson's disease. *Brain*, *104*, 167-186.

Flowers, K.A. (1976). Visual 'closed-loop' and 'open-loop' characteristics of voluntary movement in patients with Parkinsonism and intention tremor. *Brain*, *99*, 269-310.

Flowers, K.A., & Robertson, C. (1985). The effect of Parkinson's disease on the ability to maintain a mental set. *Journal of Neurology, Neurosurgery, and Psychiatry*, *48*, 517-529.

Forno, L.S. (1982). Pathology of Parkinson's disease. In C.D. Marsden & S. Fahn (Eds.), *Movement disorders* (pp. 25-40). London: Butterworths.

Frischer, M. (1989). Voluntary vs autonomous control of repetitive finger tapping in a patient with Parkinson's disease. *Neuropsychologia*, *27*, 1261-1266.

Frith, C.D., Bloxham, C.A., & Carpenter, K.N. (1986). Impairments in the learning and performance of a new manual skill in patients with Parkinson's disease. *Journal of Neurology, Neurosurgery, and Psychiatry*, *49*, 661-668.

Gentner, D.R. (1987). Timing of skilled motor performance: Tests of the proportional duration model. *Psychological Review*, *94*, 255-276.

Girotti, F., Carella, F., Grassi, M.P., Soliveri, P. Marano, R., & Caraceni, T. (1986). Motor and cognitive performances of Parkinsonian patients in the on and off phases of the disease. *Journal of Neurology, Neurosurgery, and Psychiatry*, *49*, 657-660.

Girotti, F., Marano, R., Soliveri, P., Geminiani, G., & Scigliano, G. (1988). Relationship between motor and cognitive deficits in Huntington's disease. *Journal of Neurology, 235*, 454-457.

Goldenberg, G. (1990). Performance of concurrent non-motor tasks in Parkinson's disease. *Journal of Neurology, 237*, 191-196.

Goodman, D., & Kelso, J.A.S. (1980). Are movements prepared in parts? Not under compatible (naturalised) conditions. *Journal of Experimental Psychology: General, 109*, 475-495.

Gordon, W.P., & Illes, J. (1987). Neurolinguistics of language production in Huntington's disease: A preliminary report. *Brain and Language, 31*, 1-10.

Gotham, A-M., Brown, R.G., & Marsden, C.D. (1986). Depression in Parkinson's disease: A quantitative and qualitative analysis. *Journal of Neurology, Neurosurgery, and Psychiatry, 49*, 381-389.

Graybiel, A.M. (1989). Dopaminergic and cholinergic systems in the striatum. In A.R. Crossman & M.A. Sambrook (Eds.), *Neural mechanisms in disorders of movement* (pp. 3-15). London: John Libbey.

Gresty, M.A., & Findley, L.J. (1981). Tremors in Parkinson's disease. In F.C. Rose & R. Capildeo (Eds.), *Research progress in Parkinson's disease* (pp. 75-87). Bath: Pitman Press.

Gunilla, R., Oberg, E., & Divac, I. (1985). Levels of motor planning: Cognition and the control of movement. In E.V. Evarts, S.P. Wise, & D. Bousfield (Eds.), *The motor system in neurobiology* (pp. 284-287). Amsterdam: Elsevier.

Hallett, M. (1983). Analysis of abnormal voluntary and involuntary movements with surface electromyography. *Advances in Neurology, 39*, 907-914.

Hallett, M., & Khoshbin, S. (1980). A physiological mechanism of bradykinesia. *Brain, 103*, 301-314.

Hallett, M., Shahani, B.T., & Young, R.R. (1977). Analysis of stereotyped voluntary movments at the elbow in patients with Parkinson's disease. *Journal of Neurology, Neurosurgery, and Psychiatry, 40*, 1129-1135.

Hayden, M.R. (1981). *Huntington's chorea*. Berlin: Springer-Verlag.

Hefter, J., Homberg, V., Lange, H.W., & Freund, H-J., (1987). Impairment of rapid movement in Huntington's disease. *Brain, 110*, 585-612.

Henry, F.M. & Rogers, D.E. (1960). Increased response latency for complicated movements and a "memory drum" theory of neuromotor reactions. *Research Quarterly, 31*, 448-458.

Hoehn, M.M., & Yahr, M.D. (1967). Parkinsonism: Onset, progression, and mortality. *Neurology, 17*, 427-442.

Homberg, V., & Lange, H.W. (1990). Central motor conduction to hand and leg muscles in Huntington's disease. *Movement Disorders, 5*, 214-218.

Hornykiewicz, O. (1982). Brain neurotransmitter changes in Parkinson's disease. In C.D. Marsden & S. Fahn (Eds.), *Movement disorders* (pp. 41-58). London: Butterworths.

Huttunen, J. & Homberg, V. (1990). EMG responses in leg muscles to postural perturbations in Huntington's disease. *Journal of Neurology, Neurosurgery, and Psychiatry*, *53*, 55-62.

Jankovic, J. (1987). Pathophysiology and clinical assessment of motor symptoms in Parkinson's disease. In W.C. Koller (Ed.), *Handbook of Parkinson's disease* (pp. 99-126). New York: Marcel Dekker.

Josiassen, R.C., Curry, L.M., & Mancall, E.L. (1983). Development of neuropsychological deficits in Huntington's disease. *Archives of Neurology*, *40*, 791-796.

Klapp, S.T., Wyatt, E.P., & Lingo, W.M. (1974). Response programming in simple and choice reactions. *Journal of Motor Behavior*, *6*, 263-271.

Knight, R.G., Godfrey, H.P.D., & Shelton, E.J. (1988). The psychological deficits associated with Parkinson's disease. *Clinical Psychology Review*, *8*, 391-410.

Lakie, M., & Mutch, W.J. (1989). Finger tremor in Parkinson's disease. *Journal of Neurology, Neurosurgery, and Psychiatry*, 52, 392-394.

Lasker, A.G., Zee, D.S., Hain, T.C., Folstein, S.E., & Singer, H.S. (1987). Saccades in Huntington's disease: Initiation defects and distractibility. *Neurology*, *37*, 364-369.

Lebrun-Grandie, Ph., Kien, P., Tison, F., Henry, P., Caille, J.M., & Bioulac, B. (1989). A magnetic resonance imaging evaluation of movement disorders. In A.R. Crossman & M.A. Sambrook (Eds.), *Neural mechanisms in disorders of movement* (pp. 433-443). London: John Libbey.

Lee, R.G., & Tatton, W.G. (1978). Long loop reflexes in man: Clinical applications. In J.E. Desmedt (Ed.), *Cerebral motor control in man: Long loop mechanisms* (pp. 320-333). Basel: Karger.

Lees, A.J. (1989). The on-off phenomenon. *Journal of Neurology, Neurosurgery, and Psychiatry, Special Supplement*, 29-37.

Lees, A.J. & Smith, E. (1983). Cognitive deficits in the early stages of Parkinson's disease. *Brain*, *106*, 257-270.

Levin, B.E., Llabre, M.M., & Weiner, W.J. (1988). Parkinson's disease and depression: Psychometric properties of the Beck Depression Inventory. *Journal of Neurology, Neurosurgery, and Psychiatry*, 51, 1401-1404.

Lohr, J.B. & Wisniewski, A.A. (1987). *Movement disorders: A neuropsychiatric approach*. Chichester: John Wiley.

Ludlow, C.L., Connor, N.P., & Bassich, C.J. (1987). Speech timing in Parkinson's and Huntington's disease. *Brain and Language*, *32*, 195-214.

Margolin, D.I. (1984). The neuropsychology of writing and spelling: Semantic, phonological, motor, and perceptual processes. *Quarterly Journal of Experimental Psychology*, *36A*, 459-489.

Marsden, C.D. (1980). On-off phenomena in Parkinson's disease. In U.K. Rinne, M. Klinger, & G. Stamm (Eds.), *Parkinson's disease: Current progress, problems and management* (pp. 241-254). Amsterdam: Elsevier.

Marsden, C.D. (1982). The mysterious motor function of the basal ganglia: The Robert Wartenberg Lecture. *Neurology*, *32*, 514-539.

Marsden, C.D. (1984). Function of the basal ganglia as revealed by cognitive and motor disorders in Parkinson's disease. *Canadian Journal of Neurological Science*, *11*, 129-135.

Marsden, C.D. (1985). Defects of movement in Parkinson's disease. In P.J. Delwaide & A. Agnoli (Eds.), *Clinical neurophysiology in Parkinsonism* (pp. 107-115). Amsterdam: Elsevier.

Marsden, C.D., Obeso, J.A. & Rothwell, J.C. (1983). Clinical neurophysiology of muscle jerks: Myoclonus, chorea, and tics. *Advances in Neurology*, *39*, 865-881.

Marsden, C.D., Rothwell, J.C., & Day, B.L. (1983). Long-latency automatic responses to muscle stretch in man: Origin and function. *Advances in Neurology*, *39*, 509-539.

Martin, W.R.W. & Calne, D.B. (1986). Imaging techniques and movement disorders. In C.D. Marsden & S. Fahn (Eds.), *Movement disorders 2*. (pp. 4-16). London: Butterworths.

Mayeux, K., Williams, J.B.W., Stern, Y., & Cote, L. (1984). Depression and Parkinson's disease. *Advances in Neurology*, *40*, 241-251.

McLellan, D.L. (1981). Rigidity. In F.C. Rose & R. Capildeo (Eds.), *Research progress in Parkinson's disease* (pp. 88-97). Bath: Pitman Press.

Meulenbroek, R.G.J., & Van Galen, G.P. (1989). The production of connecting strokes in cursive writing: Developing co-articulation in 8 to 12 year-old children. In R. Plamondon, C.Y. Suen, & M.L. Simner (Eds.), *Computer recognition and human production of handwriting* (pp. 273-286). Singapore: World Scientific Publishing Co.

Myers, R.H., & Falek, A. (1979). Quantification of muscle tremor of Huntington's disease patients and their offspring in an early detection study. *Biological Psychiatry*, *14*, 777-789.

Nakamura, R., Nagasaki, H., & Narabayashi, H. (1978). Disturbances of rhythm formation in patients with Parkinson's disease: Part I. Characteristics of tapping response to the periodic signals. *Perceptual and Motor Skills*, *46*, 63-75.

Noth, J., Podoll, K., & Friedmann, H.H. (1985). Long-loop reflexes in small hand muscles studied in normal subjects and in patients with Huntington's disease. *Brain*, *108*, 65-80.

Obeso, J.A., Grandas, F., Vaamonde, J., Luquin, M.R., Artieda, J., Lera, G., Rodriguez, M.E., & Martinez-Lage, J.M. (1989). Motor complications associated with chronic levodopa therapy in Parkinson's disease. *Neurology*, *39 (supplement 2)*, 11-19.

Parkinson, J. (1817). *An essay of the shaking palsy*. London: Sherwood, Neely, and Jones.

Phillips, J.G., Muller, F., & Stelmach, G.E. (1989). Movement disorders and the neural basis of motor control. In S.A. Wallace (Ed.), *Perspectives on the coordination of movement* (pp. 367-413). Amsterdam: North-Holland.

Phillips, J., Stelmach, G., & Teasdale, N. (1989). Preliminary assessment of spatio-temporal control of handwriting in Parkinsonians. In R. Plamondon, C.Y. Suen, & M.L. Simner (Eds.), *Computer recognition and human production of handwriting* (pp. 317-331). Singapore: World Scientific Publishing Co.

Phillips, J.G., Stelmach, G., & Teasdale, N. (1991). What can indices of handwriting quality tell us about Parkinsonian handwriting? *Human Movement Science, 10,* 301-314.

Podoll, K. Caspary, P. Lange, H.W. & Noth, J. (1988). Language functions in Huntington's disease. *Brain, 111*, 1475-1503.

Poizner, H., Mack, L., Verfaellie, M., Gonzalez Rothi, L.J., & Heilman, K.M. (1990). Three-dimensional computergraphic analysis of apraxia. *Brain, 113*, 85-101.

Posner, M.I., Pea, R., & Volpe, B. (1982). Cognitive-neuroscience: Developments toward a science of synthesis. In J. Mehler, M. Garrett, & E. Walker (Eds.), *Perspectives on mental representation: Experimental and theoretical studies of cognitive processes and capacities* (pp. 251-276). Hillsdale, NJ: Lawrence Erlbaum Associates.

Rafal, R.D., Inhoff, A.W., Friedman, J.H., & Bernstein, E. (1987). Programming and execution of sequential movements in Parkinson's disease. *Journal of Neurology, Neurosurgery, and Psychiatry*, *50*, 1267-1273.

Rosenbaum, D.A. (1980). Human movement initiation: Specification of arm, direction, and extent. *Journal of Experimental Psychology: General*, *109*, 444-474.

Schmidt, R.A. (1985). The search for invariance in skilled movement behavior. *Research Quarterly for Exercise and Sport*, *56*, 188-200.

Sheridan, M.R., Flowers, K.A., & Hurrell, J. (1987). Programming and execution of movements in Parkinson's disease. *Brain*, *110*, 1247-1271.

Stahl, S.M. (1986). Neuropharmacology of movement disorders: Comparison of spontaneous and drug-induced movement disorders. In M.S. Shah & A.G. Donald (Eds.) *Movement disorders* (pp. 275-292). New York: Plenum Press.

Starkstein, S.E., Esteguy, M., Berthier, M.L., Garcia, H., & Leiguarda, R. (1989). Evoked potentials, reaction time and cognitive performance in on and off phases of Parkinson's disease. *Journal of Neurology, Neurosurgery, and Psychiatry*, *52*, 338-340.

Stelmach, G.E., & Diggles, V. (1982). Control theories in motor behavior. *Acta Psychologica*, *50*, 83-105.

Stelmach, G.E., Garcia-Colera, A., & Martin, Z.E. (1989). Force transition control within a movement sequence in Parkinson's disease. *Journal of Neurology*, *236*, 406-410.

Stelmach, G.E. & Phillips, J.G. (1991). Movement disorders: Limb movements and the basal ganglia. *Physical Therapy, 71,*60-67.

Stelmach, G.E., Phillips, J.G., & Chau, A.W. (1989). Visuo-spatial processing in Parkinsonians. *Neuropsychologia*, *27*, 485-493.

Stelmach, G.E., Teasdale, N., Phillips, J., & Worringham, C.J. (1989). Force production characteristics in Parkinson's disease. *Experimental Brain Research*, *76*, 165-172.

Stelmach, G.E. & Worringham, C.J. (1988). The preparation and production of isometric force in Parkinson's disease. *Neuropsychologia*, *26*, 93-103.

Stelmach, G.E., Worringham, C.J., & Strand, E.A. (1986). Movement preparation in Parkinson's disease: The use of advanced information. *Brain*, *109*, 1179-1194.

Stelmach, G.E., Worringham, C.J., & Strand, E.A. (1987). The programming and execution of movement sequences in Parkinson's disease. *International Journal of Neuroscience*, *36*, 55-65.

Stern, Y., & Mayeux, R. (1986). Intellectual impairment in Parkinson's disease. *Advances in Neurology*, *45*, 405-408.

Still, C.N., & Goldschmidt, T.J. (1986). The effects of neuroleptics on longevity in Huntington's disease. In N.S. Shah & A.G. Donald (Eds.), *Movement disorders* (pp. 293-306). New York: Plenum Press.

Swerdlow, N.R., & Koob, G.F. (1987). Dopamine, schizophrenia, mania, and depression: Toward a unified hypothesis of cortico-striato-pallido-thalamic function. *Behavioral and Brain Sciences*, *10*, 197-245.

Taylor, A.E., Saint-Cyr, J.A., Lang, A.E., & Kenny, F.T. (1986). Parkinson's disease and depression: A critical re-evaluation. *Brain*, *109*, 279-292.

Teasdale, N., Phillips, J., & Stelmach, G.E. (1990). Temporal movement control in patients with Parkinson's disease. *Journal of Neurology, Neurosurgery, and Psychiatry, 53,* 862-868.

Teulings, H-L. & Stelmach, G.E. (1991). Control of stroke size, peak acceleration, and stroke duration in Parkinsonian handwriting. *Human Movement Science, 10,* 315-334.

Thompson, P.D., Berardelli, A., Rothwell, J.C., Day, B.L., Dick, J.P.R., Benecke, R., & Marsden, C.D. (1988). The coexistence of bradykinesia and chorea in Huntington's disease and its implications for theories of basal ganglia control of movement. *Brain*, *111*, 223-244.

Wallesch, C-W., & Fehrenbach, R.A. (1988). On the neruolinguistic nature of language abnormalities in Huntington's disease. *Journal of Neurology, Neurosurgery, and Psychiatry*, *51*, 367-373.

Wann, J.P. & Nimmo-Smith, I. (1990). Evidence against the relative invariance of timing in handwriting. *Quarterly Journal of Experimental Psychology*, *42A*, 105-119.

Wing, A.M. (1989). A comparison of the rate of pinch grip force increases and decreases in Parkinsonian bradykinesia. *Neuropsychologia*, *26*, 479-482.

Wing, A.M., & Miller, E. (1984). Basal ganglia lesions and the psychological analyses of the control of voluntary movement. *Ciba Foundation Symposium 107: Functions of the basal ganglia* (pp. 242-257). London: Pitman.

Worringham, C.J. & Stelmach, G.E. (1990). Practice effects on the preprogramming of discrete movements in Parkinson's disease. *Journal of Neurology, Neurosurgery, and Psychiatry, 53,* 702-704.

Wright, M.J., Burns, R.J., Geffen, G.M., & Geffen, L.B. (1990). Covert orientation of visual attention in Parkinson's disease: An impairment in the maintenance of attention. *Neuropsychologia*, *28*, 151-159.

Young, A.B., Albin, R.L., & Penney, J.B. (1989). Neuropharmacology of basal ganglia functions: Relationship to pathophysiology of movement disorders. In A.R. Crossman & M.A. Sambrook (Eds.), *Neural mechanisms in disorders of movement* (pp. 17-27). London: John Libbey.

Young, R.R. (1985). Tremor in Parkinson's disease. In P.J. Delwaide & A. Agnoli (Eds.), *Clinical neurophysiology in Parkinsonism* (pp. 139-162). Amsterdam: Elsevier.

Zetusky, W. J., Jankovic, J., & Pirozzolo, F. J. (1985). The heterogeneity of Parkinson's disease: Clinical and prognostic implications. *Neurology*, *35*, 522-526.

Approaches to the Study of Motor Control and Learning
J.J. Summers (Editor)

Chapter 17

ADAPTIVE MODEL THEORY: APPLICATION TO DISORDERS OF MOTOR CONTROL

Peter D. Neilson, Megan D. Neilson, & Nicholas J. O'Dwyer
University of New South Wales

Adaptive Model Theory (AMT) is a computational theory of the information processing performed by the human central nervous system during control of purposive movement. We begin with an overview of AMT which incorporates sensory analysis, response planning, and response execution stages of information processing, the concept of intermittency in movement control, and the notion of a Basic Unit of Motor Production or BUMP. We develop the idea that a finite interval of time, typically 100-200 ms, is required to preplan a response as a trajectory of desired reafference. This sensory trajectory is transformed in real time into appropriately coordinated motor commands via an adaptive internal model of the inverse dynamic relationships between outgoing motor commands and their resulting sensory consequences. A detailed description of the principles of adaptive modelling of multivariable nonlinear dynamic systems is provided and we overview an AMT-based computer simulation of human operator performance of a pursuit tracking task. We discuss possible neural implementation of adaptive modelling circuitry and focus in particular on the cerebellum where the sagittal zones appear well suited for the implementation of adaptive neural filters. Lastly we explore the implications of AMT for disorders of motor control as diverse as cerebral palsy and stuttering.

Aims and Scope

We present in this chapter a description of computational processes which provide a technological basis for emulating and elucidating the function of central neural mechanisms in the control of purposive human movement. At one level this formulation is broadly conceptual and addresses issues in motor behaviour such as the role of feedback, the process of adaptive control of movement, and the notion of central intermittency. At another level it is highly specific in describing circuitry which lends itself to the distributed parallel processing of neural networks and which is credible in terms of what neuroscience currently tells us of the structure and function of the central nervous system (CNS). At both levels our aim is to coalesce the mathematical theory of signals and systems with a theory of human movement control in keeping with established neurobiological and psychobiological findings.

We call our formulation Adaptive Model Theory (AMT). Adaptive internal models are the essence of adaptive control techniques in technological systems but the term is also used in reference to the cognitive basis of perception and performance. Indeed, the notion of the CNS forming an updatable "image" or "internal model" of the world was expressed at least as early and as diversely as Craik (1943) and Sokolov (1960). The name, therefore, appropriately reflects the diverse knowledge base on which the theory grew. Before presenting AMT we will first outline the influence of that background and, in keeping with our title, highlight the formative role played by our investigations of motor disorders. In so doing we seek to emphasise the way in which AMT derives from interests equally vested in the understanding of normal and abnormal sensorimotor control processes. The fact that we devote the main part of this chapter to normal processes in no way reflects lack of involvement with motor disorders. That involvement is both long standing and continuing (Nash, Neilson, & O'Dwyer, 1989; Neilson, 1973; Neilson, 1980; Neilson & Neilson, in press; Neilson & O'Dwyer, 1984; O'Dwyer, 1988). We strongly believe that the effective study of a disorder involves the double task of understanding the normal system in tandem with the abnormal. Which brings us to the beginnings of AMT.

The Genesis of Adaptive Model Theory

We began in the 1960s with good basic training in physics (PDN & MDN) and engineering (PDN), very little biology or psychology, and a consuming interest in working at the interface. There was little in the way of formal interdisciplinary education but, guided by Wiener's cybernetics (1948) and the pioneering studies of Stark (see Stark, 1968), we began to tackle the literature of living control systems. Working at technical jobs within a medical school facilitated postgraduate study of two particular systems in relation to disorders of those systems. These were respectively the system of long loop reflexes in relation to cerebral palsy and the feedback control of speech in relation to stuttering.

Both projects led quickly to experiments on human tracking behaviour. In one case knowledge of the limits of kinaesthetic tracking performance offered a way of separating responses that could well be voluntary from those that could only be reflex. In the other, an auditory-motor tracking task offered a means of characterising the supposed servocontrolled speech-hearing system which, by analogy to the disfluencies observed under delayed auditory feedback, was thought to become unstable in stuttering (see Yates, 1963).

The literature on tracking came from two streams which had, and still have, limited confluence. There was firstly and familiarly the engineering approach where tracking was the basis of modelling the human operator, usually as a continuous mechanism. But there was also the motor behaviour approach which was entirely new to us. Here there was preoccupation with central intermittency and the role of response feedback and, in looking beyond tracking studies per se, we found these were the concerns of the many studies on discrete movements and movement sequences (see Glencross & Barrett, 1988). In the disparity between these approaches we found the seeds of one of the conceptual problems that AMT attempts to address: How can the successful models of human operator tracking performance, achieved without reference to intermittency (e.g., Kleinman, Baron, & Levison, 1970; McRuer & Krendel, 1959a, 1959b, 1974; see also McRuer, 1980), be reconciled with psychological refractoriness? In such models the inter-response interval for a continuously responding system equals the inter-stimulus interval and there is no refractory period.

With this problem on hold, the course of our own investigations soon made the motor behaviour literature increasingly relevant to us. In the study of cerebral palsy it became apparent that despite the clear modulation of long loop reflexes from above, and some limited ability of subjects to control such modulation (Neilson & Lance, 1978), the fundamental dysfunction went beyond the province of abnormal reflexes. While problems with purposive movement control had not gone unmentioned, the view prevailed that hyperexcitable reflexes constrain or disrupt purposive movement in the spastic and athetoid forms of cerebral palsy respectively. Yet quite apart from disruptive reflexes, it seemed that cerebral palsied subjects know exactly what they want to do but are unable to do it efficiently or appropriately. To us the difficulty seemed more to be with the central processes of sensorimotor translation. With stuttering too it became clear that we had to understand normal and abnormal fluency in terms of central sensorimotor processes. Lane and Tranel (1971) had denounced an already dying servotheory of speech control and our experimental work showed likewise (Neilson, 1973). Meanwhile MacNeilage (1970), in his influential paper on the serial ordering of speech, introduced us headlong to the central vs. peripheral controversy among other theoretical problems concerning the transition from sensory goal to motor implementation.

MacNeilage and the literature he pointed to made it clear that an adequate theory of control of purposive movement must address not only the question of motor program (open loop) control vs. feedback (closed loop) control but also tackle how sensory plans give rise to motor acts to fulfil those plans. That this process must be adaptive if performance is to remain consistent and effective was clear from studies on sensorimotor rearrangement (e.g., Held & Freedman, 1963; Smith & Smith, 1962) and from the well-established ability of the human operator to adapt to a wide range of control-display characteristics (e.g., McRuer &

Krendel, 1974). Indeed, this latter literature served only to reinforce our inherently cybernetic view that the control process between sensory plan and motor implementation must be able to deal with a multiple input, multiple output, nonlinear dynamic time-varying system.

By the time we were beginning to formalise what has become AMT, a psychologist (NJO'D) keen to widen into neuroscience had joined the cerebral palsy project.

Adaptive Model Theory in Overview

We identified above three issues addressed in developing AMT: (a) the role of open loop versus closed loop control, (b) the process of adaptive control of sensorimotor performance, and (c) the basis of central intermittency. We believe these issues are best dealt with in terms of an adaptive controller which transforms an intermittently planned sensory trajectory into a set of motor commands by means of an inverse internal model of the system which lies between those motor commands and the sensory events desired. In later sections we give a specific description of how such a controller can be implemented to drive a robot using digital parallel processing. We also indicate how this might be accomplished in the CNS. In those respects AMT is unique. In broad terms, however, AMT is philosophically akin to numerous accounts of sensorimotor and/or robotic control (Arbib, 1972, 1981; Bahill & McDonald, 1983; Broadbent, 1977; Greene, 1982; Grossberg & Kuperstein, 1986; Gurfinkel & Levik, 1979/1980; Hinton, 1984; Kleinman et al., 1970; Kuperstein, 1988; Miyamoto, Kawato, Setoyama, & Suzuki, 1988; Moray, 1981; Pellionisz & Llinas, 1979; Pew, 1974; Raibert, 1978; Saltzman, 1979; Young, 1969). This list is not exhaustive and it is fast increasing with the surge of interest in the new field of neural network modelling (see Kohonen, 1988). The point is, there is now ample support for this general approach. We will now look at how AMT deals with the issues raised.

Open Loop versus Closed Loop Control

This old dissension fades once it is recognised that sensorimotor performance can be controlled by both central and peripheral influences operating interactively (e.g., Abbs & Cole, 1982; Summers, 1981). A formulation incorporating both open and closed loop processes can accommodate Lashley's renowned pianist (Lashley, 1951) and Taub's deafferented monkeys (Taub & Berman, 1968) while also allowing feedback to be operative in the regulation, correction, adaptation, and disruption of performance. Once we conceptualise there being various functional levels at which performance can be controlled, we see that much of the original controversy arose because different investigators were theorising about different things. At one level movement proceeds open loop, at another level it is influenced intermittently by feedback from previous movements while at a further level it is under the continuous control of reflex mechanisms.

The lifting of a jar full of mercury provides a good example of each level operating together within the one movement. Since most people grossly misjudge the weight, the first lifting movement will not achieve the expected result and at that level will be open loop without correction. At the next level the same movement can be considered as part of a closed loop in that the feedback will be used in modifying the wrongly judged relationship between the efferent and afferent signals involved. The reflex adjustment level will also be operative and the muscle control systems will act correctively in terms of assisting and protecting but they will not succeed in bringing the movement to its intended conclusion.

In AMT we recognise these multiple levels of control and the interactions between them. For the moment we will be concerned mainly with the evaluative, intermittent level where efferent and reafferent signals from a movement segment can be used to establish, monitor and adapt the relationship which characterises the system that lies between them.

Adaptive Control of Sensorimotor Performance

Determining the relationship between the input and output of a system is known in control theory as system identification. If the characteristics of a system change, a given input may no longer produce the same output as before, a consequence which is usually undesirable. Corrective feedback can reduce the error between what occurred and what was required but it cannot adjust for the basic problem of change in the controlled system. This is the task of adaptive control where feedback from the controlled system and the input which produced it are used to identify or "model" the current system characteristics. As soon as the changed characteristics have been modelled accurately, the correct output can be obtained. To do this, the desired output signal must be passed through a "controller" which has precisely the inverse characteristics of the controlled system. In other words, the controller must contain the inverse of the forward model. Given the forward model it is easy to calculate the inverse and the control problem is solved. The correct output will be obtained provided the models remain accurate, which will be the case if feedback is available to adapt the models whenever the system changes.

Figure 1 illustrates the concept of adaptive modelling in the control of purposive movement. We begin with the preplanned specification of an output, the desired response trajectory R^*. For the moment we will ignore how the desired response is planned and consider it simply as a signal specified across a time interval in terms of high level sensory features. This signal forms the input to a neural adaptive controller which has the task of generating the set of motor command signals M which will activate the controlled system to produce an actual response R identical to R^*. To do this the characteristics of the controller H^{-1} must be exactly the inverse of the characteristics of the controlled system H. In the later section on response execution we discuss the constituents of the controlled system which may include components external to the body (e.g., a pen in the case of a written response *R*). Here we say only that *H* defines the muscle control, biomechanical and possible external systems that lie between the origin of the motor commands and whatever response they generate.

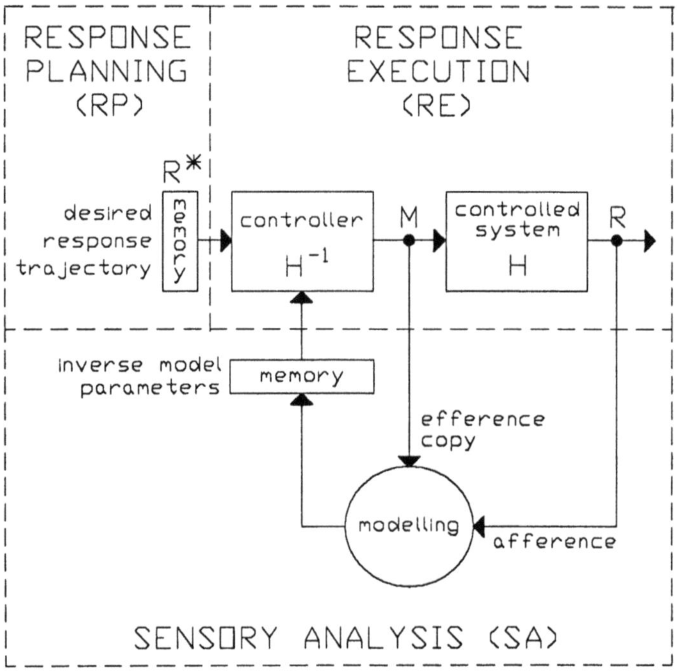

Figure 1. Flow diagram illustrating the formation and implementation of an internal model of the inverse dynamics H^{-1} of a controlled system *H* relative to sensory analysis, response planning, and response execution stages of information processing. Only modelling is illustrated and flow of information from SA to RP stages is not shown.

A response *R* consists of some combination of visual, auditory, and kinaesthetic information. This is processed by the sensory receptors and fed back through sensory analysers where it is condensed and integrated with the motor command signals which generated it. This condensation and integration is detailed in later sections. Here we say simply that the sensory and motor signals which arise in association with a response are modelled by specialised neural networks, the result being a set of parameters which define the prevailing sensorimotor relationships. Because the adaptive controller requires an inverse model to generate future sets of motor commands, the final parameters produced by the modelling networks define the relationship which transforms desired afference into efference.

We have here a means by which movement can be controlled adaptively with feedback from previous responses determining the characteristics of the system. If the controlled system changes, as happens for instance when a reaching response is viewed through prisms, the parameters specifying the inverse model must be changed to accommodate the new relationship between the efference which generated the response and the visual and kinaesthetic reafference. It is important to note the generality of the relationship defined by the parameters of the inverse model. Novel responses can be performed, the correct motor commands being generated by passing the desired sensory signal through the controller, even though that particular sensory event has not previously occurred. Provided the parameters are resident in memory, there is also no bar to skilled motor performance continuing under feedback deprivation. If no feedback is present the internal model cannot be checked or updated; movement will continue but there will be no adaptation if a change in sensorimotor relationships occurs. In normal circumstances a well-entrenched model will need minimal updating, but this ability to monitor and when necessary amend, gives the CNS the adaptive capability to deal with both internal and external change.

Central Intermittency and the Basic Unit of Motor Production

In Figure 1 we illustrated adaptive modelling and its role in the control of purposive movement. We have not yet discussed the partition of that diagram into three sections labelled sensory analysis (SA), response planning (RP), and response execution (RE). We will now identify these sections as processing stages in an intermittent three stage representation of purposive movement control.

According to AMT, the SA-stage operates continuously and in real-time. Its task is to condense afferent information and efferent information into high level feature signals and to model the relationships between these signals. Likewise the RE-stage operates continuously and in real-time reading whatever desired response signals R^* it finds in its input memory buffer and transforming them through the controller and the controlled system to generate a matching response signal R. The time required for the SA- and RE-stages to operate is only the time for transmission of the signals through the neural circuits, analogous to the flow of electrical signals through filters. This is not the case with the RP-stage. The RP-stage operates discretely rather than continuously and requires a finite interval of time to preplan a desired response trajectory R^* which it stores in a short-term memory buffer ready for execution. The planning process is then free to determine the next R^*, and so on. Unlike the continuous operation of the other two stages, the computational task of the RP-stage has a defined beginning and end and the information it provides is not available to the rest of the system until the task is complete. We propose that this is what introduces central intermittency into movement control.

Stage models are the backbone of the information processing approach to motor behaviour (e.g., Requin, 1980; Welford, 1980) and are used in accounting for the results of double stimulation reaction time experiments (see Welford, 1980). By incorporating intermittency in AMT we believe we provide a theoretical bridge between results from discrete stimulus response studies and the human operator studies mentioned previously. Indeed we have shown (Neilson, Neilson, & O'Dwyer, 1988) that gain and phase frequency response characteristics of the human operator derived from the assumptions of AMT parallel those based on continuous models of the human operator.

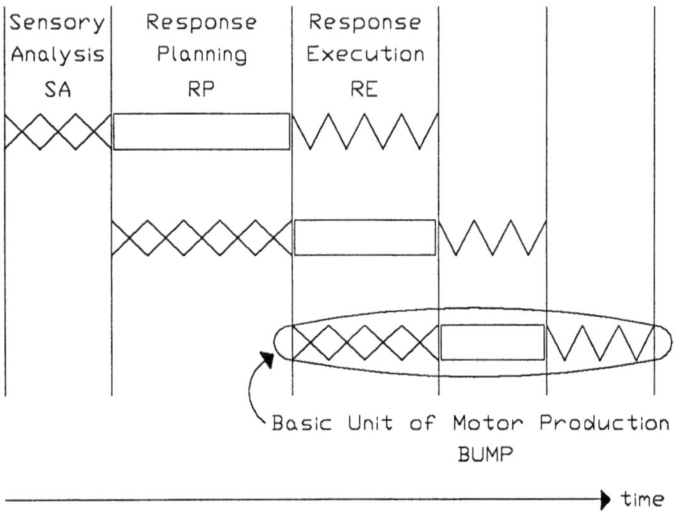

Figure 2. Diagram illustrating how the sequential operation of SA, RP, and RE stages can represent a Basic Unit of Motor Production (BUMP) while at any one point in time all three stages can operate independently and in parallel.

Like many stage formulations, AMT asserts that all three processes are working independently and in parallel. This is depicted in Figure 2. Nevertheless, a sequential operation of SA-, then RP-, then RE-stages is required to produce a particular response. In other words, all purposive movements can be seen as comprised of a concatenated sequence of submovements, each submovement planned in advance by the RP-stage and executed in an open-loop mode by the RE-stage. The three stage sequence of SA, RP, and RE processing defines what we consider a Basic Unit of Motor Production (BUMP) employed for discrete responses in reaction time experiments as well as for continuous responses in tracking tasks. The acronym BUMP is appropriate because the intrinsic intermittency of the BUMP seems sometimes to produce "bumps", particularly in the velocity profiles of movements. The velocity records of monkey tracking movements during dentate cooling (Brooks & Thach, 1981; Miall, Weir, & Stein, 1987) give an excellent example.

From Concepts to Specificity

Thus far we have introduced a number of basic features of AMT. Before we can deal with it in more detail we need to outline some of the technical basis on which it rests. There are good reasons for considering the nature of the computational tasks that the theory takes as its building blocks. If AMT is to be useful in understanding purposeful sensorimotor performance we must first be able to see those building blocks as tasks that neural circuitry might achieve. We therefore have to know what the tasks involve. It is one thing to say that the CNS has the capability of setting up an adaptive relationship between sensory and motor signals; it is another thing to say exactly how it might do it and what it might do it with. At another level, we need a wide base on which to test the theory. Knowledge of the behaviour of both normal and pathological human and animal systems is an obvious part of that base, but the ability to simulate such systems with adaptive control in robots is also useful and in some respects more flexible. If we can enhance or impede the various processing components of such a robot, it may tell us much about normal and abnormal human sensorimotor systems.

In the sections which follow we give a computational basis for implementing adaptive control technologically and then go on to consider the viability of those processes in terms of known neurobiology. We then return to a more detailed discussion of the processing elements of a BUMP and the implications for disorders. Since much of these later sections depends on some understanding of the computational aspects of AMT we have endeavoured to make that information, which is necessarily mathematical, as accessible as possible.

PRINCIPLES OF ADAPTIVE MODELLING

During the 1980s considerable advances have been made in the development of mathematical theories concerned with design of adaptive filters and adaptive control systems (see Astrom & Wittenmark, 1989; Goodwin & Sin, 1984; Widrow & Stearns, 1985). Many of the algorithms can be implemented in real-time using physically realisable computational machines employing distributed parallel processing. The computational components required to construct such machines are the four mathematical operations of addition, subtraction, multiplication, and division plus memory for storing and retrieving information. Storage and retrieval of information after a small interval of time (say 50 ms) is equivalent to introducing a 50 ms time delay into the system. Such time delays are so important in the construction of computer models of dynamic systems that they are regarded as computational elements in their own right and are known as "delayers". Delayers are represented mathematically by the symbol z^{-1}. Using only these five basic operators we will ultimately describe the design of a distributed parallel processing machine able to compute and adaptively maintain the accuracy of inverse models of multivariable, nonlinear, dynamic systems. Prior to that it will be helpful to consider some fundamental concepts.

Modelling a Dynamic System

The Nature of Dynamic Systems

The Impulse Response Function of a Pendulum. Let us begin with a brief discussion of dynamic systems and the properties of linearity and nonlinearity. The essential feature of a dynamic system is its ability to absorb energy from a short-duration input (stimulus) signal - a signal being any variable which changes as a function of time - and then to release that energy slowly so the response signal $y(t)$ outlasts the duration of the stimulus signal $u(t)$. This can be illustrated by considering the dynamic relationship between the force applied to a pendulum and the resulting angular displacement of the pendulum. Suppose that a pendulum at rest is struck a blow with a hammer applying an impulse of force. The pendulum swings vigorously due to an absorption of energy, but then continues to swing back and forth for some time with only a slowly decreasing amplitude of oscillation (Figure 3). The rate of reduction in amplitude is determined by the rate of loss of energy to the environment by frictional losses. Such a response is known as the impulse response function of the pendulum and completely characterises the response of the pendulum to any input function of force.

Memory in Response of Dynamic System. In a sense, a dynamic system has a form of memory since its output continues to respond to the stimulus after the stimulus has ceased. This is the nature of causal dynamic relationships. The response $y(t)$ of a dynamic system at time t is determined not only by the value of the stimulus $u(t)$ at time t but also by values of the stimulus at past times $u_{t-1}, u_{t-2}, \ldots, u_{t-n}$. To explain the notation employed here, imagine the input signal $u(t)$ sampled at unit intervals of time $t, t-1, \ldots, t-n$. Similarly, imagine the impulse response function of a dynamic system sampled at unit intervals of time as illustrated in Figure 3. The impulse response of a dynamic system can be represented, therefore, by its sampled values or impulse response function weights $h_0, h_1, h_2, \ldots, h_n$.

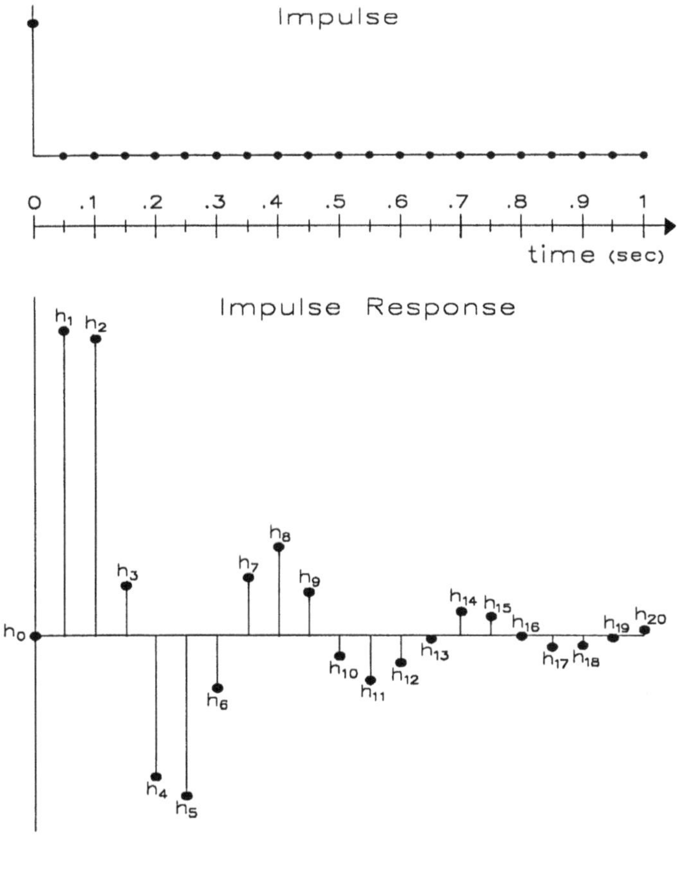

Figure 3. Top graph illustrates an impulse of force applied to a pendulum at time = 0. The bottom graph illustrates a swinging response of the pendulum to the applied force. The response long outlasts the duration of the applied force.

Linearity. The essential property of a linear dynamic system is that the response of the system to a sequence of input impulses is equal to the summation of the impulse responses of the system to each impulse delivered separately. Since any input signal $u(t)$ can be represented as a sequence of impulses, it follows that the response of a linear dynamic system to any arbitrary input signal $u(t)$ can be computed, given the impulse response function weights $h_0, h_1, \ldots, h_n$ of the system, as a linear combination of past inputs as shown in equation (1):

$$y_t = h_0 u_t + h_1 u_{t-1} + \ldots + h_n u_{t-n} \tag{1}$$

Nonlinearity. If the response of a system to a sequence of impulses deviates from the sum of the responses to each impulse applied separately, the system is said to be nonlinear. The deviation of the response from superposition of the individual impulse responses is attributed to nonlinear interactions between present and past values of the input signal. In the following we will focus on adaptive modelling of a single input, single output linear dynamic system. This will not limit the value of our discussion, however, because we will show that a parallel expansion of the basic circuit is all that is needed for adaptive modelling of multivariable nonlinear dynamic systems.

Adaptive Filters and Adaptive Models

Digital Filter Model of Dynamic System. The distributed parallel processing circuitry in Figure 4 simulates the input-output relationship of any linear dynamic system; that is, it functions as a model of the input-output relationship of any system with impulse response function weights $h_0, h_1, \ldots, h_n$. If an input signal $u(t)$ is applied to both a linear dynamic system and to the digital model, the output signal y_t' from the digital model will reproduce or simulate the output from the actual system. If a unit impulse is applied to the input of the circuit in Figure 4, it

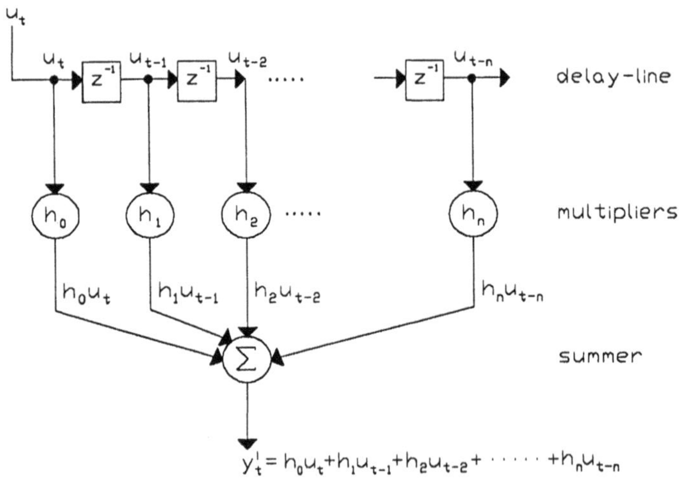

Figure 4. Schematic diagram of a transversal digital filter which simulates the linear dynamic relationship described by the impulse response function weights $h_0, h_1, \ldots, h_n$ between an input signal u_t and an output signal y_t.

will take n sample intervals to move along the delay-line. As the unit impulse travels along the delay-line, the output y_t' from the digital filter will first be h_0, then h_1, then h_2, and so on along the line. It follows that the digital model has the same impulse response function weights as the dynamic system. From the property of linearity, the digital model will simulate the response of the linear dynamic system to any arbitrary input signal $u(t)$.

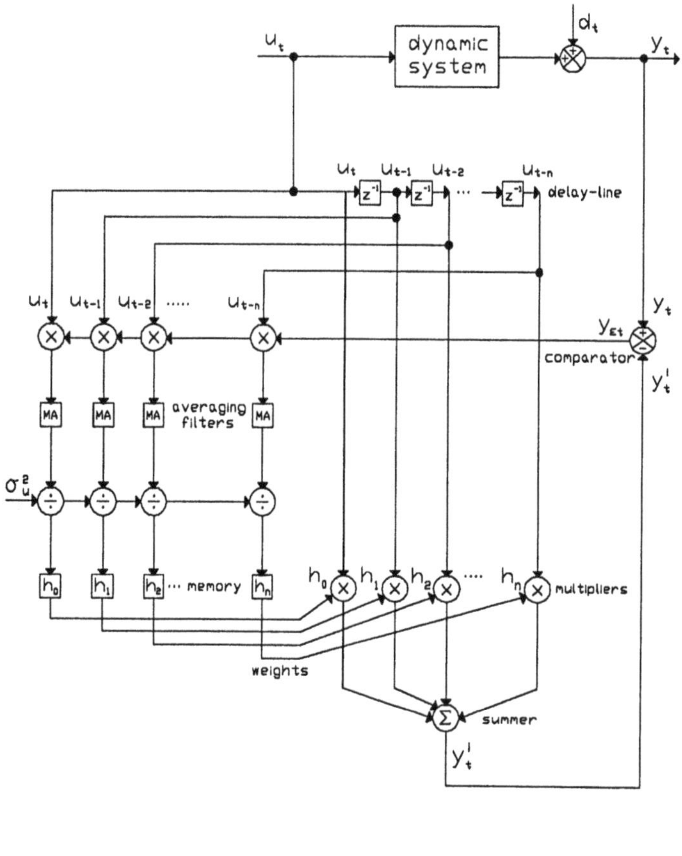

Figure 5. Schematic diagram of adaptive modelling circuitry employing distributed parallel processing to tune the h-weights of a digital filter. Feedback action in the circuit automatically adjusts the h-weights to match the impulse response function weights of the dynamic system. It is assumed here that the input signal u_t is white noise.

Adaptive Model. The digital model in Figure 4 can be incorporated into the adaptive parallel processing circuit shown in Figure 5. This circuit automatically tunes its h-weights to model accurately the input-output relationship of the linear dynamic system. As shown in Figure 5, the input signal u_t is fed to both the dynamic system and to the digital model. The output y_t' from the model is computed as a linear combination of present and past values of the input signal $h_0u_t + h_1u_{t-1} + \ldots + h_nu_{t-n}$ using h-weights retrieved from memory and implemented via an array of multipliers as shown in Figure 5. The output y_t from the dynamic system is compared with the output y_t' from the model in a comparator and the output from the comparator is the discrepancy signal $y_{\varepsilon t}$. If the h-weights exactly match the impulse response function weights of the dynamic system, the discrepancy signal $y_{\varepsilon t}$ at the output of the comparator will be either zero or equal to the disturbance signal d_t added to the output of the dynamic system (the disturbance signal d_t represents all fluctuations in the output signal y_t from the dynamic system not correlated with the input signal u_t). The discrepancy signal $y_{\varepsilon t}$ is fed to a row of multipliers, each of which also receives a delayed input signal u_t, $u_{t-1}, \ldots, u_{t-n}$ from the delay-line. Each multiplier is part of a correlator circuit and many correlator circuits operate independently and in parallel. By smoothing the lagged-product at the output of each multiplier (averaging filters in Figure 5) and normalising by the variance of the input signal (dividers in Figure 5), each correlator computes a regression coefficient between the discrepancy signal $y_{\varepsilon t}$ and its particular delayed input signal. If the h-weights in the model are the same as the impulse response function weights of the dynamic system, the computed regression coefficients will be zero and no correction will be applied to the stored h-weights. On the other hand, if the h-weights do not match the impulse response function weights of the dynamic system, the computed regression coefficients will be exactly the corrections required to increment the stored h-weights and update the model. Thus the circuit maintains an accurate internal model of the impulse response characteristics of the external dynamic system. If the response characteristics of the external system change, the model automatically tunes its h-weights to track such changes.

Temporal Characteristics of Input Signal. The h-weights in Figure 5 converge rapidly to their correct values when the input signal u_t is a sequence of random numbers. Such a random signal is known as a "white noise" signal because it has a flat spectrum analogous to the frequency spectrum of white light. The most important property of a white noise signal is that its value at one point in time is completely uncorrelated with its value at any other point in time. In other words, its autocorrelation function (correlations with lagged values of itself) is zero at all lags and the signal is completely unpredictable. If the input signal in Figure 5 deviates from white noise, however, the rate of convergence of the model h-weights is slower and there are interactions between the weights (i.e., if one weight is detuned from its correct value, it will disturb the other weights). The larger the autocorrelations within the input signal $u_t, u_{t-1}, \ldots, u_{t-n}$, the more poorly conditioned is the numerical computation performed by the adaptive circuit and the slower the convergence of the h-weights to their equilibrium values. The equilibrium values occur when the correlations (regression coefficients) between the discrepancy signal $y_{\varepsilon t}$ and delayed values of the input signal are reduced to zero. These correlations are influenced, however, by the presence of autocorrelations between present and past values of the input signal. Thus, although the model will converge to reduce the mismatch (in a least mean square sense) between y_t and y_t', the h-weights do not match the impulse response function weights of the dynamic system because they also include the influence of the autocorrelations in the input signal. In other words, the h-weights are sensitive not only to the impulse response function weights of the dynamic system but also to the statistical characteristics of temporal variations (stochastic properties) of the input signal.

Stochastic Signal Modelling. The problem described above can be overcome by prefiltering the input signal u_t through an adaptive filter to remove the autocorrelations and transform u_t into a white noise signal a_t. Such a filter is called a "prewhitening filter". As described in detail by Box and Jenkins (1976) and Ljung (1987), a stochastic signal u_t can be represented as a "moving average" of present and past values of a sequence of random (white noise) shocks $a_t, a_{t-1}, \ldots, a_{t-n}$ as in equation (2):

$$u_t = a_t + \theta_1 a_{t-1} + \theta_2 a_{t-2} + \ldots + \theta_n a_{t-n} \tag{2}$$

Apart from the fact that $\theta_0 = 1$, equation (2) has the same form as equation (1) and can be implemented using a parallel adaptive filter circuit similar to that in Figure 5. The circuit has to be rearranged, however, because it must operate in the inverse direction. Given the signal u_t, the adaptive filter must generate the prewhitened signal at its output. Equation (2) can be rearranged to locate a_t on the left hand side as shown in (3):

$$\begin{aligned} a_t &= u_t - [\theta_1 a_{t-1} - \theta_2 a_{t-2} - \ldots - \theta_n a_{t-n}] \\ &= u_t - \hat{u}_{t-1}(1) \end{aligned} \tag{3}$$

The term $\hat{u}_{t-1}(1)$ in (3) can be regarded as a one-step ahead prediction of the value of u_t made at time $t-1$ (the term inside the square bracket in (3) involves only past values $a_{t-1}, a_{t-2}, \ldots, a_{t-n}$). From (3) it can be seen that the white noise signal a_t is the one-step ahead prediction error signal equal to the difference between the actual value of u_t at time t and the prediction $\hat{u}_{t-1}(1)$ of u_t made at time $t-1$.

Adaptive Prewhitening Filter. A parallel processing adaptive filter circuit capable of tuning its θ-weights to prewhiten an input signal u_t into a white noise signal a_t is shown in Figure 6. The circuit is almost exactly the same as that shown in Figure 5 except that only past values $a_{t-1}, a_{t-2}, \ldots, a_{t-n}$ along the delay-line are used in generating the filter output $\hat{u}_{t-1}(1)$ and the input to the delay-line is the one-step ahead prediction error a_t derived from the output of the comparator. The parallel correlators adjust the θ-weights to reduce the correlations between a_t and past values of itself $a_{t-1}, a_{t-2}, \ldots, a_{t-n}$ to zero. In other words, the circuit tunes itself until the one-step ahead prediction errors have zero autocorrelations and hence are themselves unpredictable.

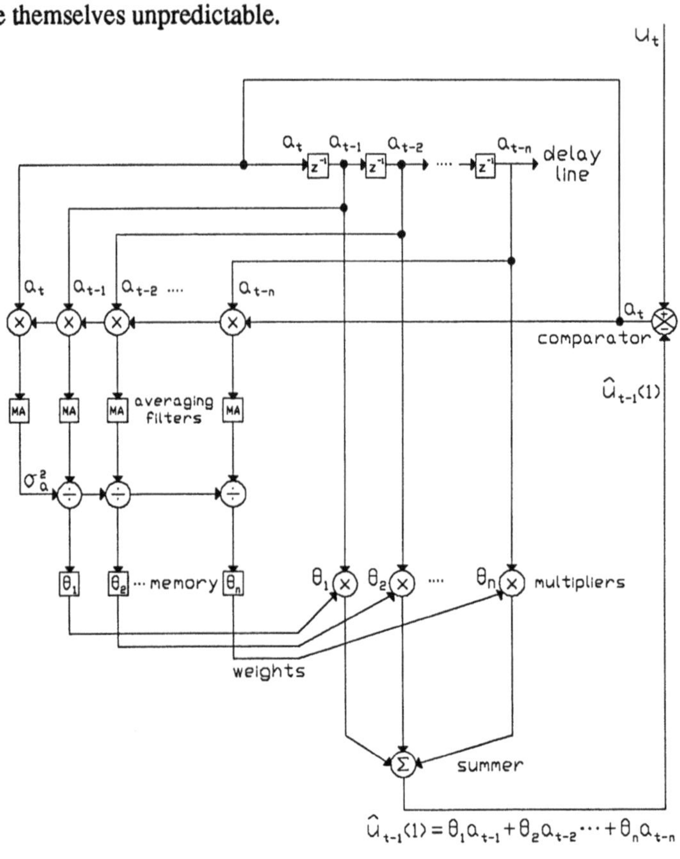

Figure 6. Schematic diagram of an adaptive prewhitening filter employing distributed parallel processing to tune automatically the θ-weights of a moving average digital filter so that the output $\hat{u}_{t-1}(1)$ from the filter represents the best possible one-step ahead prediction of the input signal u_t.

Input Signal Predictor. Best possible predictions can only occur when the prediction errors are themselves unpredictable; that is, when a_t is white noise. Thus, not only does the adaptive filter in Figure 6 automatically tune itself to prewhiten the input signal u_t, but the θ-weights are tuned to exactly the values required to generate the best possible predictions $\hat{u}_t(k)$ of future values of the input signal k steps ahead, as illustrated in equation (4) (see Box & Jenkins (1976) for detailed derivation):

$$\hat{u}_t(k) = \theta_k a_t + \theta_{k+1} a_{t-1} + \ldots + \theta_n a_{t-n+k} \quad (4)$$

The circuit in Figure 6 can be used, therefore, not only as an adaptive prewhitening filter but also to provide the θ-weights required to generate k-step ahead predictions of future values of the input signal.

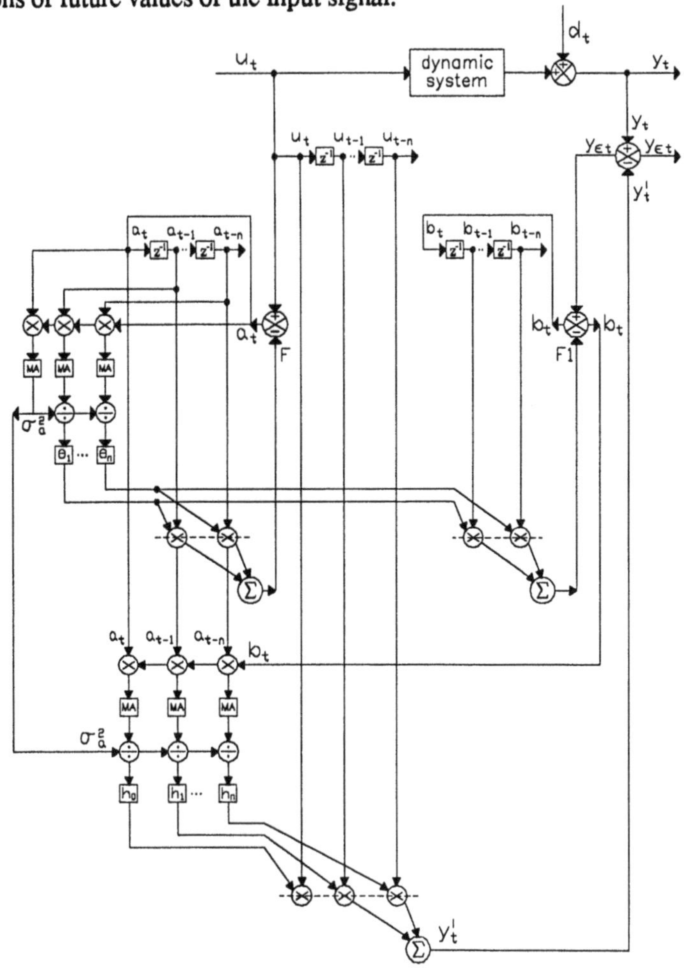

Figure 7. Schematic diagram of adaptive modelling circuitry which combines the circuits in Figures 5 and 6. The circuit prewhitens the input signal u_t and applies the same transformation to the output error signal y_{et}. Parallel cross correlation between the prewhitened input signal a_t and the transformed output error signal b_t automatically updates the h-weights of the digital filter to track the changing impulse response function weights of the dynamic system.

Combined Adaptive Modelling Circuit. The adaptive model circuit in Figure 5 and the adaptive prewhitening filter in Figure 6 can be combined, as shown in Figure 7, to obtain a parallel processing circuit able to compute and adaptively maintain an accurate internal model of the impulse response characteristics of the linear dynamic system and, at the same time, to generate predictions of future values of the input signal. The same prewhitening transformation applied to the input signal u_t to obtain a_t is also applied to the discrepancy signal $y_{\varepsilon t}$ to obtain b_t. Thus the dynamic relationship between a_t and b_t remains the same as that between u_t and $y_{\varepsilon t}$, so the *h*-weights can be updated by computing the regression coefficients between the prewhitened input a_t and the prewhitened discrepancy signal b_t. The circuit has two adaptive models, one converges to the stochastic properties of the input signal and the other converges to the impulse response characteristics of the dynamic system.

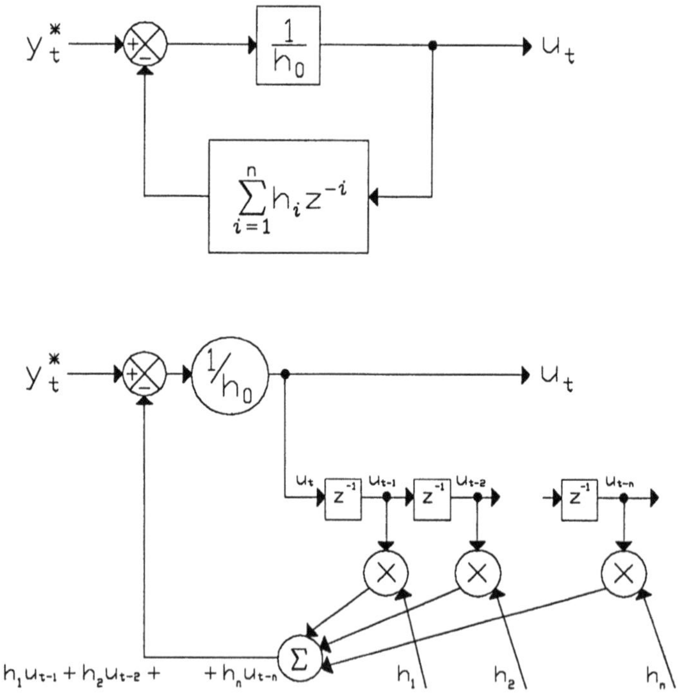

Figure 8. Schematic diagram illustrating the structure of a digital filter model of the inverse dynamic relationship between an input signal u_t and an output signal y_t. Given the impulse response function weights $h_0, h_1, \ldots, h_n$ computed by the circuit in Figure 7, the filter shown here transforms the desired response y_t^* into an appropriate input signal u_t.

Inverse Dynamic Model. Once the *h*-weights describing the impulse response characteristics of a dynamic system have been computed by the adaptive modelling circuitry in Figure 7, they can be employed as shown in Figure 8 to construct an internal model of the *inverse* of the input-output dynamic relationship of the system. That is, given the output signal y_t, the inverse model computes the input signal u_t by implementing equation (5):

$$u_t = [y_t - h_1 u_{t-1} - h_2 u_{t-2} - \ldots - h_n u_{t-n}]/h_0 \qquad (5)$$

Modelling Multiple-Input Systems

Independent Inputs

A parallel expansion of the modelling circuitry described above can be employed to establish internal models of multiple input systems. Consider, for example, the two-input, one-output system illustrated in Figure 9. If the input signals u_{1t} and u_{2t} vary independently of each other (i.e., u_{1t} and u_{2t} are not cross correlated), then the

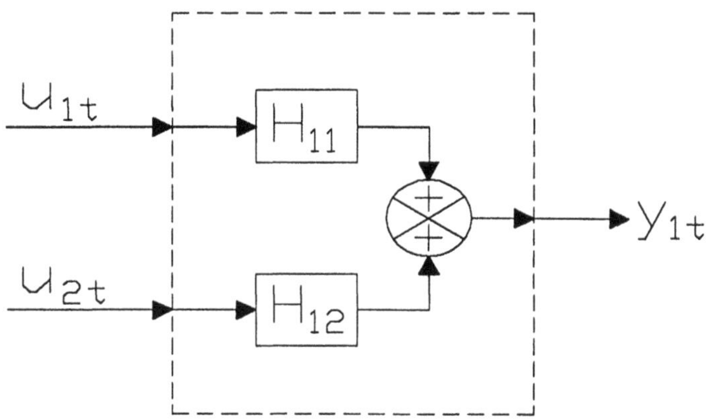

Figure 9. Block diagram illustrating a linear 2-input 1-output system.

impulse response function weights describing the linear dynamic relationships H_{11} and H_{12} in Figure 9 can be estimated independently of each other and in parallel. Each relationship can be computed in parallel using the same adaptive modelling circuitry described above in Figure 7. Providing the two input signals vary independently of each other, the impulse response function weights describing the linear dynamic relationship H_{11} can be computed by cross correlating y_{1t} with u_{1t}

and the relationship H_{12} can be computed in parallel by cross correlating y_{1t} with u_{2t}. Providing multiple input signals vary independently of each other, the input-output characteristics of a multiple input-multiple output system can be computed in parallel by a parallel expansion of the basic circuit shown in Figure 7.

Nonindependent Inputs

Problem of Perfectly Correlated Inputs. A problem occurs in modelling multiple input systems if the input signals do not vary independently of each other. Consider, for example, the two-input system discussed above in Figure 9. Imagine the two inputs u_{1t} and u_{2t} to be perfectly cross correlated with each other. This implies that there exists a dynamic relationship R_{21} between u_{1t} and u_{2t} such that $u_{2t} = R_{21}u_{1t}$ and there are no fluctuations in u_{2t} uncorrelated with fluctuations in u_{1t}. If we proceed with the two-input modelling procedure described above, the cross correlation between y_{1t} and u_{1t} will provide an estimation of the impulse response function weights not of H_{11} but of H_{11} in parallel with $R_{21}H_{12}$. Similarly, the cross correlation between y_{1t} and u_{2t} will not estimate H_{12} but H_{12} in parallel with $R_{21}^{-1}H_{11}$. Because of the perfect cross correlation between u_{1t} and u_{2t}, as far as modelling is concerned the system reduces to a virtual one-input system. It is not possible to identify the relationships H_{11} and H_{12} separately.

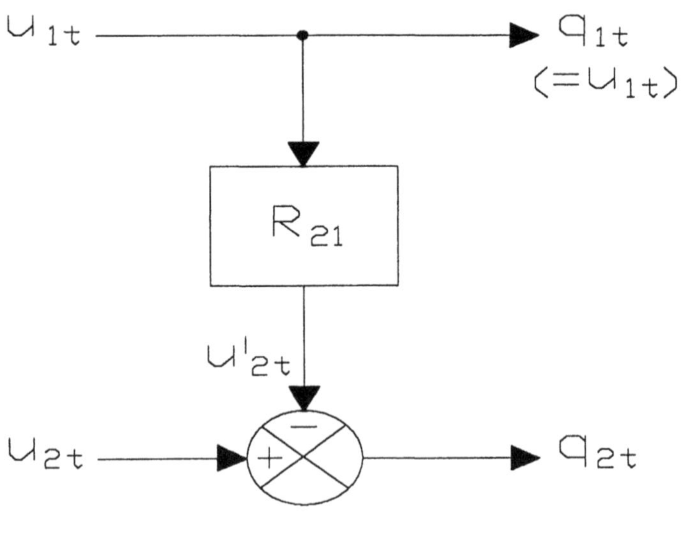

Figure 10. Block diagram showing model of dynamic relationship R_{21} between input signals u_{1t} and u_{2t} in Figure 9. R_{21} is employed to generate orthogonal signals q_{1t} and q_{2t}.

Partially Correlated Inputs. Suppose the two input signals u_{1t} and u_{2t} are correlated with each other but not perfectly; that is, there are fluctuations q_{2t} in u_{2t} not correlated with changes in u_{1t} as well as fluctuations u'_{2t} in u_{2t} that are correlated with u_{1t}. Two signals such as u_{1t} and q_{2t} which are uncorrelated with each other are said to be "orthogonal". As illustrated in Figure 10, the adaptive modelling circuitry of Figure 7 can be employed to establish a model of the linear dynamic relationship R_{21} between u_{1t} and u_{2t}. This model is represented by the block labelled R_{21} in Figure 10. By transforming the input signal u_{1t} through this model, the fluctuations u'_{2t} can be obtained. By subtracting u'_{2t} from u_{2t}, the fluctuations q_{2t} in u_{2t} not cross correlated with u_{1t} can be obtained. Thus the adaptive modelling circuitry of Figure 7 has been employed in Figure 10 to partial out the correlations between u_{1t} and u_{2t} and to obtain the orthogonal signals $q_{1t} = u_{1t}$ and q_{2t}. Once the input signals have been orthogonalised in this manner, the two-input one-output model shown in Figure 11 can be computed using the cross correlation method outlined above for independent inputs. In other words, the basic adaptive modelling circuitry of Figure 7 can be employed in parallel (3 times) to establish a model of a two-input one-output linear dynamic system shown in Figure 11. It is important to notice that the model R_{21} of the dynamic relationship between the inputs u_{1t} and u_{2t} is an essential part of the overall two-input one-output model in Figure 11.

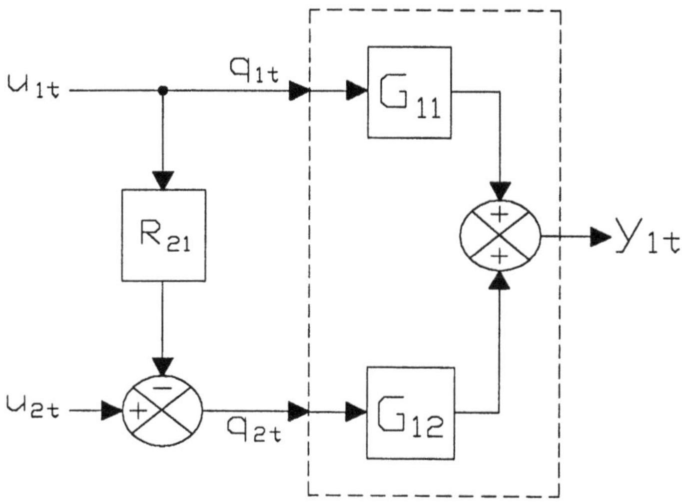

Figure 11. Block diagram showing use of orthogonalising circuit in Figure 10 to produce a model of the 2-input 1-output system shown in Figure 9 when u_{1t} and u_{2t} are partially correlated.

Adaptive Models as Orthogonalising Network. The argument developed above for a two-input one-output system can be generalised to a multiple-input multiple-output system, as illustrated for a four-input two-output system in Figure 12. A network of dynamic models of interrelationships between the input signals, labelled R_{ij} in Figure 12, can be established using a parallel expansion of the basic adaptive modelling circuitry of Figure 7. The partially correlated input signals u_{1t}, u_{2t}, u_{3t}, u_{4t} are passed through this network and a set of orthogonalised signals q_{1t}, q_{2t}, q_{3t}, q_{4t} emerge at the other end. In addition, the prewhitening filters incorporated in Figure 7 produce prewhitened versions of each of the orthogonalised signals. We will refer to this network of adaptive models, therefore, as an "orthogonalising network". The prewhitened, orthogonalised signals produced at the output of the orthogonalising network can be employed to model the multiple-input multiple-output part of the relationship as shown in Figure 12. This method of orthogonalising a set of interrelated signals is well known in signals analysis literature and is known mathematically as Gram-Schmidt orthogonalisation or QR factorisation.

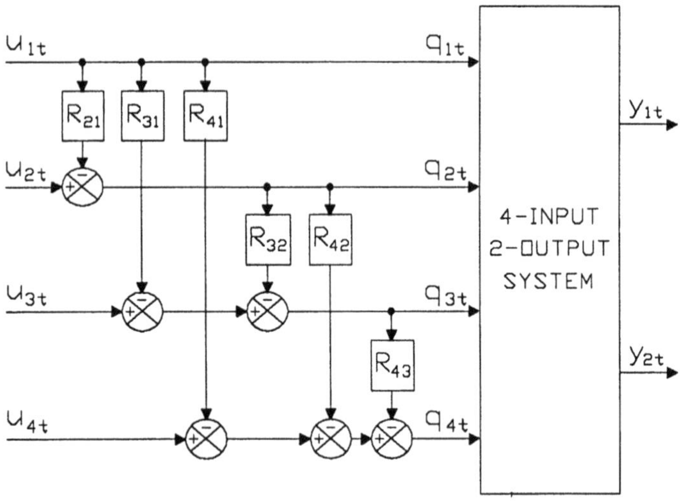

Figure 12. Block diagram showing use of a network of dynamic models R_{ij} to orthogonalise intercorrelated input signals u_{1t}, u_{2t}, u_{3t}, and u_{4t} and hence to compute a model of a 4-input 2-output system.

Degrees of Freedom of Input Signals. The orthogonalising network in Figure 12 can be expanded in parallel to orthogonalise large numbers of input signals, say 20,000. If these signals are highly intercorrelated, the expansion of the adaptive modelling circuitry might not be excessive because most of the orthogonalised signals might be negligible in magnitude. Suppose, for example, that u_{1t} and u_{2t} in Figure 12 are perfectly correlated; thus $q_{2t} = 0$. The models R_{32} and R_{42}, which have q_{2t} as an input, can therefore be eliminated from the network and the number of orthogonalised output signals reduced. This process of reduction could be quite dramatic. The 20,000 highly correlated signals could be reduced to, say, 10 orthogonal signals. Any of the 20,000 signals could be reconstructed using a combination of the 10 orthogonal signals. The 20,000 signals are said to be highly redundant and to have only 10 degrees of freedom.

Vector Analogy for Orthogonalisation of Signals. Using a vector analogy for the signals, 20,000 vectors are contained within a 10-dimensional vector space. The 10 orthogonalised signals span the vector space and represent an orthogonal coordinate system for that space. As far as modelling is concerned, the multiple-input multiple-output part of the model is reduced to a virtual 10-input system.

Inverse Orthogonalisation. An important property of the orthogonalising network in Figure 12 is the ability to reverse the direction of flow through the network. By reversing the direction of the arrows and changing minus signs to plus signs in the comparators in Figure 12, the models R_{ij} can be used to transform the orthogonalised signals q_{jt} back into the highly intercorrelated signals u_{it}.

Modelling of Nonlinear Multivariable Dynamic Systems

Using the Volterra-Wiener approach to nonlinear systems described by Marmarelis and Marmarelis (1978) and Marmarelis (1989), and employing higher order cross correlation functions to compute Wiener kernels (Lee & Schetzen, 1965) rather than impulse response function weights, it can be shown that a multivariable nonlinear dynamic system can be modelled using a parallel expansion of the basic modelling circuitry in Figure 7. Just as the output of a linear dynamic system can be expressed as a linear combination of present and past values of the input signal with coefficients known as impulse response function weights, the output from a nonlinear system can be expressed as a *linear* combination of every possible combination of products of present and past values of input signals as illustrated for a one input system in equation (6):

$$\begin{aligned} y_t = \; & h_0 u_t + h_1 u_{t-1} + \;.\;\;.\;\;.\; + h_n u_{t-n} \\ & + h_{00} u_t u_t + h_{01} u_t u_{t-1} + \;.\;\;.\;\;.\; + h_{0n} u_t u_{t-n} \\ & + h_{11} u_{t-1} u_{t-1} + \;.\;\;.\;\;.\; + h_{1n} u_{t-1} u_{t-n} \\ & + h_{21} u_{t-2} u_{t-2} + \;.\;\;.\;\;. \\ & + \;.\;\;.\;\;. \\ & + \;.\;\;. \\ & + h_{nn} u_{t-n} u_{t-n} \\ & + \text{higher order terms} \end{aligned} \tag{6}$$

The h_{ij} coefficients are known as Wiener kernels and can be computed using linear regression between the output signal y_t and the product signals $u_{t-i}u_{t-j}$, i & $j = 1, 2, \ldots, n$. This argument can be extended to higher order terms in the Volterra-Wiener series and to cross-kernel terms required to describe nonlinear interactions between different inputs in a multi-input system. Thus, apart from needing an array of multipliers to compute the products $u_{t-i}u_{t-j}$, the Wiener kernels describing the dynamics of a multivariable nonlinear system can be estimated using a parallel expansion of the basic adaptive modelling circuitry in Figure 7.

Adaptive Control System Simulation

Using the parallel computational circuits described above, we have constructed a computer simulation of an adaptive optimum control system which can control any single-input single-output linear dynamic system causing its output (or response) to track an externally applied target signal. This is achieved in the presence of a disturbance signal added to the output of the controlled system. Three computational systems are involved which operate independently and in parallel. These systems communicate through independent read and write memory buffers. The first and third systems are comprised entirely of the distributed parallel processing circuitry described above. They operate continuously and in real-time.

The first system processes the externally applied target signal as well as feedback signals from the input and output of the controlled system. It adaptively maintains accurate internal models of the stochastic variations of the signals and of the input-output relationship of the controlled system. The *h*-weights or parameters of these models are stored in memory. Using the models, the first system also generates predictions of future values of target, response, and disturbance signals and stores them in memory.

The second system introduces intermittency into control behaviour because it requires a pre-specified interval of time to (a) read from memory the predicted trajectories of target, response, and disturbance signals computed by system one, (b) preplan a standard S-shaped desired output trajectory to move the output from its predicted path into alignment with the predicted future motion of the target and (c) to store the preplanned trajectory in memory ready for execution in real-time by the third system. Because that execution takes much longer than the time taken to plan it, only the early part of the trajectory will have been executed by the time the second stage has an updated response plan ready.

The third system operates in real-time. It reads the preplanned trajectory of desired output from memory and transforms it through an internal model (computed by the first system) of the inverse dynamics of the controlled system. A signal is thus generated at the output of the inverse model which, when applied to the input of the controlled system, causes its output to match the desired response.

We regard this simulation as a computer model of the human operator performing a tracking task. The responses it generates simulate the behaviour of human subjects performing the same task (Neilson, Neilson, & O'Dwyer, 1988; Neilson, O'Dwyer, & Neilson, 1988). We will go on to equate these three parallel computing systems with the SA, RP, and RE information processing stages basic to AMT. Prior to that we examine the more fundamental proposition that the CNS has the necessary distributed parallel processing neural circuitry to implement the adaptive modelling circuitry described above.

ADAPTIVE MODELLING IN SENSORIMOTOR CONTROL

Neural Implementation of Adaptive Modelling Circuitry

The basic uniformity in the intrinsic structure of the neocortex across different cortical areas (Powell, 1981) lends itself to the implementation of distributed parallel processing, as does the functional organisation of the cortex into a columnar arrangement. Indeed, as we will now show, by regarding the cortical column as a basic computational module and by considering the connectivity of cortical and subcortical structures, a possible neural implementation of the processes described in the preceding section can be suggested, consistent with known neuroanatomy and neurophysiology.

Thalamo-Cortical and Cortico-Cortical Connections

Anatomical techniques based on axon transport staining methods have revealed a rod to column organisation in thalamo-cortical pathways. Rod-like aggregations of cells in the thalamus running horizontally from front to back and cutting across many of the anatomically identified thalamic nuclear regions, project fibres to vertical columns of cells in the cortex. Cortical columns are about 300 μm in diameter and contain about 4000 neurons (Eccles, 1984). Each column receiving excitatory input from the thalamus makes reciprocal excitatory connections back to the same rod in the thalamus (Darian-Smith, Darian-Smith, & Cheema, 1990; Jones, 1985). Goldberg (1985) has suggested that each of these excitatory cortico-thalamo-cortical loops can be viewed as giving rise to an oscillatory limit cycle process. The flow of subcortical information through to the cortex could be controlled, therefore, by modulation of the oscillation at both the thalamic and cortical ends of the loop.

Double staining techniques in the cortex have revealed a similar columnar organisation in cortico-cortical connections. Vertical columns of cells in the prefrontal and parietal regions, for example, not only have reciprocal connections with each other, but share mutual reciprocal connections with at least 15 other columns widely separated throughout the cortex (Goldman-Rakic, 1987). This suggests the existence of networks of columns distributed throughout the cortex.

Cortical Columns

Structure of Cortical Columns. The human cortex has a six layer structure. There are about 20,000 neurons/mm^3 and about 60-70% of these are pyramidal cells which send axons either to other cortical columns (cortico-cortical connections) or to subcortical centres such as basal ganglia, thalamus, brainstem, or spinal cord. Pyramidal cells also have collaterals which make synaptic contact with neighbouring cortical cells in all six layers. Indeed, it has been estimated that the number of intrinsic synaptic connections outnumber the extrinsic connections by as many as 100:1. This indicates there is a massive amount of intrinsic local interconnection between neurons in all six layers of the cortex.

Underdamped Impulse Response of Cortical Columns. As described by von Seelen, Mallot, Krone, and Dinse (1986) and by Braitenberg (1986) and others, local interconnectivity creates multiple excitatory and inhibitory feedback pathways between cells in all six layers of the cortex. As a consequence, a common response to a discrete stimulus delivered to layer IV for example, consists of a lightly damped 20 Hz oscillation of activity in a large numbers of neurons above and below the site of stimulation. These oscillations have been demonstrated in computer models of cortical circuitry (see von Seelen et al., 1986) and in post-stimulus histograms of actual recordings from cortical units in cats and monkeys (see von Seelen et al., 1986; Shaw & Silverman, 1988). The waves of cortical activity excited by a discrete stimulus can be likened to the concentric ripples which spread out from the point of impact of a raindrop on a puddle. Unlike ripples on a puddle, however, the oscillatory activity does not propagate very well horizontally through the cortex and is more or less confined to a vertical minicolumn of cells about 100-200 μm wide.

Code for Cortical Processing. As argued cogently by Shaw and Silverman (1988), the bursting response of hundreds of neurons in each layer of a cortical column to a discrete stimulus applied to layer IV suggests that the single neuron is not the appropriate unit to examine in attempting to decode higher cortical processing; the output of a single cortical neuron cannot fire another. They propose that the burst response of 50-100 neurons in each layer of a minicolumn defines an appropriate temporal and spatial separation for recording cortical signals. For such recording they suggest employing an array of say, 7x7 electrodes with about 100 μm spacing between electrodes, the activity from each electrode being summed over 50 ms time intervals (for background see Shaw & Silverman, 1988).

Cortical Delay-Lines. Lightly damped 20 Hz bursts of activity observed in cortical columns could provide a mechanism for a type of short-term memory based on reverberation. Since a discrete stimulus applied to a column causes bursts of activity of neurons in each layer at 50 ms intervals, it follows that the column could function as a short duration (50 ms) sample-and-hold memory unit. When an input (burst of activity from another column for example) excites a cortical column, it evokes an impulse response with a lightly damped 20 Hz oscillation. Consequently, repeat bursts of activity at 50 ms intervals are communicated to neighbouring columns, thereby introducing 50 ms time delays into the system. It does not seem unreasonable to suggest that 30 or more such units might be connected in series to function as a "cortical delay-line" requiring about 1.5 s for bursts of neuronal activity to pass along the line.

Basal Ganglia and Cerebellar Side-Loops

Many cortico-cortical pathways have parallel side-loops through parts of either the cerebellum or basal ganglia. Subcortical loops project from all over the cortex to the caudate and from sensorimotor cortex to the putamen, thence to globus pallidus and back to supplementary motor area (SMA) and premotor areas of the cortex via ventro-anterior nuclei in the thalamus (DeLong & Georgopoulos, 1981; DeLong, Georgopoulos, & Crutcher, 1983). Large numbers of fibres (30×10^6) descend from sensorimotor cortex through the internal capsule and cerebral peduncles to the pontine nuclei and inferior olive in the brainstem. This represents about 3/4 of the descending white matter from the cortex. Millions of mossy fibres (120×10^6) originating in pontine nuclei enter the cerebellum through the middle cerebellar peduncles. About 2×10^6 climbing fibres from cells in the inferior olive enter the cerebellum via the inferior cerebellar peduncles. Output fibres from the cerebellum connect to centres in the brainstem and tegmentum - such as vestibular nuclei, reticular formation and red nucleus at the heads of descending tracts into the spinal cord. About 1.6×10^6 fibres return from the cerebellum via the superior cerebellar peduncles to nucleus X and ventro-lateral nuclei in the thalamus which in turn project to the premotor and motor cortex respectively, thereby completing a cortico-cerebellar-thalamo-cortical loop. We propose that subcortical loops through parts of the basal ganglia and cerebellum function as adaptive internal models of multivariable dynamic relationships between sensory and motor neural signals. Because little is known about the detailed neuronal circuitry of the basal ganglia relative to knowledge about the anatomy and physiology of the cerebellum, we focus our discussion on the cerebellum. This information is based largely on Ito (1984) but see also Llinas (1981), Brooks and Thach (1981), Bloedel, Dichgans, and Precht (1985).

Anatomy of the Cerebellum

Purkinje Cells. The only output fibres from the cerebellar cortex are axons of Purkinje cells which converge on to target cells in deep cerebellar nuclei. Purkinje cells are large cells which lie in a single layer about 400 µm beneath the highly convoluted surface of the cerebellar cortex. There are about 30 million Purkinje cells in the cerebellum and they have a density of about 400/mm^2. Each Purkinje cell has an extensive dendritic tree which extends up into the 400 μm thick molecular layer at the surface of the cerebellar cortex. The dendritic trees are flattened into the plane running across the folia and extend for about 400 μm in this direction. Beneath the Purkinje cell layer there is a thick dark band known as the granular layer. Small granule cells forming this dark band in the cerebellum are probably the most densely packed neurons in the CNS. It has been estimated that there are about 40-50 billion of them.

Mossy Fibres. As mentioned above, there are two types of input fibres to the cerebellar cortex, mossy fibres and climbing fibres. Many millions of mossy fibres enter the cerebellum and each one makes complex synaptic connections with about 400 granule cells. Mossy fibres also make excitatory connections with cells in the deep cerebellar nuclei. The axon of each granule cell passes up through the Purkinje cell layer into the molecular layer at the surface of the cerebellar cortex. Once in the molecular layer the axon divides in a T-junction and runs for several millimeters in both directions parallel to the long axis of the folium. These closely packed billions of fibres are known as "parallel fibres". In running along this course, each parallel fibre passes through and makes excitatory synaptic contacts with the flattened dendritic trees of hundreds of Purkinje cells lying in a line along the long axis of the folium, like telephone wires stringing along telegraph poles. The dendritic tree of each Purkinje cell receives excitatory synaptic inputs from 100,000-200,000 parallel fibres. Thus 50-100 fibres descending from the cortex to the pontine nuclei communicate with single Purkinje cells via about 200 mossy fibres and 100,000 to 200,000 granule cells and parallel fibres. Continuous high frequency activity is recorded in these pathways.

Climbing Fibres. In contrast with the massive divergence and convergence in the mossy fibre system, climbing fibres from the inferior olive, entering the cerebellum through the inferior cerebellar peduncle, make one to one connections with individual Purkinje cells. Each fibre divides in the deep white matter of the cerebellum and sends branches into different folia in remote parts of the cerebellar cortex. At the level of the Purkinje cell layer, each branch loses its myelin sheath and forms fine tendrils which wind about the lower 2/3 of the dendritic tree of a single Purkinje cell forming multiple (400 or more) excitatory synaptic connections with it. Climbing fibres discharge at only a very low rate of about 2-10/s, but a single burst discharge in a climbing fibre has a powerful influence on the single Purkinje cell it innervates. Not only does it cause a complex multiple-spike discharge of the Purkinje cell, but it opens calcium ion gates and causes a long-term alteration in the sensitivity of the Purkinje cell to its parallel fibre synaptic input (Bloedel & Ebner, 1985; Ito, 1984; Rawson & Tilokskulchai, 1982). In other words, activity in climbing fibres can cause short-term alterations of the gains of the Purkinje cells to their parallel fibre synaptic input.

Microzone Circuit. The basic circuit of the cerebellum is thought to be the "microzone circuit" which consists of a line of Purkinje cells lying across the folium at right angles to the parallel fibres. The axons of Purkinje cells in a microzone converge on to common target cells in a deep cerebellar nucleus. Each Purkinje cell axon has an inhibitory influence on about 35 target cells while each target cell receives an inhibitory convergent input from about 900 Purkinje cells. This creates the basic cortico-nuclear complex of the cerebellum.

The Microzone Circuit as an Adaptive Model

Output signals from microzone target cells in deep cerebellar nuclei consist of weighted combinations of signals delivered to Purkinje cells in microzone circuits via mossy fibres and parallel fibres. The weights correspond to the gains of the Purkinje cells and are set by climbing fibre input. As pointed out by Fujita (1982), each microzone circuit has appropriate connectivity to function as an adaptive filter. Therefore, if the parallel fibre input signals to a microzone circuit were derived from a cortical delay line, the resulting cortico-cerebellar circuit would be identical to the adaptive modelling circuit in Figure 4 with the microzone circuit functioning as the linear combiner and the h-weights being set as gains of Purkinje cells via descending control through the inferior olive and climbing fibre input.

Cerebellar Model of a Multivariable System

The fact that parallel fibres make synaptic contacts with multiple microzone circuits lying at right angles across the parallel fibres gives the cerebellar cortex exactly the circuitry required to function as an adaptive model of a multiple-input multiple-output dynamic system. Multiple input signals are applied through beams of parallel fibres to multiple microzone circuits. The gains of the Purkinje cells in each microzone circuit are set individually by climbing fibre inputs. The outputs from each microzone circuit converge to a cluster of target cells in the cerebellar nucleus and are then relayed to the rest of the CNS. Thus the cerebellum has exactly the structure required to function as an adaptive model of a multiple-input multiple-output system. The discrepancy between the large number of mossy fibres entering the cerebellum and the relatively small number of fibres returning from the cerebellum is also consistent with adaptive modelling circuitry. It is particularly true for models of nonlinear systems which not only require present and past values of each input signal but also require products of combinations of present and past values of input signals to be directed to microzone circuits.

The Processing Stages of the Basic Unit of Motor Production

The sequential operation of SA, RP, and RE processes in the performance of a BUMP implies a flow of information through the CNS. We argued earlier that each of these processing stages operates independently and in parallel and this is consistent with their being physically located in separate parts of the CNS. We now extend our discussion of cortico-cortical and cortico-subcortical connectivity in developing a fuller picture of the possible roles of the computational processes we see as comprising the SA, RP, and RE information processing stages. For convenience we have couched much of the following description didactically rather than hypothetically and the section should therefore be read with that in mind.

Sensory Analysis

The sensory analysers occupy the posterior part of the brain in occipital, temporal and parietal lobes. Processing of sensory signals occurs continuously and in real-time with central events correlated in time with events at the periphery. Hundreds of millions of sensory receptors throughout the body encode stimuli into pulse frequency modulated trains of nerve impulses. These signals converge through specialised neural networks such as those in the spinal cord, cochlea and retina. These networks extract sensory feature signals by behaving like arrays of temporo-spatial filters. Although many of these sensory signals are employed by local reflex circuits, most if not all are communicated via the thalamus to primary projection regions in the posterior cortex.

Redundancy in Sensory Signals. Despite the convergence of sensory signals through specialised neural networks and the extraction of sensory feature signals by temporo-spatial filtering, many tens of thousands of sensory signals must enter cortical columns in the primary sensory projection regions of the cortex. There is almost certainly a high level of redundancy in these signals, however, as can be appreciated by considering the number of sensory channels involved in communicating a single degree of freedom of movement, such as rotation about the elbow, to the cortex. Such redundancy greatly improves the reliability of information transmission from receptors to cortex but would greatly increase the central workload if each signal were to be analysed separately as if it contained exclusive information.

Orthogonalisation of Sensory Signals. Sensory analysers can remove redundancy from sensory signals using an orthogonalising network of adaptive modelling circuits similar to that shown in Figure 12 to extract a set of orthogonal sensory feature signals. Since these signals vary independently, each orthogonal signal encodes unique information and together, the orthogonalised signals encode all the information encoded by the input signals. The number of non-zero orthogonal signals equals the number of degrees of freedom contained by the original set of intercorrelated input signals. This number is the minimum number of signals required to encode the input information and for highly intercorrelated input signals it may, as discussed above, be considerably less than the number of input signals.

Multivariable Modelling and Synergy Generator. Not only does an adaptive orthogonalising network remove redundancy and produce an efficient high level encoding of sensory information but, as shown above, orthogonalisation is necessary if the nervous system is to compute adaptive models of multivariable systems. Moreover, the orthogonalising network can operate in the reverse direction to transform any set of orthogonalised input signals back into a larger number of intercorrelated output signals. This is exactly what is required for the formation of "coordinative structures" or "functional synergies". Thus the orthogonalising network can function in reverse as a synergy generator and can provide essential information required for coordinating multiple muscles and controlling highly redundant movements of the human body.

Prediction of Sensory Signals. There are two types of time delays that affect human movement and need to be compensated. The first is due to inertial lag in the biomechanical system and can be compensated by introduction of inverse dynamics. A phase lag in the controlled system is compensated by a corresponding phase lead introduced by the inverse model. The second type of time delay is not so easily compensated. It is caused by pure time delay (transmission time and central planning time) in the system. The only way a backward-shift in time can be compensated is by the introduction of a corresponding forward-shift. A filter or neural circuit able to introduce such a forward-shift in time is, however, physically unrealisable because it requires the circuit to respond before the stimulus is applied. The best that can be done is to construct a predictor that generates an estimate of the most probable future value of the input based on a statistical analysis of its past variations. This is exactly the computation performed within the adaptive modelling circuitry described. Using the prewhitening filters in the adaptive modelling circuitry, the SA-stage generates predictions of future values of the orthogonalised sensory feature signals.

Separation of Reafference and Exafference. In an influential paper concerned with the optokinetic reaction, Von Holst and Mittelstaedt (1950/1973) stressed the importance of the ability of the CNS to separate sensory signals (afference) into (a) feedback signals produced by the body's own motor actions (reafference) and (b) signals generated by external inputs (exafference). A similar idea was proposed by Sperry (1950) who argued that outgoing motor commands evoke activity (corollary discharge) in sensory parts of the brain which correspond to the expected sensory consequences of the motor commands. Formation of adaptive models by the SA-stage provides a mechanism which accounts for both these proposals. As well as being signalled to muscles, copies of outgoing motor commands are transformed in real time via internal models into expected reafference signals. Comparison between afference and expected reafference provides a measure of the external disturbances or exafference. This separation of afference into reafference and exafference is part of the modelling circuitry illustrated in Figure 7 and is vitally important in the formation of adaptive models and in compensating for external disturbances.

Response Planning

Response planning is most likely performed by the frontal lobes of the brain. These regions have tight reciprocal coupling with columns of cells in the parietal and temporal regions and consequently have access to the sensory feature signals at the output of the SA-stage. The orbitofrontal cortex receives a major projection from the mediodorsal thalamic nucleus which plays a role in emotional functions (LeDoux, 1987). The prefrontal cortex projects to the mesencephalic reticular formation involved in control of arousal and to the thalamic reticular nucleus which controls selective attention by gating sensory input to the cortex (Watson, Valenstein, & Heilman, 1981). The prefrontal cortex connects in a loop through the limbic system via the cingulate cortex, hippocampus, mediodorsal nucleus of thalamus and back to prefrontal cortex. This loop is involved in the storage and retrieval of information in long-term memory (Kornhuber, 1973).

Prefrontal Cortex and Planning for the Future. The role of the prefrontal cortex suggested by the above anatomical connections is consistent with the observed behaviour of monkeys and humans with prefrontal cortex injury. Monkeys with prefrontal cortex removed can move about and feed themselves. Similarly, the movement control of human patients with prefrontal damage appears intact. This is consistent with the fact that the prefrontal cortex has no direct anatomical connections with the motor system. When tested on a delayed response task requiring memory of more than a few seconds, however, behaviour is greatly impaired (see Goldman-Rakic, 1987). Patients with frontal lobe lesions undergo a change of personality, have fluctuating moods and seem unable to control emotions and level of arousal. They are hyperactive and easily distracted, switching attention from one stimulus to another. They are unable to plan for the future. If sent to the corner shop to buy a sandwich, for example, they are likely to become confused and forget what they are doing. As argued by Goldman-Rakic, the prefrontal cortex seems to be required whenever behaviour is guided by concepts and plans stored in long-term memory rather than by sensory input directly.

Hierarchical Structure of Goals. In line with the above, we propose that response planning is performed by the prefrontal cortex using long-term memory to establish hierarchical structures of goals, each goal leading to the next. For example, to obtain qualification some years from now a student may plan to pass an exam at the end of the year, attend today's lecture, drive to college, reverse the car out of the driveway, start the engine, place the key in the ignition and so on. In getting out of a chair to walk across the room and switch on a light, the very first movement of getting out of the chair may be already directed towards the long-term goal of switching on the light. This is consistent with the hierarchy of cortical processing performed by the frontal lobes described by Fuster (1985).

Preplanning a Desired Response. At the level of the most immediate subgoal the RP-stage requires a finite interval of time to preplan a desired response to achieve the goal and to store it in short-term memory ready for execution by the RE-stage. The time required to preplan a desired response is typically 100-200 ms but this time can expand or contract depending on the current mental workload. The response is preplanned as a trajectory of desired perceptual consequences in terms of the same high level orthogonalised sensory feature signals in which feedback from the movement will eventually be encoded by the SA-stage. Central images of intended and actual movements are thus encoded in the same high level sensory feature code and can be compared directly, thus obviating the sensory versus motor language problem discussed by Schmidt (1976).

Intermittency in Movement Control. The RP-stage preplans only one response at a time and does not commence planning a second response until it has completed planning the first. This is an important aspect of AMT because, as discussed earlier, it introduces intermittency into control of movement. Unlike most other systems theory oriented accounts of sensorimotor performance, AMT offers direct links with the behavioural literature concerning variable allocation of capacity, economy of processing resources, and mental workload (e.g., Hancock & Meshkati, 1988; McLeod, 1977; Moray, 1979; Navon & Gopher, 1979). We emphasise that the notion of preplanning one response at a time should not be interpreted as a single channel theory (Welford, 1980) since AMT conceptualises response planning as involving a number of independently varying desired sensory feature signals planned independently and in parallel. As discussed previously, the number of orthogonalised desired sensory feature signals will equal the number of degrees of freedom of movement in the desired response.

Graphical Illustration of Response Planning. In Figure 13 we illustrate graphically the processes involved in preplanning a desired response trajectory. Similar processing is required for each desired sensory feature signal but since these signals are orthogonal, each can be planned independently and in parallel. In Figure 13 time is represented along the horizontal axis and the magnitude of the sensory feature signal is plotted on the vertical axis. The time axis is divided into segments of duration T_p, being the time required for the RP-stage to preplan a desired response trajectory. This time can expand or contract from response to response depending on mental workload. The time intervals associated with SA, RP, and RE processing for the particular response being considered are designated respectively by crosses, a rectangular box, and zigzags.

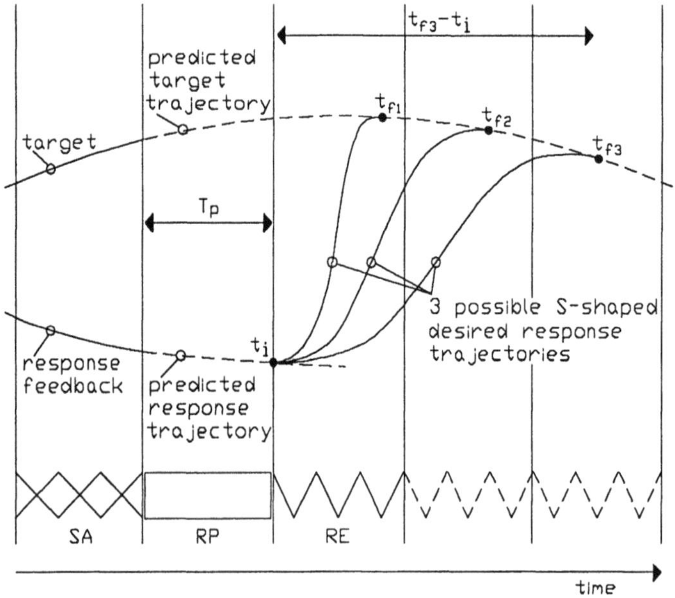

Figure 13. Graphical illustration of three possible S-shaped desired response trajectories R^* with different durations which could be preplanned by the RP-stage during a single planning interval T_p to move the response cursor from its predicted path into alignment with the predicted motion of the target.

Consider the processing performed by the RP-stage during a single planning time interval marked by the rectangular box. Motivated by a hierarchical structure of goals, the RP-stage produces a target trajectory of the desired sensory feature signal. In the case of speech, or hand writing, or other self-paced tasks, the target trajectory could be a template waveform retrieved from long-term memory and scaled in both time and magnitude to suit the task. The concept of template waveforms has been used in discussing why, for example, some features of hand writing trajectories remain invariant despite tenfold changes in writing speed (Viviani & Terzuolo, 1983). In tasks requiring coordination with a moving environment, such as catching a ball, the target trajectory will be based on a prediction of future values of sensory feature signals derived from sensory input. In a pursuit tracking task (Figure 13) the target trajectory is formed as a prediction of the future motion of the target on the screen.

By reading information from the output of the sensory analysers, the RP-stage has access to the most recent values of response feedback. The RP-stage generates a predicted response trajectory to take into account any preplanned movement already in the pipeline, so to speak, (i.e., any movement currently being executed by the RE-stage in parallel with the response planning). The predicted response can easily be computed by aligning the previously planned response trajectory with the most recently available response feedback. This effectively incorporates an intermittent feedback error correction (one correction per planning interval) for deviations between intended response and feedback of the actual response. Thus, as observed in compensatory tracking, the system functions as an intermittent feedback control system with a reaction time delay in the loop.

S-Shaped Desired Response Trajectory. Once the predicted response trajectory has been computed, the RP-stage must preplan a desired response trajectory to move the response from its predicted pathway into alignment with the predicted trajectory of the target. The S-shaped trajectories and velocity triangles often observed in kinematic data during ballistic movements, discrete responses and tracking data suggest that the desired response trajectory might consist of a standard S-shaped curve. This could involve a stereotyped computation to generate an S-shaped desired response trajectory having continuity in both position and slope at the junctions with the predicted response and the predicted target waveforms, as illustrated in Figure 13.

Variable Duration of S-Curve. The initial and final times for the S-shaped curve, t_i and t_f in Figure 13, must be specified by the RP-stage. This allows a variety of different movement strategies to be employed depending on the duration of the preplanned S-curve. It is well known that fast human movements have a fixed duration independent of the amplitude of the movement (up to intermediate amplitude at least). This is the so-called isochrony principle (Viviani & Terzuolo, 1982). The duration of a fast movement is typically about 100 ms and is thought to be limited by the duration of the biphasic EMG bursts observed in agonist and antagonist muscles during fast ballistic movements (Freund, 1983). The first burst accelerates the limb and the second burst decelerates the limb, causing it to move along a more or less S-shaped trajectory. For a fast ballistic movement the entire S-shaped curve must be executed in an open-loop mode because there is insufficient time for intermittent feedback error correction.

There is no limit, however, on the maximum duration of the S-shaped curve. As the duration of the movement is increased the accuracy of final placement improves because there is time for multiple intermittent feedback error corrections. This illustrates a type of speed-accuracy tradeoff described by Fitts' law. Final position accuracy is achieved, however, at the expense of introducing a low-pass filter between the target trajectory and the desired response trajectory (Neilson, Neilson, & O'Dwyer, 1988). As the duration of the S-shaped curve is increased the subject is unable to follow fast changes in target position.

Speed-Accuracy Tradeoff. Increasing the duration of the S-shaped curve is a strategy often adopted by people who are unskilled at a task or who have a neurological deficit which affects the accuracy of purposive movement. The slower the movement the smaller the execution error and the more time for intermittent feedback error correction. Such improved control can only be achieved, however, at the expense of high speed performance. In alien tasks, such as mirror drawing, subjects often experience a degree of compulsiveness in the readily demonstrated slowing, repetition, and blocking of hand movements. They may also report feeling as though they do not own or control their own movement (Smith & Smith, 1962).

Optimum Control Strategy. Changing the duration of the S-shaped curve is equivalent to selecting a different compromise in a speed-accuracy-effort tradeoff. The shorter the duration of the S-curve the smaller the area between the target trajectory and the desired response trajectory (Figure 13) and so the greater the accuracy (in the least mean square sense) of the movement. On the other hand, a large muscular effort is required for rapid acceleration of the desired response, so accuracy is achieved only at the cost of increased energy expenditure. Varying the speed-accuracy-effort compromise by altering the duration of the S-curve is equivalent, therefore, to altering the cost function in an adaptive optimum controller.

Response Execution

Recordings of neural activity in the basal ganglia, cerebellum, premotor cortex, motor cortex, and descending pathways reveal time-locked correlations with motor events at the periphery. This indicates that, like the SA-stage, the RE-stage operates continuously and in real-time.

Basal Ganglia Side-Loops. There is now considerable evidence that side-loops through parts of the basal ganglia are involved in control of movement. Based on a review of the neuroanatomical connections of the basal ganglia (DeLong & Georgopoulos, 1981), it has been argued that a topographically organised loop concerned with motor control passes from the sensory motor cortex to the putamen, to the ventral two-thirds of the globus pallidus, then to the nucleus ventralis lateralis pars oralis (VLo) in the thalamus and back to area 6 of the cortex (DeLong, Georgopoulos, & Crutcher, 1983). The somatotopic motor representation present in this loop suggest that there exist segregated pathways through the basal ganglia for the control of movement of different body parts

(DeLong et al., 1983). Alexander, DeLong, and Strick (1986) describe a "motor" circuit through the basal ganglia comprised of somatotopically organised influences arising from the SMA, the arcuate premotor area, the motor cortex, and the somatosensory cortex which are transmitted largely to the putamen, thence to the internal segment of the globus pallidus, to VLo and back to the SMA. In contrast, the caudate nucleus receives projections from all over the cortex. Signals from widely dispersed areas are funnelled through the caudate nucleus, globus pallidus, and ventro-anterior nuclei of the thalamus to the SMA and premotor cortex (Schneider & Lidsky, 1987).

Neurophysiological evidence for the predominant motor function of segregated side-loops through the basal ganglia comes from the relationship of the discharge of basal ganglia neurons with specific aspects of limb movements in monkeys (Allum, Anner-Baratti, & Hepp-Reymond, 1983; Crutcher & DeLong, 1984; DeLong, 1971, 1973; DeLong & Strick, 1974; DeLong & Georgopoulos, 1979, 1981; DeLong et al., 1983; Liles, 1985). The discharge of basal ganglia neurons was found to be related predominantly to the direction, amplitude, and force of movement rather than to the activity of individual muscles. Based on this evidence it has been suggested that the basal ganglia play a role in the integration of information from a variety of cortical areas and in the determination of specific parameters of movement, such as direction, amplitude, or velocity (DeLong et al., 1983).

Supplementary Motor Area. The fact that the SMA is the major site of projection of VLo of the thalamus (Schell & Strick, 1984) and thus of the output of the basal ganglia motor circuits (Alexander et al., 1986) is important because considerable evidence exists for a role of the SMA in the programming, initiation, and execution of movement. Neural recordings in monkeys have revealed instruction-induced changes in activity during preparation for a movement in SMA neurons which were not active during the movement per se (Tanji, Taniguchi, & Saga, 1980). Brinkman and Porter (1979) reported that many SMA neurons show modulation of their discharge in relation to particular movements and such modulation often precedes the onset of movement itself. Regional cerebral blood flow studies in normal human subjects (Roland, Larsen, Lassen, & Skinhoj, 1980) have shown increased blood flow (and, therefore, increased metabolic activity) in the SMA but not in other regions when subjects plan complex movement sequences but do not actually perform them. On the basis of these and other findings, it has been argued that the SMA has a role in higher motor control (Alexander et al., 1986; Brinkman & Porter, 1983; Tanji & Kurata, 1983).

Internal Model of External System. According to AMT, trajectories of desired sensory feature signals, preplanned and stored in short-term memory by the RP-stage, are read in real-time by the RE-stage and communicated via cortico-cortical connections and subcortical side-loops through parts of the basal ganglia to the SMA and premotor area 6. The subcortical side-loops function as an internal model of the multivariable relationships between sensory consequences of movement and associated proprioceptive feedback of muscle lengths and joint angle changes. The basal ganglia side-loops function, therefore, as an internal model of the inverse dynamics and kinematics of the external system being controlled. For example, when steering an automobile, the driver turns the steering wheel with his or her arms causing the vehicle to travel around a corner. As a consequence, the visual image entering the driver's eyes translates across the retina. The multivariable relationships between kinaesthetic feedback of arm movements and the associated visual consequence signals represent, as far as the driver's CNS is concerned, the dynamic steering response characteristics of the vehicle. Similarly, during speech, relationships between kinaesthetic feedback from the speech mechanism and the associated auditory feedback of speech describes the acoustic response characteristics of the speech mechanism (vocal tract shape) being controlled. Likewise, the multivariable relationships between kinaesthetic feedback of arm position and visual perception of the position of the arm provides an internal model of arm kinematics. During response execution, preplanned trajectories of desired sensory consequences are transformed through basal ganglia side-loops into appropriate trajectories of desired kinaesthetic feedback representing the muscle length and joint angle changes required to achieve them. Thus, consistent with neurophysiology, the outputs from the basal ganglia into SMA and premotor cortex are related to parameters of body movement, such as direction, amplitude and velocity of arm movement, rather than to the activity of individual muscles per se.

Cerebellar Side-Loops. Involvement of subcortical side-loops through the cerebellum in the programming and initiation of movement is now widely recognised (Arbib, 1981; Brooks, 1979; Brooks & Thach, 1981; Evarts, 1981; Wiesendanger, 1983). Evarts (1981) suggested that in the initiation of centrally programmed movements, the motor cortex would be receiving inputs both from the premotor areas (SMA and lateral area 6) via cortico-cortical inputs and from the cerebellum via the cerebello-thalamo-cortical pathways. There are well developed pathways from area 6 via the pontine nuclei to the dentate nucleus and to the lateral parts of the cerebellar hemispheres (see Brooks & Thach, 1981). The dentate projects heavily to the nucleus ventralis posterior lateralis pars oralis (VPLo) of the thalamus which, in turn, projects to the motor cortex (Asanuma, Thach, & Jones, 1983; Jones, 1983; Tracey, Asanuma, Jones, & Porter, 1980).

Evidence that cerebello-thalamo-cortical pathways are involved in the initiation of centrally programmed movements has been provided by Evarts and Tanji (1974), Thach (1975) and Strick (1978), who showed that discharges of dentate neurons associated with centrally programmed movements in the monkey occur as early as 10 ms ahead of similar activity in the motor cortex. Additional evidence for the involvement of the cerebellum in central programming of movement is provided by studies on the effects of cooling of cerebellar nuclei, which show a change in the long-latency (50-100 ms) voluntary component of motor cortex activity in response to limb displacement (Vilis, Hore, Meyer-Lohmann, & Brooks, 1976). Furthermore, Sasaki and Gemba (1983) showed that the characteristic surface-negative, depth-positive field potentials in the motor cortex preceding visually initiated hand movements in the monkey are completely eliminated following extirpation of the cerebellar hemisphere ipsilateral to the moving hand. They concluded that fast and skillful reaction time movements are initiated by impulses impinging upon the motor cortex via the neocerebellum and superficial thalamo-cortical projections. Of special interest is the work of Miall et al. (1987) who studied the visuomotor tracking performance of monkeys during reversible cooling and local anaesthetisation of the cerebellum. The nature of the tracking deficits observed gives strong support for cerebellar involvement in the prediction of the tracking target and the execution of an appropriately tuned response.

Internal Model of Biomechanical System. Consistent with the anatomical and neurophysiological evidence presented above, it is proposed in AMT that signals projected to the SMA and premotor cortex from the basal ganglia representing desired trajectories of muscle lengths and joint angles are communicated to the motor cortex via cortico-cortical connections as well as via parallel side-loops through the neocerebellum and thalamo-cortical projections. There are also subcortical connections from SMA and premotor cortex to a number of brainstem nuclei at the heads of descending tracts. These projections also have parallel side-loops through the cerebellum. We propose that the subcortical side-loops through the cerebellum function as an internal model of the multivariable relationships between kinaesthetic feedback of muscle lengths and joint angles and proprioceptive feedback of muscle tensions detected by Golgi tendon organs. Subcortical side-loops through the cerebellum function, therefore, according to AMT, as an internal model of the inverse dynamics of the biomechanical system being controlled.

Multivariable Nonlinear Biomechanical System. Tensions generated by muscles pull on bones, exert torques about joints and cause body movements detected by muscle spindles and joint receptors. Any one muscle usually operates across more than one degree of freedom of movement, however, and any one degree of freedom of movement is usually operated on by more than one muscle. The gravitational, inertial, and visco-elastic loads on a muscle vary depending on the geometric configuration of the body and its orientation in the gravitational field as well as on the level of tensions developed by other muscles. As the body moves there are reaction forces due to inertial and frictional influences as well as nonlinear interactions caused by centrifugal and coriolis forces. Loads on muscles alter as we interact with the environment and pick up and move objects and, of course, biomechanics change with growth. The biomechanical system described by relationships between tensions, muscle lengths, and joint angles is viewed, therefore, as a multivariable nonlinear changing dynamic system. Despite this complexity, it is proposed that cerebellar microzone circuits function as an internal model of the biomechanical system.

Muscle Control Systems. Desired muscle tension signals transmitted from the cerebellum to the premotor and motor cortex must be transformed into appropriate motor command signals. According to AMT, this is achieved by transforming the tension signals into motor commands via subcortical side-loops through the cerebellum. The side-loops function as an internal model of the inverse dynamics of the multivariable muscle control systems.

About five million fibres descend from motor cortex and brainstem nuclei and make synaptic connections, either directly or indirectly via interneurons, with cranial nerve motoneurons and alpha motoneurons in the spinal cord. Any one descending fibre sends collaterals to multiple levels and makes contact with motoneurons from as many as six muscles operating across different joints. Any one motoneuron receives convergent inputs from large numbers of descending fibres. Each alpha motoneuron innervates multiple muscle fibres forming a motor unit. Tensions generated by multiple motor units are sampled by Golgi tendon organs located at musculotendinous junctions. Multiple reflex pathways from Golgi tendon organs, muscle spindles, and cutaneous receptors converge on to alpha motoneurons forming multiloop feedback control systems. Clearly, there is extensive cross coupling in the descending pathways and reflex connections between upper motoneurons and Golgi tendon organs. The multivariable nature of the muscle control systems must, therefore, be taken into account. According to AMT, internal feedback of the outgoing motor commands (efference copy) and tension feedback from Golgi tendon organs drive self-tuning neural filters in cortico-cerebellar circuits. The circuits operate independently and in parallel to form internal models of the multivariable nonlinear relationships between these signals. An accurate model of the multivariable muscle control system is thus established and adaptively maintained.

Synergy Generator. The orthogonalised motor commands at the output of the muscle control system model must be transformed into a large number of intercorrelated motor commands to signal to the individual muscles. This can be achieved using a network of adaptive neural filters similar to that established by the SA-stage to orthogonalise motor command signals. The important point is that the networks of adaptive filters that orthogonalise motor command signals can be employed in reverse to transform orthogonalised signals back into a large number of intercorrelated signals. The generation of synergies requires just such an ability. Thus the operation of these networks in reverse can, in principle, translate a command with only one dimension into a richly patterned, multidimensional set of commands to muscles throughout the body. We refer to such a network of adaptive models operating in reverse as a "synergy generator".

The work of Rispal-Padel, Cicirata, & Pons (1983) supports this formulation. In a study of awake baboons with chronic electrode implants, stimulation of a rostromedial region of the dentate nucleus elicited complex movements interpreted as motor synergies. The coordinated movements produced by a single stimulation of the dentate were similar to the sum of movements induced by stimulation of each cortical point receiving excitatory projections from the same dentate focus. Moreover, the timing observed supported transmission via a cerebello-thalamo-cortical pathway. Thus the role of the neocerebellum in the execution of motor synergies is strongly endorsed.

IMPLICATIONS FOR MOTOR DISORDERS

In earlier sections we argue that cerebro-cerebellar loops are involved in establishing internal models of relationships between motor commands and their sensory consequences. The initial determination and appropriate adaptation of these relationships during growth and development depends not only on the adequacy of the basic computational circuitry but also on the integrity of the associated inputs or outputs. If any of these aspects is compromised, either by neurological insult or by intrinsic developmental anomaly or deficiency, we would expect a compromise in sensorimotor control to be manifest accordingly. These implications are explored briefly below in relation to the two disorders with which we have particular involvement, namely cerebral palsy and stuttering.

Cerebral Palsy

Cerebral palsy is a "disorder of movement and posture due to a defect or lesion of the immature brain" (Bax, 1964). Associated non-motor handicaps such as mental retardation, epilepsy, sensory and perceptual deficits, learning disabilities and behavioural disorders are common in cerebral-palsied individuals but are incidental to the diagnosis. On the basis of more than 30 population-based studies of the frequency of cerebral palsy, the prevalence rate of cerebral palsy has been estimated at 2 per 1000 live births (Paneth & Kiely, 1984). The cause of cerebral palsy cannot be identified in the majority of cases. Perinatal factors (such as birth asphyxia) traditionally have been considered the major cause but cannot account for the majority of cases. In at least half of all cases the causes antedate the labour period while about 10% of cases can be accounted for by postnatal factors. It is now apparent that the aetiology of cerebral palsy is frequently multifactorial.

Several major neuropathological studies of cerebral palsy have been reported based on autopsy examination of clinically diagnosed cases (e.g., Christensen & Melchior, 1967; Towbin, 1960). Most of the cases were severely affected, died at an earlier than average age and very often had associated mental retardation and/or epilepsy. The cerebral cortex, hemispheric white matter, basal ganglia and cerebellum were affected in varying combinations. Traditionally, the frequent involvement of the sensorimotor cortex is invoked to account for spasticity in cerebral palsy; basal ganglia lesions are associated with athetosis and other forms of dyskinesia, while abnormalities of the cerebellum are related to clinical signs of ataxia. Although their occurrence is clearly recognised, lesions of the cerebral white matter often have not received much emphasis, since attention is usually focused only on loss of neurons. Yet evidence from a variety of sources indicates that the cerebral white matter in the immature nervous system is particularly vulnerable to insult relative to other regions of the brain (e.g., DeReuck, Chattha, & Richardson, 1972; Gilles, 1977; Rorke, 1982) and in perinatal autopsies white matter damage has been reported to be far more frequent than signs of neuronal necrosis.

The importance of white matter lesions in cerebral palsy has come to be recognised increasingly following the correlation of periventricular leukomalacia with spasticity by Banker and Larroche (1962). Periventricular leukomalacia (PVL) consists of foci of necrosis (infarcts) in the white matter surrounding the lateral ventricles. Spastic quadriparesis has been demonstrated in association with PVL (DeReuck et al., 1972), a relation with spastic hemiplegia has been inferred (Armstrong & Norman, 1974) and an association with spastic diplegia has been made by many authors (e.g., Pape & Wigglesworth, 1979). Moreover, in the late 1970s and early 1980s many computed tomographic studies of the brain have been conducted in children and adolescents with cerebral palsy. The most frequent location of gross structural abnormality of the brain in these patients was the cerebral white matter, especially the periventricular region. In neonatal intensive care units during the 1980s, brain imaging was carried out on large numbers of preterm infants and asphyxiated term infants, some of whom subsequently developed cerebral palsy. Using the techniques of computed tomography (e.g., Adsett, Fitz, & Hill, 1985; Volpe, Herscovitch, Perlman, Kreusser, & Raichle, 1985), ultrasound (e.g., De Vries et al., 1985; Weindling, Rochefort, Calvert, Fok, & Wilkinson, 1985), magnetic resonance imaging (e.g., De Vries, Connell, Dubowitz, Oozeer, & Dubowitz, 1987; Wilson & Steiner, 1986) and positron emission tomography (see Volpe et al., 1985), the outstanding location of the structural abnormalities of the brain in these cerebral-palsied patients again has been shown to be the periventricular white matter (for more extensive review of the neuropathology of cerebral palsy see O'Dwyer, 1988).

We believe AMT provides a connecting link between these neuropathological observations and the syndrome of motor disabilities observed in cerebral palsy. If periventricular white matter damage of the type described above destroyed fibres on the motor side in cerebellar subcortical loops normally involved in computing internal models of relationships between motor commands and their sensory consequences then, from birth and onwards during the period of normal motor development, ability of the damaged nervous system to compute internal models of its own muscle control systems would be impaired. Consequently, normal motor development would not occur. Although such a person may be able to appreciate the desired perceptual goals of a movement, the damaged nervous system would be unable to translate this appreciation into appropriate motor commands to perform it. Inappropriate motor commands would be generated instead. Feedback from the resulting inappropriate movements would seem unrelated to outgoing motor commands and so would be experienced as involuntary movements as if caused by some external disturbance. Increased levels of muscle co-contraction and increased reflex sensitivities may, to some extent, represent the body's normal reaction to protect itself against external disturbances by stiffening.

Stuttering

The literature concerning this disorder is extensive but there are accessible overviews such as Andrews et al., (1983) and Cooper (1990) from which the following background is taken. Stuttering is defined in the International Classification of Diseases as "disorders in the rhythm of speech, in which the individual knows precisely what he wishes to say, but at the time is unable to say it because of an involuntary, repetitive prolongation or cessation of sound" (World Health Organization, 1977, p. 202). The large majority of stutterers begin to stutter in childhood, most between the ages of two and five. Three times as many boys are affected than girls and this disproportion increases with age. Typically there is no obvious cause, hence the term idiopathic or developmental stuttering. There is now good evidence that genetic factors play a significant role in the condition which has long been known to be familial, male relatives of female stutterers being at greatest risk. In keeping with this biological focus the once popular theories of stuttering as a neurotic response or a learned behaviour have gone unsupported and it is now widely acknowledged as a disorder of speech motor control.

While investigation of the neuromotor correlates of stuttering currently dominates aetiological research (e.g., Peters, Hulstijn, & Starkweather, in press), clues to the underlying neuropathology remain hard won. There are now many studies which point to functional abnormalities in developmental stutterers but as yet, knowledge of structural abnormality of the nervous system in relation to disfluency is limited to the comparatively rare cases of what is termed acquired stuttering. This may occur as one of the sequelae to brain injury, either traumatic or ischaemic, but has also been reported in association with degenerative disease of the nervous system and toxic response due to chemical agents (see McClean, 1990). The anatomical findings to date are far from homogeneous but, as discussed by McClean, this should not be surprising given that the integrity of motor control processes depends on interdependent function of several anatomically distributed systems (see earlier sections). The neural basis of stuttering, acquired or developmental, is therefore likely to be diverse.

We have argued elsewhere in terms of AMT that stutterers are deficient in the neural processing resources responsible for determining and adaptively maintaining sensorimotor models which subserve speech production (Neilson & Neilson, 1987, in press). This hypothesis is supported by our finding that while stutterers and nonstutterers have comparable performance on visual tracking, stutterers perform poorly on auditory tracking tasks. We hold that the task of transforming a body movement into the variation of an auditory tracking marker closely parallels the problem of transforming a changing vocal tract configuration into a changing speech signal. Just as the successful performance of an auditory tracking task involves the forming of an internal model of the relationship between the movement of a control and the concomitant change in an auditory signal, so the task of speech requires the modelling of the relationship between the respiratory, laryngeal, and supralaryngeal activity and the concomitant auditory feedback of the speech signal produced by that activity. In both cases we are dealing with the multivariable relationship between feedback of muscle/joint/pressure receptor information and an acoustic consequence. Both involve the forming of an internal model of an external system, in the former a tracking apparatus, in the latter the vocal tract.

In the RE-stage section we discussed the anatomical loops which may serve to implement the internal models of the three subsystems involved in response execution, namely the muscle control, the biomechanical, and the external systems. In the case of transformation according to the inverse characteristics of an external system, the relevant subcortical loop passes through parts of the basal ganglia to the SMA and premotor area 6. We might therefore expect the information flow through this loop to be in some way compromised in stutterers, either because the loop inputs are affected or because of a structural or functional problem within the loop itself. We therefore note the findings of Ludlow, Rosenberg, Salazar, Grafman, and Smutok (1987) who carried out a careful study of the site of brain lesions in war veterans who had acquired a chronic stutter after sustaining a penetrating missile wound. Comparison of CT scan data from these patients with that of nonstuttering head injured subjects showed no difference in the frequency of lesions in Broca's area or in the supplementary and primary motor areas, but significantly more frequent involvement of the frontal white matter and of subcortical areas, in particular the basal ganglia and the internal and external capsules. While studies of developmental stutterers lack the opportunity for similar anatomical probing, neurophysiological and behavioural data are frequently used as pointers to possible areas of malfunction. In this vein the supplementary motor area has received recent focus (see Caruso, in press; Caruso, Abbs, & Gracco, 1988; Webster, in press) and its importance in relation to subcortical processing is emphasised.

In terms of AMT, involvement of the basal ganglia/SMA processing loop in stuttering fits well with the concept that modelling of the vocal tract is essentially that of an external system. It must be remembered, however, that the models implemented in that loop depend on cortical as well as subcortical processing for their formation and adaptive maintainance. Therefore, satisfactory operation of the loop relies on the availability of an adequate and appropriate model. According to AMT the storage, accessibility, and integrity of the repertoire of models depends on cortical processes. We have previously discussed stuttering and the amelioration of disfluency in terms of the availability of "capacity" or "resources" in a distributed parallel processing system (Neilson & Neilson, 1987; Neilson & Neilson, in press). Certainly the variation of fluency with cognitive load points to the distribution of such resources being cortically based and there is ample neurobiological evidence suggesting functional cortical differences between stutterers and nonstutterers (e.g., see Moore, 1990). Thus a cohesive view of the disorder must tie together the role of cortical and subcortical processes in the implementation of speech motor control. We believe that AMT provides a useful framework for that task.

REFERENCES

Abbs, J. H. & Cole, K. J. (1982). Consideration of bulbar and suprabulbar afferent influences upon speech motor coordination and programming. In S. Grillner, B. Lindblom, J. Lubker, & A. Persson (Eds.), *Speech motor control.* Oxford: Pergamon.

Adsett, D. B., Fitz, C. R., & Hill, A. (1985). Hypoxic-ischaemic cerebral injury in the term newborn: Correlation of CT findings with neurological outcome. *Developmental Medicine & Child Neurology, 27,* 155-160.

Alexander, G. E., DeLong, M. R., & Strick, P. L. (1986). Parallel organization of functionally segregated circuits linking basal ganglia and cortex. *Annual Review of Neuroscience, 9,* 357-381.

Allum, J. H. J., Anner-Baratti, R. E. C., & Hepp-Reymond, M.-C. (1983). Activity of neurones in the "motor" thalamus and globus pallidus during the control of isometric finger force in the monkey. In J. Massion, J. Paillard, W. Schultz, & M. Wiesendanger (Eds.), *Neural coding of motor performance* (pp. 194-203). Berlin: Springer-Verlag.

Andrews, G., Craig, A., Feyer, A.-M., Hoddinott, S., Howie, P., & Neilson, M. (1983). Stuttering: A review of research findings and theories circa 1982. *Journal of Speech and Hearing Disorders, 48,* 226-246.

Arbib, M. A. (1972). *The metaphorical brain. An introduction to cybernetics as artificial intelligence and brain theory.* New York: Wiley.

Arbib, M. (1981). Perceptual structures and distributed motor control. In V. B. Brooks (Ed.), *Handbook of physiology: Sec. 1. The nervous system: Vol. II. Motor control, Part 2* (pp. 1449-1480). Bethesda, MD: American Physiological Society.

Armstrong, D., & Norman, M. G. (1974). Periventricular leucomalacia in neonates. Complications and sequelae. *Archives of Disease in Childhood, 49,* 367-375.

Asanuma, C., Thach, W. T., & Jones, E. G. (1983). Distribution of cerebellar terminations and their relation to other afferent terminations in the ventral lateral thalamic region of the monkey. *Brain Research Reviews, 5,* 237-265.

Astrom, K. J. & Wittenmark, B. (1989). *Adaptive control.* Reading, MA: Addison-Wesley.

Bahill, A. T. & McDonald, J. D. (1983). Model emulates human smooth pursuit system producing zero-latency target tracking. *Biological Cybernetics, 48,* 213-222.

Banker, B. Q. & Larroche, J.-Cl. (1962). Periventricular leukomalacia of infancy. *Archives of Neurology, 7,* 386-410.

Bax, M. C. O. (1964). Terminology and classification of cerebral palsy. *Developmental Medicine & Child Neurology, 6,* 295-297.

Bloedel, J. R., Dichgans, J., & Precht, W. (1985). (Eds.). *Cerebellar functions.* Berlin: Springer-Verlag.

Bloedel, J. R. & Ebner, T. J. (1985). Climbing fiber function: Regulation of Purkinje cell responsiveness. In J. R. Bloedel, J. Dichgans, & W. Precht (Eds.), *Cerebellar functions* (pp. 247-259). Berlin: Springer-Verlag.

Box, G. E. P. & Jenkins, G. M. (1976). *Time series analysis: Forecasting and control.* San Francisco: Holden-Day.

Braitenberg, V. (1986). Two views of the cerebral cortex. In G. Palm & A. Aertsen (Eds.), *Brain theory* (pp. 81-96). Berlin: Springer-Verlag.

Brinkman, C. & Porter, R. (1979). Supplementary motor area in the monkey: Activity of neurons during performance of a learned motor task. *Journal of Neurophysiology, 42,* 681-709.

Brinkman, C. & Porter, R. (1983). Supplementary motor area and premotor area of monkey cerebral cortex. In J. E. Desmedt (Ed.), *Motor control mechanisms in health and disease* (Advances in Neurology, Vol. 39, pp. 393-420). New York: Raven Press.

Broadbent, D. E. (1977). Levels, hierarchies, and the locus of control. *Quarterly Journal of Experimental Psychology, 29,* 181-201.

Brooks, V. B. (1979). Control of intended limb movements by the lateral and intermediate cerebellum. In H. Asanuma & V. J. Wilson (Eds.), *Integration in the nervous system* (pp. 321-357). Tokyo: Igaku Shoin.

Brooks, V. B. & Thach, W. T. (1981). Cerebellar control of posture and movement. In V. B. Brooks (Ed.), *Handbook of physiology: Sec. 1. The nervous system: Vol. II. Motor control, Part 2* (pp. 877-946). Bethesda, MD: American Physiological Society.

Caruso, A. J. (in press). Neuromotor processes underlying stuttering. In H. F. M. Peters, W. Hulstijn, & C. W. Starkweather (Eds.), *Speech motor control and stuttering.* Amsterdam: Elsevier.

Caruso, A. J., Abbs, J. H., & Gracco, V. L. (1988). Kinematic analysis of multiple movement coordination during speech in stutterers. *Brain, 111,* 439-455.

Christensen, E. & Melchior, J. C. (1967). *Cerebral palsy. A clinical and neuropathological study* (Clinics in Developmental Medicine, No. 25). London: Spastics Society/Heinemann.

Cooper, J. A. (Ed.). (1990). *Research needs in stuttering: Roadblocks and future directions* (ASHA Reports 18). Rockville, MD: American Speech-Language-Hearing Association.

Craik, K. J. W. (1943). *The nature of explanation.* London: Cambridge University Press.

Crutcher, M. D. & DeLong, M. R. (1984). Single cell studies of the primate putamen. II. Relations to direction of movements and pattern of muscular activity. *Experimental Brain Research, 53,* 244-258.

Darian-Smith, C., Darian-Smith, I., & Cheema, S. S. (1990). Thalamic projections to sensorimotor cortex in the newborn macaque. *Journal of Comparative Neurology, 299,* 47-63.

DeLong, M. R. (1971). Activity of pallidal neurons during movement. *Journal of Neurophysiology, 34,* 414-427.

DeLong, M. R. (1973). Putamen: activity of single units during slow and rapid arm movements. *Science, 179,* 1240-1242.

DeLong, M. R. & Georgopoulos, A. P. (1979). Motor functions of the basal ganglia as revealed by studies of single cell activity in the behaving primate. In L. J. Poirier, T. L. Sourkes, & P. J. Bedard (Eds.), *Advances in neurology* (pp. 131-140). New York: Raven Press.

DeLong, M. R. & Georgopoulos, A. P. (1981). Motor functions of the basal ganglia. In V. B. Brooks (Ed.), *Handbook of physiology: Sec. 1. The nervous system: Vol II. Motor control, Part 2* (pp. 1017-1061). Bethesda, MD: American Physiological Society.

DeLong, M. R., Georgopoulos, A. P., & Crutcher, M. D. (1983). Cortico-basal ganglia relations and coding of motor performance. In J. Massion, J. Paillard, W. Schultz, & M. Wiesendanger (Eds.), *Neural coding of motor performance* (Experimental Brain Research Supplementum 7, pp. 30-40). Berlin: Springer-Verlag.

DeLong, M. R. & Strick, P. L. (1974). Relation of basal ganglia, cerebellum and motor cortex units to ramp and ballistic limb movements. *Brain Research, 71,* 327-335.

DeReuck, J., Chattha, A. S., & Richardson, E. P. (1972). Pathogenesis and evolution of periventricular leukomalacia in infancy. *Archives of Neurology, 27,* 229-236.

De Vries, L. S., Connell, J. A., Dubowitz, L. M. S., Oozeer, R. C., & Dubowitz, V. (1987). Neurological, electrophysiological and MRI abnormalities in infants with extensive cystic leukomalacia. *Neuropediatrics, 18,* 61-66.

De Vries, L. S., Dubowitz, L. M. S., Dubowitz, V., Kaiser, A., Lary, S., Silverman, M., Whitelaw, A., & Wigglesworth, J. S. (1985). Predictive value of cranial ultrasound in the newborn baby: A reappraisal. *The Lancet, II(8447),* 137-140.

Eccles, J. C. (1984). The cerebral neocortex: A theory of its operation. In E. G. Jones & A. Peters (Eds.), *Cerebral cortex: Vol. 2. Functional properties of cortical cells* (pp. 1-36). New York: Plenum Press.

Evarts, E. V. (1981). Role of motor cortex in voluntary movements in primates. In V. B. Brooks (Ed.), *Handbook of physiology: Sec 1. The nervous system: Vol II. Motor control, Part 2* (pp. 1083-1120). Bethesda, MD: American Physiological Society.

Evarts, E. V. & Tanji, J. (1974). Gating of motor cortex reflexes by prior instruction. *Brain Research, 71*, 479-494.

Freund, H.-J. (1983). Motor unit and muscle activity in voluntary motor control. *Physiological Reviews, 63*, 387-436.

Fujita, M. (1982). Adaptive filter model of the cerebellum. *Biological Cybernetics, 45*, 195-206.

Fuster, J. M. (1985). The path to action. *Behavioral and Brain Sciences, 8*, 589-591.

Gilles, F. H. (1977). Lesions attributed to perinatal asphyxia in the human. In L. Gluck (Ed.), *Intrauterine asphyxia and the developing fetal brain* (pp. 99-107). Chicago: Year Book.

Glencross, J. & Barrett, N. (1988). *The programming and amendment of skilled movements.* Paper presented at the XXIV International Congress of Psychology, Sydney, Australia, Aug 28 - Sep 3.

Goldberg, G. (1985). Supplementary motor area structure and function: Review and hypotheses. *Behavioral and Brain Sciences, 8*, 567-616.

Goldman-Rakic, P. S. (1987). Circuitry of primate prefrontal cortex and regulation of behavior by representational memory. In F. Plum (Ed.), *Handbook of physiology: Sec 1. The nervous system: Vol. V. Higher functions of the brain, Part 1* (pp. 373-417). Bethesda, MD: American Physiological Society.

Goodwin, G. C. & Sin, K. S. (1984). *Adaptive filtering prediction and control.* Englewood Cliffs, NJ: Prentice-Hall.

Greene, P. H. (1982). Why is it easy to control your arms?. *Journal of Motor Behavior, 14*, 260-286.

Grossberg, S. & Kuperstein, M. (1986). *Neural dynamics of adaptive sensory-motor control: Ballistic eye movements* (Advances in Psychology, 30). Amsterdam: North-Holland.

Gurfinkel, V. S. & Levik, Yu. S. (1980). Sensory complexes and sensomotor integration. *Human Physiology, 6*, 269-281 (Translated from Fiziologiya Cheloveka, 1979, 5, 399-414). New York: Consultants Bureau.

Hancock, P. A. & Meshkati, N. (Eds.). (1988). *Human mental workload* (Advances in Psychology, 52). Amsterdam: North-Holland.

Held, R. & Freedman, S. J. (1963). Plasticity in human sensorimotor control. *Science, 142*, 455-462.

Hinton, G. (1984). Some computational solutions to Bernstein's problems. In H. T. A. Whiting (Ed.), *Human motor actions: Bernstein reassessed* (Advances in Psychology, 17, pp. 413-438). Amsterdam: North-Holland.

Holst, E. von & Mittelstaedt, H. (1973). The reafference principle. Interaction between the central nervous system and the periphery. In *Selected papers of Erich von Holst: The behavioural physiology of animals and man* (Vol. 1, pp. 139-173). London: Methuen. (Transl. from German by R. Martin, originally published 1950).

Ito, M. (1984). *The cerebellum and neural control.* New York: Raven Press.

Jones, E. G. (1985). *The thalamus.* New York: Plenum Press.

Kleinman, D. L., Baron, S., & Levison, W. H. (1970). An optimal control model of human response, Part I: Theory and validation. *Automatica, 6,* 357-369.

Kohonen, T. (1988). An introduction to neural computing. *Neural Networks 1,* 3-16.

Kornhuber, H. H. (1973). Neural control of input into long-term memory: Limbic system and amnestic syndrome in man. In H. P. Zippel (Ed.), *Memory and transfer of information* (pp. 1-22). New York: Plenum Press.

Kuperstein, M. (1988). Neural model of adaptive hand-eye coordination for single postures. *Science, 239,* 1308-1311.

Lane, H. & Tranel, B. (1971). The Lombard sign and the role of hearing in speech. *Journal of Speech and Hearing Research, 14,* 677-709.

Lashley, K. S. (1951). The problem of serial order of behavior. In L. A. Jeffress (Ed.), *Cerebral mechanisms in behavior* (pp. 112-136). New York: Wiley.

LeDoux, J. E. (1987). Emotion. In F. Plum (Ed.), *Handbook of physiology: Sec. 1. The nervous system: Vol. V. Higher functions of the brain, Part 1* (pp. 419-459). Bethesda, MD: American Physiological Society.

Lee, Y. W. & Schetzen, M. (1965). Measurement of the Wiener kernels of a nonlinear system by cross-correlation. *International Journal of Control, 2,* 237-254.

Liles, S. L. (1985). Activity of neurons in putamen during active and passive movements of the wrist. *Journal of Neurophysiology, 53,* 217-236.

Ljung, L. (1987). *System identification: Theory for the user.* Englewood Cliffs, NJ: Prentice-Hall.

Llinas, R. (1981). Electrophysiology of the cerebellar networks. In V. B. Brooks (Ed.), *Handbook of physiology: Sec. 1. The nervous system: Vol. II. Motor control, Part 2* (pp. 831-876). Bethesda, MD: American Physiological Society.

Ludlow, C. L., Rosenberg, J., Salazar, A., Grafman, J., & Smutok, M. (1987). Site of penetrating brain lesions causing chronic acquired stuttering. *Annals of Neurology, 22,* 60-66.

MacNeilage, P. F. (1970). Motor control of serial ordering of speech. *Psychological Review, 77,* 182-196.

Marmarelis, P. Z. & Marmarelis, V. Z. (1978). *Analysis of physiological systems: The white-noise approach.* New York: Plenum Press.

Marmarelis, V. Z. (1989). Volterra-Wiener analysis of a class of nonlinear feedback systems and application to sensory biosystems. In V. Z. Marmarelis (Ed.), *Advanced methods of physiological system modeling, Vol. 2* (pp. 1-52). New York: Plenum Press.

McClean, M. D. (1990). Neuromotor aspects of stuttering: Levels of impairment and disability. In J. A. Cooper (Ed.), *Research needs in stuttering: Roadblocks and future directions* (ASHA Reports 18, pp. 64-71). Rockville, MD: American Speech-Language-Hearing Association.

McLeod, P. (1977). Parallel processing and the psychological refractory period. *Acta Psychologica, 41,* 381-396.

McRuer, D. T. (1980). Human dynamics in man-machine systems. *Automatica, 16,* 237-253.

McRuer, D. T. & Krendel, E. S. (1959a). The human operator as a servo system element, Part I. *Journal of The Franklin Institute, 267,* 381-403.

McRuer, D. T. & Krendel, E. S. (1959b). The human operator as a servo system element, Part II. *Journal of The Franklin Institute, 267,* 511-536.

McRuer, D. T. & Krendel, E. S. (1974). *Mathematical models of human pilot behavior* (AGARDograph No. 188). Neuilly sur Seine, France: North Atlantic Treaty Organization, Advisory Group for Aerospace Research and Development.

Miall, R. C., Weir, D. J., & Stein, J. F. (1987). Visuo-motor tracking during reversible inactivation of the cerebellum. *Experimental Brain Research, 65,* 455-464.

Miyamoto, H., Kawato, M., Setoyama, T., & Suzuki, R. (1988). Feedback-error-learning neural network for trajectory control of a robotic manipulator. *Neural Networks, 1,* 251-265.

Moore, W. H. Jr. (1990). Pathophysiology of stuttering: Cerebral activation differences in stutterers vs. nonstutterers. In J. A. Cooper (Ed.), *Research needs in stuttering: Roadblocks and future directions* (ASHA Reports 18, pp. 72-80). Rockville, MD: American Speech-Language-Hearing Association.

Moray, N. (Ed.). (1979). *Mental workload: Its theory and measurement* (NATO conference series: III. Human factors; v.8). New York: Plenum Press.

Moray, N. (1981). Feedback and the control of skilled behaviour. In D. Holding (Ed.), *Human skills* (pp. 15-39). Chichester: Wiley.

Nash, J., Neilson, P. D., & O'Dwyer, N. J. (1989). Reducing spasticity to control muscle contracture of children with cerebral palsy. *Developmental Medicine & Child Neurology, 31,* 471-480.

Navon, D. & Gopher, D. (1979). On the economy of the human processing system: A model of multiple capacity. *Psychological Review, 86,* 214-255.

Neilson, M. D. (1980). *Stuttering and the control of speech: A systems analysis approach.* Unpublished doctoral dissertation, University of New South Wales, Sydney, Australia.

Neilson, M. D. & Neilson, P. D. (1987). Speech motor control and stuttering: A computational model of adaptive sensory-motor processing. *Speech Communication, 6,* 325-333.

Neilson, M. D. & Neilson, P. D. (in press). Adaptive model theory of speech motor control and stuttering. In H. F. M. Peters, W. Hulstijn, & C. W. Starkweather (Eds.), *Speech motor control and stuttering.* Amsterdam: Elsevier.

Neilson, P. D. (1973). *Cerebral palsy: A neurophysiological and systems theory analysis.* Unpublished doctoral dissertation, University of New South Wales, Sydney, Australia.

Neilson, P. D. & Lance, J. W. (1978). Reflex transmission characteristics during voluntary activity in normal man and in patients with movement disorder. In J.

E. Desmedt (Ed.), *Cerebral motor control in man: Long loop mechanisms* (Progress in Clinical Neurophysiology, Vol. 4, pp. 263-289). Basel: Karger.

Neilson, P. D., Neilson, M. D., & O'Dwyer, N. J. (1988). Internal models and intermittency: A theoretical account of human tracking behavior. *Biological Cybernetics, 58*, 101-112.

Neilson, P. D. & O'Dwyer, N. J. (1984). Reproducibility and variability of speech muscle activity in athetoid dysarthria of cerebral palsy. *Journal of Speech and Hearing Research, 27*, 502-517.

Neilson, P. D., O'Dwyer, N. J., & Neilson, M. D. (1988). Stochastic prediction in pursuit tracking: An experimental test of adaptive model theory. *Biological Cybernetics, 58*, 113-122.

O'Dwyer, N. J. (1988). *Control of speech muscles in human and cerebral-palsied speakers: An electromyographic analysis*. Unpublished doctoral dissertation, University of New South Wales, Sydney, Australia.

Paneth, N. & Kiely, J. (1984). The frequency of cerebral palsy: A review of population studies in industrialised nations since 1950. In F. Stanley & E. Alberman (Eds.), *The epidemiology of the cerebral palsies* (Clinics in Developmental Medicine, No. 87, pp. 46-56). Oxford: Spastics International/Blackwell.

Pape, K. E. & Wigglesworth, J. S. (1979). *Haemorrhage, ischaemia and the perinatal brain* (Clinics in Developmental Medicine, No. 69/70). London: Spastics International Medical Publications/Heinemann.

Pellionisz, A. & Llinas, R. (1979). Brain modeling by tensor network theory and computer simulation. The cerebellum: Distributed processor for predictive coordination. *Neuroscience, 4*, 323-348.

Peters, H. F. M., Hulstijn, W., & Starkweather, C. W. (Eds.). (in press). *Speech motor control and stuttering*. Amsterdam: Elsevier.

Pew, R. W. (1974). Human perceptual-motor performance. In B. H. Kantowitz (Ed.), *Human information processing: Tutorials in performance and cognition* (pp. 1-39). Hillsdale, NJ: Lawrence Erlbaum Associates.

Powell, T. P. S. (1981). Certain aspects of the intrinsic organisation of the cerebral cortex. In O. Pompeiano & C. Ajmone Marsan (Eds.), *Brain mechanisms and perceptual awareness* (pp. 1-19). New York: Raven Press.

Raibert, M. H. (1978). A model for sensorimotor control and learning. *Biological Cybernetics, 29*, 29-36.

Rawson, J. A. & Tilokskulchai, K. (1982). Climbing fiber modification of cerebellar Purkinje cell responses to parallel fiber inputs. *Brain Research, 237*, 492-497.

Requin, J. (1980). Toward a psychobiology of preparation for action. In G. E. Stelmach & J. Requin (Eds.), *Tutorials in motor behavior* (Advances in Psychology, 1, pp. 373-398). Amsterdam: North-Holland.

Rispal-Padel, L., Cicirata, F., & Pons, J.-C. (1983). Neocerebellar synergies. In J. Massion, J. Paillard, W. Schultz, & M. Wiesendanger (Eds.), *Neural coding of motor performance* (Experimental Brain Research Supplementum 7, pp. 213-223). Berlin: Springer-Verlag.

Roland, P. E., Larsen, B., Lassen, N. A., & Skinhoj, E. (1980). Supplementary motor area and other cortical areas in organization of voluntary movements in man. *Journal of Neurophysiology, 43*, 118-136.

Rorke, L. B. (1982). *Pathology of perinatal brain injury*. New York: Raven Press.

Saltzman, E. (1979). Levels of sensorimotor representation. *Journal of Mathematical Psychology, 20*, 91-163.

Sasaki, K. & Gemba, H. (1983). Premovement cortical potentials associated with self-paced and reaction time movements. In J. Massion, J. Paillard, W. Schultz, & M. Wiesendanger (Eds.), *Neural coding of motor performance* (Experimental Brain Research Supplementum 7, pp. 88-96). Berlin: Springer-Verlag.

Schell, G. R. & Strick, P. L. (1984). The origin of thalamic inputs to the arcuate premotor and supplementary motor areas. *Journal of Neuroscience, 4*, 539-560.

Schmidt, R. A. (1976). The schema as a solution to some persistent problems in motor learning theory. In G. E. Stelmach (Ed.), *Motor control. Issues and trends* (pp. 41-65). New York: Academic Press.

Schneider, J. S. & Lidsky, T. I. (Eds.). (1987). *Basal ganglia and behavior: Sensory aspects of motor functioning*. Toronto: Hans Huber.

Seelen, W. von, Mallot, H. A., Krone, G., & Dinse, H. (1986). On information processing in the cat's visual cortex. In G. Palm & A. Aertsen (Eds.), *Brain theory* (pp. 49-79). Berlin: Springer-Verlag.

Shaw, G. L. & Silverman, D. J. (1988). Simulations of the trion model and the search for the code of higher cortical processing. In R. M. J. Cotterill (Ed.), *Computer simulation in brain science* (pp. 189-209). Cambridge: Cambridge University Press.

Smith, K. U. & Smith, W. M. (1962). *Perception and Motion. An analysis of space-structured behavior*. Philadelphia: W. B. Saunders.

Sokolov, E. N. (1960). Neuronal models and the orienting reflex. In M. A. B. Brazier (Ed.), *The central nervous system and behavior* (pp. 187-276). New York: Josiah Macy, Jr. Foundation.

Sperry, R. W. (1950). Neural basis of the spontaneous optokinetic response produced by visual neural inversion. *Journal of Comparative and Physiological Psychology, 43*, 482-489.

Stark, L. (1968). *Neurological control systems*. New York: Plenum Press.

Strick, P. L. (1978). Cerebellar involvement in 'volitional' muscle responses to load changes. In J. E. Desmedt (Ed.), *Cerebral motor control in man: Long loop mechanisms* (Progress in Clinical Neurophysiology, Vol. 4, pp. 85-93). Basel: Karger.

Summers, J. J. (1981). Motor programs. In D. Holding (Ed.), *Human skills* (pp. 41-64). Chichester: Wiley.

Tanji, J. & Kurata, K. (1983). Functional organization of the supplementary motor area. In J. E. Desmedt (Ed.), *Motor control mechanisms in health and disease* (Advances in Neurology, Vol. 39, pp. 421-431). New York: Raven Press.

Tanji, J., Taniguchi, K., & Saga, T. (1980). The supplementary motor area: Neuronal responses to motor instructions. *Journal of Neurophysiology, 43,* 60-68.

Taub, E. & Berman, A. J. (1968). Movement and learning in the absence of sensory feedback. In S. J. Freedman (Ed.), *The neuropsychology of spatially oriented behavior* (pp. 173-192). Homewood, IL: Dorsey.

Thach, W. T. (1975). Timing of activity in cerebellar dentate nucleus and cerebellar motor cortex during prompt volitional movement. *Brain Research, 88,* 233-241.

Towbin, A. (1960). *The pathology of cerebral palsy.* Springfield, IL: Charles C. Thomas.

Tracey, D. J., Asanuma, C., Jones, E. G., & Porter, R. (1980). Thalamic relay to motor cortex: Afferent pathways from brainstem, cerebellum and spinal cord in monkeys. *Journal of Neurophysiology, 44,* 532-554.

Vilis, T., Hore, J., Meyer-Lohmann, J., & Brooks, V. B. (1976). Dual nature of the precentral responses to limb perturbations revealed by cerebellar cooling. *Brain Research, 117,* 336-340.

Viviani, P. & Terzuolo, C. (1982). Trajectory determines movement dynamics. *Neuroscience, 7,* 431-437.

Viviani, P & Terzuolo, C. (1983). The organization of movement in handwriting and typing. In B. Butterworth (Ed.), *Language production, Vol. 2* (pp. 103-146). London: Academic Press.

Volpe, J. J., Herscovitch, P., Perlman, J. M., Kreusser, K. L., & Raichle, M. E. (1985). Positron emission tomography in the asphyxiated term newborn: Parasagittal impairment of cerebral blood flow. *Annals of Neurology, 17,* 287-296.

Watson, R. T., Valenstein, E., & Heilman, K. M. (1981). Thalamic neglect: The possible role of the medial thalamus and nucleus reticularis thalami in behavior. *Archives of Neurology, 38,* 501-507.

Webster, W. G. (in press). Hurried hands and tangled tongues: Implications of current research for the management of stuttering. In E. Boberg (Ed.), *The neuropsychology of stuttering.* Edmonton, Alberta: University of Alberta Press.

Weindling, A. M., Rochefort, M. J., Calvert, S. A., Fok, T.-F., & Wilkinson, A. (1985). Development of cerebral palsy after ultrasonographic detection of periventricular cysts in the newborn. *Developmental Medicine & Child Neurology, 27,* 800-806.

Welford, A. T. (1980). The single-channel hypothesis. In A. T. Welford (Ed.), *Reaction times* (pp. 215-252). London: Academic Press.

World Health Organization (1977). *Manual of the international statistical classification of diseases, injuries, and causes of death (Vol. 1).* Geneva: World Health Organization.

Widrow, B. & Stearns, S. D. (1985). *Adaptive signal processing.* Englewood Cliffs, NJ: Prentice-Hall.

Wiener, N. (1948). *Cybernetics.* New York: John Wiley & Sons.

Wiesendanger, M. (1983). Cortico-cerebellar loops. In J. Massion, J. Paillard, W. Schultz, & M. Wiesendanger (Eds.), *Neural coding of motor performance* (Experimental Brain Research Supplementum 7, pp. 41-53). Springer-Verlag: Berlin.

Wilson, D. A. & Steiner, R. E. (1986). Periventricular leukomalacia: Evaluation with MR imaging. *Radiology, 160*, 507-511.

Yates, A. J. (1963). Recent empirical and theoretical approaches to the experimental manipulation of speech in normal speakers and stammerers. *Behaviour Research and Therapy, 1*, 95-119.

Young, L. R. (1969). On adaptive manual control. *Ergonomics, 12*, 635-675.

PART V

EPILOGUE

Approaches to the Study of Motor Control and Learning
J.J. Summers (Editor)

Chapter 18

MOVEMENT BEHAVIOUR: A FIELD IN CRISIS?

Jeffery J. Summers
University of Melbourne

The general themes which have emerged from the chapters in this book are examined in an attempt to assess the current status and possible future direction of research on motor control and learning. The motor-action controversy, molecular versus molar research, and movement outcome versus movement process are issues that appear in a number of chapters. An argument is put forward that the field is moving towards a reconciliation between the motor systems and action systems approaches to motor control, rather than a further polarisation of the competing views.

The aim of this volume was to illustrate the diversity of approaches and techniques currently being taken by researchers in the movement behaviour field. Part of this diversity stems from the fact that movement control is now an important research area in a number of disciplines (e.g., engineering, human movement science, neuroscience, physiology, psychology). As Laszlo (chap. 2) points out, the academic background of the researcher exerts a strong influence on the topics examined, and the methods and techniques employed. It is also clear, however, that researchers within a discipline are becoming increasing aware of work in other fields relevant to motor function. In the present volume, for example, researchers with a backgound in psychology, are incorporating findings from neurophysiology and biomechanics into their models (e.g., Thomassen & Van Galen, chap. 4). Likewise, neuroscientists in their attempt to establish the links between neuronal activities (microscopic events) and behaviour (macroscopic events) are drawing on contributions from engineering, physiology, psychology, and robotics (e.g., Haggard, chap. 7; Neilson, Neilson, & O'Dwyer, chap. 17).

Although the amalgamation of knowledge from related fields is clearly necessary for the development of coherent theories of motor control and learning, it does pose the theorist with a dilemma. Stelmach and Hughes (1987), for example, suggest that the movement scientist is caught "between deciding whether we should focus more on (neuro) motor control or on (psycho) motor behavior, trying to understand the jargon of each, and all the while wondering whether there cannot be a middle ground where the views might profitably converge" (p. 190).

A similar dilemma to that faced in integrating findings across disciplines is evident within the discipline of psychology in the debate between the information processing and ecological approaches to the study of human behaviour. In the movement area this debate has been designated the motor systems - action systems controversy (Meijer & Roth, 1988). Not only are there deep conceptual and philosophical differences between the two viewpoints, but they use different 'languages'. The motor systems approach uses the terminology of information theory and cognition, whereas the action systems perspective employs the language of physics and mathematics. To add to the confusion each approach is referred to by a variety of labels (see Abernethy & Sparrow, chap. 1, table 1).

In the first chapter of the present volume Abernethy and Sparrow examined historical developments in the field of motor control and learning from a Kuhnian perspective. Content and citation analyses from the *Journal of Motor Behavior* were used to plot paradigm shifts over the period 1969 - 1989. The authors conclude that the battle between the motor systems and action systems approaches has placed the motor control and learning field "in the midst of a true paradigm crisis" (p. 27). Abernethy and Sparrow further argue that the current paradigm crisis will not be resolved by reconciliation of the two views. The conceptual and philosophical differences between the two positions are seen as being too great to allow a hybridisation to occur. Rather the authors predict that the field is entering a long period of bitter and intense conflict from which one of the competing views will emerge as dominant.

In this final chapter I will attempt to evaluate Abernethy and Sparrow's conclusions in the light of the themes emerging from the chapters in the present volume. The contributors were selected to provide a blend of researchers with established reputations in the movement behaviour field and younger researchers in the early stages of their career. As Abernethy and Sparrow note, it is the young scientists who have little invested interest in the survival of the existing paradigm that are usually the instigators of a paradigm shift. The present volume, therefore, should provide an indication of the current status and, perhaps, future direction of research on motor behaviour.

GENERAL THEMES

Motor-Action Controversy

The debate between the computational/prescriptive approach and the ecological/emergent properties approach to motor control and learning is the central theme of several chapters in the present volume (e.g., Whiting, Vogt, & Vereijken, chap. 3; Savelsbergh, Whiting, & Pijpers, chap. 11; Abernethy & Burgess-Limerick, chap. 12). Of particular relevance to the view that the movement field is in the midst of a paradigm crisis is that other authors, adopting a more prescriptive approach, also express dissatisfaction with the incumbent information processing paradigm (e.g., Laszlo, chap. 2; Williams, chap. 8). Laszlo (chap. 2), for example, argues that the molecular research (e.g., lever positioning and reaction time studies) typical of the information processing perspective has contributed little to our understanding of perceptuo-motor function.

Other authors have clearly abandoned the cognitive prescriptive (top-down) approach to motor control in favour of the emergent properties (bottom-up) approach (e.g., Parker, chap. 6; Savelsberg, Whiting, & Pijpers, chap. 11). It is also noteworthy that the 'defection' of influential figures in the field from the existing paradigm to the new emerging paradigm is a further sign of paradigm crisis. In the present volume John Whiting's shift in his work on motor learning (chap. 3) and 'catching behaviour' (chap. 11) to an action systems perspective is a good example of this phenomenon.

Finally, the influence of the action systems perspective can be seen in the research issues being examined by contributors. Perception-action coupling and the mechanisms underlying movement coordination are key issues within the ecological framework and are the topics examined in several chapters (although not necessarily from an action system perspective) of the present volume (Sparrow, chap. 5; Parker, chap. 6; Haggard, chap. 7; Kerr, chap. 9; Savelsberg, et al., chap. 11; Abernethy & Burgess-Limerick, chap. 12). On the other hand, continuing interest in the information processing approach and central control/representation issues is also clearly evident in the contributions by Thomassen and Van Galen (chap. 4), Williams (chap. 8), Glencross and Barrett (chap. 10), Anson (chap. 13), Charlton (chap. 15), and Phillips and Stelmach (chap. 16).

Molecular versus Molar Research

Laszlo in Chapter 2 argues strongly that motor researchers should move away from the molecular approach in which small, well-defined bits of behaviour are studied under ‘contrived’ laboratory conditions, and toward molar research focusing on "broadly based ‘representative’ chunks of behaviour" (p. 49). Although the control of discrete unidimensional movements remains an important topic within the motor domain (e.g., Williams, chap. 8; Kerr, chap. 9; Glencross & Barrett; chap. 10; Anson, chap. 13), research involving tasks more related to every-day functioning is also clearly evident in the present volume. Some of the ‘real-world’ tasks being studied by contributors include: video-games (Laszlo, chap. 2), slalom ski-type movements (Whiting, et al., chap. 3), handwriting (Thomassen & Van Galen, chap. 4), creeping (Sparrow, chap. 5), jumping-jacks (Parker, chap. 6), catching (Savelsberg, et al., chap. 11), running, hopping, and jumping (Larkin & Hoare, chap. 14), and reaching and grasping (Charlton, chap. 15).

The increased interest in the study of real-world tasks is another example of the influence of the ecological approach which advocates the use of more natural research settings. However, there is no reason why information processing principles cannot be applied to the analysis of ‘real-world’ tasks, as the chapters by Charlton, and Thomassen and Van Galen illustrate. In fact, for some time the information processing approach has been, and still continues to be, the dominant paradigm for the study of the so-called ‘cognitive motor skills’ (Colley, 1989a), such as writing, drawing, typing, musical performance, and speech.

Movement Outcome versus Movement Process

Another theme that emerges from several chapters in this volume is the call for researchers to focus on the movement process itself rather than just on movement outcomes (e.g., reaction time, errors). It is argued that a better understanding of the processes underlying movement control may be gained from examining the events and regularities evident in the kinematic, kinetic, and electromyographic (EMG) profiles of movement. The use of kinematic measures, for example, can provide valuable information for the assessment of motor dysfunction and the recovery process (Larkin & Hoare, chap. 14; Charlton, chap. 15; Phillips & Stelmach, chap. 16).

The description of movement at several levels (e.g., reaction time, kinematic, muscular) is a feature of a number of chapters (e.g., Williams, chap. 8; Kerr, chap. 9; Anson, chap. 13; Phillips & Stelmach, chap. 16). Furthermore, the action systems view that movement can be modelled by the principles of non-linear, limit cycle oscillators has provided researchers with the techniques from synergetics for analysing interlimb coordination, such as phase portrait analysis (see Sparrow, chap. 5; Parker, chap. 6).

Although the increasing interest in the examination of real-world tasks and movement processes reflects the influence of the action systems approach, it should also be acknowledged that the recent development of sophisticated motion analysis technology has contributed to the shift in research emphasis by movement scientists of all theoretical orientations.

FUTURE DIRECTIONS

Reconciliation or Confrontation?

The general themes evident in the present volume clearly indicate that aspects of the ecological approach to perception and action have gained considerable acceptance amongst movement researchers. However, many authors appear to be advocating a merging of the motor systems - action systems views, rather than the overthrow of the incumbent information processing approach.

As Sheridan (1988) points out ecological theorists have been guilty of setting up Keele's (1968) definition of a motor program as a 'straw man'. Few, if any, information processing theorists still adhere to the notion of a single level of control specifying every detail in the response. Rather the current view is of a multi-level system incorporating a high level cognitive system responsible for the planning, representation, and strategic control of action and a lower level dynamic system responsible for the execution of movement (e.g., Colley, 1989a,b; Summers, 1989a). Recent conceptions of the organisation of the higher premotoric levels suggest a system of independent *modules* performing specialised functions (see Keele, Cohen, & Ivry, 1990; Thomassen & Van Galen, chap. 4). According to this view, therefore, motor systems and action systems theories are not incompatible but, rather, are addressing different levels within a multi-level motor system.

The notion of distributed control is also a feature of most multi-level hybrid models, thereby allowing control to shift from one level to another depending on such factors as the task demands, environmental constraints, and intention of the performer. Such a system allows for motor activities to be executed by self-organising task-specific ensembles of coordinative structures and controlled through a direct linkage between perception and the motor system. The evidence for this latter mode of control appears to be strongest in natural actions, (e.g., locomotion, stairclimbing, reaching for objects) and in the execution of highly overlearned simple cyclic actions (e.g., finger oscillation tasks). In activities, however, involving the translation of a symbolic code into a sequence of movements (e.g., writing, drawing, dance, musical performance) and sport skills where the performer is engaged in continual decision making regarding shot selection, tactics etc., the involvement of cognitive processes is undeniable.

In hybrid models the cognitive system is able to override lower-level dynamic systems when necessary and is involved in the construction of new coordinative structures (Colley, 1989b; Summers, 1989b; Summers & Burns, 1990). The interaction between the cognitive and dynamical systems is nicely illustrated in a study by Mulder and Geurts (1989) on the control of balance. In the normal healthy adult the maintenance of an upright posture requires little or no cognitive processing being regulated by the activation of lower-level coordinative structures. However, for patients who have had a lower limb amputation standing with a prosthesis requires the reorganisation of their motor system, that is, new coordinative structures have to established. Mulder and Geurts argued that this relearning process involves cognitive resources. To test this hypothesis they examined the effect of concurrent performance of a cognitive task (Stroop test) on balance (standing upright on a force platform) in lower limb amputees and matched control subjects. For the control subjects dual task performance did not differ from single task (standing only) performance. For the amputees, however, performance of the cognitive task interferred with the ability to stand upright, producing a large increase in fore-aft sway, particularly at the start of the rehabilitation period (one to two days after the first prothesis fitting). By the end of rehabilitation, however, there was no difference between single and dual task conditions, suggesting that lower-level control had been reestablished.

Another example of cognitive override of lower-level systems comes from the work we have been doing in our laboratory on bimanual coordination (see Summers, 1990, for a review of this work). Some of the strongest evidence for the nonlinear oscillator model of control has come from the entrainment effects observed when subjects are asked to move the two index fingers (or two hands) at different frequencies (see Jeka & Kelso, 1989; Turvey, 1990). In our work we have examined the production of polyrhythms (e.g., 3 against 2; 5 against 3). Polyrhythms require the simultaneous production of two conflicting but isochronous movement sequences, one with each hand. Successful performance of polyrhythms, therefore, would seem to require central control to be exerted over lower-level coupled oscillatory mechanisms.

In one experiment, for example, we examined the effects, on the production of a 5 against 3 polyrhythm, of learning the motor pattern for each hand separately before combining them (Summers & Kennedy, in press). When unskilled subjects (nonmusicians) attempted to perform the two rhythms concurrently strong entrainment between the hands was observed. Skilled (musically trained) subjects, in contrast, 'solved' the concurrent task by interleaving the movements of the two hands. In particular, these subjects appeared to adopt the strategy of focusing attention on producing regular beats with the fast hand and 'slotting in' the movements of the slow hand, in a more automatic fashion.

The above examples and others in the literature (see Abernethy & Sparrow, chap. 1; Hughes & Stelmach, 1986) are consistent with the notion that the cognitive system can influence lower-level dynamic systems. In the present volume, multi-level distributed processing models underlie, explicitly or implicitly, the work of several authors (Anson, chap. 13; Charlton, chap. 15; Haggard, chap. 7; Kerr, chap. 9; Larkin & Hoare, chap. 14; Neilson, et al., chap. 17; Phillips & Stelmach, chap. 16; Thomassen & Van Galen, chap. 4; Williams, chap. 8).

At the present time the hybrid view is being advocated primarily by information processing theorists. As Abernethy and Sparrow (chap. 1) point out, multi-level hybrid models incorporating some form of cognitive processes/representation "would directly violate the philosophical base of the 'action-systems' approach" (p. 33). However, the notion of high-level controllers capable of starting, stopping, and modifying lower-level oscillator mechanisms has been proposed by some adherents to the dynamical approach (e.g., Craske & Craske, 1986; Yaminishi, Kawato, & Suzuki, 1980).

A growing willingness of proponents of the action system approach to acknowledge cognitive processes is also apparent in the present volume. Parker, in Chapter 6, for example, adopts a systems dynamic approach to the study of the development of multi-limb rhythmic action. Males aged 7, 9, and 18+ years were required to perform starjumps at their preferred tempo and at metronome-paced rates. Children's starjumping at self-selected tempos could be described by coupled, nonlinear oscillator mechanisms with limit cycle properties. However, dynamical control was less apparent on the metronome-paced trials. Parker concludes that:

> ... to perform rhythmic matching tasks also demands some level of cognitve constraint over the self-organising system dynamics with regard to correcting the mismatch between the beat and the response (p. 189).

Abernethy and Burgess-Limerik (chap. 12) in their review of visual processes underlying skilled movement also indicate that some integration of direct and indirect views of visual perception may be beneficial to both sides. Likewise, Whiting, et al., (chap. 3) suggest that, with regard to motor control, convergence between the motor system and action system approaches, rather than a further polarisation, is likely in the future.

The acceptance of some form of cognition by ecological theorists seems more likely as they begin to model more complex culturally-determined skills, and, in particular, address the problem of skill acquisition. Beek (1989), for example, in his analysis of the act of juggling acknowledges that dynamics alone cannot provide a complete explanation of skilled performance.

Motor Learning

The ultimate test for any theory of motor behaviour lies in its ability to explain the process of learning, that is, how well-coordinated temporally ordered patterns of movement are achieved in spite of the multitude of degrees of freedom to be controlled and constantly changing contextual conditions (Whiting, et al., chap. 3).

Although much of the early work in the movement behaviour field was concerned with motor learning, since the 1970's movement researchers have been primarily concerned with the mechanisms underlying the control of skilled performance rather than the acquisition of skill. Whiting, et al. (chap. 3), in fact, argue that the concept of a template or internal model is "one of the few contributions" (p. 89) to our understanding of motor skill acquisition arising from the information processing perspective. Certainly the view that the central nervous system forms an updatatable image or internal model of the world has been a key concept in neuroscience approaches to movement control (e.g., Adaptive Model Theory, Neilson et al., chap. 17) and robotics.

Recently there has been a rekindling of interest in skill acquisition by information processing theorists. On the one hand, 'old' issues in the motor learning literature, such as knowledge of results, are being revisited (e.g., Salmoni, Schmidt, & Walter, 1984; Winstein & Schmidt, 1990). On the other hand, researchers are beginning to study the knowledge base underlying the acquisition and performance of sport skills (e.g., Allard & Burnett, 1985; Thomas, French, & Humphries, 1986). The latter area has as its foundations the work in cognitive psychology on expert-novice differences in the structure and representation of domain-specific knowledge (e.g., chess, physics, mathematics, medicine, computer programming), the distinction between different types of knowledge (i.e., declarative, procedural, strategic), and the notion of production systems (see Anderson, 1985; Chi, Glaser, & Farr, 1988 for review). The basic premise behind this work is that success in sporting situations is due partly to the individual's sport-specific knowledge base which allows the athlete to anticipate and rapidly select the most appropriate reponse for a particular situation.

A related development in the field of cognitive psychology which may have important implications for understanding motor skill acquisition are connectionist or neural network models of cognition. In these models networks of simple processing units (nodes) take on activation levels and send excitatory and inhibitory signals to each other (Stelmach & Hughes, 1987). MacKay (1985), for example, has developed an activation theory of action in which the nodes are organised into two general systems that can operate independently: a mental system containing cognitive units representing the components of a skill and the relationship between them, and a muscle movement system which specifies muscle-specific patterns of movement. The attractiveness of such models is that they have the potential for mapping psychological constructs (e.g., the executive) onto physiological constructs (neural networks). In the present volume this general approach to the modelling of motor behaviour is evident in the chapters by Haggard (chap. 7) and Neilson, et al. (chap. 17).

The recent developments in cognitive science promise much for an understanding of the higher level planning and programming processes in motor control and learning. This approach, however, says little about the implementation of higher level processes at the muscle movement level (Colley, 1989a).

The ecological approach to motor behaviour has also begun to address the issue of skill acquisition. The challenge for ecological psychologists is to explain motor learning with minimal resort to intelligent operations (Newell, 1991). Important concepts within this approach to learning are perception-action coupling and the distinction between the terms control, coordination, and skill (see, Whiting et al., chap 3; Sparrow, chap. 5). According to this view skill acquisition should be considered "to be the problem of how both coordination and control of the system, in providing solutions to a particular problem posed by the environment, are achieved" (Whiting et al., chap 3, p. 93). The learner is seen as searching (exploring) the perceptual-motor workspace to find the optimal solutions to the motor problem (see Whiting, et al., chap. 3, for a discussion of search strategies). Learning, is achieved when the perceptual environment and the action environment are coordinated in a way consistent with the task demands (Newell, 1991).

The identification of the critical perceptual and kinetic variables in the perceptual-motor workspace that are used by the learner are the crucial issues for the action system approach to motor learning. The role of information in the motor learning process is also very different to that used by cognitive theorists (e.g., feedback). Information in the ecological approach is "the means via which the learner channels the mapping of information and movement dynamics in the perceptual-motor workspace" (Newell, 1991, p. 231). The idea of exploration - the search for the optimal solution to a motor problem - is nicely illustrated by the research on the learning of slalom ski-type movements reported in Chapter 3 by Whiting, Vogt, and Vereijken.

The motor systems - action systems debate, therefore, appears to be shifting to the arena of skill acquisition. The action systems perspective offers a new and exciting approach to the study of motor learning. However, the extent to which concepts such as 'smart' perceptual systems (Runeson, 1977) will allow this approach to account for skill acquisition without recourse to 'cognitive' concepts such as internal models, remains to be seen. It may be that learning issues will provide the catalyst for a reconciliation between the competing views.

CONCLUDING REMARKS

In this chapter I have argued that the resolution of the current paradigm crisis within the field of motor behaviour (Abernethy & Sparrow, chap. 1) lies in the hybridisation of the action systems and motor systems approaches. One of the early goals of the ecological approach was to 'trim down the homunculus' in explanations of motor control and learning. To a large extent this has been achieved, certainly in natural activities (e.g., locomotion) and coincident-timing skills (see Abernethy & Burgess-Limerick, chap. 12; Savelsbergh, et al., chap. 11). As a consequence most information processing theorists now acknowledge that much of movement control can be accomplished through self-organising dynamic systems. Action system theorists, on the other hand, are beginning to acknowledge that in modelling more complex culturally-determined skills (e.g., juggling) more than dynamics may be needed to explain all aspects of skilled performance.

If the above analysis is correct then the challenge for motor behaviour theorists lies at the interface between knowledge and lower-level dynamical driven systems. At the present time all we have are demonstrations that knowledge and intentions can affect movement processes. To gain an understanding of the interaction between levels, however, will require not only some reconciliation of conceptual and philosophical differences between the two approaches but the adoption of a common language to describe the interface. The translation of so-called cognitive processes into the language of dynamics, for example, will not be an easy task for as Beek (1989) states "the issue of intentionality constitutes the ultimate bottleneck for a physical account of action (as well as for any other theory of movement production)" (p. 194). In the present volume the work of Haggard (chap. 7) and Neilson, Neilson, and O'Dwyer (chap. 17) offer promising approaches to the modelling of the multi-level motor system.

The field of motor control and learning does appear to be destined for a further period of turbulence, but the prospect that a coherent theory of motor behaviour will emerge through an integration of the competing paradigms "should be worth the battle" (Whiting, et al., chap. 3, p. 105).

REFERENCES

Allard, F., & Burnett, N. (1985). Skill in sport. *Canadian Journal of Psychology, 39,* 294-312.

Anderson, J.R. (1985). *Cognitive psychology and its implications.* New York: Freeman.

Beek, P.J. (1989). *Juggling dynamics.* Amsterdam: Free University Press.

Chi, M.T.H., Glaser, R., & Farr, M.J. (Eds.) (1988). *The nature of expertise.* Hillsdale, NJ: Lawrence Erlbaum Associates.

Colley, A.M. (1989a). Cognitive motor skills. In D.H. Holding (Ed.), *Human skills, 2nd edition* (pp. 229-248). Chichester: Wiley.

Colley, A.M. (1989b). Learning motor skills: integrating cognition and action. In A.M. Colley & J.R. Beech (Eds.), *Acquisition and performance of cognitive skills* (pp. 166-189). Chichester: Wiley.

Craske, B., & Craske, J.D. (1986). Oscillator mechanisms in the human motor system: investigating their properties using the aftercontraction effect. *Journal of Motor Behavior, 18,* 117-145.

Hughes, B.G., & Stelmach, G.E. (1986). On Bernstein as a contributor to cognitive theories of motor behavior. *Human Movement Science, 5,* 35-45.

Jeka, J.J. & Kelso, J.A.S. (1989). The dynamic pattern approach to coordinated behavior: A tutorial review. In S.A. Wallace (Ed.), *Perspectives on the coordination of movement* (pp. 3-45). Amsterdam: North-Holland.

Keele, S.W. (1968). Movement control in skilled motor performance. *Psychological Bulletin, 70,* 387-403.

Keele, S.W., Cohen, A., & Ivry, R. (1990). Motor programs: Concepts and issues. In M. Jeannerod (Ed.), *Attention and Performance XIII* (pp. 77-110). Hillsdale. NJ: Lawrence Erlbaum Associates.

MacKay, D.G. (1985). A theory of the representation, organization and timing of action with implications for sequencing disorders. In E.A. Roy (Ed.), *Neurological studies of apraxia and related disorders* (pp. 267-308). Amsterdam: North-Holland.

Meijer, O.G., & Roth, K. (Eds.) (1988). *Complex movement behaviour: 'The' motor-action controversy.* Amsterdam: North-Holland.

Mulder, T. & Geurts, S. (1989, October). *The assessment of motor dysfunctions: Preliminaries to a disbility oriented approach.* Paper presented at the round-table conference on Clinical Assessment of Motor Dysfunctions, Ancona, Italy.

Newell, K.M. (1991). Motor skill acquisition. *Annual Review of Psychology, 42,* 213-237.

Runeson, S. (1977). On the possibility of 'smart' perceptual mechanisms. *Scandinavian Journal of Psychology, 18,* 172-179.

Salmoni, A.W., Schmidt, R.A., & Walter, C.B. (1984). Knowledge of results and motor learning: A review and reappraisal. *Psychological Bulletin, 95,* 355-386.

Sheridan, M. (1988). Movement metaphors. In A.M. Colley & J.R. Beech (Eds.), *Cognition and action in skilled behaviour.* Amsterdam: North-Holland.

Stelmach, G.E., & Hughes, B.G. (1987). The cognitivist orientation: The problem of system reduction. *European Bulletin of Cognitive Psychology, 7,* 190-194.

Summers, J.J. (1989a). Motor programs. In D.H. Holding (Ed.), *Human skills, 2nd edition* (pp. 49-69). Chichester: Wiley.

Summers, J.J. (1989b). Temporal constraints in the performance of bimanual tasks. In D. Vickers and P.L. Smith (Eds.), *Human information processing: Measures, mechanisms, and models* (pp. 155-168). Amsterdam: Elsevier.

Summers, J.J. (1990). Temporal constraints on concurrent task performance. In G.E. Hammond (Ed.), *Cerebral control of speech and limb movements* (pp. 661-680). Amsterdam: North-Holland.

Summers, J.J. & Burns, B.D. (1990). Timing in human movement sequences. In R.A. Block (Ed.), *Cognitive models of psychological time* (pp. 181-206). Hillsdale, NJ: Lawrence Erlbaum Associates.

Summers, J.J. & Kennedy, T.M. (in press). Strategies in the production of a 5:3 polyrhythm. *Human Movement Science.*

Thomas, J.R., French, K.E., & Humphries, C.A. (1986). Knowledge development and sport skill performance: Directions for motor behavior research. *Journal of Sport Psychology, 8,* 259-272.

Turvey, M.T. (1990). Coordination. *American Psychologist, 45,* 938-953.

Winstein, C.J., & Schmidt, R.A. (1990). Reduced relative frequency of knowledge of results enhances motor skill learning. *Journal of Experimental Psychology: Learning, Memory, and Cognition, 16,* 677-691.

Yaminishi, J., Kawato, M., & Suzuki, R. (1980). Two coupled oscillators as a model for coordinated finger tapping by both hands. *Biological Cybernetics, 37,* 219-225.

INDEXES

Subject Index

Author Index

www.ingramcontent.com/pod-product-compliance
Ingram Content Group UK Ltd.
Pitfield, Milton Keynes, MK11 3LW, UK
UKHW020224290926
15470UKWH00001B/369

9 780444 884558